The Fitness

The Fitness Blueprint

Evidence-based practice for optimising body composition

Samuel Dicken

Disclaimer:

You should always consult your GP before attempting any lifestyle changes or starting a new diet or exercise plan. The author of this book is not a qualified medical professional. The author accepts no liability for any damages or harm as a result of any recommendations made in this book.

This book is for healthy individuals without pre-existing disease. The recommendations provided are not intended to treat, cure or help any disease.

Cover design and illustrations: Rob Dicken (www.strikethree.co.uk)

Acknowledgements

A big thank you goes to everyone who has given up their time to help proof-read different chapters and provided support and feedback on designing the book, including Catherine Redshaw, Jessica Greaves, Rosa Sulley, Matthew Bradley, Matt Teale, Joe Miller, Will Chisholm, Jack Maullin, Anna Cooke and Jim Dicken.

I am especially thankful to Rob Dicken for the time and support he has given in designing the cover and graphical content of the book, and for putting up with my amendments!

To Mum and Dad,

You'll probably never read this book but at least give it a dust every once in a while

About the author

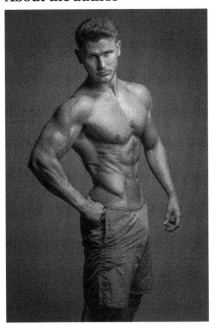

Sam Dicken is currently a Clinical Scientist at Guy's and St Thomas' NHS Foundation Trust on the NHS Scientist Training Programme, specialising in vascular science. Sam has a degree from Cambridge University in Natural Sciences with a focus on physiology, development and neuroscience. He is studying for a Master's in Clinical Science at Newcastle University, and will begin a Medical Research Council Funded Master's in Research and PhD in experimental and personalised medicine at UCL in September 2020, with a focus on cardiovascular disease.

He has experience of working in the sports nutrition industry, a wealth of clinical experience during his time in hospital, and a passion for sports and exercise, representing Cambridge University at varsity rugby and as a keen weightlifter with a focus on strength and body composition.

Sam has a career focus on how diet, exercise and lifestyle influence metabolism, body composition and development of cardiovascular disease. He has fostered an interest in the continuum between health and disease, and how the very factors that may lead to disease and mortality are the same factors that allow individuals to become elite athletes or live long and healthy lives.

This book combines his passion for physical training and exercise with his career skills, research interests and the evidence-based approach of his clinical training. This book will dispel common fitness myths and set the truth straight about how to eat and train to build muscle and lose fat.

Table of Contents

1. Introduction

Welcome to The Fitness Blueprint!

This book will provide a thorough discussion on what we currently know about diet and exercise to lose fat, gain muscle or to maintain current body shape. There are basic principles that underpin achieving these goals. However, numerous plans and methods lead to the same end goal, and there is no perfect route to meet these basic principles for everyone. The best plan for an individual is often purely down to personal preference. What this means is that there is not just one, but a wide range of potential plans (or *blueprints*, as such). It is down to you to decide which blueprints you think will best suit your lifestyle and goals.

Who is this book for?

This book is suitable for anyone looking to improve their *body composition* (this is considered to be a reduction in body fat, an increase in muscle mass, or both). The book is also suitable for anyone looking to maintain their current body composition (in other words, to maintain similar levels of muscle and fat mass). This book is not suitable for those with a medical condition. This book does not provide any recommendations or support for preventing or treating diseases. It is purely to aid normal, healthy individuals without pre-existing disease to achieve body composition related goals.

The Fitness Blueprint aims to:

- Outline the key points you need to focus on regarding diet and exercise for muscle gain or weight loss, as supported by scientific research.
- Outline what we still do not know about diet and exercise for muscle gain or weight loss, and as such requires further scientific research.
- Outline some of the incorrect information commonly held as true in the fitness community about diet and exercise for muscle gain or weight loss, as shown by scientific research (or the lack of).

This book will allow you to understand how to train and eat to achieve changes in body composition. The book will also give you the knowledge to decide *how* to achieve this personally, and how to move forward when you reach a sticking point. Knowing what *does* and *doesn't* matter is a powerful tool to allow you to devote your time and energy to the factors that are most important, and save time by not concerning yourself with the factors that are less important. Plenty of information is already available regarding fitness, muscle growth and weight loss. However, most of it lacks explanation, is purely anecdotal, or just plain incorrect. Many approaches to fitness thus far have been purely experiential, with little consideration for any evidence.

What is optimal, is personal.

There is no perfect body composition for everyone. What is considered optimal will depend on what your goal is and what you consider to be your target body composition. You may *already* be at what you perceive to be your optimal body composition, and your main concern may be in *maintaining* it. What is considered an ideal body composition also varies greatly between sports. The ideal amount of muscle and fat mass for a footballer, tennis player, boxer or rugby player will differ greatly. Adding some muscle as a boxer may be catastrophic in failing to meet a weight class. Adding some muscle as a rugby player may improve match performance. Also, most evidence-based recommendations are of optimum ranges rather than exact values. Variation exists in the findings of research and between individuals. People will respond and adhere better to slightly different plans. In other words, the exact same diet and training plan will *not* be optimal for two different people, but those plans will sit within the general principles for the desired goal. This book will provide these recommendations and discuss how you can find your optimum based on your personal preferences.

2. Should I alter my body composition? The exam analogy

Your qualifications nor your job define who you are. Similarly, neither does the way you look. No one should feel pressured or guilty into altering the way they look. Altering body composition is a choice. Determine your reasons for doing so. Decreasing fat mass or increasing muscle mass won't necessarily make you happier. Whether you choose to attempt change or not, is up to you.

Should you alter your body composition? Consider the fact that many reading this book will have been through the trials and tribulations of studying for and sitting exams. This may have been at school, sixth form, university, work or in many other areas of life, regardless of whether there was a want to or not. Many of us spend countless hours preparing to do as well as possible in these exams, which can be incredibly stressful for some.

Your exam performances or your career do not define who you are as a person. Despite this, we still put in a lot of effort and devote large parts of our lives to them. For some they can be highly demanding and lead to stress and health issues. For others, they are relatively stress free, not time consuming and can often be largely enjoyable experiences. Your body composition similarly does not define who you are. For some people, the process of losing fat or gaining muscle can be very stressful and lead to health issues. For others, they are relatively stress free, not time consuming and can often be largely enjoyable experiences.

Even without an exam or a specific reason to study, some people still like to study or learn. This could be a new skill, perfecting a craft or just reading. Some people enjoy trying to improve themselves. Even if there is no explicit end goal (e.g. a beach holiday or a professional sport) some people still like to exercise and eat *'well'* to lose fat, gain muscle or improve general fitness. Some people enjoy the process of trying to improve themselves, some don't.

Sometimes people do not want to study, but they have exams they must sit if they want to further their career. Studying and exams may not be the primary goal.

Career progression may also not be the primary goal. Career progression may just be a mechanism through which to increase financial earnings. Some people do not care about altering body composition but realise that in order to improve in their sport, they need to change the relative amount of fat and muscle they carry. This may be the case for sports such as rugby, boxing or football. Improving body composition may not be the primary goal.

Some people sit exams and study because they are forced to (e.g. at school) and never attempt to study or sit exams again. They may pursue other career paths and become very successful or find motivation to study in other ways. The nature of how some people study or have previously been examined may not have suited them. Some people change their diet and exercise because they were told to, or they had previously been changed in a way that was not enjoyable to the individual, such that they never attempt any change again. However, some people may find greater enjoyment in playing sports or other activities, or later in life find their own diet and exercise strategies that allow them to succeed. Previous experiences with diet and exercise can influence people's relationships with diet and exercise[1]. Different people like to eat different things and exercise in different ways.

Some people may choose a certain career because they believe it will make them happier. This is not always the case. Similarly, some people may choose to change their body composition as they think it will make them happier. This is not always the case.

The number of exams or qualifications, and therefore the amount of studying you may need (or not need) depends on the individual. Some people may not need any exams for their job or lifestyle and are perfectly happy. Some people may need a vast number of qualifications to reach their goals and therefore spend a lot of time studying. The exams sat and qualifications needed can vary greatly between people. The amount of work required for different people to achieve their desired body composition varies greatly. Some people may have no desire to change, some may have a great desire. If little to no change in body composition is desired, then little work may be required. If large changes in body composition are desired, then more work may be required.

Some people enjoy exercising and eating well, some people hate it. Some people care about changing their body composition and some people don't. Some people want to change their body composition as a primary outcome. Some people want to change their body composition to facilitate another primary outcome. Work out *why* you want to change your body composition, or even if you *need* to.

References

1   Myers VH, McVay MA, Champagne CM, Hollis JF, Coughlin JW, Funk KL et al. Weight loss history as a predictor of weight loss: results from Phase I of the weight loss maintenance trial. *J Behav Med* 2013; 36. Available from: doi:10.1007/s10865-012-9450-0.

3. Evidence-based practice

Research reveals many insights. Metabolisms are not slow or fast; you cannot 'damage' your metabolism. No diet is superior for weight loss when you consume the same amount of energy. Superfoods do not exist, this is just a marketing tool. And how would you define a superfood, lots of vitamins and minerals? This definition would make many plant-based and animal-based foods a superfood. Sugar is not inherently 'bad'. No food in itself is inherently fattening or causes weight gain. You don't need to avoid specific foods because the latest influencer said they're 'bad' for you. Exclude foods because you're allergic, have ethical or environmental concerns regarding its production or consumption, or have a personal preference not to consume that food (i.e. you don't like the taste). Organic food is not more nutritious than conventional food. Detox diets don't work. Most supplements have no evidence that they actually have any benefit. Wearing a waist slimming belt does not make your waist smaller. Sweat is not your fat burning. Aerobic exercise does not increase your lung capacity. Muscle soreness the day after a weight session does not mean more muscle growth. You don't have to lift 'heavy' weights to build muscle. You don't need to exercise to lose weight. Fasted exercise does not result in greater fat loss. More on this later.

Medicine in the last 100 years has progressed rapidly from decision making based purely on the opinion and experiences of doctors, to combining first-hand knowledge and patient preferences with evidence from research studies. This evidence-based approach in medicine, or *'evidence-based medicine'* (EBM) is defined as the *"integration of the best research evidence with clinical expertise and patient values."* (Thoma and Eaves, 2015[1]). David Sackett amongst others, pioneered this systematic approach to medical care, due to many medical decisions and treatments being based on old and outdated textbooks. Information to treat patients was routinely being passed down from senior colleagues without question, very much like fitness related information is passed on without question today[2]. Since the birth of evidence-based medicine, many treatments that had previously been strongly *'believed'* to be beneficial, have been proven to be quite useless, and even detrimental to patient health[3].

Evidence-based medicine involves three components:

1. The recommended evidence-based options for the condition a patient has, based on **high-quality research**.
2. The combined **expertise** of healthcare professionals.
3. The **personal preferences** of the patient.

This relatively new approach in how to achieve positive outcomes has enabled advancements in health and improvements in patient care. It establishes what works in what scenario, what doesn't work (or worse, causes harm), and what is still unknown. Even so, healthcare is still far from being completely evidence-based. Unfortunately, despite large amounts of research into diet and exercise, the fitness world is still caught up in anecdotes, recommendations from experience and subjective opinion. There is little consideration for any quantitative evidence, but even when it is used, it is mis-used to reinforce incorrect ideologies. Indeed, professional fitness athletes have been shown to rarely utilise evidence-based information or scientific knowledge, and often rely on information from other professional fitness athletes[4]. Yet, these are the people that many of the general public look up to for training and nutritional advice. Evidence-based approaches to body composition are all but *non-existent*.

Multidisciplinary meetings

I have been lucky enough to spend several years working in National Health Service (NHS) hospitals alongside doctors, nurses and other healthcare professionals. The NHS uses evidence-based recommendations developed by government institutions such as the *National Institute of Health and Care Excellence* (NICE)[5]. During this time, I was able to observe several *multi-disciplinary meetings* (MDMs). Multi-disciplinary meetings are excellent examples of evidence-based practice. Here, a group of doctors, nurses and other healthcare professionals discuss complex patient cases under their care. They do this because the most suitable management and treatment of a patient's disease or condition is not always clear. Do we operate? Do we give medication? Do we leave it be and monitor the patient closely? When discussing a patient in these meetings, the final decision on how to manage the patient combines:

1. The recommended evidence-based options for the patient's condition (from research).
2. The combined clinical expertise of the professionals in the meeting (from professional experience).

3. The personal preferences of the patient (from open discussions between the patient and healthcare professionals).

For example, the *aorta* (the blood vessel that carries blood from the heart to the rest of the body) can become enlarged and increase in diameter (called an *aneurysm*) at the level of the belly button. Part of my role in hospital was to measure the diameters of aortas. Enlarged aortas rarely cause any pain or symptoms, but if they rupture, they can be life threatening. Only 20% of people with an aneurysm rupture survive. Older men are screened in the community to see if they have an aneurysm. If they do, they are kept on a surveillance programme to keep an eye on the aorta size. When the diameters get too big, the patient is put forward to repair the aneurysm (the decision of what is *'too big'* is determined from research, finding when the risk of a rupture outweighs the risk of the repair). Repair is possible either by keyhole access or by open surgery where the abdomen is cut open. Both options have their risks and benefits. But with recent evidence, it has become apparent that open surgery is the most effective option, and NICE guidelines will soon be updated to recommend this to NHS Trusts and hospitals[6]. Using *just* the evidence from research to decide the correct treatment does *not* always result in the best outcome. Aneurysms are not universally repaired whenever they exceed the diameter deemed *'too big'*, as being suitable for repair. For example, if the patient has expressed a reluctance to have open surgery, or perhaps the patient has other health problems (e.g. they are overweight, diabetic or old and frail), this can increase the chances of complications with open repair. The surgeon might look at the patient's scans and decide that the operation may also be technically too difficult and high risk. Thus, by considering expert opinion and patient preference, it may mean that the best option is actually conservative management, leaving the aneurysm as it is. The risks of intervening for this particular patient are greater, and the wishes of the patient have been respected. This is a real-life example of evidence-based practice in medicine and the power of considering all three perspectives in achieving the best outcome.

Evidence-based practice in fitness

It struck me after attending these multi-disciplinary meetings and seeing the success of evidence-based medicine in practice with NICE guidance, that there is an incredible lack of research or evidence to support what was being claimed or advertised by *'influencers'* and some experts or coaches in the *fitness* world. These claims and recommendations rarely consider individual preferences or lifestyles. The definition of evidence-based practice is *not* limited to medicine. We can modify this definition for evidence-based practice in fitness. Fitness broadly covers diet and training, and is defined in this context as *"the condition of being physically strong and healthy."* (Cambridge Dictionary[7]). This is not some revolutionary new approach. However, it is very much in its infancy. It is with this knowledge and perspective that has provided the motivation for me to write this book[8].

Evidence based-practice in fitness therefore combines:

- The current best available evidence, using **high-quality reviews and research**.
- The **expertise** and first-hand evidence from experts in the fields of exercise and nutrition.
- The specific **needs, preferences and lifestyle choices** of individuals.

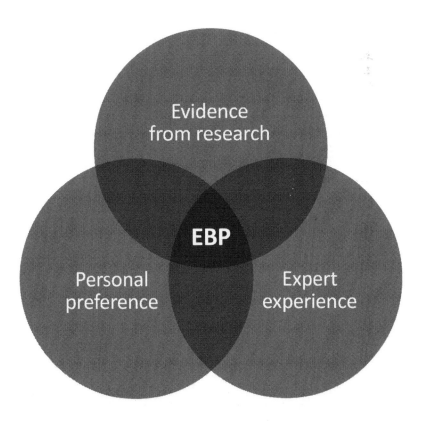

Evidence-based practice (EBP) combines the evidence from research, the personal preference of the individual and expert opinion.

The current best evidence from research

Scientific research has been defined as:

"the neutral, systematic, planned, and multiple-step process that uses previously discovered facts to advance knowledge that does not exist in the literature."
Erol, 2017[9].

In the last 20 to 30 years, lots of research has been conducted into how what we eat, how we exercise and how we live can affect our health, body fat levels, and muscle mass. Despite this growing body of knowledge, mainstream media is often completely *unaware* of these findings, and continues to churn out content that is outdated or just wrong.

For research to be used in the real-world, it requires coaches, personal trainers, dieticians, and individuals to stay up to date with new findings and incorporate them into their current understanding. It can be many years before even clinical research gets put into practical use. Many clinical guidelines are several years out of date and can conflict each other in terms of their recommendations. For example, narrowing of the *carotid artery* (the blood vessel in the neck supplying blood to the brain) increases the risk of a future *stroke* (a lack of blood to the brain). One treatment option is an invasive surgery where the artery is widened to improve blood flow. Some guidelines say that individuals with this narrowing without any symptoms *should* receive invasive treatment, while other guidelines recommend that individuals with this narrowing without any symptoms *should not* receive invasive treatment[10]. Even some medical-related recommendations still do *not* use the best available evidence, let alone any fitness-related recommendations. The problem is that many people do not have the ability to read or interpret scientific research, and therefore it may never get seen in practice. Another issue is that very little research is freely available nor well publicised, which makes it difficult to even access it.

Pseudoscience is not science

Pseudoscience is the art of using scientific language, quoting select scientific articles and using anecdotes to back-up an agenda that does not follow the current lines of thinking. It can be difficult to define and has been suggested to exist on a continuum with science[11,12]. Evidence-based practice is an important tool to prevent the occurrence of pseudoscience[11].

Pseudoscience typically[11]:

- Does not use peer-review processes (getting other researchers to check the validity of your work).
- Relies on *confirming* findings rather than *refuting* findings (confirmation biases).
- Relies heavily on anecdote.
- Develops new *hypotheses* when they are needed, when research results are not confirmatory. In other words, collecting lots of data and looking for links *after* data collection, not generating a hypothesis *before* data collection[9].

It is very easy to cherry-pick studies, *'evidence'* or anecdotes to create any narrative you want[13]. Many high-profile individuals use this technique (both knowingly and unknowingly) in order to seemingly validate their apparently sound scientific and theoretical claims, which often supports the rationale behind a product they may be selling. Detox diets rely heavily on anecdotes and case studies of individuals that have used such products. I recommend reading Ben Goldacre's *'Bad Science'*, which covers pseudoscience in great and interesting detail, with some real-life examples[14].

Prominent figures in fitness commonly promote novel training methods, specific diets or a range of supplements as part of their secrets to success. It therefore may not be in their interest to show that evidence does not support their method as being superior, or show that there is no evidence at all to support what they are claiming. They can often also be completely unaware that any evidence may exist. It is often the case that those writing about or promoting medical information or general health and fitness in the media often have little to no scientific experience, meaning much of the current fitness literature is not evidence-based.

Being able to understand and read scientific papers should not be left to only those who conduct research. There are some great resources available, such as those by Trisha Greenhalgh[15]. These resources explain how to make sense of a research paper, how to critically judge if its conclusions are in line with its results and if its results are reliable. I hope this book provides sufficient detail, but I have provided references to all the studies I mention so should you wish, you can critique these papers yourself.

The expertise and first-hand evidence from experts in the fields of exercise and nutrition

Despite all this evidence, there are many areas yet to be studied and many others that are difficult to quantify. As much as evidence can help lead us to what works, years of *professional* knowledge and experience is, and always will have value in the fitness world, as it does in the medical world. To clarify, this isn't some guy down the local gym advocating his weird exercise or workout. This refers to an experienced coach or researcher understanding how the evidence may apply to a specific person, based on their needs. As an example, sports coaches often publish books of their training methods and how they have turned their athletes into champions. Additionally, experienced coaches have a wealth of tips and tricks that research studies would struggle to demonstrate. Such as, advice on how to correctly perform an exercise to target a muscle or convenient approaches to meal planning are often developed through coaches and their clients. Also, the majority of research conducted so far in fitness has been on young males who have never trained before or are relatively new to training. There are massive gaps in our research knowledge base. Fewer studies are conducted in groups such as people who have been training for a long time, or in females. The expertise and experience of experts can help to fill these gaps and place this evidence into a real-world context. The opinion of some of the leading evidence-based coaches have been incorporated into this book.

The needs and lifestyles of individuals embarking on a fitness journey

For changes in body composition to occur, there are basic principles that *must* be met. But, there are a wide range of options to adhere to that achieve these principles. Which of these options you choose is down to your lifestyle and preferences. Find what personally suits you and whether you can adhere to it.

There is a recurring theme that will routinely be mentioned throughout the book: '*it depends on your personal preference*'. Contrary to popular belief, there are no '*magic pills*', no '*shortcuts*' and no newly discovered health fixes. The recommended guidance for diet, exercise and lifestyle is quite broad. For example, to lose weight a calorie deficit is important. But low-carbohydrate, low-fat or ketogenic diets for example, are all effective for weight loss if they generate a *calorie deficit*.

The final piece to the jigsaw of evidence-based practice is that it is continually evolving. With new evidence, greater experience and changes to individual lifestyles, the best approach may change, incorporating this new information into the existing framework. This book is a guide with the current information we have. Although the basic underlying principles in this book will remain largely unchanged, over time, the guidance will slowly become stronger as new information becomes available which answers the unknown questions.

Useful resources and recommended experts in the field

If you want to read and discover more about evidence-based fitness, there are some great resources available. Searching academic literature can be a minefield, but there are *position stands* and *consensus statements* (get the best expert minds on a particular topic to write a critical review and create recommendations based on the current literature) available from several leading exercise and nutrition organisations:

- International Society of Sports Nutrition (ISSN)[16].
- Academy of Nutrition and Dietetics (AND)[17].
- National Strength and Conditioning Association (NSCA)[18].
- American College of Sports Medicine (ACSM)[19].

Many of these position stands and consensus statements have been incorporated into this book.

There are also numerous academic authorities and personalities with vast amounts of useful freely available information on the internet. Their research and expert opinions have also been included into this book:

Alan Aragon https://alanaragon.com/aarr/
Brad Schoenfeld http://www.lookgreatnaked.com
James Krieger https://weightology.net/free-content/
Layne Norton https://www.biolayne.com
Menno Henselmans https://mennohenselmans.com
Eric Helms https://3dmusclejourney.com
Bret Contreras https://bretcontreras.com
Mike Israetel https://renaissanceperiodization.com
John Rusin https://drjohnrusin.com
Chris Beardsley https://www.strengthandconditioningresearch.com
Martin MacDonald https://www.martin-macdonald.com
Stephan Guyenet

https://www.stephanguyenet.com
Gab Fundaro   https://vitaminphdnutrition.com/about/
Greg Nuckols   https://www.strongerbyscience.com
Andy Morgan   https://rippedbody.com/
Bill Campbell   https://www.usf.edu/education/faculty/faculty-profiles/bill-campbell.aspx
Jackson Peos   https://www.jpshealthandfitness.com.au/author/jackson-peos/
Grant Tinsley   http://granttinsley.com
Jacob Schepis   https://www.jpshealthandfitness.com.au
Jorn Trommelen   https://www.nutritiontactics.com
Examine.com   https://examine.com
Brad Dieter   http://sciencedrivennutrition.com/about/

I highly recommend looking up some of these leading authorities and science communicators in the field of fitness from time to time. I will mention some of their works and their articles outlining their viewpoints, which will form part of the evidence-based approach to this guide, providing views of leading experts and coaches in fitness. This list is not exhaustive, with many other individuals with invaluable information and insights.

References

1   Thoma A, Eaves FF. A Brief History of Evidence-Based Medicine (EBM) and the Contributions of Dr David Sackett. *Aesthet Surg J* 2015; 35: NP261–NP263.

2   Sackett DL, Rosenberg WM, Gray JA, Haynes RB, Richardson WS. Evidence based medicine: what it is and what it isn't. *BMJ* 1996; 312: 71–72.

3   Evans I, Thornton H, Chalmers I, Glasziou P. *Testing Treatments: Better Research for Better Healthcare*. 2nd ed. Pinter & Martin: London, 2011 Available from: http://www.ncbi.nlm.nih.gov/books/NBK66204/ (accessed 4 Feb 2020).

4   Helms E, Prnjak K, Linardon J. Towards a Sustainable Nutrition Paradigm in Physique Sport: A Narrative Review. *Sports* 2019; 7: 172.

5   NICE. *The National Institute for Health and Care Excellence.* Available from: https://www.nice.org.uk/ (accessed 14 Feb 2020).

6   NICE. *Abdominal aortic aneurysm: diagnosis and management.* Available from: https://www.nice.org.uk/guidance/indevelopment/gid-cgwave0769/documents (accessed 14 Feb 2020).

7   Cambridge English Dictionary. *Fitness - meaning in the Cambridge English Dictionary.* Available from: https://dictionary.cambridge.org/dictionary/english/fitness (accessed 14 Feb 2020).

8   English KL, Amonette WE, Graham M, Spiering BA. What is "Evidence-Based" Strength and Conditioning? *Strength Cond J* 2012; 34: 19–24.

9   Erol A. How to Conduct Scientific Research? *Noro Psikiyatri Arsivi* 2017; 54: 97–98.

10   Abbott AL, Paraskevas KI, Kakkos SK, Golledge J, Eckstein H-H, Diaz-Sandoval LJ et al. Systematic Review of Guidelines for the Management of Asymptomatic and Symptomatic Carotid Stenosis. *Stroke* 2015; 46: 3288–3301.

11   Lee CM, Hunsley J. Evidence-Based Practice: Separating Science From Pseudoscience. *Can J Psychiatry Rev Can Psychiatr* 2015; 60: 534–540.

12   McNally R. *Is the pseudoscience concept useful for clinical psychology? The demise of pseudoscience.* Available from: https://emdria.omeka.net/items/show/16817 (accessed 14 Feb 2020).

13   Kumar D. Battling pseudoscience in the era of medical misinformation – rising role of health advocacy. *J Fam Community Med* 2019; 26: 67–68.

14   Goldacre B. *Bad Science.* Available from: https://www.badscience.net/books/bad-science/ (accessed 14 Feb 2020).

15   The BMJ. *How to read a paper.* Available from: https://www.bmj.com/about-bmj/resources-readers/publications/how-read-paper (accessed 14 Feb 2020).

16   ISSN. *International society of sports nutrition position stands.* Available from: https://www.biomedcentral.com/collections/ISSNPosP (accessed 14 Feb 2020).

17   AND. *Position Papers.* Available from: https://www.eatrightpro.org/practice/position-and-practice-papers/position-papers (accessed 14 Feb 2020).

18   NSCA. *Position Statements.* Available from: https://www.nsca.com/about-us/position-statements/ (accessed 14 Feb 2020).

19   ACSM. *Position Stands.* Available from: https://www.acsm.org/acsm-positions-policy/official-positions/ACSM-position-stands (accessed 14 Feb 2020).

4. Research is research, right?

Research findings are not definitive, and not all evidence is of the same quality.

Imagine looking for evidence to support eating a certain diet for weight loss. There are lots of studies, comparing different diets, in different people, with different study designs. This means there can be many different conclusions. One small scale *observational* study demonstrating a slight benefit is fairly weak evidence. Several, large scale *randomised controlled trials* with a low risk of bias showing a large, meaningful benefit is strong evidence. *No study is perfect.* Every study has some flaw or limitation. How well the study was designed, conducted and analysed can all heavily influence the reliability and repeatability of the results. It can be difficult to know what's high-quality or low-quality evidence without some knowledge of study design and without spending hours sifting through pages of scientifically dense text. This is a problem, because despite individual studies being *informative*, in themselves they are usually *not definitive*. They are often misused. Consider a football match, a football league and a football knockout tournament, such as a Premier League match, the Premier League and the FA cup. The FA cup is renowned for its upsets. On any given day, any team has a chance of beating another team, even those who are several divisions below. The classic *'giantkillers'*; as a Herefordian I think of the Ronnie Radford 30-yard screamer where Hereford United beat top division Newcastle United in the 1971-72 FA Cup. In the Premier League, even the team at the top of the league can lose to the team at the bottom of league. Clearly, every now and then there are results which seem to go against the grain or the prevailing view. However, a football league is far less cut-throat than a knockout tournament. Losing a match is not the end of the road. Instead, points are awarded based on whether a team wins, draws or loses. Adding together the points each team collects from every match in a season results in definitive winners, losers and those who perform similarly in mid-table. In research, any one study can create unexpected and surprising results. This can be from a poor study design, or how the study is conducted or analysed. Imagine the top football team having their star players injured, playing on a less than perfect pitch and performing badly. In other words, there are underlying factors which may impair identifying the true result. I am writing this book the season after Manchester

City achieved a record breaking 101 points in the premier league. However, in the 2018-2019 season, Manchester City lost to Newcastle United who were in the relegation zone whilst they were in 2nd place. Now, if someone were to come up to you and tell you because of that result, Newcastle United are definitively a better team than Manchester City, you would laugh at the claim, considering their overall league positions and your pre-existing knowledge on the topic. Similarly, it can be very easy for someone to cherry-pick research studies which confirm their pre-existing ideas regardless of any flaws, and ignore studies which do not agree. This is called *confirmation bias*, and it is very common. If someone believed Newcastle United were better than Manchester City and wanted to prove it, they may only mention the games that Newcastle win, and they may ignore the games that they lose. They may point out any flaws in the matches that don't agree with their belief. Perhaps some key players were injured or there were poor refereeing decisions. If you had no idea about English football, you may be *convinced* into thinking Newcastle United are better than Manchester City if the case were well argued. If you had no idea about a research topic, you may be *convinced* into thinking whatever narrative is claimed based on the studies cited, is true. Fortunately, we can get around this by putting all the studies on a particular topic together and analyse all the data at once, much like a football league table where the points each team has collected are added up, producing winners, losers and those in between. These *studies of studies* are called *systematic reviews* and *meta-analyses*. However, systematic reviews and meta-analyses are not widely available for every single topic, because there may be limited research available (a bit like the start of a football season where teams have only played a few matches, and league positions do not mean much). As such, we need a hierarchy to determine the relative quality of individual studies, so that we can put their findings in context.

The evidence pyramid

Evidence-based practice uses research to help make decisions. However, not all research is of the same quality. There is a general hierarchy of what is considered strong evidence, through to weak evidence. This is roughly based on the study design that the research uses and its methodological quality[1].

An overview of different types of research is important for when we come to discuss the research on diet and exercise for body composition. How well the study was designed, conducted and analysed should always be considered and can heavily impact the reliability and repeatability of the results. More weight can be placed in the findings of a higher quality study than a poorer quality study. I recommend reading Trisha Greenhalgh's '*How To Read A Paper*' for learning how to read research and understand if it is well designed[2].

The quality of existing research on a topic affects the influence that any future research on the topic may have, and therefore our confidence in current findings.

The quality of evidence can be understood with our football league analogy. At the start of the season when a few matches have been played, the result of the next match and the points awarded can significantly influence the position of a team in the league. Teams can jump several places up or down the table with a win or a loss. However, near the end of the season with a few games left, the majority of teams will be within one or two positions of their final league standing, and the result of a subsequent match has less of an effect on the overall standing. Similarly, with more studies on a topic, more is known about the outcome, such that any new studies would have less of an impact on the understanding of the topic:

- **Many high quality studies** = high confidence. A new study is unlikely to change our opinion or recommendation.
- **Some moderate quality studies** = moderate confidence. A new study could change our opinion or recommendation.
- **Few low quality studies** = low confidence. A new study could likely change our opinion or add a lot more confidence to our view.

With no research, the best available evidence is that of professional expert opinion, such as from coaches or from researchers in relevant scientific fields. Often, the first human research on a topic may be *observational*, which can provide useful insights. It may well be that by the time that several *randomised controlled trials* have been conducted on a topic, the results of the higher levels of evidence (a randomised controlled trial) differ to that of the lower levels of evidence (expert opinion and observational evidence). And hence, evidence-based practice requires a continual search for the *best available evidence* with which to inform decision-making.

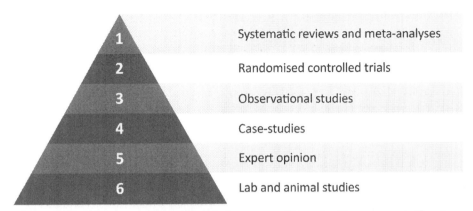

The evidence pyramid. The highest quality studies are at the top, and the lowest quality studies are at the bottom. Systematic reviews and meta-analyses of randomised controlled trials and randomised controlled trials are used to inform best practice in health and medicine. Case-studies, expert opinion, lab and animal studies and theory guide are what guides the majority of mainstream fitness information.

The types of human studies we can use to generate evidence

There are different types of studies we can use in research. Each has its own benefits and drawbacks which affects how confident we can be in drawing conclusions from them.

Generally, the more evidence on a topic at the top of the pyramid and the more conclusive the results (several studies with similar findings), the stronger support and confidence we can make for a recommendation. The less evidence on a topic at the top of the pyramid, and the more inconclusive the results are (repeat studies with different outcomes), the less support and confidence we have on a recommendation[3].

In short, *no* study exists that is completely flawless or exempt from any bias or limitation. The question therefore is not *whether* bias exists, but *how much* bias there may be, and as a result, how much reliance can we place on the results[4].

Systematic review and meta-analysis

The highest quality evidence is not primary research itself, but the synthesis of many high-quality studies into one analysis.

A *review* is where a leading academic in a scientific field writes an overview on a topic, referencing specific studies to back up what they say. They are useful but can be open to interpretation and bias. By cherry-picking studies, a review may not portray the general consensus, by emphasising some studies that agree and excluding other studies that disagree with the authors' points. Think of an article you might read in a newspaper or website on any topic. These can be very biased (e.g. a political article), depending on who they are written by and the organisation it is written for. Scientific reviews however, go through a *peer-review* process, where other leading researchers proof-read their work to check for errors and ensure its scientific quality[5]. This would in theory remove any bias. But, usually there will always be some bias to an extent[5]. This is in part because different research labs and researchers will have slightly different viewpoints and interpretations on a topic. However, a *systematic review* requires a methodical approach to searching and analysing the research on a given topic. This search process must be clearly stated at the start of the review. This means that systematic reviews are less biased and therefore more reliable than narrative reviews, including all relevant research, providing an excellent evaluation. For example, when assessing whether a particular diet affects weight loss, a review may focus more on certain studies, such as the ones which show it works, and less on others, which show it to be less effective. Whereas, a systematic review would include all relevant papers on that diet and weight loss.

As mentioned in the football league analogy, we can put all the studies on a particular topic together and clump all the data into one and analyse it. This is much more informative than analysing the individual studies in isolation. *Meta-analyses* can be of *randomised controlled trials* or *observational studies*, but other studies can be analysed together. The data collected in a systematic review is used to conduct the meta-analysis. Meta-analyses are about as good as it gets in terms of evidence. However, the quality of a meta-analysis is highly dependent on the quality of the studies they assess. We can look at each of the individual studies included in the overall analysis to determine the amount of bias or flaws that may be present, and factor this into our findings and recommendations. By assessing the quality of the individual studies, we can thus determine the quality of the meta-analysis. The risk of bias and confidence in the findings is usually part of the meta-analysis, helping to provide an insight into how robust the results are.

Sometimes, new individual studies may provide higher quality information if they are of a much higher quality than the numerous low-quality studies used in the meta-analysis, such as an incredibly well conducted randomised controlled trial with many participants, compared to a meta-analysis using high-risk-of-bias observational data (a thought to bear in mind)[3].

There are two main ways of analytically studying humans. Studies can be *interventional (i.e. experimental),* where we can either give people something or do something to them, and monitor outcomes[7]. Or, studies can be *observational,* where we watch and see what people already do and monitor outcomes[7]. In both of these types of research, we can compare the outcomes between different groups of people.

Interventional studies

Randomised controlled trials

Randomised controlled trials are the *'gold standard'* for research. Participants are prospectively randomly allocated into:

- a *treatment* group that will receive an *intervention* of interest (such as a being made to eat a certain food, follow a specific diet, consume a certain supplement, or follow a specific training plan or exercise).
- a group that receives a different treatment or intervention for comparison (such as a different food, a different diet, a different supplement, or a different training plan or exercise).
- a group that receives no treatment at all for comparison[8].

Randomised controlled trials provide strong evidence to suggest *cause and effect* between an intervention and an outcome (e.g. protein intake and muscle growth), and one of the best study designs to minimise forms of bias[2]. Even so, the quality of a randomised controlled trial can differ depending on several factors. Bias can occur through systematic errors in the study. Biases that may occur in randomised controlled trials can include[2,7]:

- **Recruitment.** For example, if you advertise a study by email only, then you are systematically biasing the study to only include people who use (or check) emails and only those who use or own a computer.
- **Inclusion and exclusion criteria.** For example, say you only want to study females between the age of 20 and 30, those would be your inclusion criteria. But, how specific should your criteria be? The more specific the criteria required for someone to be eligible to take part, the less generalisable the findings are to the wider population. But, the wider the criteria for someone to be eligible to take part, the more likely that there will be confounding factors and significant differences between the groups of people being studied. Inclusion criteria can be based on almost

any variable, but typically consider age, gender, training experience, dieting history, smoking history and body mass index.

- **Blinding and randomisation** are very important in randomised controlled trials as sources of bias.
- **Blinding.** Participants (*single-blind*), or participants and researchers (*double-blind*) can be masked from knowing who receives what treatment. This helps to make sure researchers do not consciously or unconsciously influence the study. Knowing which group is on a certain training plan or diet may influence how the researchers treat them. As a researcher, if you know a participant is taking the supplement of interest for weight loss, you might motivate them that little bit extra during their training sessions or get them to step on the scales a second time as their weight wasn't quite as low as you had expected.
- **Randomisation.** To ensure that the groups of people you study are the same (e.g. age, gender or training experience), except for whatever diet or training plan you give them. Not all controlled studies are randomised, which lowers their quality. The method used to randomise participants is also important.
- **Study design.** Compare the intervention to a *placebo* or a suitable *control*. The study may not have suitable or meaningful controls, or no control at all, which lowers the study quality and its real-life meaningfulness.
- **Expectation bias.** If you are told you are being given something that is expected to work better, it can make you perform better. This relates to whether participants are blinded to the intervention.
- **Performance bias.** Did groups perform workouts correctly or follow the intended protocol? Did a researcher push one group to train hard, and another group not so much? Did a researcher give more diet advice to one group than another for weight loss? Was the study protocol adhered to?
- **Exclusion bias.** Did people drop out from the study because an intervention (e.g. the test diet or training plan) was too difficult to adhere to, or too time-consuming to commit? A high dropout rate may suggest that whatever is being studied may be hard to follow, or caused other issues.
- **Outcome bias.** Were measurements taken in exactly the same way between two groups? For weight loss, did both groups have their weight measured at the same time every day, were measures of fat mass conducted in the same way? For muscle gain, were measurements of muscle size measured in the same way, at the same place? Were the tools used to measure outcomes accurate?
- **Outcomes.** Are the outcomes of the study relevant to what we are interested in? Does the study measure a direct or indirect marker of muscle growth or fat loss? Are they the same outcomes as originally described?

- **Discussion.** The results of a study are objective, but the discussion and interpretation of those results is subjective. The discussion helps to put the research into the wider context of the subject area and is in the hands of the authors. There will always be some subjective measure to this discussion, and similarly, people who read and use research can take a subjective interpretation of this discussion and the findings, meaning the claims made from the study may not be what was found. A third party reporting a study may draw very different conclusions. For example, a study assessing weight loss with a pill may find that the group taking the pill lost 3kg in one month. This may be used as a marketing tool for the pill showing it to be beneficial for weight loss. However, if the study was well conducted it would have a control or placebo group. Most likely (based on current research), the placebo or control group also lost a comparable and *non-significantly* different amount of weight to the pill group (i.e. the weight loss pill has no effect on weight loss), but this may be omitted from marketing campaigns[8].

Pretty much any aspect of fitness (diet, exercise and other lifestyle variables) and its effect on body composition can be assessed with a randomised controlled trial. We know who we are studying (healthy, non-obese people), we know what we want to compare (A vs B; high vs low protein intake, high vs low training volume, supplement A vs placebo, diet A vs diet B) and we know what we want to assess (fat loss or muscle gain). Therefore, we can see if one intervention is better than the other, or equivalent.

For example, you could conduct a randomised controlled trial to see if diet 'A' is better for weight loss than diet 'B'. If the outcomes from the group on diet A were significantly different from the outcomes in the group on diet B, there would be evidence to suggest it could have a greater effect on weight loss. Even so, other factors such as the duration of the study, the number of people studied, adherence to the diet, participant training status, amount of weekly training, ethnicity, smoking, alcohol intake (the list goes on) could affect the strength and usefulness of the findings.

A useful study design to overcome this is to get each participant to receive *all* the interventions in a study, called a *cross-over design*. Cross-over trials are where a participant undergoes each treatment or intervention with a break in between interventions (a *washout* period). Cross-over studies can increase the strength of the study findings because each participant acts as their own control. This can reduce many biases and variabilities that may explain differences in results between groups.

Interventional studies can also be *non-randomised*. This introduces a risk of bias, but in certain scenarios it can be more practical and suitable than randomisation, which can sometimes be impossible.

As good as randomised controlled trials are, they are expensive and difficult to conduct. Also, randomised controlled trials are not always the best design for measuring some outcomes, and therefore other study designs can be very useful. For example, when assessing dietary patterns or long-term outcomes, this can be very difficult and expensive to do with a randomised controlled trial, because it requires participants to adhere to the intervention for a long time. This can increase the rate of people dropping out of the study, and can become impractical to implement[3].

Funding for diet and exercise research in health

There is generally far less funding from corporations, charities or governments for studies that do not involve treating a disease, do not involve giving people drugs, or do not involve procedures and treatments that may be of financial interest, On one hand, the greater the financial interest from corporations, the less likely any significant findings in a study are actually true (*commercial bias*)[7]. On the other hand, a lack of funding immediately limits the quality and quantity of research regarding diet and exercise conducted within healthy populations.

With fewer resources, lower quality studies must be performed with less strict methodologies. Reducing biases is both expensive and time consuming[9,10].

Standards have been created for how randomised trials should be reported, to improve consistency and accurately report findings. The *Consolidated Standards of Reporting Trials* (CONSORT) is a set of recommendations that have been produced for improving the reporting and quality of randomised controlled trials[11]. In sports nutrition, it has been shown that many journals that publish articles often fail to adhere to robust CONSORT recommendations[12]. The lower the quality and reporting of the research, the less reliable the findings.

Observational studies

We can learn a lot by watching what people do and what happens to them as a result. Observing what happens is a way of seeing *correlations* or *associations*. However, it cannot show us cause and effect. In other words, observational studies can show that when '*A*' increases, '*B*' also increases. Such that, we can say that an increase in A is associated with an increase in B. But, it *cannot* be used alone to show that A *causes* B. Examples include studying the amount of fruit and vegetables people eat and their body mass index or waist circumference, to see if there is a relationship. *Observational studies* give useful insights on many topics. Data can be produced very quickly and they are often much easier to perform and cheaper than randomised controlled trials[7]. *Longitudinal studies* are where researchers observe people over a period of time. For example, studying the effects of a diet on weight loss with *cohorts* of people on different diets. Data can be collected from a given point onwards (*prospective*) or collected from the past (*retrospective*). Prospective studies are higher quality forms of evidence[7]. *Cross-sectional studies* are a snapshot in time. They look at a group of people at a particular point in time and observe them, which can include taking measurements and asking about their lifestyle, diet and exercise history. For example, a survey may look at people's food intakes and exercise habits to see if the types of food people eat varies with how much exercise they do. We can also find people (*cases*) who have successfully gained muscle mass, or who have successfully lost weight on a diet and compare them to *controls* (such as the general population) and ask them what they do to compare and gain insights into what might work.

Observational studies are often used to identify relationships between variables (such as eating certain foods and changes in body weight) to generate hypotheses, which can then be rigorously studied and quantified in randomised controlled trials[3]. Observational studies by themselves usually do *not* constitute strong evidence for making recommendations. This is an important point to remember when we come to discuss the evidence on certain topics, especially diet.

Descriptive studies

Descriptive studies are lower forms of evidence than analytical studies, describing the characteristics of a person or persons who may differ from the general population[7].

In a *case study*, we can find someone who has gained lots of muscle mass or someone who has successfully lost weight on a diet. We can ask them what they did (or do), to gain insights into what might work. These studies have high levels of bias and can be misinterpreted. If you wanted to run fast, you might ask Usain Bolt what he does. He ate chicken nuggets on the day he broke the 100m world record at the 2008 Olympics in Beijing. This doesn't mean that eating chicken nuggets will make you run faster. A *case series* is simply a description of multiple case studies. For example, studying multiple elite level sprinters, rather than just Usain Bolt. Case studies and case series are primarily used for very rare phenomena (i.e. a rare disease or elite athletes)[7]. Much in the same way that anecdotes can be highly biased, the nature of descriptive studies means that there is much room for bias, especially confirmation bias (looking for relationships that support an agenda).

Expert opinion

Any human research is considered higher quality evidence than the opinion of an expert. The opinion of an expert is not research. It is the least important piece of evidence, because opinion can be heavily driven by bias. When there are no studies on a topic, expert opinion can be useful to drive hypotheses and new ideas for future research. There is a *difference* between expert opinion to help determine the optimum choice for an individual based on evidence from research and personal preference (the evidence-based approach), and the opinion that a particular diet is undeniably better than another for weight loss, despite evidence opposing this opinion or with no evidence at all.

Lab studies

Lab studies in cells or animals are important for mechanistic and preliminary evidence. They can provide initial evidence to support the rationale for human studies and provide an explanation for any findings from randomised controlled trials or observational studies.

When we can't conduct randomised controlled trials or long-term studies, lab studies can actually be very useful to try and find a link between two variables, such as protein intake and satiety, or resistance training and muscle growth. They are very useful for identifying the mechanism behind a process which cannot be achieved with observational or interventional studies. For example, we might know that mechanical tension is the primary driver of muscle growth in human studies. But with lab studies, we can see how this tension leads to cellular changes that cause muscle growth. This extra knowledge can help us to work out whether a causal relationship truly exists, and how to train better for muscle growth.

Animal studies are the lowest quality form of evidence and should only be used to drive hypotheses in human studies. No lab or animal study is used to drive recommendations in healthcare. They should *not* be used by themselves to generate recommendations in humans, and should supplement higher quality evidence. This is another important point to remember when we discuss the evidence on certain topics.

Quality of evidence

The hierarchy of evidence in this book will follow the consensus of the scientific medical bodies; the *Grading of Recommendations Assessment, Development and Evaluation* (GRADE) approach, opting for higher quality evidence first, before referring to lower quality evidence as outlined above in the evidence pyramid[1,3,13,14].

When meta-analyses (studies of studies) aren't available on a topic, I'll use systematic reviews. If neither are available, I'll discuss individual studies and reviews starting with randomised controlled trials, before working through observational studies. At some point any new research topic will have minimal evidence. This is common in fitness. In these scenarios, the individual study evidence is still useful, but should be interpreted with caution.

Very rarely are recommendations of a high certainty. Even if a significant result is found e.g. *'doing X leads to significantly more weight loss than doing Y'*, there is often a cautionary note saying there is a *'low certainty of* evidence' or *'more research is needed to confirm findings'*. This refers to the evidence pyramid and the risks of bias, indicating the quality of the research studies and the number of people being studied is fairly low. So, even though an effect was seen, it would be hard to fully support recommendations without further evidence to confirm it. This isn't being pessimistic or shooting down evidence, but *critically appraising* research to identify potential gaps in the knowledge where more research is needed to confirm or refute findings. *Critical appraisal* is an integral component of scientific research and the evidence-based process. Media can damage and warp the view of research by taking a low-quality study and reporting its findings as 100% fact rather than what it is, which is one tiny piece of a very large jigsaw[15]. Higher-quality large-scale studies are more expensive, complex and time consuming than more basic, lower quality studies with fewer participants. It often requires numerous basic, lower quality studies to justify funding a higher quality study. Small initial studies are needed to work out what the higher quality studies need to measure, in whom, and over what time frame. This is why initial studies on new topics are very insightful and useful to consider, but at the same time they should not be used to draw definitive conclusions or strong recommendations.

"The media does not seem to have much room for reporting of in-process findings and loves short sound bites. In many articles, the result is: reporting on every new study as if it were definitive, complete with comments from detractors or other scientists who recite well-known and well-accepted caveats. This practice treats science as if it were politics and adds to public confusion."
Jacobs and Tapsell, 2013[15].

It's not as clear as black and white

The world of research and evidence-based practice is rarely *'yes'* or *'no'*, or *'do this'* or *'don't do that'*. There are many grey areas and topics that don't appear to be that important for body composition. Often the outcome of research can fall heavily upon the interpretation of the authors and the reader. In this book I have tried to remain as impartial as possible, taking a neutral stance on topics, basing recommendations from the general academic consensus whilst trying to include a range of expert opinions. However, if you disagree or find evidence that opposes what this book covers (or supports!) then please get in touch and let me know. Evidence-based practice is about shifting best practice and recommendations based on new evidence that comes to light, and factoring this into the current knowledge base.

Averages: the importance of individuality

Use research findings as a guide, and then use trial and error to work out what works best for you.

Research findings report what happens *on average*. Individual results can differ massively from this average, as we will see later. Some people may do slightly better and some people may do slightly worse. Even fewer might do much much better or much much worse. But, the majority of people will have results near to the average. Say there were two training plans, 'A' and 'B'. A results in more muscle growth than B. If you studied (using a randomised controlled trial) a large group of people and gave them plan A or B, the average outcome would be that A results in more muscle growth; a given individual has better results with plan A than with plan B (person Y). However, although on average plan B is worse than plan A, some individuals may have better results with plan B than plan A (person X). We can use personal preference and the experience of professionals to understand when certain options may be more suitable for certain people.

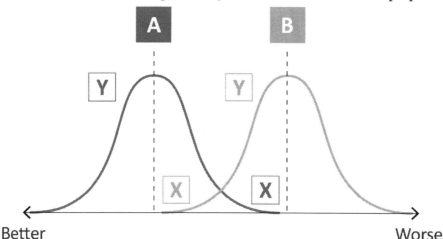

Better   Worse

Most people will be like person Y; they have better results with plan A than plan B. But, some people will be like person X and have better

results on plan B than plan A, even though on average B is not as good as A.

Who is the study on?

This will be mentioned specifically in different chapters, but in general:

- The majority of research looking at muscle growth is on *young, untrained males*. The minority of research is on trained males and trained or untrained females.

- The majority of research on weight loss is on *overweight* and *obese, sedentary individuals*.

- Dietary studies are often without any training plan, and training studies are often without a dietary plan.

Research regarding body composition exists for particular populations, such as those with other diseases. Caution should be taken when generalising findings from a study on a specific group of people onto another group of people, especially if one population is healthy and the other has disease. The greater the difference between the studied population and population of interest to apply the study findings to, the more caution that needs to be applied. A study in young, untrained, healthy males is more applicable and relevant than a study of obese, sedentary, elderly females to young, untrained, healthy males.

Biology is noisy, and signals can be small

Unlike mathematics or physics, biology can be highly variable. The response from a certain action cannot be predicted as accurately[16]. For example, the normal ranges of many molecules in the blood can be huge, yet still be considered normal. And, whenever we measure something, there is *error* in the measurement. Often, measurement tools can only be as accurate as within a few percent of the *true value*. Variability and error are everywhere; how we measure things (such as muscle size or body fat levels), weight changes, individual responses to diets, meals and macronutrients, and even in things such as how accurately people record the food they eat and the exercise they do. This means that when we look at the results, we see large *variances**. Even without giving any intervention (e.g. changing people's diets or changing their training), there may be slight differences in serial measurements of the same thing, such as weighing yourself on the scales from day to day.

* *Variance refers to the amount of variation about the mean. If the average height in the population is 170cm, then if height varied from 1cm above and below 170cm, this would be seen as a fairly small variability and low variance. If height varied from 50cm above and below 170cm, this would be a large variability and high variance; there are people as short as 120cm and as tall as 220cm, but still an average height of 170cm.*

P-values

In research, we use *statistics* to formally determine whether differences exist. In controlled trials, this is often used to compare before and after an intervention or compare between groups receiving different interventions. However, rather than trying to prove there is a difference, we try to *disprove* there is *no* difference. In other words, instead of confirming what we think may happen, we try and invalidate the opposite view. We start with a *null hypothesis,* which states that there is no difference between whatever is being measured (e.g. a comparison between before and after, or between two groups). We then test this hypothesis to see how similar the data is to our null hypothesis '*model*'. The result (called a *P-value*) can provide information on if the differences between whatever is being measured can be best explained just by *chance,* or if the difference is so large that chance alone does not explain the difference very well. This is called a *significant difference.* If a result is significant, we *reject* the null hypothesis and accept the *alternative hypothesis,* which usually states that there *is* a difference between whatever is being measured.

Statistical testing assesses not just the data, but the *assumptions* made about the data[17]. A P-value lies between 0 and 1. A value of 1 means that the data fits our null hypothesis and assumptions perfectly. A P-value of 0 means the data does not fit our null hypothesis or assumptions at all. A null hypothesis could be that no difference in body composition exists between two training plans, A and B. If the study was well conducted and there truly was no difference, we would expect to see a p-value closer to 1. If either the study was poorly conducted, or there was a true difference, we would expect the P-value to be closer to 0. In summary, if we think plan A is better than plan B, rather than trying to *prove* plan A is better than plan B, we try and *disprove* they are the same.

We use an *arbitrary cutoff* in the statistical test to determine how well the data observed matches the assumptions and the null hypothesis model, which are considered to be true for the analysis (i.e. there is no true difference between A and B)[17]. If the P-value is below the arbitrary cutoff, you would reject the null hypothesis, that there is no difference between the groups. You would then accept the alternative hypothesis, that there is a difference. If the P-value is above the arbitrary cutoff, you would accept the null hypothesis, that there is no difference between the groups. This does *not* mean that we reject the alternative hypothesis. It just means that the data conforms with our null hypothesis and assumptions, so there is no reason to reject it[17].

P-values are a contentious area in statistics, because they can be misused and misinterpreted. Other statistical techniques such as *effect sizes* (intervention X increases muscle size by 20% compared to intervention Y) and *confidence intervals* (intervention X increases muscle size on average by 20% compared to intervention Y, but most likely the average lies somewhere between 5% and 35%) have been suggested to improve reporting and to give results a real-life context[17]. Even so, small effect sizes indicate that any finding may also be less likely to actually be true, and just be by chance[10]. P-values assume that all the assumptions made in the study are correct, which is not necessarily the case. As such, a small P-value might mean there is a difference between two groups, or it could mean some of the study design assumptions were incorrect. Similarly, a large P-value might occur even when a true difference exists between two groups, but some assumption of the study design is incorrect (i.e. biases or the type of data being analysed). Hence, poor study design (e.g. biases in how people are recruited or whether randomisation was used to place people into groups) can result in apparent differences when none truly exist (called a *type I error*) or result in no apparent difference when one truly exists (called a *type II error*)[7,10,17]. A highly significant finding may just be representative of large amounts of bias[10]. To summarise, a statistically significant finding may not be true, and a statistically non-significant finding may actually be true.

The P-value tells us how plausible the data is if the null hypothesis model and any assumptions made to calculate it were true. P-values do not tell us whether our hypothesis is true or not, nor does it tell us the probability that the difference observed occurred by chance alone. Unless all the assumptions made are known to be correct, it cannot actually tell us anything specifically about that hypothesis[17].

It is easier to identify a significant difference between two things when there is a large difference between the two means (the average), and lots of measurements (a bigger sample size) are taken of each outcome (lots of values used to calculate the means). We can do a *power* calculation to work out how many things or people we need to generate a significant difference for the outcome of interest, by predicting the expected difference (usually from previous smaller scale studies). Therefore, any good study should be designed to find a statistically significant difference, if there is one to be found. A bigger sample size can reduce the probability of error[7].

Variable responses and the importance of individuality in fitness

The variability in response to a stimulus is huge between people.

The fact that studies can show high variability in outcomes despite using rigorous and tightly controlled study designs highlights how individual responses to the same stimulus can vary wildly. The responses of people from an intervention follows a normal distribution.

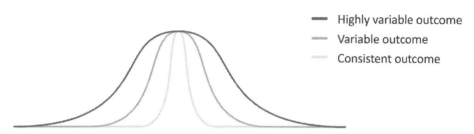

— Highly variable outcome

— Variable outcome

— Consistent outcome

The more variable the outcome, the greater the spread of possible values around the average value. The less variable the outcome, the smaller the spread of possible values around the average value. The outcomes from diet and exercise studies tend to be highly variable.

There is far more variability *between* people, compared to the variability *within* a person in response to a change or given exposure (eating a certain food, diet or using a certain training plan, for example). In response to the same training programme, some people can increase muscle mass by 40%, some by 5-10%, and some may not even grow at all. As such, many well-designed exercise and diet studies may find no differences between groups due to the similar averages in the outcomes from interventions, coupled with the large variabilities in the outcomes from interventions[10].

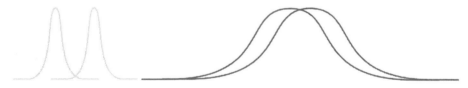

Smaller variabilities in outcomes makes it much easier to identify smaller differences in outcomes between groups, if one exists. Left: small variability and large differences between groups makes it easier to find a difference. Right: large variability and small differences between groups makes it harder to find a difference.

When studying muscle gain and fat loss, often the effects are very small and therefore any differences are small. This means that if we have a lot of variability, it makes it difficult to spot this small effect. In some cases, a study may find an effect that is the opposite to what was expected. Such a result should be interpreted in the context of the quality of the study that generated the finding, and other studies on the topic.

Imagine a study where we placed people into two diet groups; 'A' and 'B'. Participants in both groups are similar for important variables (age, gender, lifestyle etc.), and both are taking part in the same resistance training programme to build muscle, but they are on different diets. We measure important values such as initial muscle mass and fat mass and compare this with the same measurements at the end of the study. We can then see if diet A or diet B leads to greater muscle growth. Let's say that diet A genuinely leads to greater muscle growth. In fact, let's say that diet A leads to twice as much muscle growth as diet B. This high-quality study might show a 2% increase on average in muscle mass in diet A from the start of the study, and a 1% increase on average in diet B. We then use the previously mentioned statistics to identify whether intervention A and B are different. This means that we can see whether the difference we find between the two groups is best explained by chance, or the difference is too large to be best explained by chance alone, and they are *significantly different*. However, this result may or may not be statistically significant (i.e. considered an important difference and not a negligible difference) if the variability around the means are large. This could happen if some people build little muscle (e.g. a 0.1% increase) and some people build a lot of muscle (e.g. a 10% increase) in both groups. Muscle growth can be slow and incredibly variable between people. Therefore, it could be that the study was too short to generate a significant difference (possibly not enough time for meaningful muscle growth), or it can be because the responses of individuals in each group varied so much that no difference was found between the groups.

Studies are short

Conducting research is expensive. It can be hard to recruit people to take part. Even more so when you start asking them to eat certain foods and tell them to follow a specific training programme for weeks on end. This means that diet and training studies are often relatively short in duration, often 6 to 12 weeks in length. The longer a study is, the harder it is to recruit people, the greater the risk of participants dropping out, and the more expensive it is. If small but significant differences do exist, it may be that they cannot be identified in shorter duration studies due to the high variability in measurements. If longer duration studies are not feasible, we can use more people in the shorter duration studies which gives the statistical analysis more *power*, meaning we can find smaller significant differences in the results. Smaller studies not only result in less power, but also increase the risk that any significant finding is less likely to actually be a true finding, and just be by chance[10]. The implications of small, short duration studies will become more apparent later on in studies assessing body composition, especially in trained individuals.

This is also why the experience of expert coaches and trainers are important, as they can provide insights into what can work well or not so well over time periods much longer than can be conducted in studies, over years and decades.

Insignificantly significant

P-values can be a useful tool to formally compare the findings of studies. But, they can be misinterpreted[10]. Two studies could have significant findings, one with very significant findings (the statistical result is well below the arbitrary cut off), and another having only just reached significance (just below the arbitrary cut off). Even if a study finds a significant result, it might not be as important as the authors might like to think, which can make interpreting research slightly trickier[17].

For example, some studies have such weak statistical significance that if one or two participants had the opposite result in a 'Yes' or 'No' style study (e.g. whether or not participants lost 3kg of weight on a particular diet), then the results would no longer be significant (i.e. the probability the differences were due to chance rises above the arbitrary cut off)[18]. People also drop out of studies, such as if they fail to follow the study protocol, lose interest, get injured, or have other commitments. In these borderline studies, often more people drop out than are needed to influence the significance of the result. If one or two participants had the opposite result, the results would no longer be significant. Yet, *more* than 1 or 2 people dropped out of the studies[18].

Flip a coin enough times and you will get 5 heads in a row.

Another point to consider is that the authors of studies may also conduct many statistical analyses. If you conduct enough, just by chance alone you'll get a significant finding. If you flip a coin enough times, you will get 5 heads in a row, even though this is statistically unlikely. The more analyses that a study conducts, the less likely any significant findings are actually true[10]. It is becoming common practice that randomised controlled trials are registered to a database prior to its completion (such as *Clinicaltrials.gov*[19]), to improve transparency and so that researchers analyse what they originally intended to analyse[10].

Statistical significance vs real-life significance: putting research into practice

Statistical significance does not necessarily mean real-life meaningful significance.

So, we've conducted a study on two groups of people, group A and group B. We found that the diet in group A had significantly increased muscle mass compared to the diet in group B, as measured by our statistical tests. Great, so now we can tell the world about our amazing new diet for muscle growth that is so much better than any other diet? Well, no. First, a study like this *only* shows our diet is significantly better than the diet given to group B. The diet in group B may be a poor diet to build muscle. This is a trick used in studies to make one intervention look much better than it is, by comparing the intervention of interest to a control intervention that isn't very good in the first place. Even if it is a high-quality study that was well designed and conducted so that any biases are minimised, we need to consider the practical real-life meaningfulness of the results[17]. For example, was the extra muscle gain of meaningful benefit? And how much extra effort was required to achieve the differences found? Meaningfulness can be *subjective* and *objective*.

Let's use an example of weight loss to explain subjective meaningfulness. This time, people in group A and B are on different diets, but everything else is the same. Say over the course of 16 weeks, the people in group A lost 4kg in weight. The people in group B lost 3kg. We did the statistics and the differences were significant, but only just lower than our arbitrary *by chance* threshold. So, by following the diet in group A, on *average*, people lost an extra 1kg of weight, or 33% greater *relative* weight loss than those in group B. However, the dietary intervention in group A was very difficult, very expensive and many participants complained of feeling hungry, agitated, and tired during the study. On the other hand, group B reported high levels of satiety, feeling well-rested and energised. Therefore, was the extra 1kg of weight lost over the course of 16 weeks worth the extra effort? Fortunately or unfortunately (depending on your viewpoint), there isn't a right or wrong answer. Some people might prefer to go through the large amount of extra effort for the small additional benefit in weight loss, while others might prefer the easier option (which for most would be much easier to adhere to) for marginally less, but still meaningful weight loss. Subjective meaningfulness will become apparent in the diet and training sections, with some variables requiring much more effort for less benefit. Some individuals may subjectively consider these topics to be important enough to consider doing, to 'cover all bases'.

A real-life example of statistical versus objectively meaningful significance was demonstrated in a randomised controlled trial assessing coffee consumption on fat mass[20]. One group of people consumed normal coffee and another group consumed coffee with added *chlorogenic acid* (a substance usually found in coffee). After 12 weeks, there was significantly greater weight loss in the group where people drank coffee with added chlorogenic acid. However, this statistical significance was of a 0.1kg reduction in weight over 12 weeks compared to a 0.0kg weight change in the control coffee group. This statistical difference has no real-life significance. Step on the scales and weigh yourself. Then step off and repeat the measurement. It will probably vary by 0.1kg. Increasing the sample size of a study increases its power, which increases the ability to identify a significant difference that may not actually be a meaningful difference[10].

In contrast, a meaningful result may actually be *smaller* than the smallest statistically significant finding that the study can be powered to find[17]. The issue arises when the difference we are looking for is small and we only have a limited number of people willing to participate. This is true for many studies on muscle growth and weight loss. In trained individuals, muscle growth is slow, highly variable and there are far fewer trained than untrained people. This makes it difficult to prove differences in studies on trained individuals. Trained individuals also have highly variable training histories and ways of training, which creates added variability in the groups being studied. However, it should be known beforehand how many people are needed in the study (with a *power* calculation), such that enough people are recruited anyway[7]. Even so, the findings may be smaller than expected, so no significant differences are found. A review on a particular topic may therefore appear to be as though there is no significant effect, as many small studies find no difference. However, there could still be an important effect, but the studies were *underpowered* to find it. This is where meta-analyses can be very useful, by combining data from similarly designed studies to increase the effective sample size. This enables identification of smaller, significant differences, and why they are incredibly useful in the world of evidence-based fitness[8].

As briefly mentioned earlier, *confidence intervals* are another useful statistical tool. They are a measure of *interval estimates* – the probability that the true value (the average) lies within a certain range of values. Imagine conducting lots of hypothesis tests to generate P-values for lots of possible differences between two groups. For example, to test how well the data conforms to a difference between A and B of 0, of 0.5, of 1, of 2, and so on. At certain differences above and below the true difference, the P-value will cross the significant arbitrary cut-off value. A confidence interval means that if we repeated the study many times, we can have a certain level of confidence that the true value would lie within this range of values[17]. In other words, confidence intervals are a way of saying that the true value likely lies within a range, rather than stating a specific value. But, confidence intervals do not guarantee the true value lies within this range, and they again also assume that the hypothesis and assumptions are true, like P-values[17]. The smaller that range, the more confident we can be in that specific mean value estimate. In the example above, diet A results in 4kg of weight loss,

33% more than group B (3kg of weight loss). Confidence intervals could be used to say that the true average effect size of using the diet in group A would be between say, 15% and 50%, or 1.15 and 1.50 times greater than the diet in group B. You can be pretty confident the true average lies between these values. The smaller the range of the intervals, the more precise the estimation can be. An interval from 25% to 35% is more precise than 15% to 50% (or 1.25-1.35 compared to 1.15-1.50)[17]. If the confidence intervals do not cross the no difference *null* value (in this case, 1.00), then it provides good confidence that there *is* a true difference between groups. Confidence intervals and P-values are *related*. Confidence intervals are important tools to determine whether a significant difference has real-life, meaningful significance, by considering the possible effect size, and not just its significance (the P-value)[7,17].

Using statistical tools such as confidence intervals can help to show *trends* in findings. Regardless, *non-significant trends* in the data do not form the basis for a strong scientific argument for recommendation, and should be used to guide further research[8].

Confounding and mediation

A major issue with research especially in observational studies, is *confounding*[21]. We think there is an association between two variables, but actually this association is explained by another variable. Say we conduct a study and measure three variables, '*A*', '*B*' and '*C*'. After conducting the analysis, we find there is an association between the two variables, A and C. However, it turns out that A is also linked to the variable B, and B is also linked to C. A and B are confounded when:

1.   A and B are related to C.
2.   A and B are associated, but B *is not caused* by A[21].

Say a study shows an association between A and C. When A increases, C increases. But, when B increases, C also increases. We can remove the influence of B on C (in statistics, we can *adjust* for this variable). With this adjustment, the association between A and C is reduced. Now, when A increases, C does not increase as much as before, but it still increases. B is a *confounding variable*. B explained some of the changes seen in C, but not as a result of changes in A. We see this very often in human studies. Sometimes, the effect of confounding can be so great that after adjusting for the confounding variable B, the association between A and C can be completely lost. In this case, when A increases, C does not increase at all. There is *no* direct association between A and C. This is why common confounders such as age and gender are controlled for between study groups in randomised controlled trials or adjusted for in observation studies.

We can draw this out:

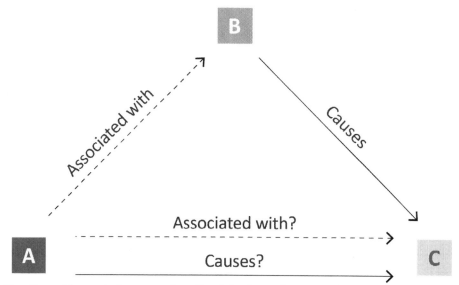

Confounding: A is associated with C. B is associated with C. A is associated with B, but *does not* cause B.

An example of confounding in an observational study is comparing the body mass index (weight divided by height[2]) (C) of people who do not eat meat (A), versus people who do eat meat. Non-meat eaters generally have a lower body mass index than people who eat meat[22]. People who eat meat are more likely to do less physical activity and eat less fruit and vegetables (B)[22]. Consuming more meat does not cause people to do less exercise or eat less fruit or vegetables, but both are associated with a higher body mass index. Non-meat eaters also tend to consume less energy and less protein than meat eaters, which can influence weight change and muscle growth[22,23]. In other words, there are differences between people who do or do not eat meat other than just their meat consumption, that can explain differences in body mass index and body composition. These confounders amongst many others (such as socioeconomic status, alcohol intake and smoking history) need to be accounted for.

    A.   Meat consumption.
    B.   Physical activity and fruit and vegetable intake.
    C.   Body mass index.

    1.   A and B are related to C.
    2.   A and B are associated, but B *is not caused* by A.

An example of confounding in a randomised controlled trial could be the effect of two different resistance training plans (A) on muscle growth (C), and the protein intake of each group (B). Resistance training results in muscle growth but in itself does not cause greater protein intake. However, protein intake also influences muscle growth. If protein intake is not controlled for in a training study, it may appear as though one resistance training programme is better than another for muscle growth, when in fact it may just be that all the people in one group consumed optimal amounts of protein and the other group ate much less protein.

    A.   Resistance training.
    B.   Protein intake.
    C.   Muscle growth.

    1.   A and B are related to C.
    2.   A and B are associated, but B *is not caused* by A.

Mediation

Very importantly, *mediation* is similar, but different to confounding. B is a mediator of A when:

    1.   A and B are related to C.
    2.   A and B are associated, but B *is caused* by A[21].

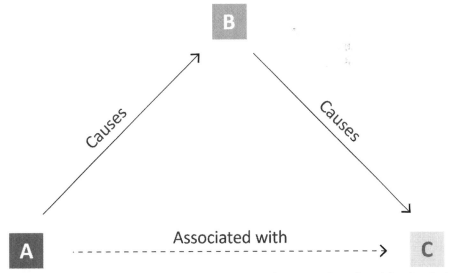

Mediation: A is associated with C. B is associated with C. A is associated with B, but *does* cause B.

An example of mediation is excess sugar or fat consumption (A), weight gain (C) and a daily calorie surplus (eating more energy than you expend) (B). Excessive sugar or fat consumption causes weight gain[24]. However, this is as a result of excess calorie consumption. Therefore, the association between sugar or fat consumption and weight gain is explained by any excess calorie consumption. When there is no calorie surplus, fat or sugar consumption does not result in weight gain. Excess calorie consumption mediates weight gain as a result of the calorie content of sugar and fat consumed. This will be discussed in much greater detail later on.

A. Excess sugar and/or fat consumption.
B. Calorie surplus.
C. Weight gain.

1. A and B are related to C.
2. A and B are associated, but B *is caused* by A.

Another example of mediation would be going to the gym twice per week (A), leg muscle growth (C), and performing a leg resistance training workout twice per week (B). Going to the gym is associated with leg muscle growth. However, this is entirely explained and mediated by the leg workout that takes place during the gym. Controlling for the leg workout results in no association between going to the gym and leg muscle growth. Going to the gym in itself, does not build muscle. But, a leg workout occurs from going to the gym.

A. Going to the gym every week.
B. Leg workout every week.
C. Leg muscle growth.

1. A and B are related to C.
2. A and B are associated, but B *is caused* by A.

Sometimes, the difference between a confounder or mediator is obvious. At other times, it can be very difficult to determine. How do you know if a variable is a confounder or a mediator? This can get even more tricky when there is a mediator that partially explains the relationship between A and C, and a confounder that is unrelated to A, but has the same mediator relating to C. As discussed in the training chapters, mechanical tension, metabolic stress and muscle damage are proposed mechanisms of muscle growth. The close relationship between mechanical tension, metabolic stress and muscle damage makes it difficult to determine whether metabolic stress and muscle damage are confounders or mediators, or partial confounders or mediators of mechanical tension and muscle growth, or even if they are relevant at all. This is critical, because it influences evidence-based recommendations.

Health and fitness in the media

It is pretty hard to avoid fitness in the media. Every day, new articles and ads boast about the latest miracle diet, the best training plans to get you 'lean' and 'toned', or new 'research' about a miracle food, cure or remedy. A typical headline may read: *'study shows amazing new findings that revolutionise the way we think about fitness'*. In reality, new research makes tiny baby steps building on the knowledge that we already have. Sudden miracle findings that radically change our viewpoint are incredibly rare, and if they do, should be carefully examined. The problem is that immediate solutions and fixes make for great headlines that sell. *'New study confirms findings and strengthens what we already suspected about losing weight'* is far less catchy.

Most information regarding fitness is poorly interpreted or incorrect in the media. This doesn't mean all articles are poor or unreliable. High-quality information is often written by impartial organisations or by guest authors who are scientists themselves. But, this ultimately makes the issue of working out how to improve body composition a minefield when there is so much conflicting or incorrect information available. I will refer to some excellent, publicly available online articles from leading experts in the field of diet and exercise.

Want to know how easy it is for information to be misreported in the media? John Bohannon made up a study about how eating chocolate promotes greater weight loss than not eating chocolate*. This was an actual study, but purposely designed to be a very low-quality study to generate significant findings. For example, there were few participants, participants were not matched between study groups for age or gender and there were many study endpoints, increasing the probability that a statistically significant finding would be found in at least one measurement by chance. The study managed to get onto the front cover of *Bild*, and numerous online websites including *The Huffington Post* and the *Daily Mail*[25].

* Note: it is entirely possible to eat chocolate and lose weight, and not eat any chocolate and gain weight, by increasing or decreasing total daily calorie intake.

Why do conflicting views and findings exist in research?

Research can be largely positive, largely negative, or largely neutral in outcomes across studies. In some topics, there are clear differences and a consensus agreement. However, often there are both positive and negative results, and conflicting views from the interpretations of researchers. Study quality is an important factor as discussed. Differences in outcomes can also be due to comparing studies with fundamental differences which are not necessarily obvious in the *abstract* (a short summary of the study), or because of confounding variables that have not been considered or differ between studies. A prime example is the debate between low carbohydrate or low fat diets and weight loss (discussed in chapter 8). Some studies conclude that low carbohydrate diets are better. Some studies conclude that low fat diets are better. Some say they are equal. However, when we control for factors that we know affect weight change, such as total calorie intake and protein intake, studies show low fat or low carbohydrate diets are equally effective. Neither is superior. Therefore, studies not equating calorie intake or protein intake are not actually directly *comparable*, which can lead to incorrect conclusions about results if such studies are compared. This applies to many research areas where study designs appear to be the same or similar, but actually are assessing different things with different study designs. Assessing a diet where energy intake is unrestricted (i.e. people can eat as much as they like) is very different to assessing a diet where energy intake is controlled (i.e. people can only consume a given number of calories per day). This is where the critique of research papers to determine the strength and quality of each study, and also whether important factors have been considered is important to determine what is the best current available evidence on a topic.

Publication Bias

People tend to tell people when they 'have' found something. People don't tend to tell people when they 'haven't' found something.

Positive or significant findings are more likely to be published than non-significant findings (called *publication bias*). This results in a bias in the research database, showing something to apparently be beneficial, but actually when considering all the studies that were conducted but *not* published in a peer-reviewed journal, the positive studies may actually be outweighed by the unpublished negative studies. Plotting the study outcome against the study size (see graph below) can show if the results are biased towards a larger or smaller effect. It would be expected that less precise, smaller studies would have outcomes greater or smaller than the more precise, larger studies. If for example, smaller studies showing a smaller effect are not present, but smaller studies showing a larger effect are present, then the results give the impression of a larger effect than there probably is. This would indicate publication bias.

This can be due to underhand tactics to only publish data supporting a benefit (e.g. a drug to treat a disease or a supplement to aid muscle growth). However, it is often just due to the fact that people conducting research are more likely to put in the effort required to prepare a research study for publication when they find an effect or a difference. However, a study showing no difference is *equally* as important as a study showing a difference[10].

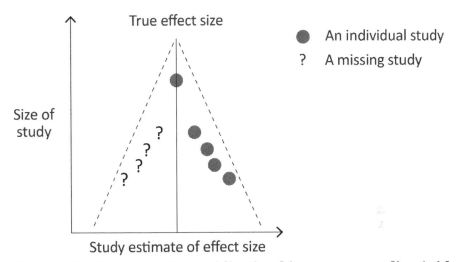

A *funnel plot* demonstrating publication bias. **Larger studies (with more participants) will have less-variable outcomes that are nearer to the true value. Smaller studies will have more-variable outcomes that will be greater and smaller than the true value.**

Summary

There is a hierarchy of evidence, based on study design and methodology.

A positive (a significant difference) result may not actually be true.

A neutral (no significant difference) result may not actually be true.

A positive result is more likely to be published. A neutral or negative result is less likely to be published.

Human studies have high levels of variability. Individual responses can be lost within the average of a population.

A significant finding is not necessarily a meaningful finding.

Stronger recommendations can be made when[10]:

- *Systematic reviews and meta-analyses exist for a topic, based on well-designed randomised controlled trials.*
- *Trials involve a large number of participants.*
- *Trials use accurate tools to measure directly relevant endpoints.*
- *Trials assess a small selection of measures which result in highly significant, large effect sizes.*
- *There are minimal corporate interests or private funding.*

Very few research areas have a strong level of evidence, and very few will ever achieve this level of evidence.

The probability that findings are actually true decreases further with smaller meta-analyses, greater bias in randomised controlled trials, and decrease even further in observational studies.

The more research labs working on a topic, the more likely any significant finding is also unlikely to actually be true.

References

1   Harbour R, Miller J. A new system for grading recommendations in evidence based guidelines. *BMJ* 2001; 323: 334–336.

2   Greenhalgh T. *How to Read a Paper: The Basics of Evidence-based Medicine and Healthcare*, 6th Edition. Wiley 2019. Available from: https://www.wiley.com/en-us/How+to+Read+a+Paper%3A+The+Basics+of+Evidence+based+Medicine+and+Healthcare%2C+6th+Edition-p-9781119484745 (accessed 4 Feb 2020).

3   Johnston BC, Seivenpiper JL, Vernooij RWM, de Souza RJ, Jenkins DJA, Zeraatkar D et al. The Philosophy of Evidence-Based Principles and Practice in Nutrition. *Mayo Clin Proc Innov Qual Outcomes* 2019; 3: 189–199.

4   McClements DJ. *Nutraceuticals: Superfoods or Superfads? In: Future Foods.* SpringerLink 2019. Available from: https://link.springer.com/chapter/10.1007/978-3-030-12995-8_6 (accessed 4 Feb 2020).

5   Smith R. Peer review: a flawed process at the heart of science and journals. *J R Soc Med* 2006; 99: 178–182.

6   Evans I, Thornton H, Chalmers I, Glasziou P. *Testing Treatments: Better Research for Better Healthcare.* 2nd ed. Pinter & Martin: London, 2011 Available from: http://www.ncbi.nlm.nih.gov/books/NBK66204/ (accessed 4 Feb 2020).

7   Çaparlar CÖ, Dönmez A. What is Scientific Research and How Can it be Done? *Turk J Anaesthesiol Reanim* 2016; 44: 212–218.

8   Kerksick CM, Wilborn CD, Roberts MD, Smith-Ryan A, Kleiner SM, Jäger R et al. ISSN exercise & sports nutrition review update: research & recommendations. *J Int Soc Sports Nutr* 2018; 15. Available from: doi:10.1186/s12970-018-0242-y.

9   Ludwig DS, Ebbeling CB, Heymsfield SB. Improving the Quality of Dietary Research. *JAMA* 2019; 322: 1549–1550.

10   Ioannidis JPA. Why Most Published Research Findings Are False. *PLOS Med* 2005; 2: e124.

11   Consort. *Welcome to the CONSORT Website.* Available from: http://www.consort-statement.org/ (accessed 4 Feb 2020).

12   Proceedings of the Fifteenth International Society of Sports Nutrition (ISSN) Conference and Expo. *J Int Soc Sports Nutr* 2018; 15: 1-37. Available from: https://jissn.biomedcentral.com/articles/10.1186/s12970-018-0256-5 (accessed 6 Feb 2020).

13   Grade Working Group. Grading quality of evidence and strength of recommendations. *BMJ* 2004; 328: 1490.

14   Burns PB, Rohrich RJ, Chung KC. The Levels of Evidence and their role in Evidence-Based Medicine. *Plast Reconstr Surg* 2011; 128: 305–310.

15   Jacobs DR, Tapsell LC. Food synergy: the key to a healthy diet. *Proc Nutr Soc* 2013; 72: 200–206.

16   Hall KD. Modeling metabolic adaptations and energy regulation in humans. *Annu Rev Nutr* 2012; 32: 35–54.

17   Greenland S, Senn SJ, Rothman KJ, Carlin JB, Poole C, Goodman SN et al. Statistical tests, P values, confidence intervals, and power: a guide to misinterpretations. *Eur J Epidemiol* 2016; 31: 337–350.

18   Pędziwiatr M, Mizera M, Wysocki M, Małczak P, Stefura T, Gajewska N et al. The fragility of statistically significant results from clinical nutrition randomized controlled trials. *Clin Nutr* 2019. Available from: doi:10.1016/j.clnu.2019.05.024.

19   ClinicalTrials.gov. *ClinicalTrials.gov.* Available from: https://clinicaltrials.gov/ (accessed 4 Feb 2020).

20   Watanabe T, Kobayashi S, Yamaguchi T, Hibi M, Fukuhara I, Osaki N. Coffee Abundant in Chlorogenic Acids Reduces Abdominal Fat in Overweight Adults: A Randomized, Double-Blind, Controlled Trial. *Nutrients* 2019; 11. Available from: doi:10.3390/nu11071617.

21   Babyak MA. Understanding confounding and mediation. *Evid Based Ment Health* 2009; 12: 68–71.

22   Papier K, Tong TYN, Appleby PN, Bradbury KE, Fensom GK, Knuppel A et al. Comparison of Major Protein-Source Foods and Other Food Groups in Meat-Eaters and Non-Meat-Eaters in the EPIC-Oxford Cohort. *Nutrients* 2019. Available from: doi:10.3390/nu11040824.

23   Clarys P, Deliens T, Huybrechts I, Deriemaeker P, Vanaelst B, De Keyzer W et al. Comparison of Nutritional Quality of the Vegan, Vegetarian, Semi-

Vegetarian, Pesco-Vegetarian and Omnivorous Diet. *Nutrients* 2014; 6: 1318–1332.

24   Hall KD, Ayuketah A, Brychta R, Cai H, Cassimatis T, Chen KY et al. Ultra-processed diets cause excess calorie intake and weight gain: A one-month inpatient randomized controlled trial of ad libitum food intake. *Cell Metab* 2019. Available from: doi:10.31232/osf.io/w3zh2.

25   Bohannon J. *I Fooled Millions Into Thinking Chocolate Helps Weight Loss. Here's How.* 2015. Available from: https://io9.gizmodo.com/i-fooled-millions-into-thinking-chocolate-helps-weight-1707251800 (accessed 5 Feb 2020).

5. Body composition and health

Body composition is not synonymous with health. Health is much more than just body composition.

With all else the same, increasing muscle mass or decreasing fat mass aligns with improved physical health outcomes.

The focus of this book is on body composition. For our purposes, body composition simply refers to how much fat and how much muscle you have. An improvement in body composition is regarded as a relative decrease in body fat, and/or an increase in muscle mass. What someone considers to be an optimum balance of fat and muscle mass is personal. Indeed, someone may already be at their perceived optimal body composition. However, regardless of the amount of fat someone wants to lose or how much muscle someone wants to gain, if any at all, there are basic weight loss and muscle gain principles that apply to all.

Health is more than just body composition. Improving health should also consider general physical, mental and social health and wellbeing.

"A healthy diet should optimize health, defined broadly as being a state of complete physical, mental and social well-being and not merely the absence of disease."
EAT-Lancet Commission, 2019[1].

Body weight is less important than *body composition* for health[2]. In people eating a well-structured diet with no deficiencies, participating in exercise and with no pre-existing disease, then with all else being equal, an increase in muscle mass and/or a decrease in fat mass within the normal healthy range is associated with improved health outcomes. Excluding the extremes of body composition (very low body fat percentages, and/or increasing muscle mass through the use of anabolic steroids), markers of physical health improve, and disease risk is reduced with lower levels of body fat and with increased muscle mass[3–6]. As an absolute minimum, body fat levels should not drop below 5% for males, and not below 12% for females to maintain health[7]. Neither is it recommended nor necessary to drop anywhere near as low as these body fat levels as a generally active, healthy individual.

The largest influence of diet on physical health is via its effect on body composition.

"There appears to be little weight loss advantage or difference in metabolic health outcomes between dietary approaches and improvements in health are relative to degree of weight loss."
Thom and Lean, 2017[8].

Losing weight does not mean better health.

Weight loss is *not* synonymous with improved health. Weight lost from muscle mass is detrimental to health, such as in starvation or with aging. Weight loss to the detriment of health can occur in elite athletes, such as boxers rapidly dropping weight for a fight, or bodybuilders reaching very low levels of body fat. Similarly, such divergences between health and body weight occur in the general population, where people try to achieve weight loss by following poor quality diets, exercise plans and lifestyles. Very low levels of body fat and muscle mass are detrimental to health[9,10]. For the vast majority of the population, there is *no* reason to make body composition changes to the detriment of health. This book will discuss body composition in the context of improving or maintaining general health, not to the detriment of health.

Muscle mass is important for many aspects of health. Skeletal muscle (the muscles that attach to the skeleton, such as biceps or calves) provides an important role in regulating blood sugar levels[11]. Very low levels of muscle mass can be to the detriment of health. Low levels of muscle mass can be particularly problematic in older age, where total body muscle mass naturally decreases after the age of 30 by 4-5% per decade[12]. This can increase the risk of falls, bone loss and fractures, frailty and immobility[12,13]. Increasing muscle strength has been associated with maintenance of long-term health[12]. Maintaining or improving strength is linked to maintaining or increasing muscle mass. However, increasing muscle mass with the aid of anabolic steroids again results in a divergence between muscle mass and health. Anabolic steroid use increases the risk of mortality and leads to a range of health complications including problems with the heart and blood vessels, skin, liver and cognitive changes to name a few[14,15].

Sex differences in body composition

Women generally have more fat mass and less muscle mass than men. The amount of muscle that women can build is less than men due to lower levels of circulating testosterone.

Males and females differ in body composition from genetics, but both genders vary across a continuum. Males usually have lower body fat percentages, averaging around 15% of body weight as fat mass compared to around 25-27% in females. This includes essential fat stores found in the central nervous system as well as fat stored under the skin (*subcutaneous fat*) and around organs (*visceral fat*). Body composition also varies between males and females in terms of where fat may be stored – the gynoid '*pear-shaped*' pattern is found in females with fat stored around the hips and thighs, and the android '*apple-shaped*' pattern in males, with fat stored around the abdomen[11]. These are generalisations. Where fat is stored will vary on an individual basis, such that for the same body fat percentage, someone may store more fat around their abdomen compared to someone else who may store more fat around the hips, or another part of the body.

In terms of muscle mass, females generally carry less muscle than men. The difference is greater in the upper body than the lower body[11]. As will be discussed later, the primary driver of muscle growth is resistance training. The increase in *muscle protein synthesis* over the course of a day after a resistance training session is the same in males and females. Meaning, resistance training results in the same muscle building stimulus for females as for males[16]. But in reality, females will not be able to build as much muscle as men because of lower levels of circulating *testosterone* (an important hormone in muscle growth). Even with similar and adequate nutrition, good genetics and an optimal resistance training programme, women do not build as much muscle as men[17].

What determines body weight?

Your body weight depends on three main factors:

- your *genetics.*
- your *environment.*
- your *behaviour.*

You cannot change your *genetics*, but it is possible to change your *environment* and *behaviours,* to an extent[8]. There are factors outside of your control that influence your body weight.

Genetics influences body composition, but we know far too little to make any recommendations based on the genes someone has.

Genes are specific DNA sequences that code for proteins. The ways in which genes are activated and the subsequent ways in which proteins can interact and exert an effect are highly complex. We know that our genes influence our body weight. But, genes do not act by themselves in isolation. Genetics can explain 65% of the population variation in body mass index (BMI), which likely involves 1000s of genes that all influence energy intake, energy expenditure and physical activity[18]. This is complicated further when considering that genes interact with other genes, and genes interact with the environment. You may have seen in the news about modern *genotyping* studies where people have had their genes scanned to see which genes may predispose them to gaining (or losing) weight. This is an exciting and very new area of research. However, at this stage there is not enough evidence to advise a particular diet based on someone's genes[19]. Therefore, the role of genetics will not be discussed further. Who knows, maybe in 20 to 30 years' time we might be able to recommend certain diets to some people with a specific genotype (the genes you have). But right now, there's *no* evidence to support this. A study of 609 adults found no influence of genotype on the success of weight loss. People with a genetic make-up suited to a low fat diet lost as much weight on a high fat diet as people genetically suited to a high fat diet, and vice versa[20]. Genotype had no association with dietary changes on weight loss. Another study found similar short-term weight loss when in a calorie deficit, regardless of whether a participant had certain variants of a gene that are associated with an increased risk of obesity (the *FTO* gene)[21]. It is also important to point out that this genetic research is primarily focussed on body weight and not body composition. The gene-based diets also relate to body weight and waist circumference and therefore would not necessarily be designed for muscle growth or reducing fat mass whilst preserving muscle mass.

So now we know that genetic, environmental and behavioural factors influence our body weight. But what causes our body weight to change?

How to lose weight, how to maintain weight, and how to gain weight

Weight change is determined by the long-term balance between calories consumed and calories expended.

Above all other factors such as the amount of protein, carbohydrates or fat in your diet, meal timing, meal frequency or even food source and quality, if you eat more calories than you expend, you will gain weight. Eat less than you expend, and you will lose weight.

Body weight consists of *fat mass* and *fat-free mass*. Fat-free mass includes organs, bones, blood and muscle. Muscle is also known as *lean muscle mass*[22].

There is the only equation you need to learn if you want to lose, maintain or gain weight:

Calorie (energy) intake – Calorie (energy) expenditure = ± Weight change[2,8]

This means that weight gain is highly correlated with calorie intake[23]. A calorie is a unit of energy*. Consume more energy than you need, and there will be weight gain. Consume less energy than you need, and there will be weight loss. Consume the same amount of energy as you need, and there will be no change in weight[2]. Weight change can occur through changes in both fat mass and fat-free mass.

* The terms 'calorie' and 'energy' will be used interchangeably in this book.

The relative difference between the calories you consume and the calories you expend dictates weight change. It follows the *first rule of thermodynamics*, you cannot destroy or create energy, only change its form[2,19].

Losing weight is theoretically simple. Losing weight is practically very difficult.

Although the difference between what you expend and what you consume dictates weight change, many factors inside *and* outside of your control influence how much energy you expend and how much energy you consume. Despite the common belief that body weight is simply a case of how much you choose to eat and how much you choose to exercise, this is *not true*. As simple and correct as the *'calories in, calories out'* concept is, it only tells us *why* we lose (or gain) weight. It doesn't help us to work out *how* to lose weight (or gain weight). Telling someone they need to eat less food and move more to lose weight is like telling a football team that to win matches, they need to score more goals and concede fewer goals to win a match. As correct as it may be, it provides no help in achieving the desired outcome. Losing weight and maintaining weight loss is difficult because of the complex changes that have to take place in order to achieve a long-term change in body composition *and* because of the factors outside our control. A long-term change in body composition requires a long-term shift in *behaviour* and *habits*. It is influenced by the environmental, behavioural and genetic factors mentioned before. Some of which we can alter, and some of which we cannot[24]. Some people struggle to lose weight. Conversely, some people struggle to gain weight. No matter how much some people think they are eating, they cannot add weight and build muscle.

Genetics, environment and behaviour influence both calorie intake and calorie expenditure.

Factors within all three can either promote or suppress energy intake and expenditure[24]. What this means is that genetics do not *cause* weight gain, but instead influence energy intake and expenditure, such that it may make it harder or easier to gain weight. This is also partially why some people, even with the best of behavioural intentions and motivation, struggle to induce meaningful weight change.

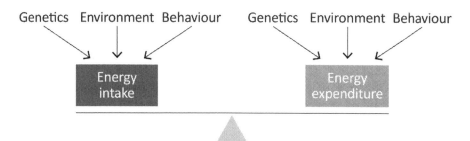

Genetics, environment and behaviour influence our energy intake and energy expenditure. The long-term balance between energy intake and expenditure determines our body weight.

Your environment can influence energy balance, including factors such as the people you surround yourself with, your home, your neighbourhood and food availability. Behavioural choices can positively or negatively influence weight change. Regular physical activity and consuming high levels of dietary fibre have convincingly strong evidence that they may protect against weight gain. A sedentary lifestyle and high intakes of energy-dense, micronutrient-poor food have convincingly strong evidence that they may promote weight gain[25]. The more you move (resulting in a tendency to increase the number of calories you expend) and the fewer calories you eat (therefore the less energy you consume), the more likely you are to be in a calorie deficit and lose weight. The less you move (resulting in a tendency to decrease the number of calories you expend)), and the more calories you eat (therefore the more energy you consume), the more likely you are to be in a calorie surplus and gain weight.

The overwhelming and prevailing view amongst academics is that energy balance determines weight gain and weight loss (energy consumed – energy expended: the energy balance model)[2].

The energy balance model is simply what has been described above. Weight change is the result of differences between energy intake and energy expenditure. There are some sceptics that believe weight gain is the result of carbohydrate consumption, and the resulting rise in *insulin* causes fat storage (the *carbohydrate-insulin model*), leading to weight gain[26,27]. This is discussed in more detail in chapter 8. Layne Norton has written an excellent publicly available summary on why the carbohydrate-insulin model does not make sense, how it has been disproven from the research we have, and why the energy balance model fits the data incredibly well[27,28].

How much weight you gain or lose will then depend on the *size* and *duration* of the calorie difference and to a lesser extent, other factors. Which means, you can lose weight on a diet of just doughnuts or cake. Is this healthy or optimal? No. But it highlights how simple (theoretically) weight loss can be. The difficult bit of course is achieving and sticking to this calorie restricted diet. In other words, *consistency* and *adherence*.

Adherence: forming new habits and sticking to them

Regardless of the chosen diet, weight loss correlates with dietary *adherence*. Greater weight loss is seen in people who adhere to being in the predetermined calorie deficit[29,30]. If you didn't lose as much weight as you'd expected or didn't lose any weight at all, it's probably because your calorie deficit wasn't as big as you thought, or because you weren't even in a calorie deficit in the first place. It has been repeatedly shown in studies that participants grossly underreport energy intake[31–33].

Adherence and the formation of new habits required for changes in body composition will not be discussed in this book but will be assumed to be present. Discussions of how to progress or improve when plateauing will assume that there is adherence to the plan of choice.

It would be short-sighted to write a book about lifestyle changes without providing resources on how to successfully bring about changes and enforce new habits. This is way beyond the scope of this book. For some great resources that include how to create habits that you stick to in the long term, I recommend reading '*Atomic Habits*' by James Clear[34], and literature on the concept of *self-determination theory*[35].

Metabolism, appetite and weight change: how does the body balance energy in and energy out?

We know that genetic, environmental and behavioural factors influence our body weight by affecting how much energy we expend and how much energy we consume. This difference between calories in and calories out causes our body weight to change. But things get more complicated, as it is clear that body weight is regulated[36]. What causes our intake and expenditure to be matched? What drives us to eat or to stop eating food, and what does our body do when we eat more or less food than we need?

American adults gain on average 0.5-1kg of weight per year, which is around 2500 extra kilocalories (kcal, referred to as *'calories'*, but this is actually 1000x smaller in magnitude) consumed over the course of an approximate 1,000,000kcal annual calorie intake. If this were from a daily calorie surplus, it would mean overfeeding by just under 7kcal per day[36]. Weight gain is usually the result of brief periods of overfeeding without subsequent periods of underfeeding, rather than a tiny daily calorie surplus (i.e. 7kcal per day) for long durations[36]. People put on *'holiday weight'*, but then never lose it again[18]. Therefore, there are regulatory mechanisms that to try to balance energy intake with expenditure, but they can be breached.

Basal metabolic rate

The body is resistant to change. It wants to keep things as they are (the concept of homeostasis). The body will act to keep things the same and will adjust accordingly, depending on whether you eat more than you need, or less than you need. Your metabolism is not fixed. If you lose weight your metabolism will decrease. If you gain weight your metabolism will increase. No matter your previous weight change history, your metabolism will be the very similar at a given body composition, you cannot 'damage' it.

Metabolism refers to chemical processes that take place within the body to generate energy from food. This energy is then used to carry out any active function within the body, including breaking down food, building new tissue or fuelling muscles[37]. The rate at which we use energy to fuel these processes varies depending on what we are doing (such as exercising, eating or sleeping). At the most basic level, there is a minimum rate of metabolism that is required for us to stay alive[38].

This is our *resting metabolic rate (RMR)*, or *basal metabolic rate (BMR)*. BMR and RMR actually have minor technical differences in calculation, but are negligible for our discussion. It is the largest component of our *total daily energy expenditure (TDEE)*. Basal metabolic rate varies between individuals, but not as much as people think. A 5"1' female weighing 50kg will indeed have a much lower basal metabolic rate than a 6"0' male weighing 90kg. But, the basal metabolic rate of people with a comparable height, weight, gender and age, is quite similar[2,39]. The *standard deviation* of resting metabolic rate for a given body composition is around 300kcal. This means that 68% of people with the same muscle mass and fat mass will have a metabolic rate within 300kcal of each other. 95% of people with the same muscle mass and fat mass will have a metabolic rate within 600 kcal of each other[2]. Therefore, even the most extreme resting metabolic rates will only be around 300kcal smaller or larger than the average for their body composition. The largest portion of our metabolic rate is the result of fuelling our organs and tissues. The most energy demanding tissues per unit weight are the heart and kidneys[40]. Muscle and fat are both active tissues that contribute to basal metabolic rate. Fat mass is not completely inactive, playing a role in hormone production, but is less metabolically active than muscle. The effect of increasing muscle mass actually has a fairly limited effect on basal metabolic rate. Adding 5kg of muscle mass would only increase basal metabolic rate by around 65 kcal per day. Adding 5kg of fat mass would increase basal metabolic rate by around 23 kcal per day[40]. However, this excludes any additional energy expenditure from increased muscle mass during exercise, which can start to become meaningful. We can calculate basal metabolic rate using fancy equipment where we measure the rate that someone is breathing in oxygen. This can tell us how many calories someone is burning after making a few assumptions (called *indirect calorimetry*). Obviously, this is impractical for you and I. Fortunately, there are formulae that have been developed from human studies that can be used to roughly calculate our basal metabolic rate. Chapter 7 will discuss calculating your energy needs.

Total daily energy expenditure

Unless you spend your whole life lying completely still, the amount of energy your body uses is greater than your basal metabolic rate. Our overall daily metabolic rate, or *total daily energy expenditure* (TDEE) includes not just our basal metabolic rate, but other energy requiring processes:

1. **Non-exercise activity thermogenesis (NEAT)**: the energy used during movement not associated with exercise (e.g. fidgeting, cooking, cleaning).
2. **Exercise activity thermogenesis (EAT):** the energy used during conscious physical activity (exercise).
3. The **thermic effect of food (TEF):** the energy cost of eating, digesting, absorbing, using and storing ingested food.

The variation in NEAT and EAT between people can be very large, and are major factors influencing weight change or weight maintenance.

And so,

$$TDEE = BMR + NEAT + EAT + TEF$$

At weight maintenance,

Total daily energy intake = Total daily energy expenditure (TDEI) = (TDEE)

Component of total daily energy expenditure (TDEE)	Proportion of total daily energy expenditure (TDEE)
Basal metabolic rate (BMR)	60-70%
Non-exercise activity thermogenesis (NEAT)	15-50%
Exercise activity thermogenesis (EAT)	15-30%
Thermic effect of food (TEF)	8-15%

The relative contributions of the components of total daily energy expenditure. From Aragon et al., 2017[40].

It is important to note that the components of total daily energy expenditure are not independent of each other, and not independent of energy intake. Components of the energy balance model (energy intake – energy expenditure) are related, such that changes in one may result in compensation in another component[37].

Despite popular belief, obese individuals have a *higher basal metabolic rate* and a *higher total daily energy expenditure* than lean individuals[2,41].

Appetite: the drive to eat

If we haven't eaten for a while, we start to *feel* hungry, and have a desire to consume food. Similarly, during and after a meal, we start to *feel* full, and no longer have a desire to consume food. These feelings help to regulate acute food intake.

- **Appetite** is the presence of hunger and feeling the need to consume food. Appetite is driven by orexigenic (increasing appetite) mechanisms[22].
- **Satiation** is when we stop eating food due to a reduction in appetite, which is specific to taste[42]. A reduction in appetite is driven by anorexigenic (decreasing appetite) mechanisms. We are *satiated* when

we are no longer hungry. *Satiety* is the mechanism after a meal that determines how much time passes before our next meal[42].

The balance between orexigenic and anorexigenic mechanisms (increasing or decreasing appetite) determines the balance between hunger and satiety and the drive to eat.

When we are hungry, we seek out food. Eating food provides us with a reward (people like eating food), which is coordinated by the brain[18]. The reward centre of the brain ensures we eat so that we consume the energy and nutrients needed to live. We can learn to eat rewarding foods with certain qualities, associating sight, taste and environmental-based cues with food reward (e.g. good looking food being more appealing, nice tasting food being more appealing, and food presented in a nice location being more appealing).

- **Palatability** is how enjoyable and pleasant a certain food is to eat. Palatability can be influenced by how much energy is in the food, its texture and what is in the food (e.g. the fat, sugar, starch, salt and other content of the food). Palatability is not a quality of a food itself, but of how it is perceived by a person. The same meal can have a different palatability for two people[42]. The palatability of a food source also influences the size of a meal[43]. As we eat, palatability decreases as satiety increases. The first bite of a meal will be more pleasing than the subsequent bites after it[42].

The food we eat also affects satiety, including the type of macronutrient consumed, the volume of the food, its energy density and the food matrix. Different foods of equal calories can provide very different levels of satiety[44].

Food intake at a particular meal can vary greatly, but food intake across the day for a given individual is largely consistent, indicating there are compensatory mechanisms that increase energy intake when smaller meals have been consumed, and decrease energy intake when larger meals have been consumed[37]. Other factors can influence food intake. Just changing the size of the plate that food is served on can influence portion size perception[45-47].

A part of our brain called the *hypothalamus* collects lots of different appetite stimulating and appetite suppressing signals from around the body and determines our overall desire to eat or not to eat. Some of the signals it receives and integrates includes[22]:

- **Hormones** (including leptin, ghrelin and insulin).
- **Neural signals** from the stomach, and gut peptides (of which there are many) such as cholecystokinin and peptide $YY_{3\text{-}36}$.
- **Blood glucose** (sugar) levels.
- **Social, psychological** and **environmental** factors.

These factors are then also influenced by the underlying genetics of the individual.

Our levels of body fat can modulate satiety signals that are generated when eating a meal. With lower body fat, your body is less sensitive to these satiety factors generated from eating a meal, which promotes a tendency to consume more energy. Similarly, with higher body fat, your body is more sensitive to these satiety factors generated from eating a meal, which promotes a tendency to consume less energy[43,48,49].

Weight maintenance

Long term maintenance of weight appears to be controlled. There is a homeostatic resistance to weight change. Whether this acts to maintain body weight at a given weight, within a range, or just to minimise change, is inconclusive.

Energy intake and expenditure are interrelated. Along with evidence that there are dynamic changes that act to promote weight gain after weight loss, it has been suggested that the body must aim to maintain some level of body weight[41]. The *control-theory* of body weight regulation is based on the concept that negative feedback loops act to maintain body weight[22]. Changes in body weight are the result of mismatches in energy intake and expenditure. So, by monitoring body weight, the body can adjust intake and expenditure to control body weight.

Long-term regulation of body weight is hotly debated, and several mathematical *control-theory models* exist to try and explain how weight regulation may be controlled[22]. Three of the most common models are the *static, set point* and *settling point* models of body weight[22,41]:

- **Static.** Energy intake and expenditure are independent of body weight. The static model does not explain research findings and is unlikely to be true.
- **Settling point.** A negative feedback model of weight change[18,22]. The most common form of the settling-point model is where energy expenditure increases with increasing body weight, and energy intake is

independent of body weight. The settling-point model is proposed to explain body fat regulation[18].

- **Set point.** The *lipostatic model* of body fat regulation[18]. Energy intake and expenditure depend on body weight. There is a target level of body weight, and feedback control of body weight occurs through both energy intake and expenditure[22]. The set point model has been proposed to explain the findings in research, in that when people lose or gain weight, they tend to return to their previous weight[18].

However, the set point theory fails to explain why there is an obesity epidemic and many of the social and behavioural aspects of energy intake and expenditure[18]. In Western societies, individuals tend to increase body weight year on year[18]. Indeed, the settling point can explain phenomena that the set point cannot[18]. But also, there are other phenomena that the settling point cannot explain. The set point model addresses primarily physiological and genetic factors, whereas the settling point model addresses primarily environmental and societal factors. However, this is a superficial separation because of the interrelation between these factors; genes interact with the environment, and vice versa[18]. As a result, other more complex models have been proposed, such as a *hybrid set and settling point* model (the *dual-intervention point model*) whereby body weight is regulated to stay within a range, rather than at a specific value[18,22].

Increasing evidence suggests there is less of a set point and more of a narrow optimum range that the body aims to keep within. There appears to be strong opposition to a reduced body weight, with strong mechanisms to oppose weight loss. However, there appears to be a weaker opposition to increased body weight, with less strong mechanisms to oppose weight gain. The fact that there is an increasing obesity epidemic within the population suggests that negative feedback mechanisms may be surpassed or may not be as strong to prevent weight gain[18,36,41,50]. Obesity may be better explained by the hybrid set and settling point model than either model alone, with a strong resistance to weight loss, but a weaker resistance to weight gain[18].

When body weight changes, there are changes in the mechanisms that influence energy intake and expenditure, but how these changes are coordinated in relation to body weight is still largely unknown.

Long term regulation of metabolism and maintenance of weight is a complex network involving multiple regions of the brain (especially the hypothalamus). These brain regions integrate multiple signals and communicate with each other. They then act upon various compartments of the body. The factors influencing energy balance are highly integrated, with compensatory mechanisms[48]. There is no *single* dominating factor that *prevents* or *promotes* weight change in healthy individuals. For example, there isn't a particular *hormone* that causes or prevents weight change by itself[49].

Even though the body aims to balance energy intake and expenditure, it is clear there is a relative energy imbalance across a period of hours and across the day. Averaging over a longer period of days and weeks, energy expenditure and intake begin to be better matched[37]. For example, intake exceeds expenditure during a meal, and expenditure exceeds intake during exercise. But over many days, small variations will be averaged and there will be a similar balance of intake and expenditure, when weight remains consistent[18].

Hormones

Certain hormones influence energy intake and energy expenditure, but they do not in themselves prevent weight loss or promote weight gain.

Knowledge of hormones is *not* necessary for weight change, weight maintenance, or health. However, due to widespread media attention of specific hormones and how they may affect your appetite and long-term weight change, it is important to briefly mention them. This means you can understand their role and relative importance in body composition. This overview will cover the main hormones involved in weight regulation, weight change and appetite.

A *hormone* is a molecule produced by a specific tissue in the body and transported via the blood to act in another tissue of the body.

Insulin

Insulin is produced by the pancreas and is released into the blood circulation. It acts upon many cells including muscle and fat. Long-term insulin levels in the blood increase with increasing levels of fat mass. Short-term blood insulin levels vary with what and how much is eaten in a given meal. This means that insulin levels give information about the current energy state (*fed* or *fasted*) of the body in relation to the overall long-term energy status of the individual (body fat levels)[51]. Between meals (fasted), there is a certain level of sugar in the blood that the body aims to keep relatively constant. When you eat a meal, any carbohydrate from the meal is broken down and absorbed in the gut which then enters the bloodstream as sugar. This elevates blood sugar levels above resting (fasted) levels. To return blood sugar levels back to resting levels, the *pancreas* increases production of insulin, which promotes the use and storage of blood sugar (glucose) and suppresses the usage of already stored energy (such as fat). Insulin levels also increase as a result of signals from the gut which are activated when you eat a meal (kind of like the gut telling your body that it's just eaten and preparing it to use the incoming energy). Between meals, insulin levels drop as blood sugar (glucose) levels drop back down to resting levels from being used, or stored in cells. Between meals, other hormones promote stored energy to be utilised to provide energy to cells (such as muscles) and to help maintain resting blood sugar levels (glucose), so that blood sugar levels do not drop too low. Across the day, the body fluctuates between storing consumed energy (fat storage) and using stored energy through fat *lipolysis* (fat utilisation) and fat *oxidation* (fat burning). Fluctuations align with periods of consuming meals and the periods between consuming meals.

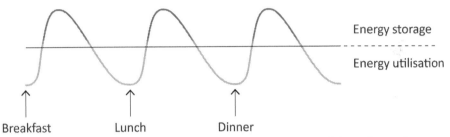

Consumption of a meal results in the body switching from its own energy stores to using the energy stores within the meal. After a period of time, the body slowly reverts back to using its own energy stores. Depending on whether the energy within the meals is equal to, greater than, or less than the energy needs of the individual, will determine whether energy stores stay the same, decrease, or increase.

Leptin

Leptin is a hormone produced by *fat cells* and released into the blood. When there is a large amount of fat mass, more leptin is produced and therefore more leptin is in the blood[36]. When fat mass is reduced, there is less circulating leptin in the blood. Leptin acts to *reduce* food intake. Therefore, when fat mass falls, leptin levels fall, resulting in a relative increase in the drive to eat. Leptin is a long-term signal in humans. This means that it isn't a driving factor to eat a particular meal, but it can influence the general overall feeling of hunger across the day[18,51]. Leptin gives information about the overall long-term energy status in the body. Low leptin levels can increase the feeling of cravings. Leptin also has the action of promoting *thyroid hormone* production. Thyroid hormone stimulates metabolism. This makes sense. As the body's energy stores fall (less fat mass) due to calorie restriction, leptin levels fall, reducing thyroid hormone production along with increasing feelings of hunger. These mechanisms aim to reduce energy expenditure (through metabolism) and increase the overall feeling of hunger to increase energy intake in an attempt to match energy intake to expenditure, and return the body to its original weight (to maintain homeostasis). As the body's energy stores increase (more adipose tissue), mechanisms are in place to increase the metabolism of the body and reduce the overall feeling of hunger[18].

Leptin, insulin and probably other hormones act to set the overall long-term feeling of being hungry or satiated across the day. However, it is important to remember that *when* and *what* we eat is also heavily influenced by our *environment*. For example, the cultural tendency to eat set meals (*'breakfast'*, *'lunch'* and *'dinner'*), and with *whom* or *where* we eat can all influence intake. Stress can also affect hunger levels and food intake (such as comfort eating), as well as habits. Other hormones also influence the acute drive to eat.

Ghrelin

Ghrelin is the *hunger* hormone[51]. Ghrelin is the only hormone that *promotes* appetite (remember, leptin *suppresses* appetite, but its effects are when levels are low. When fat stores are reduced, leptin levels are lower, resulting in a reduction in appetite suppression). Ghrelin is released from the *stomach* and levels rise between meals in response to being in a fasted state. It tells the hypothalamus (part of the brain) that it is time to eat.

Testosterone

Testosterone is a well-known hormone involved in increasing muscle mass. It may also influence body fat levels.

Cortisol

Cortisol has a range of functions including regulating blood sugar (glucose) levels, anti-inflammatory properties and influencing mood. Cortisol can also influence food intake[52]. Like testosterone, its levels vary across day and night (it follows a *circadian rhythm*). Cortisol levels peak early in the morning and slowly drop across the day. Cortisol forms part of the *general adaptation syndrome* concept originally developed by Hans Selye[53]. This is discussed in chapter 18. In short, cortisol levels can be elevated after an acute *stress* is placed on the body. This provides a *signal* to the body to *adapt* to this stress. Confusion around the role of cortisol on body composition exists because cortisol is seen as a marker of general stress levels. High levels of stress for long periods of time can impair favourable changes in body composition, resulting in muscle breakdown and fat storage. Indeed, cortisol can promote muscle break down, prevent storage of energy in fat stores, and promote the utilisation of fat stores[51]. However, the issue to address is not elevated cortisol but the *reasons* causing chronically elevated stress, which could be work-related stresses, family stress or sleep deprivation. As mentioned, acute elevations in cortisol have an important adaptive role.

Thyroid hormones

Thyroid hormones can *influence* our metabolic rate by acting on cells around the body[36]. The body can alter the rate at which it burns energy. Basal metabolic rate is not a fixed entity but constantly in flux. Signals from the hypothalamus can alter metabolic rate by increasing or decreasing the production of thyroid hormones. Again, this is part of the homeostatic mechanism in response to when our body weight changes.

When do we know it is time to stop eating a meal?

Signals from the stomach including stretch receptor signals (when the volume of food you eat literally stretches the stomach) and gut hormones indicate on a short timescale when we are full. It can take several hours for a meal to be absorbed and for insulin levels in the blood to rise in response to increased blood sugar levels. If we did not have short-term signals, we would keep on eating for hours! These signals tell the hypothalamus (part of the brain) that you are full and to stop eating. Signals to stop eating include:

- The **taste** of food.
- **Cholecystokinin**, a hormone released from the gut when you eat. It acts to promote satiety (feeling full).
- **PYY** and **obestatin** are hormones relating to satiety and hunger that have recently been discovered. It is likely there are further hormones and other signals that have yet to be identified.

Hormones do not prevent you from losing weight. Hormones influence weight change through energy intake and energy expenditure, but do not dictate weight change. Regardless of your hormones, if you are in a calorie deficit, you will lose weight. If you are in a calorie surplus, you will gain weight.

Total daily energy intake and expenditure can vary due to hormonal activity. This has been misinterpreted by some to mean that hormones *cause* weight gain or are the reason for being unable to lose weight. At first glance, it would appear that hormones might prevent losing weight or promote gaining weight. Insulin levels in the blood rise after eating a meal (rising after consuming carbohydrates and protein), and insulin suppresses fat oxidation (burning fat), and promotes the storage of energy (including storing energy as fat). Similarly, you might think that once you start to lose some weight, the reduction in adipose tissue (your fat stores) will lower leptin levels, resulting in severe hunger and overconsumption. Based on this reasoning, some people have promoted diets *'designed'* to work because they address these *'hormonal issues'*. Examples include *'underactive thyroids'* reducing metabolic rate, or *'insulin preventing fat loss and promoting weight gain'*. Similar concepts exist with cortisol or leptin. This is *not true*. Hormones play a role in regulating appetite and satiety, but they are *not* the driving factors behind weight loss or weight gain.

The discussion above is only a brief introduction into the complexity of metabolism and weight regulation. Considering the effect of a single hormone grossly oversimplifies the factors determining weight change. For example, there are other hormones that influence appetite and satiety (some of which have only recently been discovered, and probably many more will be discovered in the future), as well as influences from the sympathetic and parasympathetic nervous systems (*'fight or flight'*), neural signalling, signalling from the gut, and psychological and social factors amongst many others. These factors influence energy intake and expenditure, not weight loss or gain themselves. The difference between energy intake and expenditure determines weight change. It is the integration of the factors discussed (and many others) that affect how easy (or not so easy) it is to achieve a calorie deficit or surplus[41].

In overweight and obese people, a range of metabolic changes can occur. This includes having high levels of resting (fasted) blood sugar (glucose) and insulin. There is a relative inability of insulin to promote the use and storage of blood sugar (glucose). This is called *insulin resistance*. Insulin resistance is not the cause of obesity. Insulin resistance is mainly the result of being overweight or obese; having extended periods of being in a calorie surplus and therefore net energy storage.

Basal metabolic rate changes as body weight changes

Your basal metabolic rate and total daily energy intake are dynamic, not static entities. You do not have a set metabolism that is fast, normal or slow. Your metabolism is constantly shifting depending on your overall energy intake and changes in your body composition.

In the general population, metabolism is determined by body composition and total daily calorie intake (relative to energy needs). It is not determined by previous dieting history, or how much weight has previously been gained or lost.

A change in body composition results in a change in basal metabolic rate. *Adaptive thermogenesis* (or *metabolic adaptation*) is a term used to describe the change in metabolic rate and energy expenditure that is larger than expected based on body composition changes alone[51]. When you lose weight, your metabolic rate decreases because there is less of you. Adaptive thermogenesis is a further reduction of your metabolic rate beyond this expected reduction. The extent of the reduction in energy expenditure due to adaptive thermogenesis when losing weight differs greatly between people. In some people it does not shift much, in others it can change a lot. Adaptive thermogenesis can be explained by changes in factors contributing to total daily energy expenditure outside of basal metabolic rate. For individuals who have lost weight, a large proportion of adaptive thermogenesis actually appears to be from a reduction in energy expenditure due to moving less. They expend less energy via exercise and non-exercise activity thermogenesis (EAT and NEAT)[40]. When using larger calorie deficits without any resistance training programme and with lower protein intakes, adaptive thermogenesis can lead to significant reductions in energy expenditure. Increasing protein intake and resistance training can help to limit adaptive thermogenesis even when in a large calorie deficit[40,41]. Optimising weight loss is discussed in chapter 7.

The body adapts to changing calorie intake. Energy expenditure does not remain constant if you eat too much (and gain weight) or eat too little (and lose weight)[41,54,55]. One mechanism by which the body achieves this is by changing how much you move around during the day, called non-exercise activity thermogenesis (NEAT)[56]. Sometimes you might fidget around, move your legs or tap your foot. Perhaps your job involves being on your feet for large parts of the day. This low-level movement can actually account for a fairly large amount of daily energy expenditure. Ever notice how you fidget more when you have been inactive all day, but after hard exercise you seem to sit quite still? With increases in calorie intake, the body tends to move more. With a decrease in calorie intake, the body tends to move less. How much more you move when you increase calorie intake and how much less you move when you decrease your calorie intake varies between people, which is a factor which can make weight change easier or harder for different people. Weight loss can result in a significant reduction in NEAT and therefore result in a lowering of total daily energy expenditure. This can make further weight loss or weight maintenance more difficult[36].

Just fidgeting more or less throughout the day can have a significant impact on energy expenditure. People will increase or decrease NEAT to a different extent

65

depending on over or underfeeding. But, not only does NEAT change; exercise-activity thermogenesis (EAT) can also decline with weight loss. People tend to perform less exercise because of greater feelings of fatigue and tiredness when in a calorie deficit[51]. Also as the body weighs less, less energy is required to perform the same physical task. This is compounded by the fact that *skeletal muscles* (the muscles we use to move around) become more efficient with weight loss; they use less energy to perform the same amount of work[36,51]. With weight loss, people exercise less, with less body weight and with more efficient muscles. This means a reduction in EAT and therefore a reduction in total daily energy expenditure. Despite performing less exercise, obese individuals can have greater energy expenditure from a lower level of physical activity because of the greater energy cost associated with moving the greater body mass[2].

NEAT and EAT can account for up to 90% of the changes in energy expenditure beyond what is expected from changes in body composition alone[36,51].

The *relative* amount of energy expended from the thermic effect of feeding (TEF) will not change. But, because less food is being consumed during calorie restriction, the *absolute* amount of energy required to access and use the energy within food is reduced. But, this is fairly insignificant[51].

When you lose weight[37,51,54]:

- **Total daily energy expenditure** (TDEE) decreases.
- **Basal metabolic rate** (BMR) decreases.
- **The thermic effect of food** (TEF) is relatively unchanged (except for the fact you are eating less food).
- **Non-exercise activity thermogenesis** (NEAT) decreases.
- **Exercise-activity thermogenesis** (EAT) decreases.
- Skeletal muscle efficiency increases.

Changes in energy intake influences changes in energy expenditure. Changes in energy expenditure influences changes in energy intake.

Adaptive thermogenesis may explain why people struggle to lose weight or struggle to maintain any weight loss[51].

Adaptive thermogenesis contributes to the homeostatic mechanism to maintain body weight. People often regain the weight they have lost during a calorie deficit by not considering that their basal metabolic rate and total daily energy expenditure are now *lower* than before the weight loss. People then return to their original behaviours and calorie intake from before. This therefore generates a calorie surplus and weight regain. Repeated over many cycles (e.g. January resolutions or summer holidays) results in *yoyo dieting*; intermittent periods of

weight loss and weight gain from reverting between the habitual lifestyle and the short-term energy restricted regime.

Similarly, metabolic rate can increase beyond what is expected from increases in body mass alone when in a calorie surplus (an adaptive increase in energy expenditure is known as *luxuskonsumption*)[2]. However, the adaptive mechanisms that act to prevent weight gain appear to not be as strong as the mechanisms acting to prevent weight loss[2,48]. The body strongly resists a reduction in weight, but does not appear to resist increases in weight to the same extent. The size of the increase in adaptive thermogenesis from increasing food intake and body weight will again differ between people. An overfeeding study found that overall, adaptive thermogenesis was not meaningfully significant (metabolic rate whilst sleeping increased by an additional 43kcal per day) in participants eating 40% more calories than their maintenance intake (40% is a large surplus). However, there was very large variability within this non-significant increase[57]. Some people had large positive changes (+396kcal per day), and some had large negative changes (-211kcal per day). Individual responses to the same calorie surplus varies widely[58]. Studies of overfeeding in non-obese individuals who are so called *'hardgainers'* (people who struggle to gain weight despite reportedly consuming excess calories) found that overfeeding led to an increase in NEAT. An increase in NEAT increased total daily energy expenditure, reducing the size of the calculated caloric surplus and therefore reducing the rate of weight gain[40,56]. In one study, 12 *monozygotic male twins* (twins from the same egg, meaning they are genetically identical) were overfed by 1000kcal per day. The average weight gain was 8.1kg (5.4kg as fat, 2.7kg as muscle) after 100 days[59]. However, weight gain varied from 4.3kg to 13.3kg. There was 6-fold greater variation *across* pairs of twins than *within* pairs of twins. The authors concluded that there is a large genetic component explaining the adaptive response to overfeeding[59]. On the whole, research on changes in energy expenditure and adaptive thermogenesis when overfeeding (increased energy expenditure with a caloric surplus) is not as clear cut as it is with a calorie deficit and reduced energy expenditure[58]. However, differences may be as a result of the study designs used, measurement errors, and the huge person-to-person variability in response to overfeeding (as seen in the *'hardgainer'* example above), such that individual metabolic responses can be lost in the averages of studies[58,60].

Slow and fast metabolisms

Slow and fast metabolisms are a myth, people with similar body compositions have similar basal metabolic rates[37]. However, people with similar body compositions can have very different total daily energy expenditures depending on their levels of exercise and non-exercise activity thermogenesis (EAT and NEAT).

People sometimes think that the reason they cannot lose weight or why they have gained weight is because they have a *'slow'* metabolism. However, people of a similar body shape have a similar basal metabolic rate. The number of calories consumed, and the number of calories expended increase with body fat levels[41]. Obese people have higher a total daily energy expenditure than lean people from an increased basal metabolic rate, EAT and NEAT. Despite a commonly seen reduction in the amount of EAT performed in obese people, the increased energy cost of moving the extra body weight and the extra energy required during breathing to move the additional weight offsets this reduction[2,41]. But, obese people also eat more. Long-term substantial weight loss can be very difficult, but this is due to other factors that limit the ability to generate a calorie deficit or prevent a calorie surplus (i.e. the long-term balance of satiety and appetite to match energy expenditure, and any changes in EAT, NEAT or adaptive thermogenesis with weight change), rather than because metabolism is slow in the first place[36,37].

Similarly, people do not have *'fast'* metabolisms, and neither can you speed up your metabolism by eating specific foods. There are currently no methods or specific foods that are conclusively proven to permanently increase or decrease your rate of metabolism, beyond just altering your total daily energy intake or body composition.

You may see friends, family or colleagues regularly consume high energy density, ultra-processed foods (see chapter 12 regarding energy and nutrient density) and remain at a low body fat percentage without any noticeable weight gain. This is not because they have a fast metabolism. It is because although they may eat these foods regularly, their food intakes throughout the rest of the day or the week are at a level such that their total calorie intake is not excessive. They may also have higher levels of EAT and NEAT. Meaning, that although they have a similar basal metabolism to someone of a similar height and weight, they expend what they consume because their total daily energy expenditure is much higher.

People think they have slow metabolisms. In reality, people tend to just overestimate how much energy they expend and tend to eat more than they actually expend[61].

Metabolic damage

In the general population, metabolisms cannot be 'damaged'. They do not drastically drop and never recover back to a previous 'normal range'. Metabolism fluctuates with changes in body weight and food intake.

With reductions in weight, metabolic adaptation will occur. However, to say that the metabolism is now *'damaged'* is incorrect. Numerous studies show that basal metabolic rate does not drastically drop after weight loss and is not disproportionately lower than expected when weight loss is maintained[62,63]. A large part of this is due to changes in EAT and NEAT during periods of weight loss, which can account for significant changes in total daily energy expenditure. NEAT and EAT can account for as much as 90% of the reduction in total daily energy expenditure beyond what is expected from changes in body composition alone after weight loss. Part of this is due to the increased efficiency of skeletal muscle with weight loss, meaning the same volume of physical activity will result in less energy expended[36]. Total daily energy expenditure has fallen from moving less, not because basal metabolic rate has been *'damaged'* and is now severely reduced. People who are successful in long-term weight loss tend to have a higher total daily energy expenditure because they move more, as seen from higher levels of EAT in people who maintain weight loss[63].

Studies show decreases or increases in metabolism in non-obese individuals who undergo weight loss are not permanent[64]. If you stay at a lower body weight, your basal metabolism will be slightly lower, but if you return to your original weight, it will return to a similar original level.

Summary

Your metabolism is not fixed. It is also not slow or fast.

Weight change is determined by the difference between energy intake and energy expenditure.

Lots of factors influence your energy intake and energy expenditure.

Factors influencing energy intake and energy expenditure may make it relatively harder or easier to achieve a calorie surplus or deficit, which varies greatly between people.

When in a calorie deficit or a calorie surplus, weight will be lost or gained regardless of any influencing factors.

No single factor influencing energy intake and energy expenditure can stop weight change when energy expenditure does not match energy intake.

After losing weight, your original calorie intake before losing weight is no longer your maintenance calorie intake. Your total daily energy expenditure will be lower. Your new maintenance energy intake needs to take into account the changes in your body composition.

The role of adaptive thermogenesis and weight change is a developing topic and not fully understood. Most research is currently in animals or sedentary, overweight and obese people[51].

References

1   Willett W, Rockström J, Loken B, Springmann M, Lang T, Vermeulen S et al. Food in the Anthropocene: the EAT–Lancet Commission on healthy diets from sustainable food systems. *The Lancet* 2019; 393: 447–492.

2   Hall KD. Modeling metabolic adaptations and energy regulation in humans. *Annu Rev Nutr* 2012; 32: 35–54.

3   Di Angelantonio E, Bhupathiraju SN, Wormser D, Gao P, Kaptoge S, de Gonzalez AB et al. Body-mass index and all-cause mortality: individual-participant-data meta-analysis of 239 prospective studies in four continents. *The Lancet* 2016; 388: 776–786.

4   Böhm A, Heitmann BL. The use of bioelectrical impedance analysis for body composition in epidemiological studies. *European Journal of Clinical Nutrition 2013;* Available from: https://www.nature.com/articles/ejcn2012168 (accessed 5 Feb 2020).

5   Westerterp-Plantenga MS, Lemmens SG, Westerterp KR. Dietary protein – its role in satiety, energetics, weight loss and health. *Br J Nutr* 2012; 108: S105–S112.

6   Lee DH, Keum N, Hu FB, Orav EJ, Rimm EB, Willett WC et al. Predicted lean body mass, fat mass, and all cause and cause specific mortality in men: prospective US cohort study. *BMJ* 2018; 362. Available from: doi:10.1136/bmj.k2575.

7   American Dietetic Association, Dieticians of Canada, American College of Sports Medicine, Rodriguez NR, Di Marco NM, Langley S. American College of Sports Medicine position stand. Nutrition and Athletic Performance. *Med Sci Sports Exerc* 2009; 41: 709–731.

8   Thom G, Lean M. Is There an Optimal Diet for Weight Management and Metabolic Health? *Gastroenterology* 2017; 152: 1739–1751.

9   Maffetone PB, Rivera-Dominguez I, Laursen PB. Overfat and Underfat: New Terms and Definitions Long Overdue. *Front Public Health* 2017; 4. Available from: doi:10.3389/fpubh.2016.00279.

10   Lorem GF, Schirmer H, Emaus N. What is the impact of underweight on self-reported health trajectories and mortality rates: a cohort study. *Health Qual Life Outcomes* 2017; 15. Available from: doi:10.1186/s12955-017-0766-x.

11   Bredella M. Sex Differences in Body Composition. In: Mauvais-Jarvis F (ed.) *Sex and Gender Factors Affecting Metabolic Homeostasis, Diabetes and Obesity.* SpringerLink. Available from: https://link.springer.com/chapter/10.1007%2F978-3-319-70178-3_2 (accessed 5 Feb 2020).

12   McLeod M, Breen L, Hamilton DL, Philp A. Live strong and prosper: the importance of skeletal muscle strength for healthy ageing. *Biogerontology* 2016; 17: 497–510.

13   Wolfe RR. The underappreciated role of muscle in health and disease. *Am J Clin Nutr* 2006; 84: 475–482.

14   Horwitz H, Andersen JT, Dalhoff KP. Health consequences of androgenic anabolic steroid use. *J Intern Med* 2019; 285: 333–340.

15   Hoffman JR, Ratamess NA. Medical Issues Associated with Anabolic Steroid Use: Are They Exaggerated? *J Sports Sci Med* 2006; 5: 182–193.

16   West DWD, Burd NA, Churchward-Venne TA, Camera DM, Mitchell CJ, Baker SK et al. Sex-based comparisons of myofibrillar protein synthesis after resistance exercise in the fed state. *J Appl Physiol Bethesda Md* 2012; 112: 1805–1813.

17   Ivey FM, Roth SM, Ferrell RE, Tracy BL, Lemmer JT, Hurlbut DE et al. Effects of age, gender, and myostatin genotype on the hypertrophic response to heavy resistance strength training. *J Gerontol A Biol Sci Med Sci* 2000; 55: M641-648.

18   Speakman JR, Levitsky DA, Allison DB, Bray MS, de Castro JM, Clegg DJ et al. Set points, settling points and some alternative models: theoretical options to understand how genes and environments combine to regulate body adiposity. *Dis Model Mech* 2011; 4: 733–745.

19   Martinez AJ, Navas-Carretero S, Saris WHM, Astrup A. Personalized weight loss strategies—the role of macronutrient distribution. *Nature Reviews Endocrinology.* Available from: https://www.nature.com/articles/nrendo.2014.175 (accessed 5 Feb 2020).

20   Gardner CD, Trepanowski JF, Gobbo LCD, Hauser ME, Rigdon J, Ioannidis JPA et al. Effect of low-fat vs low-carbohydrate diet on 12-month weight loss in overweight adults and the association with genotype pattern or insulin secretion the DIETFITS randomized clinical trial. *J Am Med Assoc* 2018; 319: 667–679.

21   Antonio J, Knafo S, Kenyon M, Ali A, Carson C, Ellerbroek A et al. Assessment of the FTO gene polymorphisms (rs1421085, rs17817449 and

rs9939609) in exercise-trained men and women: the effects of a 4-week hypocaloric diet. *J Int Soc Sports Nutr* 2019; 16: 36.

22   Geary N. Control-theory models of body-weight regulation and body-weight-regulatory appetite. *Appetite* 2020; 144: 104440.

23   Hall KD, Ayuketah A, Brychta R, Cai H, Cassimatis T, Chen KY et al. Ultra-processed diets cause excess calorie intake and weight gain: A one-month inpatient randomized controlled trial of ad libitum food intake. *Cell Metab* 2019. Available from: doi:10.31232/osf.io/w3zh2.

24   González-Muniesa P, Mártinez-González M, Hu F, et al. Obesity. *Nat. Rev. Dis. Primer* 2017. Available from: doi:10.1038/nrdp.2017.35.

25   WHO. *Diet, nutrition and the prevention of chronic diseases.* Available from: https://www.who.int/dietphysicalactivity/publications/trs916/en/ (accessed 5 Feb 2020).

26   Hall KD, Guyenet SJ, Leibel RL. The Carbohydrate-Insulin Model of Obesity Is Difficult to Reconcile With Current Evidence. *JAMA Intern Med* 2018; 178: 1103–1105.

27   Hall KD. A review of the carbohydrate-insulin model of obesity. *Eur J Clin Nutr* 2017; 71: 323–326.

28   Norton L. *Science, Stories, and Side-Stepping: The Stephan Guyenet vs. Gary   Taubes   Debate.*   Biolayne.   Available   from: https://www.biolayne.com/articles/research/science-stories-and-side-stepping-the-stephan-guyenet-vs-gary-taubes-debate/ (accessed 5 Feb 2020).

29   Clifton PM, Condo D, Keogh JB. Long term weight maintenance after advice to consume low carbohydrate, higher protein diets--a systematic review and meta analysis. *Nutr Metab Cardiovasc Dis NMCD* 2014; 24: 224–235.

30   Alhassan S, Kim S, Bersamin A, King AC, Gardner CD. Dietary adherence and weight loss success among overweight women: results from the A TO Z weight loss study. *Int J Obes* 2005 2008; 32: 985–991.

31   Hill RJ, Davies PS. The validity of self-reported energy intake as determined using the doubly labelled water technique. *Br J Nutr* 2001. Available from: doi:10.1079/BJN2000281.

32   Carlsen MH, Lillegaard ITL, Karlsen AS, Blomhoff R, Drevon CA, Andersen LF. Evaluation of energy and dietary intake estimates from a food frequency questionnaire using independent energy expenditure measurement and weighed food records. *Nutr J.* 2010 Available from: doi:10.1186/1475-2891-9-37.

33   Schoeller DA. How accurate is self-reported dietary energy intake? *Nutr Rev* 1990; 48: 373–379.

34   Clear J. *Atomic Habits: An Easy & Proven Way to Build Good Habits & Break Bad Ones.* Available from: https://jamesclear.com/atomic-habits (accessed 5 Feb 2020).

35   Selfdeterminationtheory.org. *An approach to human motivation & personality.* Available from: https://selfdeterminationtheory.org/ (accessed 5 Feb 2020).

36 Rosenbaum M, Leibel RL. Adaptive thermogenesis in humans. *Int J Obes* 2010; 34: S47–S55.

37 Hall KD, Heymsfield SB, Kemnitz JW, Klein S, Schoeller DA, Speakman JR. Energy balance and its components: implications for body weight regulation. *Am J Clin Nutr* 2012; 95: 989–994.

38 Lessan N, Ali T. Energy Metabolism and Intermittent Fasting: The Ramadan Perspective. *Nutrients* 2019; 11: 1192.

39 McMurray RG, Soares J, Caspersen CJ, McCurdy T. Examining Variations of Resting Metabolic Rate of Adults: A Public Health Perspective. *Med Sci Sports Exerc* 2014; 46: 1352–1358.

40 Aragon A, Schoenfeld B, Wildman R, Kleiner S, VanDusseldorp T, Taylor L et al. International society of sports nutrition position stand: Diets and body composition. *J Int Soc Sports Nutr* 2017; 14. Available from: doi:10.1186/s12970-017-0174-y.

41 Hall KD, Guo J. Obesity Energetics: Body Weight Regulation and the Effects of Diet Composition. *Gastroenterology* 2017; 152: 1718-1727.e3.

42 Pribic T, Azpiroz F. Biogastronomy: Factors that determine the biological response to meal ingestion. *Neurogastroenterol Motil* 2018; 30: e13309.

43 Guyenet SJ, Schwartz MW. Regulation of Food Intake, Energy Balance, and Body Fat Mass: Implications for the Pathogenesis and Treatment of Obesity. *J Clin Endocrinol Metab* 2012; 97: 745–755.

44 Holt SH, Miller JC, Petocz P, Farmakalidis E. A satiety index of common foods. *Eur J Clin Nutr* 1995; 49: 675–690.

45 Penaforte FRO, Japur CC, Diez-Garcia RW, Hernandez JC, Palmma-Linares I, Chiarello PG. Plate size does not affect perception of food portion size. *J Hum Nutr Diet Off J Br Diet Assoc* 2014; 27 Suppl 2: 214–219.

46 Öner C, Özdemir M, Telatar B, Yeşildağ Ş. Does Plate Size Used in Food Service Affect Portion Perception? *Turk J Fam Med Prim Care* 2016; 10: 182–187.

47 Peng M. How does plate size affect estimated satiation and intake for individuals in normal-weight and overweight groups? *Obes Sci Pract* 2017; 3: 282–288.

48 Morton GJ, Cummings DE, Baskin DG, Barsh GS, Schwartz MW. Central nervous system control of food intake and body weight. *Nature* 2006; 443: 289–295.

49 Woods SC, Seeley RJ, Porte D, Schwartz MW. Signals That Regulate Food Intake and Energy Homeostasis. *Science* 1998; 280: 1378–1383.

50 Benton D, Young HA. Reducing Calorie Intake May Not Help You Lose Body Weight. *Perspect Psychol Sci* 2017; 12: 703–714.

51 Trexler ET, Smith-Ryan AE, Norton LE. Metabolic adaptation to weight loss: implications for the athlete. *J Int Soc Sports Nutr* 2014; 11: 7.

52 Gali Ramamoorthy T, Begum G, Harno E, White A. Developmental programming of hypothalamic neuronal circuits: impact on energy balance control. *Front Neurosci* 2015; 9. Available from: doi:10.3389/fnins.2015.00126.

53   Selye H. Stress and the General Adaptation Syndrome. *Br Med J* 1950; 1: 1383–1392.

54   Leibel RL, Rosenbaum M, Hirsch J. Changes in Energy Expenditure Resulting from Altered Body Weight. *N Engl J Med* 1995; 332: 621–628.

55   Müller MJ, Enderle J, Bosy-Westphal A. Changes in Energy Expenditure with Weight Gain and Weight Loss in Humans. *Curr Obes Rep* 2016; 5: 413–423.

56   Levine JA, Eberhardt NL, Jensen MD. Role of nonexercise activity thermogenesis in resistance to fat gain in humans. *Science* 1999; 283: 212–214.

57   Johannsen DL, Marlatt KL, Conley KE, Smith SR, Ravussin E. Metabolic adaptation is not observed after 8 weeks of overfeeding but energy expenditure variability is associated with weight recovery. *Am J Clin Nutr* 2019; 110: 805–813.

58   Joosen AM, Westerterp KR. Energy expenditure during overfeeding. *Nutr Metab* 2006; 3: 25.

59   Bouchard C, Tremblay A, Després JP, Nadeau A, Lupien PJ, Thériault G et al. The response to long-term overfeeding in identical twins. *N Engl J Med* 1990; 322: 1477–1482.

60   Giroux V, Saidj S, Simon C, Laville M, Segrestin B, Mathieu M-E. Physical activity, energy expenditure and sedentary parameters in overfeeding studies - a systematic review. *BMC Public Health* 2018; 18. Available from: doi:10.1186/s12889-018-5801-2.

61   Willbond SM, Laviolette MA, Duval K, Doucet E. Normal weight men and women overestimate exercise energy expenditure. *J Sports Med Phys Fitness* 2010; 50: 377–384.

62   Ostendorf DM, Melanson EL, Caldwell AE, Creasy SA, Pan Z, MacLean PS et al. No consistent evidence of a disproportionately low resting energy expenditure in long-term successful weight-loss maintainers. *Am J Clin Nutr* 2018; 108: 658–666.

63   Ostendorf DM, Caldwell AE, Creasy SA, Pan Z, Lyden K, Bergouignan A et al. Physical Activity Energy Expenditure and Total Daily Energy Expenditure in Successful Weight Loss Maintainers. *Obes Silver Spring Md* 2019; 27: 496–504.

64   Zinchenko A, Henselmans M. Metabolic Damage: do Negative Metabolic Adaptations During Underfeeding Persist After Refeeding in Non-Obese Populations? *Med Res Arch* 2016; 4. Available from: https://journals.ke-i.org/mra/article/view/908 (accessed 5 Feb 2020).

6. The fuel for life

Macronutrients: protein, carbohydrate and fat

Our energy to live comes from the food and drink we consume. Some of this energy is used to build new cells or structures. Some of this energy is used to fuel the cells of our body. Whatever is left over is stored. Humans obtain energy from *macronutrients* (nutrients we need in large amounts): protein, carbohydrate and fat. We don't usually consume these in isolation, but in a combined *matrix* in the form of food. Different macronutrients have both similar and distinct uses in the body. Only fat and protein are *essential* to human life as they are both required to build new structures in the body. Carbohydrates are used as an energy source and are the primary and preferred fuel source for cells in a typical diet.

Protein

Protein contains 4kcal per gram. Protein is essential for life as the body is continually breaking down proteins and rebuilding itself, such as hair, nails, skin and even the gut lining. Some of the protein that is broken down is reused, but some is lost daily. Proteins are required to produce hormones and enzymes which need to be made on a daily basis. Hence, lost protein needs to be replaced every day through dietary protein consumption. Protein is important to promote muscle protein synthesis, muscle growth and recovery from both aerobic and anaerobic exercise.

Proteins are made up of individual building blocks called *amino acids*. Different proteins have a specific sequence of amino acids, and a specific shape. Some amino acids can only be obtained through the diet *(essential amino acids (EAAs))*. Non-essential amino acids (NEAAs) can be obtained through the diet or made using other amino acids and glucose (sugar). Specific amino acids can have different effects on the body.

Branched-chain amino acids (BCAAs) are a specific sub-set of essential amino acids. The three BCAAs are leucine, isoleucine and valine. Their relative importance in muscle protein synthesis will be discussed later in chapter 9, and BCAA supplementation in chapter 25.

Protein sources can be complete or incomplete. *Complete protein sources* contain all the essential amino acids in sufficient quantities. Examples include meat, poultry, dairy, eggs, soy and fish. *Incomplete protein sources* do not contain all of the essential amino acids. Examples include plant protein sources such as legumes and pulses. The relative importance of this is discussed in chapter 9.

Humans do not have a dedicated protein *'store'* as such, where we can access protein for growth or energy. Excess protein can be broken down and used as energy, or chemically converted to fat and stored in adipose tissue (fat stores). Usually proteins in the body are continually broken down and rebuilt such that protein levels are maintained. However, the body can further break down muscles and other protein structures for energy use, without subsequent re-building. This results in a reduction in total protein levels. This is more likely to happen in a calorie deficit or with insufficient protein intake. Long-term muscle wasting and loss of protein in the body is detrimental to health[1].

Carbohydrate

Carbohydrates contain 4kcal per gram. Although not essential, they are the primary fuel source of cells. Carbohydrates can be *simple* (sugar) or *complex* (such as *starch* in plants or *glycogen* in animals). Complex carbohydrates are long chains of simple sugars. Simple sugars are used to *transport* energy. Complex carbohydrates are used to *store* energy.

Sugar exists in different forms. The basic building blocks include *glucose*, *fructose* and *galactose*. The basic building blocks can be joined together to build other sugars including *sucrose* (two glucose molecules) and *lactose* (a glucose and a galactose molecule). The blood sugar we refer to in humans is glucose. Glucose and fructose are found naturally in a range of foods including fruit and vegetables, but are also added to ultra-processed foods as *high-fructose corn syrup*. Sucrose is what we typically use as *'sugar'* in tea and coffee. Lactose is found in dairy products. Different types of sugar are found in different food sources, and are digested, absorbed and used in slightly different ways.

Starch and glycogen are complex carbohydrates. In plants, carbohydrates are stored as *starch*. In animals, carbohydrates are stored as *glycogen*. Some glycogen is stored in your liver and some in your muscle. For a 70kg man, around 400kcal (100g) of glycogen is stored in the liver, and 1600kcal (400g) is stored in muscle[2]. This is a very small amount compared to the potential amount of fat that can be stored in the body. When carbohydrates are ingested, they are digested and then absorbed through the gut. The carbohydrates are then either used in cells or stored. Once liver and muscle glycogen stores are full, any excess carbohydrates are chemically converted to fat and stored in adipose tissue (fat stores). Plants also have carbohydrates that function for structural purposes, called *cellulose*. We cannot break down cellulose or other parts of plants (including some forms of starch). This forms part of our diet called *dietary fibre*.

We can obtain carbohydrates from many plant-based foods (e.g. cereals, fruits, legumes and vegetables) and some animal-based foods (e.g. dairy). Simple sugars rapidly enter the bloodstream after being absorbed from the gut. Complex carbohydrates are broken down in the gut before entering the bloodstream as sugar, which is a slower process. Food sources usually contain a mixture of simple and complex carbohydrates and rarely contain only simple or complex carbohydrates. This means that carbohydrate food sources are absorbed and utilised at different rates. The idea of *'fast'* and *'slow'* digesting carbohydrates is an oversimplification, but good enough for our purposes of understanding of carbohydrates.

Glycaemic index and glycaemic load (GI and GL)

GI and GL are measures of the type and amount of the simple and complex carbohydrates in a food source. Both concepts are not necessary for fat loss or muscle gain in healthy people. GI and GL also oversimplify the effects of a food and ignores other important food components. These include total energy density, nutrient density, fibre, micronutrients, phytonutrient content and the effect of the food on satiety.

The *glycaemic index* (GI) and *glycaemic load* (GL) are measures of assessing the carbohydrate content in food. GI and GL can be useful tools to use in certain diseases, but they are *unimportant* for regulating body composition in *healthy* people.

The glycaemic index is a measure of how quickly a carbohydrate you eat gets broken down in the gut, absorbed and enters the bloodstream as glucose (a type of sugar)[3]. It is a 0-100 scale, with glucose (a type of sugar) scoring 100. It is a measure of the *quality* of carbohydrate in a food[3]. *Bananas* are a low *energy density*, high *nutrient density* food source. This means that for its volume, it contains a relatively low number of calories and a relatively high amount of nutrients. The carbohydrates within a banana are predominately sugars, yet bananas have a moderately low glycaemic index of 51[4]. This is because the sugars in a banana (and any fruit) are primarily *fructose* and *sucrose*. Fructose and sucrose each have low glycaemic indexes of 15 and 65, respectively[4]. Despite being types of sugar, they do not cause a rapid rise in the levels of glucose in the blood[4]. The glycaemic index can also be affected by other things, such as what else is consumed with the carbohydrate source. The sugars in fruit are bound within the cells of the fruit, meaning they are not easily accessible and not quickly digested. This means that they are more slowly absorbed than a pure source of sugar. The glycaemic index also does not consider *how much* carbohydrate you ate. This is where glycaemic load comes in. The glycaemic load considers the glycaemic index (*quality*) of the food, and how much carbohydrate (*quantity*) is in the food[3]. Taking our banana example, bananas have a moderate glycaemic index, but a glycaemic load of 13. Although bananas mainly contain carbohydrates in the form of sugar, there's relatively not that much in them per unit weight, so the overall 'load' of carbohydrate is quite low (low energy density). Even so, the glycaemic load is purely a measure of carbohydrate in a food source. Therefore, it is feasible to have equal glycaemic loads for a large plate of carrots, and a bar of chocolate. However, their overall effects on the body are drastically different. The former contains many nutrients, vitamins, minerals and fibre, in a much greater volume of food. The latter primarily provides calories with little nutritional content in a much smaller volume of food. The glycaemic index and glycaemic load ignore the importance of total calorie intake as the driving factor for weight change. The energy and nutrient density of foods is discussed further in chapter 12.

As a healthy individual, there is no need to consider the glycaemic index or glycaemic load of a food to lose weight or gain muscle.

Fat

Fats are essential to life and contain 9kcal per gram. Fats are a type of *lipid*[5]. They are the *most energy dense* macronutrient. Fats provide structural and functional uses and are found in cell membranes, around nerves and are needed during inflammatory responses. Fats are key components of many hormones, being required for the production of steroid hormones such as testosterone and oestrogen. Fats are needed for the absorption of fat-soluble vitamins including vitamin A, D, E and K. We can get fats from a range of sources including meat, oily fish, nuts, seeds and vegetables. Different types of fat can have different effects on the body[6].

Compared to protein and carbohydrate, fat is the *least satiating* macronutrient and has less of an effect in terms of promoting an end to food consumption (i.e. meal termination)[7]. However, fats have important dietary roles in providing taste and palatability to food[5].

Fats have different names based on their chemical structure. Their structure affects how the fat interacts with the body. Fats can be *unsaturated* or *saturated*. Saturated fats can be produced by the body[8]. *Unsaturated fat* can be *monounsaturated* or *polyunsaturated*, which again refers to the structure of the fat. Unsaturated fats and saturated fats are interchangeable in the diet. *Omega-3* and *omega-6* are sub-types of polyunsaturated fats. The number reflects the slightly different structure of the polyunsaturated fat. There are two *essential fatty acids* (we must obtain them from the diet, the body cannot make them). One of which is an omega-3 and the other is an omega-6 polyunsaturated fatty acid[5]. Both essential fatty acids can be used to build the same molecules in the body. Therefore, the type of fat consumed can alter the effect that these molecules have on the body.

Most foods contain both saturated and unsaturated fat, but in different relative proportions. High proportions of saturated fat can be found in ultra-processed foods, meat, cheese, cream and butter. Low proportions of saturated fat can be found in lean meat, poultry, fish and plant sources. Sources of monounsaturated fat include olive oil, avocado and nuts. Oily fish, such as salmon and sardines are sources of omega-3 polyunsaturated fat. Vegetable oils contain higher levels of omega-6 polyunsaturated fats. Unsaturated fats (in particular, monounsaturated and omega-3 polyunsaturated fats) have been suggested to have more beneficial effects on the body than saturated fats[6,9].

Trans fats

Trans fats are produced from partially hydrogenated oils in industrial processing. Trans fats are found in animal fat, butters, margarines and ultra-processed foods such as cakes and biscuits[8,10]. Consumption is linked with poorer health outcomes[8,10]. Their consumption is declining as they are slowly being removed from food production.

Cholesterol

Cholesterol is essential for the body and is another type of lipid alongside fat. It is important for the normal function of the brain and nervous system, and also forms part of cell membranes[5]. The majority of cholesterol inside the body is made by the liver from saturated fat (rather than being obtained directly from the cholesterol consumed in our diet), where it is transported around in the blood. Having too much cholesterol in the blood can increase the *risk* of cardiovascular disease.

Lipids (including fat and cholesterol) are insoluble in water. Therefore, they need to be transported in in the blood attached to proteins, called *lipoproteins*. There are two main forms:

- **High-density lipoprotein** (HDL), also known as the 'good' cholesterol, carries cholesterol away from cells and to the liver where it is processed. Higher levels of HDL-cholesterol are considered better and reduce the risk of cardiovascular disease.

- **Low-density lipoprotein** (LDL), also known as the 'bad' cholesterol. LDL delivers cholesterol to cells that need it. But, sometimes there can be too much circulating in the blood. LDL-cholesterol can then build up in the walls of arteries and lead to cardiovascular disease. Lower levels of LDL-cholesterol are better to reduce the risk of cardiovascular disease, but again they still play a vital role in the body. It is a bit more complex than this. Other factors such as the size of the LDL particle also have an effect[9].

The role of fat intake and health is discussed in chapter 12.

Energy stores

The amount of protein, carbohydrate and fat we can store in the body as an accessible energy source varies greatly:

- **Protein:** minimal to no storage as a functional energy source in the body.
- **Carbohydrate:** limited storage in muscle and liver as glycogen.
- **Fat:** unlimited storage in adipose tissue (fat cells).

Protein and carbohydrate storage between lean and obese people is virtually identical. Additional energy storage in obese people is as fat mass[11].

The potential to store fat is almost unlimited, and fat is the main energy store in humans. Fat reserves can constitute over 100,000kcal of stored energy in lean people, and up to 1,000,000kcal in obese people[12]. Carbohydrate can be stored in muscles and in the liver as glycogen. Even in very lean people, glycogen stores are relatively small to what can be stored as fat (2000-3000kcal). Glycogen stores are maximised after a meal containing carbohydrate[12]. In a calorie surplus, excess energy is stored in adipose tissue (fat cells) as fat. Dietary fat can readily be stored. Protein and carbohydrate are first converted to fat before being stored. Converting protein to fat is an energy inefficient process, but can still occur. Fat stores can be found under the skin (*subcutaneous fat*) and around our organs (*visceral fat*)[13].

Micronutrients: vitamins and minerals

You don't need a multivitamin, mineral pill or tablets – a balanced diet can provide all the micronutrition you need. Only in certain scenarios would vitamin or mineral supplementation be useful, such as in vegan or vegetarian diets, or during a calorie deficit when food intake may limit micronutrient consumption. Consult your GP if you believe you are micronutrient deficient.

Micronutrients are nutrients that are needed in small quantities, usually on a microgram or milligram scale. Vitamins and minerals are micronutrients. For a comprehensive, up to date overview on vitamins and minerals, I recommend the *Linus Pauling Institute* open-access resource for micronutrients[14]. However, what will be covered here should be more than enough for the purposes of body composition.

A balanced diet will provide all the vitamins and minerals in the quantities needed[15,16]. This is hard to believe, considering the increasing sales of multivitamin pills. In general, there should be no reason to be concerned about lacking in any vitamins and minerals if you are consuming a balanced diet[17,18]. A multivitamin is a sub-optimal substitute for a diet lacking in nutrient rich food sources. A diet lacking in vitamins and minerals indicates that the diet is probably of poor quality. Vitamin and mineral rich foods contain other health-related compounds such as fibre and phytonutrients. Conversely, exceeding daily recommended intakes of vitamins and minerals do not provide further benefit and can be detrimental if consumed in excess[19]. There will be certain scenarios where supplementation may be relevant (such as during a calorie deficit where food intake is limited)[20]. Micronutrient deficiencies may occur when adopting a diet that restricts food sources. Examples include a vegetarian or vegan diet, or low carbohydrate or low fat diets that limit food options[17]. The tables below outline the basics of vitamins and minerals. The sources listed below are notable sources of the vitamin or mineral, but many *food groups* contain vitamins and minerals. Fruits, vegetables, grains, nuts, legumes, meats, eggs, dairy and fish all contain vitamins and minerals, but at varying levels.

Vitamins

Vitamins are organic molecules that cannot be produced by the body and therefore must be consumed in the diet. They can be *fat-soluble* or *water-soluble*. Fat-soluble vitamins are absorbed in the gut and can lead to deficiencies or overdoses. Water-soluble vitamins are not stored and pass through the body in the urine, but require daily consumption.

Vitamin	Functions	Examples of good sources
Vitamin A (Retinol)	Supports the immune system against infection and illnesses, helps to keep skin healthy, helps vision in low light	Dairy (cheese, milk, yoghurt), eggs, oily fish
Vitamin B1 (Thiamin)	Helps the body to metabolise food, and maintain a healthy nervous system	Eggs, bread, rice, pulses
Vitamin B2 (Riboflavin)	Helps the body to metabolise food, supports the healthy function of skin, eyes and nervous system	Milk, eggs, meat, fish
Vitamin B3 (Niacin)	Helps the body to metabolise food, supports the healthy function of skin and nervous system	Meat, fish, milk, cereals, lentils
Pantothenic Acid	Helps the body to metabolise food	Most animal- and plant-based foods
Vitamin B6	Helps to release and store energy from carbohydrates and protein, used to form *Haemoglobin* (found in red blood cells which carries oxygen around the body)	Meat, fish, eggs, vegetables, milk
Vitamin B7 (Biotin)	Helps the body to break down food sources for energy	Eggs, liver, yeast
Vitamin B9 (Folate)	Help to form normal red blood cells	Vegetables (broccoli, brussels sprouts, spinach, asparagus, peas, chickpeas)
Vitamin B12*	Helps with red blood cell formation, helps to keep the nervous system healthy, helping to metabolise food and use folate	Meat, fish (salmon, cod), dairy (milk, cheese), eggs
Vitamin C (Ascorbic Acid)	Has antioxidant properties, keeping cells healthy, maintain healthy skin, blood vessels, bones and cartilage, support with healing wounds	Many fruits including oranges, kiwi, peppers, strawberries, blackcurrants, and vegetables (brussels sprouts, broccoli)

Vitamin D	Helps to keep bones, teeth and muscles healthy by regulating calcium and phosphate levels in the body, as well as other roles	Oily fish, red meat, eggs. Sunlight (between March and October). Between October and March, vitamin D needs to be obtained through the diet
Vitamin E	Helps to maintain healthy skin and eyes, support the immune system against infection	Plant oils (olive oil), nuts, seeds
Vitamin K	Helps the body form blood clots for wound healing	Green vegetables (broccoli, spinach), vegetable oils, cereals

Vitamins[14].

* Vitamin B12 is not naturally found in fruit, vegetables or grains. Therefore vitamin B12 may be lacking in a vegan or vegetarian diet[21]. See chapter 8 regarding vegan and vegetarian diets.

Minerals

Minerals are inorganic molecules that are needed for a wide range of bodily functions. They are not made by animals or organisms, but are derived from the Earth itself. Usually minerals are obtained from plants as they extract minerals from the soil, or indirectly from animals that consume plants.

A few of the main minerals are outlined below. Some others include sodium, chloride, magnesium, potassium, phosphorus and zinc.

Mineral	Function	Good Sources
Calcium	Supports strong bones and teeth, helps to regulate muscle contractions (including heart muscle), help with normal blood clotting	Dairy (milk, cheese), green vegetables (broccoli, cabbage), soya beans, nuts, bread
Iodine	A key component of *thyroid hormones*, which helps to maintain a normal metabolism	Seafood, dairy, grains (depends on the iodine content of soil)
Iron	Helps maintain healthy red blood cells and many other vital roles	Meats, beans, nuts, wholegrains, leafy vegetables

Examples of some minerals[14,22].

If you believe you have a micronutrient deficiency or you are unsure, then you should always go to your GP in the first instance before taking a vitamin or mineral supplement.

Water

Water is often overlooked when discussing nutrition and diets, but sufficient water consumption is of vital importance to achieving body composition changes. However, drinking more water does not raise your basal metabolic rate and does not result in more calories being burned[23].

The amount of water you need to drink will vary based on your physical activity levels and how much you sweat during the day, which is individual. Therefore, a specific number cannot be recommended.

Fibre

Fibre is the part of a plant that we are unable to digest. Therefore, we are unable to obtain much of the energy within them. Fibre can be *soluble* or *insoluble*. As a carbohydrate, fibre has caloric value of 4kcal per gram, although humans can usually obtain no more than 2kcal per gram.

Fibre has important health benefits[24]:

- Provides an energy source for the bacteria in our gut.
- Helps with the passage of food through the gut.
- Helps to keep us feeling full (satiated)[25].
- Helps to reduce the risk of bowel cancer.
- Reduces blood lipid levels and blood pressure[26].

Fibre makes a given food source less energy dense. Increased consumption of fibre-rich foods (plant-based foods such as vegetables, fruit and whole grains) is associated with a lower body mass index (BMI), lower body fat percentage and smaller waist circumference[27]. This effect can in part be attributed to the increase in satiety and resulting reduction in caloric intake from consuming less energy dense foods. However, the fact that people who eat more fibre-rich foods also display other healthful traits should be considered.

The *NHS* has publicly available advice on how to increase daily fibre intake[28]:

- Aim to consume at least 5 portions of fruit and veg per day*.
- Choose wholemeal and wholegrain breads and pastas.
- Eat potatoes with skins on.

- Consume more legumes, such as pulses and peas. You could try adding these to curries or tomato dishes.

Increasing the fibre content of food reduces its energy density. Altering the energy density of foods is discussed further in chapter 12.

* Note that this is an arbitrary target, and greater consumption can provide greater benefit.

Current dietary recommendations: dietary reference values

Any changes in body composition should be achieved whilst ensuring health is maintained or improved. As a starting point from a health perspective, we can look at the dietary recommendations from health organisations. The UK government has released a report on dietary recommendations. The main points are summarised below.

Dietary component	Recommended intake
Fruit and vegetables	5 a day
Red and processed meat	Less than 70g per day (490g per week)
Oily fish	One portion (140g) per week
Total fat intake	Up to 35% of daily calorie intake
Saturated fatty acid intake	Up to 10% of daily calorie intake
Sugar* (excluding naturally occurring sugar such as in fruits, vegetables and milk)	No more than 5% of daily calorie intake
Fibre	30g per day

From: Public Health England[29-31].

* "All monosaccharides and disaccharides [sugars] added to foods by the manufacturer, cook or consumer, plus sugars naturally present in honey, syrups and unsweetened fruit juices. Under this definition, lactose (milk sugar) when naturally present in milk and milk products and sugars contained within the cellular structure of foods (particularly fruits and vegetables) are excluded."
Public Health England[30].

Similar recommendations have been made by the *World Health Organisation, United States Department of Health,* and the *American Heart Association*[8]. It is important to point out that these recommendations are for the *sedentary general population*, based on data from *observational studies* (see chapter 4 regarding study design). These numbers are a minimum or maximum to prevent deficiencies and to maintain health at a *population* level. For example, high sugar and/or fat consumption is associated with weight gain, obesity and metabolic problems from excess calorie intake, not sugar and/or fat itself[32,33]. Hence, the recommendation to limit sugar or fat intake aids in preventing calorie overconsumption[32,34]. At a population scale, limiting added sugar or fat intake will limit calorie overconsumption, hence the recommendations[8]. At an *individual* scale, sugar and fat intake can be factored into total daily intake such that higher intakes do not result in calorie overconsumption. Weight loss *can* still be achieved with high sugar intake[33]. Other authorities have suggested much higher acceptable intakes of added sugars than the UK government guidelines[32]. The US and other guidelines do not place an upper limit on total fat intake[8,35,36].

What's your diet?

Diets with the aim of weight loss can manipulate macronutrients, manipulate food sources, or manipulate the timing of food consumption.

There is a never-ending list of diets. Every so often, a new fad diet seems to appear out of thin air with '*guaranteed*' results. Common diets or diet strategies include low carbohydrate, low fat, high fat, high protein, intermittent fasting, vegan, vegetarian, ketogenic or very low calorie diets. *New* diets are generally just a variant of one of the above. They *all* lead to weight loss when they are implemented with a daily calorie deficit[37]. They also *all* lead to weight gain if they are implemented with a daily calorie surplus[37]. You can lose weight on a diet purely of doughnuts and cheeseburgers. But, this would result in nutritional deficiencies and health implications. You can also gain weight on a diet of purely lettuce, if you ate enough. But again, this would also lead to nutritional deficiencies from a lack of dietary variation. Significant weight loss from muscle mass is also detrimental to health. Weight change does *not* mean health improvement.

Currently, no conclusive evidence demonstrates a significant benefit to any specific diet that makes that diet better than any another diet for weight loss.

"Our limited knowledge allows us to conclude that there is no optimally effective diet for all individuals to lose weight."
Freire, 2020[38].

People often think that a certain diet is better for weight loss because they found they lost weight following it, and didn't lose weight following an alternative diet. This is simply because the certain diet *works* for *them*, i.e. they found it easier to enter and maintain a calorie deficit with that diet compared to the other diets they tried. Different diets are easier to adhere to for different people. Whether someone finds one diet better than another will come down to personal preference[37]. It is very easy to say that a particular diet leads to greater weight loss when placed in a larger calorie deficit. At a population level, diets are equivocal for weight loss. At an individual level, certain diets can be better for weight loss, because of improved adherence.

Different diets work better for different people, because they can adhere to them better.

The majority of the calories you burn primarily come from just living and being alive. For the average person, going to the gym or going on a run typically burns a fraction of your daily calories. A 60kg woman may need 2000 kcal from living (basal metabolic rate, thermic effect of food and non-exercise activity thermogenesis). A 20-minute run may only burn 150-200kcal (exercise activity thermogenesis), the equivalent of a slice of toast without any butter. Dietary changes, not exercise should be the primary determinant as to whether you are increasing, decreasing or maintaining weight by generating a calorie surplus, deficit, or neither[39]. Dietary interventions result in greater weight loss than exercise interventions[39]. This does *not* mean exercise is unimportant; the health benefits are countless, and exercise does contribute to weight loss and weight maintenance. It just means it is not a requirement for weight change and should not be the primary tool to promote weight change (see chapter 24 regarding aerobic exercise for weight loss).

The pie charts below highlight the relative importance of diet, resistance training and aerobic exercise for weight loss (promoting fat loss but minimising muscle loss) or weight gain (promoting muscle growth but minimising fat gain) goals. The proportions are not how much time you should be devoting to each factor, but their relative importance.

These charts assume that adequate sleep, good overall nutrition (no deficiencies) and minimal stress are present. These factors significantly influence changes in body composition. For example, 5.5 hours sleep per night compared to 8.5 hours results in 55% less weight lost as fat over the course of 2 weeks whilst in a calorie deficit[40]. This means more weight is lost as muscle, which would be considered a less than optimal change in body composition[40].

Weight loss

Diet is the most important factor for weight loss. Regardless of how hard you train or how much exercise you do, you will *not* lose weight unless you are in a calorie deficit. Meta-analyses of weight loss interventions find that exercise alone does not result in as much weight loss as a dietary intervention or a combined exercise and dietary intervention[39].

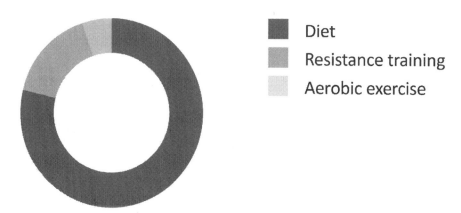

The relative importance of diet and exercise for weight loss, with fat loss as a priority.

Resistance training will be important. Once the calorie deficit is set up and weight is being lost, resistance training will help to preserve muscle mass and make sure weight loss is mainly as fat and not excessively as muscle. Additional exercise should only be considered once you have created a calorie deficit by manipulating your diet, and you have a solid training programme (consisting of resistance training and possibly aerobic exercise) in place. The rate of weight loss will slow down over time. At this point, additional aerobic exercise may help to maintain the calorie deficit without having to further reduce calorie intake. This is dependent on your current training load. This will be discussed in more detail in chapter 18 and 24.

Muscle preservation when losing weight

Preserve muscle when trying to lose weight for more successful and effective weight loss.

Often it can be very tempting to try and lose weight fast. You might have a holiday booked in a few weeks' time, so you decide to eat very little for a short period beforehand in an attempt to get *'in shape'* for your trip. Unfortunately, when we lose weight, we do not just lose fat. We also lose muscle. When the aim is weight loss, the weight we actually want to reduce is our fat mass and not our muscle mass (or more broadly, our fat-free mass). It is beneficial to minimise the amount of muscle that is lost. Excluding severely low body fat percentages, this aligns with improved physical health outcomes.

Becoming more 'toned' is a misunderstood concept. Resting muscle *tone* is the passive tension of muscles to maintain body posture. Muscle tone can also be a measure of how active the muscle is and the amount of tension it is generating, meaning you can increase muscle tone just by tensing your muscles (e.g. flexing your bicep will increase its tone). What people are actually referring to when they want to be more 'toned' is a relative reduction in fat mass, and/or a relative increase in muscle mass. Reductions in fat mass allow visualisation of muscle mass and the 'toned' appearance. If you lose weight as muscle mass, this will reduce the visibility of muscle at a given body fat percentage. For example, to see visible abs, your body fat percentage must be sufficiently low. However, losing muscle mass means it will be harder to visually see abs at a given body fat level.

Body composition has a large effect on our resting metabolic rate. As our body weight drops, our basal metabolic rate and total daily energy expenditure will also drop (discussed in chapter 5)[41]. Despite muscle mass having a fairly low resting metabolic expenditure, the energy demands of additional muscle increases during exercise. Similarly, there is an additional energy cost to moving this additional muscle mass around. Total daily energy expenditure will reduce with weight loss anyway. Excess muscle loss will only add to this reduction. This makes it harder to further lose weight and makes it more likely to lead to weight regain following cessation of the calorie deficit. A greater proportion of weight lost as muscle means we are losing proportionately *less* fat per unit of weight lost. Therefore, to lose the *same* amount of fat as someone losing relatively *more* fat per unit of weight lost would require a *longer* period of time in a deficit. This means a longer and more stressful weight loss process to achieve the same amount of fat loss, resulting in further muscle loss. Having greater muscle mass is associated with improved health outcomes[1].

Weight gain

As the primary driver to stimulate muscle protein synthesis and growth, resistance training is very important when trying to gain muscle.

Diet is still very important. Energy is required to build new muscle structures, fuel muscle building and fuel new muscle. You *can* build muscle in a calorie deficit when resistance training, however growth will be less than when in a calorie surplus. Muscle growth is optimised in a calorie surplus[37]. If you eat less than your current daily calorie needs, there will be limitations on the amount of energy available to build and fuel new muscle mass. Aerobic exercise is relatively unimportant for muscle growth. The potential influence of aerobic exercise on muscle growth is discussed in chapter 24.

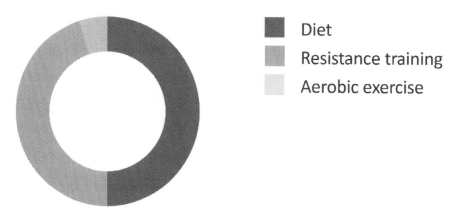

The relative importance of diet and exercise for weight gain, with muscle gain as a priority.

Weight change

It isn't a particular food or macronutrient (carbohydrate, fat or protein) that is the culprit of weight gain. It is the excess consumption of calories above total daily energy needs. This is primarily the result of brief periods of overfeeding, rather than small daily surpluses over a long period of time. Tasty foods tend to be very energy dense; usually high in fat and carbohydrate (often sugar). This means a small amount of food does little to make you feel full (satiated), whilst providing a large number of calories (i.e. high energy density). This makes it easy to eat more than you need. This can lead to the assumption of excluding specific foods or macronutrients to ensure weight loss.

No specific food is inherently fattening, nor is any specific food inherently slimming.

Links between specific foods/food groups and weight gain or health issues are from observational studies (that do not show causality) and tends to result from excessively high consumption of that food, rather than any level of consumption. Randomised controlled trials demonstrate that weight loss is dictated by energy balance, not by relative macronutrient content[11]. There is no need to exclude any foods or food groups for the reason that they cause weight gain or prevent weight loss. Any food can be included in a successful diet when consumed in moderation. Exclusion of specific foods from your diet should be due to allergies (e.g. lactose intolerance, coeliac disease (gluten intolerance) or nut allergies), and/or for ethical and environmental reasons (e.g. consumption of animal-based foods). Exclusion of specific foods should *not* be due to a belief that its complete exclusion is superior to low or moderate consumption for body composition and health.

For example, currently there is no conclusive evidence that vegan or vegetarian diets are *inherently* better for health than omnivorous diets when comparing individuals with similar characteristics, lifestyles and dietary patterns (i.e. health conscious meat eaters compared to health conscious non-meat eaters with similar socio-economic backgrounds, body mass index, physical activity and other dietary patterns)[42-51].

All diets work at a population level. Some diets work better than others at an individual level.

Check the table below for a summary of diets. Spot the recurring theme.

Dieting strategy	Can it lead to weight loss?	Can it lead to weight gain?	Calorie equated, are there any specific health or body composition benefits to this diet?
Low carbohydrate	Yes, when in a calorie deficit	Yes, when in a calorie surplus	No
Low fat	Yes, when in a calorie deficit	Yes, when in a calorie surplus	No
Any combination of fat and carbohydrate	Yes, when in a calorie deficit	Yes, when in a calorie surplus	No
High protein	Yes, when in a calorie deficit	Yes, when in a calorie surplus	Yes, up to a certain daily intake of protein
Ketogenic	Yes, when in a calorie deficit	Yes, when in a calorie surplus	No
Vegan, vegetarian, pescatarian	Yes, when in a calorie deficit	Yes, when in a calorie surplus	No
Intermittent fasting	Yes, when in a calorie deficit	Yes, when in a calorie surplus	No
Any fad diet	Yes, when in a calorie deficit	Yes, when in a calorie surplus	No, and will probably make you nutrient deficient

The main types of diets and their effects on body composition.

Is a calorie, a calorie?

There is high quality evidence to show that when it comes to weight loss or weight gain, all that matters is the energy difference between your daily energy intake and energy expenditure, regardless of the type of calorie[11].

Yes, there is variation in the proportion of calories we can obtain and use from different macronutrients and food sources, but not to the extent that it overrides total calorie intake as the primary factor determining weight change, nor does it vary so much that we cannot track calorie intake and correlate it to weight change.

There is conflicting evidence on whether certain diets are better than others for weight loss. There are comparative randomised controlled trials showing low carbohydrate diets to be superior for weight loss and fat loss than low fat diets[52,53]. But, there are also studies showing low fat diets to be superior for weight loss and fat loss than low carbohydrate diets[52,54,55]. How is this possible from such high quality studies? Besides any general study criticisms mentioned in chapter 4, there are two main reasons why. The first is that total calorie intakes have *not* been controlled between groups. Weight change is the result of energy deficits or surpluses. A bigger deficit means greater weight loss, which is more important than whether the surplus or deficit came from changing protein, carbohydrate or fat intake. A non-systematic review concluded that any macronutrient combination results in the same amount of weight loss with the same calorie deficit[7].

"Repeated meta-analyses have shown convincingly that longer-term weight losses and metabolic improvements occur independent of macronutrient composition of the diet, and greater energy restriction results in greater weight loss, regardless of whether restrictions are mainly from protein, carbohydrate, or fat."
Thom and Lean, 2017[7].

However, despite the same amount of weight loss, equating calories does not necessarily mean the same amount of muscle and fat loss. This is due to the second reason, that protein intake has *not* been controlled for. The amount of protein you consume can influence the proportion of weight change via fat mass or via muscle mass. Studies looking at diets with higher protein intake tend to result in better outcomes in body composition when in a calorie deficit (promoting muscle retention) or in a calorie surplus (promoting muscle growth) compared to a lower protein diet[56-58]. Similarly, computational modelling demonstrates that varying the macronutrient proportions in a diet (the quantity of protein, carbohydrate and fat) only has a small effect on body composition outcomes, and even less so when protein intake is controlled[2].

When calories *and* protein are controlled for, low fat or low carbohydrate diets are just as effective for weight loss and changes in body composition[11]. A meta-analysis of 32 controlled feeding studies (participants are given all of their food which is accurately measured) compared calorie-equated and protein-equated diets, where people ate differing amounts of carbohydrates or fats. The meta-analysis found that high fat diets produced marginally greater weight loss. However, although significant, the difference was *not* meaningful in a real-life context (see chapter 4 regarding differences between statistical and real-life significance)[11].

"For all practical purposes "a calorie is a calorie" when it comes to body fat and energy expenditure differences."
Hall and Guo, 2017[11].

From a weight gain perspective, a randomised controlled trial of overfeeding conducted in a metabolic ward* showed that the additional calorie intake above maintenance calorie needs predicts the increase in fat and muscle mass. But, only the increase in protein intake predicted the increase in muscle mass, not the increase in fat mass[59]. The influence of protein on body composition is discussed in chapters 8 and 9.

* *Metabolic ward studies are very useful high quality studies, because participant energy intakes and expenditures are calculated very accurately.*

"Calories are more important than protein while consuming excess amounts of energy with respect to increases in body fat... We can account for all excess energy consumed through energy stored in fat and in protein or expended in higher total energy."
Hall and Guo, 2017[11].

The thermic effect of food (TEF)

If you consume food containing 10 calories of energy, you will not actually get to *'use'* all 10 of those calories. Energy is required to ingest, digest, absorb and utilise the food we eat. How much is left over for us to use varies, based on the macronutrient content and the food itself. This is called the *thermic effect of food* (TEF) (also known as *diet-induced thermogenesis*, or *diet-induced energy expenditure*), which makes up part of our total daily energy expenditure alongside basal metabolic rate (BMR), exercise activity thermogenesis (EAT) and non-exercise activity thermogenesis (NEAT) (discussed in chapter 5). This means that some of the food you eat just ends up being lost as heat. Lab-based studies show that the energy within each macronutrient can be equated to the energy obtained within the body[11]. Each macronutrient has a slightly different thermic effect of food. However, the thermic effect of food for each macronutrient is an average. The actual value will vary depending on the specific food and type of fat, carbohydrate or protein that is consumed[37]. Protein has the highest thermic effect, meaning it requires the most energy to access those 10 calories. Different protein sources have different thermic effects, as well as protein quantity[60]. The thermic effect of fat is 0 to 3%, carbohydrate is 5 to 10%, and protein is around 20-30% (the thermic effect of alcohol is 10 to 40%)[41]. An average mixed meal has a thermic effect of around 10% (8-15%). Therefore, over the course of the day, the thermic effect of food averages out at around 10% of total calorie intake.

Other factors also affect how much energy we obtain from food. For example, blending, cooking (and variations of), cooling and the age of food can influence how much energy we obtain, as well as food processing (such as raw, processed or ultra-processed food)[37]. Despite the thermic effect of food being significant in itself for total daily energy expenditure, the overall effect of different thermic effects and variation in energy acquisition for different macronutrients and foods is significantly less important. The contribution of the thermic effect of food to energy expenditure is around 8-15% (on average 10%)[37]. Any variation in the thermic effect between foods will only affect total daily energy expenditure by at most, a few percent. When this is contrasted to the potential variation in energy expenditure that can result from exercise and non-exercise activity thermogenesis, *variation* in the thermic effect of food is *meaningless* for long-term weight change or maintenance. We can calculate how much energy we can obtain from different foods and macronutrients, which informs us of how many calories we would actually obtain. Metabolic ward studies can accurately relate energy intake to any resulting weight change from a variety of food sources[59,61]. If you consumed a range of different food sources over several days (and therefore different thermic effects), there would not be a meaningful difference in the amount of energy available for the body across those days, based purely on the variation in energy acquisition. No studies to date demonstrate that dietary composition has a greater influence on weight loss than the size of the calorie deficit. Also consider that over longer periods, the habitual dietary pattern of an individual is fairly consistent, such that daily fluctuations in the thermic effect of food would average out to a similar percentage of energy intake. From theoretical, lab and acute human studies, it is clear that foods vary in terms of their thermic effect. However, from long-term human studies on weight change, it is clear that this variation does not have practical significance.

To lose weight, eat any combination of foods and macronutrients, so long as it is less than your total daily energy expenditure[2].

Nutrition

The past 40 years has seen remarkable changes in the understanding of nutrition and weight change. The sudden rise in ultra-processed foods rich in fats in the 70's and 80's and an increase in obesity led to the idea that fats were the cause of weight gain. By the 90's, sugar was the enemy after a rapid rise in sugar consumption and obesity in the United States. However, sugar consumption is now on the decline, yet obesity rates are on the rise. People want a culprit, a scapegoat or a clear reason as to what is causing weight gain or preventing weight loss. It is generally accepted that the real cause of weight gain is due to excessive calorie consumption, and not a particular macronutrient *per se*. Historically, food was scarce. Large amounts of energy had to be expended to access or consume food (e.g. hunting, manual farming and food production). Jobs also had higher energy requirements (e.g. building, farming and mining). Nowadays, you can pop to your local high street shop and pick up a sandwich, snack and drink for lunch that could meet more than half of your daily calorie needs for under a fiver. You can even get it delivered to the desk you haven't moved from all morning for a little extra. Never have we lived in a time where food has been so readily accessible and energy dense, alongside a society that is becoming more and more sedentary. Readily accessible, highly palatable and high energy density food, combined with lower physical activity and lower general movement means consuming more calories than are expended, and therefore weight gain.

'Diets' don't work, but 'diets' do

Part of the reason why weight loss plans *'fail'* (weight loss is not maintained) is due to the fact that *'diets'* are seen as *short-term drastic weight loss interventions* with no consideration for *long-term weight loss maintenance*. People exclude foods they like because they believe it is stopping them from losing weight and include foods they don't like because they think it will make them lose weight. A major issue is the use of the word *'diet'*. In fact, the word has multiple meanings. Its primary meaning is to just describe the energy and foods you regularly consume:

"Food and drink regularly provided or consumed."
Merriam-Webster[62].

However, diet also refers to an attempt to lose weight:

"A regimen of eating and drinking sparingly so as to reduce one's weight."
Merriam-Webster[62].

As in the common phrase *'I'm going on a diet'*. The word *'diet'* is too often associated with the latter short-term drastic change in eating pattern. *'I'm going on a diet'* is synonymous with an attempt of weight loss and an attempt to be healthier, which can lead to confusion as to what a diet is. Everyone is already *'on a diet'*. When we look at the definitions it is clear to see how going *'on a diet'* for a few weeks for weight loss is not *your* diet, because it will not represent *your* regular food choices that *you* find most palatable and leave *you* feeling satiated. Going *'on'* a diet implies that at some point you will be coming *'off'* the diet and returning to the habitual eating pattern. Drastic short-term diets result in weight loss, but not weight loss *maintenance*. It is not possible to adhere to such drastic dietary changes in the long-term, resulting in a return to the original diet and regain of any lost weight. This is because drastic short-term diets do not involve sustainable behavioural changes. Long-term weight change and weight loss maintenance requires long-term *behavioural change*[2]. Diets for weight loss maintenance should involve long term, gradual transitions from your *pre-existing* diet towards a *sustainable* calorie intake with enjoyable food choices[2]. The numerous fad diets that exist, demanding the exclusion of complete food groups for weight loss only fuels the unnecessary misconception of what is required for weight loss and what constitutes successful weight loss.

Successful changes in weight loss involve short-term and moderate-term (weeks to months) minor to moderate changes to your long-term (months to years) habitual diet (primarily by decreasing total daily calorie intake by varying the quantity of your *usual* food choices). By this, a period of weight loss that could be successfully maintained would involve a diet that is largely identical to your long-term diet, however it would have a slightly lower daily calorie intake, and possibly other minor adjustments to align with what we know about diets for weight loss. Similarly, the subsequent weight maintenance period (i.e. thereafter) would involve a diet largely identical to your weight loss diet, but with a slightly higher daily calorie intake than the period of weight loss, but a lower calorie intake than before the period of weight loss. It should not involve nor require drastic changes, such as excluding any foods you like or adding any foods you do not like that leave you feeling unsatiated.

Importantly, any minor change in your diet that results in a change in body composition means that your original diet is *no longer* your long-term maintenance diet. With weight loss or weight gain, your long term diet will shift slightly in terms of the daily calorie intake required for weight maintenance, because your body composition has changed (see chapter 5 regarding changes in total daily energy expenditure with weight change)[2]. For example, if you *lose* weight, your energy expenditure will *decrease*. Therefore, your new maintenance energy intake will be *smaller* than your maintenance energy intake before weight loss[63]. This is why drastic short-term diets do not result in weight loss maintenance, because no long-term change in energy intake has occurred.

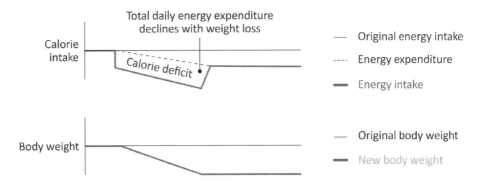

Successful weight loss and weight loss maintenance, due to a long-term change in dietary pattern.

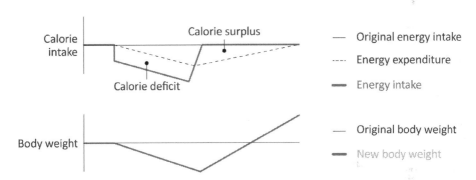

Weight loss, but unsuccessful weight loss maintenance. Returning energy intake back to the original intake before weight loss results in a calorie surplus and potentially weight regain.

Some have suggested that the concept of *'reverse dieting'* should be used as a tool to prevent weight regain after a period of weight loss. Reverse dieting involves slowly increasing energy intake from the energy intake during the weight loss period, up to the new energy intake required for weight maintenance (where calorie intake will equal calorie expenditure) at the new body weight. The idea is to slowly increase calorie intake, allowing energy expenditure and other adaptive changes that occur with weight loss to slowly return nearer to the levels they were at before weight loss[64]. In theory it makes sense to help minimise weight gain, but very little evidence exists regarding its use and efficacy (being primarily anecdotal), compared to simply increasing calorie intake immediately up to the new predicted energy intake required for weight maintenance[64].

Studies have looked at the habits of people who have successfully maintained weight loss[65-68]. Weight loss maintainers tend to adhere to a *'healthy'* eating pattern (discussed in chapter 12) and maintain their physical activity levels from the weight loss period. Weight loss maintenance requires changes in *habits* and *behaviours*.

Energy intake: the intuition-tracking continuum

Food intake can vary from purely intuitive approaches (based on appetite and satiety) to purely tracked, conscious approaches (consumption based on the calorie and macronutrient needs of the individual). A wide range of approaches fit in between these extremes.

If you have ever tried to lose weight or build muscle, you may have taken a more conscious effort to assess the food you are eating compared to when you had no body composition goals (i.e. eating to maintain weight). You may have started to take a closer interest in the number of calories in the foods you eat, observing the *'traffic light'* nutritional information on the packaging of foods which highlights the calorie, fat and sugar content. You might have even tried to guess how many calories you usually eat or try to work out how many calories you might need to eat to lose weight. Perhaps you have opted for restaurant meals that have fewer calories or tried to cook food with different ingredients. How conscious you are with your dietary energy intake at any point in time is on a *spectrum* from intuitive, habit-based eating, through to tracked, calculated eating.

Unless you blindly eat until satiated, there will be some conscious element of tracking your food intake, even though you might not think you do.

Even when you go shopping at the supermarket you may unknowingly use some element of conscious food intake. When choosing a pizza for dinner you might look at the calorie content and avoid the pizzas with the most calories. Or perhaps, you choose a smaller pizza to prevent overconsumption. You may have dinner planned at a restaurant in the evening and you want to have a starter, main and a big chocolate cake for pudding. Therefore, you *consciously* opt for low calorie options earlier in the day to prevent eating too many calories. You do this despite the fact that the low calorie options provide little satiety and you are hungry all day until dinner in the evening. Reading nutrition claims (e.g. *'low in fat'* or *'low calorie'*) on food packaging can also influence the consciousness of the consumer[69]. Such examples are very common, but are often not considered as tracking food intake. They are not purely intuitive. Even though there was no weighing of food on scales or checking the macronutrient content, there is still an element of being conscious and mindful about food intake in these examples.

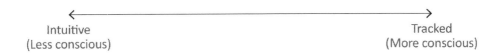

Intuitive
(Less conscious)

Tracked
(More conscious)

Habit/intuitive approach	Conscious/tracked approach
Use hunger and satiety to approximate portions, eating when hunger is present and terminating eating when satiated.	Consciousness can vary from low to high. Low consciousness may involve being aware of portion sizes or meal frequency. High consciousness may involve tracking calorie and nutrient needs.
Requires less thought.	Requires more thought.
Most ideal for long-term weight maintenance as you aim to match your energy intake to your feelings of appetite and satiety.	A useful tool to use in the short term (weeks to months) for successful body composition changes by ensuring a relative deficit or surplus by accurately measuring energy intake.
For specific short-term (weeks to months) body composition goals, it may be difficult to ensure a relative deficit or surplus or accurate measure of energy and macronutrient intake, which can result in not achieving goals.	For long term weight maintenance, intensely tracking intake can be time-consuming, stressful and largely unnecessary.

In general, research demonstrates that intuitive approaches (eating based on hunger and satiety) is associated with more stable weight maintenance, fewer eating related disorders and improved eating behaviours[70,71]. However, research also demonstrates that more conscious, tracked approaches result in greater weight loss during interventions[72]. It is important to remember that weight loss interventions are *not* long-term periods, but achieving weight maintenance *is*. The evidence of a detrimental effect from tracking food intake has not been conclusively demonstrated[70]. The positive or negative influence of more intuitive or more tracked food intake is likely to be highly affected by *how* it is implemented and *who* uses them (i.e. individual factors)[70]. For example, *intermittent fasting* (not eating for a period of the day) can be a useful tool for weight loss and help with dietary adherence for some. But, not eating for a period of the day may be from deciding to skip meals, and be detrimental to health for others. Intermittent fasting may result from a more *flexible* approach to dieting, but meal skipping may result from a more *rigid* approach to dieting. More *flexible* approaches (the inclusion of all foods at varying intakes, reducing portion sizes, allowing some variation in energy and macronutrient needs) to dieting are associated with improved long-term weight loss and weight maintenance compared to *rigid* approaches (all or nothing, eating only specific foods, excluding energy dense foods that are palatable for the individual, meeting exact energy and macronutrient needs)[70,73]. Flexible approaches can be easier to adapt to, and more sustainable than rigid approaches[70]. The *majority* of drastic short-term diets for weight loss are rigid approaches. The extent to which someone may be flexible or rigid with their diet will again be highly individual. A flexible approach can still involve tracking or being more conscious about energy intake. Tracking or being more conscious with food intake improves dietary adherence during randomised controlled trials and correlates with greater weight loss[72]. More intuitive approaches are useful for weight maintenance, but are not necessarily useful for weight loss[70]. Rigid, flexible, intuitive and tracked approaches are all relative concepts; where a given individual will lie on the two continuums will vary greatly.

Being more conscious with food intake does not mean you must track every little element of your diet. Likewise, being more intuitive with your food intake does not mean that you eat blindly until you are full.

Intuitive and conscious approaches to eating are not mutually exclusive across days, months or years. You could track intake on weekdays and not on weekends, you could track only your total calorie intake, or track your calorie intake and protein intake, or track your intake of fat, protein and carbohydrates. You might track your food intake during work and eat intuitively for dinner. You may never track at all, or track everything. There is *no superior method* and it is highly dependent on *personal preference*. Find the method that allows *you* to adhere to your plan, whether that is losing or gaining weight, or simply maintaining your weight with no specific goals. The balance of tracking and intuition for each scenario will be completely different for different people. It may also differ across the continuum depending on the goal in mind, and therefore the method used can vary over time. The intuitive approach requires less thought and time commitment and less effort to enjoy a more social lifestyle. However, it is more difficult to generate a positive change in body composition, especially when small and consistent changes in energy intake are needed.

Do I need to track my calorie intake? The saving money analogy

For weight change, tracking-based approaches work for some people at certain times and habit-based approaches work for some people at certain times. Work out the certain times when such strategies work for you.

Tracking food intake often seems like an extreme step for many people. Tracking is a more conscious approach to energy intake. However, whether it needs to be done and the extent to which it is used will depend on your goals, your current starting point, and personal preference. Despite variations in energy expenditure and energy intake, weight gain or weight loss can be predicted from the relative calorie surplus or deficit[11]. Therefore, tracking energy intake provides a *means* to ensure weight change.

A good way to understand whether or not you should consider some element of tracking calories is with the analogy of saving money. We will consider that the aim is to lose weight. In the analogy below, this is equivalent to saving money.

Let's consider that you need to save some money for a summer holiday coming up (i.e. you want to lose weight for the holiday). At the moment, you are neither saving money, nor spending too much money – your outgoings at the end of the month are the same as your salary. This is equivalent to you eating at your calorie maintenance, you are not gaining or losing weight.

We know that in order to lose weight, we need to reduce our calorie intake below maintenance energy needs. Similarly, to save money, we know we need to reduce our monthly spending to below our monthly salary. It is unlikely you will be getting a pay raise any time soon, so your monthly salary is fixed. Similarly, let's say you already exercise 3 to 4 times per week, so it is unlikely you could add in more exercise, so your energy expenditure is not going to increase. Therefore, we need to reduce food intake or reduce our monthly spending.

On most weekends you spend freely on expensive drinks, meals and other things, which you realise are quite expensive and you could easily reduce spending on them with minimal effect on your lifestyle. You consider reducing the rate at which you spend on these things. At the end of the month, you find that you have saved some money and you have not had to put too much effort into achieving this. This is the more intuitive approach, although there is still conscious thought. Rather than being highly conscious and tracking specifically what you spend, you identify the areas where you could probably limit your spending on expensive items and opt for lower cost items which provide similar satisfaction but leave you with cash left over. For example, having fewer drinks in bars and clubs on a night out, or not buying the most expensive steak at a restaurant and opting for a slightly cheaper dish. You still get to do the things you enjoy, but without the additional cost. Similarly, if your diet contains many high energy density foods (i.e. high calorie foods in a small food volume such as ultra-processed foods), then switching some of these foods for lower energy density alternatives (i.e. the same calorie content in a larger food volume, such as fruits and vegetables) can lead to a calorie deficit whilst maintaining satiety. This can often happen when people eat more fruit and vegetables because their lower energy densities can result in a reduction in daily energy intake as the greater food volume provides satiety. This can reduce total calorie intake without having to consciously consider reducing calorie intake.

On most weekends you spend freely on expensive drinks, meals and other things, which you realise are quite expensive and you could easily reduce spending on them with minimal effect on your lifestyle. You consider reducing the rate at which you spend on these things. At the end of the month, you find that you have still not saved any money. You opted for cheaper options on some weekends, but on other weekends you still spent heavily, which wiped out any money you had saved on other weekends. In this case, it may be difficult to reduce your spending without budgeting by keeping receipts and a running total of expenses. Next month, you only allow £50 to spend on each weekend. At the end of the month, you find that you have saved some money. This time in order to save money, it required conscious thinking and tracking. This is the more calculated approach. You may find that small intuitive spending changes do not impact largely on reducing your expenses, so you are not saving much. But, when given a budget and consciously tracking spending, you can save money. Similarly, if you have tried to make small dietary changes and found no weight loss over several weeks, then it may be wise to track your calorie intake to assess where you could limit your calorie intake so that you can ensure you are in a calorie deficit. Whether it is necessary to limit spending every day, on weekends or only in restaurants for example, will depend on how much tracking you find necessary to save money, and how much tracking you find feasible to adhere to. Whether it is necessary to track energy intake every day, on weekends or only in restaurants for example, will depend on how much tracking you find necessary to ensure a calorie deficit, and how much tracking you find feasible to *adhere* to.

Your relative fat mass may also affect whether you track, and how much you track. Additionally, you may consider how much you are able to reasonably lose per week. In the saving money analogy, if you have a small salary and need to save some money, then you will likely need to track your spending and can only save a small amount per month. Spending cannot fall below the expenses for essentials such as rent, food and travel. Therefore, if your monthly salary is small, the amount of money left over after all the essential expenses have been paid is small. This means that any amount of money saved will also be small without spending below the essential expenses, which cannot be sustained in the long-term without problems (e.g. losing your house). Similarly, the leaner you are, the lower your total daily energy expenditure, and therefore the smaller the calorie deficit you can generate without dropping energy intake below your basal metabolic rate, which cannot be maintained in the long-term without problems*. Therefore, in this scenario, it is more likely that you will need to track your intake with a smaller rate of weight loss per week. Also, if you have a smaller salary, then it is unlikely that you can save much money without causing significant disruption to your way of living. Trying to save a lot of money when you do not earn much money can be very tiring and hard to sustain in the long-term, and most likely unnecessary. Trying to save a small amount each week or month is much easier to do and is more sustainable. If you are lean, then large calorie deficits can be problematic in terms of leading to muscle loss instead of fat loss.

When you are lean, small calorie deficits are sustainable and result in long-term success[37].

* As discussed in chapter 5, when you are leaner your basal metabolic rate and total daily energy expenditure will also be lower. In general, as your body weight falls, changes in adaptive thermogenesis, exercise activity thermogenesis and non-exercise activity thermogenesis will mean the relative size between basal metabolic rate and total daily energy expenditure is smaller at lower body fat levels, than at higher body fat levels.

If you have a large salary and need to save some money, then you will likely be able to achieve this without much tracking and can save a larger amount per month compared to a smaller salary. Spending cannot fall lower than the total expenses for essential outgoings such as rent, food and travel. Therefore, if your monthly salary is large, the amount of money left over after the essential expenses can be large**. This means that a large amount of money can be saved without spending less than the essential expenses, which cannot be maintained in the long-term without problems (e.g. losing your house). Similarly, the more body fat you have, the higher your total daily energy expenditure, and therefore the larger the calorie deficit you can generate without dropping energy intake below your basal metabolic rate, which cannot be maintained in the long-term without causing problems*. Therefore, in this scenario, it is less likely that you will need to track your intake to ensure a calorie deficit and the more weight you can feasibly lose per week. Larger calorie deficits are feasible when you have a higher body fat percentage and can result in long-term weight loss[37].

** People with larger salaries will probably also have higher essential outgoings such as more expensive rents and extra bills, but in general will have relatively more expendable money than people with smaller salaries.

Therefore, if you do not earn much, you should aim to save a small amount to prevent major disruption to your way of living. You will probably need to track your spending to achieve this. If you earn quite a lot, then it is possible to save quite a lot without major disruption to your way of living. You may not need to track your spending to achieve this. Similarly, the leaner you are, the less weight you should lose per week to ensure fat loss and minimise muscle loss and the more likely it is you may need to track your intake to achieve this. The more fat mass you are carrying, the more weight you can sustainably lose per week, and you may not need to track your intake to achieve this. However, this is a generalisation, and the need to track will be specific to the individual.

The main point to consider with an intuitive or tracked approach is *consistency* and *adherence*. Similar to budgeting to save money, tracking provides a reliable measure that you are on target to meet your goals and keeps it realistic. However, tracking spending does *not* mean that you are saving. Tracking just allows you to see how much you are spending, and therefore allows for conscious adjustment of spending to ensure saving. Similarly, tracking food intake does not mean weight loss. It just allows you to see how much energy you are consuming, to allow for conscious adjustment of intake to ensure a calorie deficit. Just because it may be easier to not track expenses with larger salaries, it does not mean it is always the right choice. Some people regardless of their salary will prefer to save money by tracking expenses. Similarly, people with small salaries can save money effortlessly without tracking, because they might not spend much besides their essential outgoings. Some people can save money without too much thought, and some people can only save money if they track their spending. Some people may also struggle to accurately track spending or find that tracking spending is very stressful. The same is true for tracking calories. With weight loss, some people can lose weight without too much thought by making small lifestyle changes which do not require tracking of food intake, whereas some people need to track their intake. These are the two extremes on the spectrum of tracking versus intuitive approaches. It may be that you are not very good at saving on weekends, so you only track your spending on weekends to prevent overspending, or you only track your spending for evening meals as these tend to be expensive. Similarly, you may track your total calorie intake, or perhaps your total intake and protein intake, or intake of all macronutrients on weekends.

Intuitive and conscious approaches can both can be suitable and successful methods of long-term and short-term changes in body composition and weight maintenance. When considering the best approach for achieving goals in body composition, the main factor in deciding which is most appropriate for you is a behavioural one. Would you find it easier to have everything calculated, so that you know whether you are hitting your calorie and macronutrient targets? Or do you not have the time or commitment to track intake, and would find it much less stressful having more freedom in what to eat without having to think about the calories in each meal? The latter approach would come at the expense of uncertainty regarding whether your calorie and macronutrient intake is actually what you think it is. Neither strategy is definitively better than the other, being dependent on the individual and the specific scenario. Most people will probably find the intuitive approach less effort and better suited for long-term weight maintenance, but this would be of little benefit for fat loss or muscle gain if it does not result in the desired energy intake for weight change. In contrast, tracking intake can result in the desired energy intake, but people may fail to achieve their goals due to a lack of adherence to tracking. This doesn't mean the calculated approach doesn't work, nor does it mean the intuitive approach is too imprecise to work. It means that for a given individual, a given approach may not be ideal based on their circumstances. Perhaps you have very consistent and regular meals and calculating them is effortless. Or perhaps you eat when you can around work, and planning intake is near on impossible.

How to use a more intuitive approach to optimise body composition

Use it whenever it suits you.

Greater potential to use a more intuitive approach when:	Lower potential to use a more intuitive approach when:
First attempt at weight loss or weight gain for adherence or buy-in to the process.	Previous habit-based energy intake did not result in weight change.
Weight loss at a higher body fat percentage and therefore room for a larger calorie deficit with greater margin for error.	Trained individual at a lower body fat percentage looking to decrease fat mass and preserve muscle mass, and therefore a smaller calorie deficit is desirable with less margin for error.
Weight gain at a lower body fat percentage and relatively untrained and therefore room for a larger calorie surplus with greater margin for error.	Trained individual at a lower body fat percentage looking to increase muscle mass and minimise fat mass gain, and therefore a smaller calorie surplus is desirable with less margin for error.

How to use a more tracked approach to optimise body composition

Use it whenever it suits you.

Greater potential to use a more tracked approach when:	Lower need to use a more tracked approach when:
Previous habit-based energy intake did not result in weight change.	First attempt at weight loss or weight gain for adherence or buy-in to the process.
Trained individual at a lower body fat percentage looking to decrease fat mass and preserve muscle mass, and therefore a smaller calorie deficit is desirable with less margin for error.	Weight loss at a higher body fat percentage and therefore greater room for a larger calorie deficit with greater margin for error.
Trained individual at a lower body fat percentage looking to increase muscle mass and minimise fat mass gain, and therefore a smaller calorie surplus is desirable with less margin for error.	Weight gain at a lower body fat percentage and relatively untrained and therefore greater room for a larger calorie surplus with greater margin for error.

The majority of attempts to lose weight fail because they are seen as quick fixes. Successful diets are long-term lifestyle adjustments to food choices that allow people to remain full, satiated and happy with what they eat, whilst allowing maintenance of a healthy weight after a successful weight gain or weight loss period. With this in mind, it is important with both of these strategies that you carefully consider how to implement them. Even though your habitual diet may be shifted towards the intuitive end, when aiming for weight gain or weight loss your usual diet may shift towards the tracked end of the spectrum as you become more conscious about energy intake.

Suddenly jumping into a purely tracked approach from a purely intuitive approach may leave you feeling burnt out after a few weeks and could result in non-adherence. Instead, you could try calculating just one of your meals each day (e.g. lunch), or food intake for a few days per week. You could work out what an optimal meal size should be, such that you no longer need to calculate calories and simply gauge intake based on portion size. This would reduce the level of consciousness required to track, whilst maintaining accuracy with energy intake. Similarly, if you have been tracking food for a long time especially during a period of weight loss, reverting back to a purely intuitive approach may result in excess calorie consumption for some, but provide a much needed reduction in stress and freedom to enjoy food for others. There are many strategies, and no single strategy is ideal for everyone all the time.

If measuring calories is too stressful, then starting with a more habit-based approach would be suitable for a change in body composition. However, if this appears to be unsuccessful or you need the regimented routine of being held to account with numbers, then a calculated approach may suit you.

How conscious you need to be about your calorie intake will depend on your goal. For example, although you may not be tracking calories, you may find you need to eat past satiety to achieve a calorie surplus, or similarly find you may be feeling slightly less than full when eating in a calorie deficit. Likewise, if you know you need to eat more protein, you could consciously add an extra portion to a meal or have an extra protein rich snack. The remaining diet chapters will discuss in more detail specific numbers and ranges for optimising body composition.

Adherence

The most important part of your diet is consistency and adherence - meaningful and successful changes in body composition occur over longer periods of time, not after one or two days. Many factors will influence dietary adherence including food choice, food availability, social factors (e.g. events and parties) and motivations[38,74]. Don't skip breakfast if you love breakfast. Don't plan to prepare all your meals on a Sunday if you regularly have social events or plans on Sundays.

Make things as easy as possible for yourself. A sub-optimal plan that you can adhere to is always better than a more optimal plan that you are inconsistent with[38].

Greater adherence to a given diet in a calorie deficit results in greater weight loss outcomes[75]. In other words, diets work when people adhere to them.

Research shows that there are mechanisms and factors that can improve adherence. Some of these factors can be influenced and controlled by the individual[74]:

1. Choose foods that promote reductions in appetite and increase satiety.
2. Create a diet suited to you (individualised).
3. Monitor food intake (intuitive vs tracking).

These factors will be discussed in each chapter, to help you identify the dietary strategy that you can adhere to. It should be noted that the long-term diet that you will adhere to best will be one which already closely aligns to your current dietary preferences[74]. If your current diet is high in carbohydrate, it is likely that the long-term diet you can adhere to will also be high in carbohydrate.

Self-monitoring of food intake

Being *aware* of the foods you eat has been shown to be a valuable tool in providing dietary adherence. This does not mean weighing every little piece of food you eat and calculating its specific macro and micronutrient content. Raising self-awareness of food intake, even if fairly rough and inaccurate (such as measuring *'fist-sizes'* or *'thumb-tips'* of food portions) has important value[74,76]. Tracking your diet, progress and training results in improved weight loss outcomes and adherence[77]. Adherence to completing food intake records leads to greater weight loss than not completing food intake records[78]. A systematic review found self-monitoring strategies such as keeping a food diary (e.g. a paper or electronic record) was associated with greater weight loss[79]. This is proposed to improve adherence to the intended plan by being more conscious about energy intake and therefore ensuring the calorie deficit is present. On average, when making changes to diet to induce a change in body composition, not relying completely on intuition and habit to determine food intake and remaining conscious of eating can improve success.

Write a food plan. Consider the following questions:

- *Which foods do you like to eat?*
- *Which foods do you not like eating?*
- *What proportion of your food intake is derived from whole food sources (such as fruit or vegetables)?*
- *What proportion of your food intake is derived from ultra-processed food sources (such as chocolate, crisps or cakes)?*
- *At what times during the day do you prefer to eat?*
- *At what times during the day do you actually eat?*
- *How hungry do you feel across the day?*
- *Does your current food intake satisfy your appetite?*

The next chapter will discuss different types of diets and nutrition for specific goals. At this stage it would be worthwhile to keep in mind the foods you like and dislike and the types of meals you enjoy. Consider what you enjoy eating or what you could happily eat and see which diet strategy may best fit your dietary choices. Identify how your dietary choices can be used to meet the nutrition intakes for your goal of interest. After writing your lists, you might find a trend in the types of foods you like and dislike. Are your favourite foods carbohydrate rich? High in fats? How much protein are you already eating? How many fruit and vegetables do you eat? Does your current diet make you feel full through the day, or are you always hungry? It can also help to identify whether you might be eating too much or too little. Rather than choosing a plan and finding what you can fit into that plan, find the foods you like to eat and the manner in which you like to eat first. Then see what would be compatible with your personal preferences. Do you enjoy eating meat, fish or dairy? Then utilising a vegan diet may not be sustainable. Are you never hungry in the mornings but hungry later in the day? Then fasting in the morning may be a suitable strategy to promote a daily calorie deficit.

This may seem like a lot of effort, but that's because it is. If you genuinely needed to save money, you would sit down, look at your expenses and see what you could or could not live without, and how often you can have them. If you care enough about changing your body composition, then do the same.

Keep it simple

A useful strategy to ensure adherence has been developed by Andy Morgan, which allows for tracking macronutrients with minimal effort[80]. By developing a small set of meals with similar sizes, it can allow you to achieve your target calorie and macronutrient intakes by rotating across the meals during the week. This can be achieved by making meals that quickly divide your calorie and macronutrient needs between however many meals you consume per day:

- Choose a source of protein (e.g. chicken, beef, fish or plant-based sources).
- Add vegetables (e.g. carrots, cauliflower, vegetable stir fry).
- Add seasoning or flavouring as required (e.g. herbs and spices).
- Add carbohydrates and/or fats depending on calorie and macronutrient needs and personal preferences (e.g. carbohydrate rich foods such as potato and rice for higher carbohydrate diets, or fat rich foods such as nuts, oily fish or avocado for higher fat diets).
- Create a menu of 6 to 8 meals that you can conveniently rotate through across the week that meet your dietary needs.

This can minimise stress, effort and the time needed to meet the dietary requirements of your goals and help to improve adherence. This saves you having to think of new meals that are enjoyable and meet your dietary needs. An in-depth discussion of how to do this can be found on Andy Morgan's publicly available website[80].

Summary

Protein, carbohydrates and fat are major components of food we eat. Protein and fat are essential, but carbohydrates act as a main fuel source. Excess energy is primarily stored as fat.

Vitamins and minerals are minor components of the food we eat. A varied, balanced diet provides all the micronutrition that is needed. Supplementation is not necessary.

Dietary intake can vary from an intuitive approach, to a conscious, tracked approach. Different individuals will find they are more suited to different points on the spectrum. Approaches to dietary intake can shift between more intuitive and more tracked approaches.

Long term weight maintenance tends to be best achieved with a more intuitive approach.

Successful weight change tends to be best achieved with a more conscious, tracked approach.

Dietary adherence is a very important factor for successful weight change and long-term weight loss maintenance.

Make things as easy as possible for yourself. A sub-optimal diet plan that you can adhere to is always better than a more optimal plan that you are inconsistent with.

References

1   McLeod M, Breen L, Hamilton DL, Philp A. Live strong and prosper: the importance of skeletal muscle strength for healthy ageing. *Biogerontology* 2016; 17: 497–510.

2   Hall KD. Modeling metabolic adaptations and energy regulation in humans. *Annu Rev Nutr* 2012; 32: 35–54.

3   Foster-Powell K, Holt SHA, Brand-Miller JC. International table of glycemic index and glycemic load values: 2002. *Am J Clin Nutr* 2002; 76: 5–56.

4   Atkinson FS, Foster-Powell K, Brand-Miller JC. International Tables of Glycemic Index and Glycemic Load Values: 2008. *Diabetes Care* 2008; 31: 2281–2283.

5   National Research Council Committee on Diet and Health. *Fats and Other Lipids.* In: *Diet and Health: Implications for Reducing Chronic Disease Risk.* National Academies Press (US), 1989. Available from: https://www.ncbi.nlm.nih.gov/books/NBK218759/ (accessed 5 Feb 2020).

6   Di Nicolantonio JJ, O'Keefe JH. Good Fats versus Bad Fats: A Comparison of Fatty Acids in the Promotion of Insulin Resistance, Inflammation, and Obesity. *Mo Med* 2017; 114: 303–307.

7   Thom G, Lean M. Is There an Optimal Diet for Weight Management and Metabolic Health? *Gastroenterology* 2017; 152: 1739–1751.

8   Liu AG, Ford NA, Hu FB, Zelman KM, Mozaffarian D, Kris-Etherton PM. A healthy approach to dietary fats: understanding the science and taking action to reduce consumer confusion. *Nutr J* 2017; 16. Available from: doi:10.1186/s12937-017-0271-4.

9   Siri-Tarino PW, Chiu S, Bergeron N, Krauss RM. Saturated Fats Versus Polyunsaturated Fats Versus Carbohydrates for Cardiovascular Disease Prevention and Treatment. *Annu Rev Nutr* 2015; 35: 517–543.

10   Dhaka V, Gulia N, Ahlawat KS, Khatkar BS. Trans fats—sources, health risks and alternative approach - A review. *J Food Sci Technol* 2011; 48: 534–541.

11   Hall KD, Guo J. Obesity Energetics: Body Weight Regulation and the Effects of Diet Composition. *Gastroenterology* 2017; 152: 1718-1727.e3.

12   Hall KD, Heymsfield SB, Kemnitz JW, Klein S, Schoeller DA, Speakman JR. Energy balance and its components: implications for body weight regulation. *Am J Clin Nutr* 2012; 95: 989–994.

13   Jensen MD. Role of Body Fat Distribution and the Metabolic Complications of Obesity. *J Clin Endocrinol Metab* 2008; 93: S57–S63.

14   Oregon State University. *Linus Pauling Institute: Micronutrient Information Center.* 2014. Available from: https://lpi.oregonstate.edu/mic (accessed 5 Feb 2020).

15   Valavanidis A. Dietary Supplements: Beneficial to Human Health or Just Peace of Mind? A Critical Review on the Issue of Benefit/Risk of Dietary Supplements. *Pharmakeftiki* 2016; 28: 60–83.

16   Thomas DT, Erdman KA, Burke LM. Position of the Academy of Nutrition and Dietetics, Dietitians of Canada, and the American College of Sports Medicine: Nutrition and Athletic Performance. *J Acad Nutr Diet* 2016; 116: 501–528.

17   American Dietetic Association, Dieticians of Canada, American College of Sports Medicine, Rodriguez NR, Di Marco NM, Langley S. American College of Sports Medicine position stand. Nutrition and Athletic Performance. *Med Sci Sports Exerc* 2009; 41: 709–731.

18   Marra MV, Bailey RL. Position of the Academy of Nutrition and Dietetics: Micronutrient Supplementation. *J Acad Nutr Diet* 2018; 118: 2162–2173.

19   Blumberg JB, Bailey RL, Sesso HD, Ulrich CM. The Evolving Role of Multivitamin/Multimineral Supplement Use among Adults in the Age of Personalized Nutrition. *Nutrients* 2018; 10. Available from: doi:10.3390/nu10020248.

20   Helms ER, Aragon AA, Fitschen PJ. Evidence-based recommendations for natural bodybuilding contest preparation: nutrition and supplementation. *J Int Soc Sports Nutr* 2014; 11: 20.

21   Pawlak R, Parrott SJ, Raj S, Cullum-Dugan D, Lucus D. How prevalent is vitamin B12 deficiency among vegetarians? *Nutr Rev* 2013; 71: 110–117.

22   Kerksick CM, Wilborn CD, Roberts MD, Smith-Ryan A, Kleiner SM, Jäger R et al. ISSN exercise & sports nutrition review update: research & recommendations. *J Int Soc Sports Nutr 2018*; 15. Available from: doi:10.1186/s12970-018-0242-y.

23   Charrière N, Miles-Chan JL, Montani J-P, Dulloo AG. Water-induced thermogenesis and fat oxidation: a reassessment. *Nutr Diabetes* 2015; 5: e190.

24   Reynolds A, Mann J, Cummings J, Winter N, Mete E, Morenga LT. Carbohydrate quality and human health: a series of systematic reviews and meta-analyses. *The Lancet* 2019; 393: 434–445.

25   Rolls BJ, Ello-Martin JA, Tohill BC. What Can Intervention Studies Tell Us about the Relationship between Fruit and Vegetable Consumption and Weight Management? *Nutr Rev* 2004; 62: 1–17.

26   Hartley L, May MD, Loveman E, Colquitt JL, Rees K. Dietary fibre for the primary prevention of cardiovascular disease. *Cochrane Database Syst Rev* 2016. Available from: doi:10.1002/14651858.CD011472.pub2.

27   Gibson R, Eriksen R, Chambers E, Gao H, Aresu M, Heard A et al. Intakes and Food Sources of Dietary Fibre and Their Associations with Measures of Body Composition and Inflammation in UK Adults: Cross-Sectional Analysis of the Airwave Health Monitoring Study. *Nutrients* 2019; 11. Available from: doi:10.3390/nu11081839.

28   NHS. *How to get more fibre into your diet.* 2018. Available from: https://www.nhs.uk/live-well/eat-well/how-to-get-more-fibre-into-your-diet/ (accessed 7 Feb 2020).

29   GOV.UK. *NDNS: results from Years 1 to 4 (combined).* Available from: https://www.gov.uk/government/statistics/national-diet-and-nutrition-survey-results-from-years-1-to-4-combined-of-the-rolling-programme-for-2008-and-2009-to-2011-and-2012 (accessed 5 Feb 2020).

30   GOV.UK. *NDNS: results from years 7 and 8 (combined).* Available from: https://www.gov.uk/government/statistics/ndns-results-from-years-7-and-8-combined (accessed 5 Feb 2020).

31   GOV.UK. *SACN Carbohydrates and Health Report.* Available from: https://www.gov.uk/government/publications/sacn-carbohydrates-and-health-report (accessed 5 Feb 2020).

32   Rippe JM, Angelopoulos TJ. Relationship between Added Sugars Consumption and Chronic Disease Risk Factors: Current Understanding. *Nutrients* 2016; 8. Available from: doi:10.3390/nu8110697.

33   Surwit RS, Feinglos MN, McCaskill CC, Clay SL, Babyak MA, Brownlow BS et al. Metabolic and behavioral effects of a high-sucrose diet during weight loss. *Am J Clin Nutr* 1997; 65: 908–915.

34   Slavin J. Two more pieces to the 1000-piece carbohydrate puzzle. *Am J Clin Nutr* 2014; 100: 4–5.

35   Johnston BC, Seivenpiper JL, Vernooij RWM, de Souza RJ, Jenkins DJA, Zeraatkar D et al. The Philosophy of Evidence-Based Principles and Practice in Nutrition. *Mayo Clin Proc Innov Qual Outcomes* 2019; 3: 189–199.

36   Health.gov. *Report Index - 2015 Advisory Report.* Available from: https://health.gov/dietaryguidelines/2015-scientific-report/ (accessed 5 Feb 2020).

37   Aragon AA, Schoenfeld BJ, Wildman R, Kleiner S, VanDusseldorp T, Taylor L et al. International society of sports nutrition position stand: diets and body composition. *J Int Soc Sports Nutr* 2017; 14. Available from: doi:10.1186/s12970-017-0174-y.

38   Freire R. Scientific evidence of diets for weight loss: Different macronutrient composition, intermittent fasting, and popular diets. *Nutrition* 2020; 69: 110549.

39   Swift DL, Johannsen NM, Lavie CJ, Earnest CP, Church TS. The Role of Exercise and Physical Activity in Weight Loss and Maintenance. *Prog Cardiovasc Dis* 2014; 56: 441–447.

40   Nedeltcheva AV, Kilkus JM, Imperial J, Schoeller DA, Penev PD. Insufficient sleep undermines dietary efforts to reduce adiposity. *Ann Intern Med* 2010; 153: 435–441.

41   Westerterp-Plantenga MS, Lemmens SG, Westerterp KR. Dietary protein – its role in satiety, energetics, weight loss and health. *Br J Nutr* 2012; 108: S105–S112.

42   Gillman MW. Enjoy your fruits and vegetables. *BMJ* 1996; 313: 765–766.

43   Key TJ, Thorogood M, Appleby PN, Burr ML. Dietary habits and mortality in 11,000 vegetarians and health conscious people: results of a 17 year follow up. *BMJ* 1996; 313: 775–779.

44   Zeraatkar D, Han MA, Guyatt GH, Vernooij RWM, El Dib R, Cheung K et al. Red and Processed Meat Consumption and Risk for All-Cause Mortality and Cardiometabolic Outcomes: A Systematic Review and Meta-analysis of Cohort Studies. *Ann Intern Med* 2019; 171: 703.

45   Valli C, Rabassa M, Johnston BC, Kuijpers R, Prokop-Dorner A, Zajac J et al. Health-Related Values and Preferences Regarding Meat Consumption: A Mixed-Methods Systematic Review. *Ann Intern Med* 2019. Available from: doi:10.7326/M19-1326.

46   Vernooij RWM, Zeraatkar D, Han MA, El Dib R, Zworth M, Milio K et al. Patterns of Red and Processed Meat Consumption and Risk for Cardiometabolic and Cancer Outcomes: A Systematic Review and Meta-analysis of Cohort Studies. *Ann Intern Med* 2019. Available from: doi:10.7326/M19-1583.

47   Zeraatkar D, Johnston BC, Bartoszko J, Cheung K, Bala MM, Valli C et al. Effect of Lower Versus Higher Red Meat Intake on Cardiometabolic and Cancer Outcomes: A Systematic Review of Randomized Trials. *Ann Intern Med* 2019. Available from: doi:10.7326/M19-0622.

48   Han MA, Zeraatkar D, Guyatt GH, Vernooij RWM, El Dib R, Zhang Y et al. Reduction of Red and Processed Meat Intake and Cancer Mortality and Incidence: A Systematic Review and Meta-analysis of Cohort Studies. *Ann Intern Med* 2019; 171: 711.

49   Johnston BC, Zeraatkar D, Han MA, Vernooij RWM, Valli C, El Dib R et al. Unprocessed Red Meat and Processed Meat Consumption: Dietary Guideline Recommendations From the Nutritional Recommendations (NutriRECS) Consortium. *Ann Intern Med* 2019; 171: 756.

50   Appleby PN, Crowe FL, Bradbury KE, Travis RC, Key TJ. Mortality in vegetarians and comparable nonvegetarians in the United Kingdom. *Am J Clin Nutr* 2016; 103: 218–230.

51   Zeraatkar D, Han MA, Guyatt GH, Vernooij RWM, El Dib R, Cheung K et al. Red and Processed Meat Consumption and Risk for All-Cause Mortality and Cardiometabolic Outcomes: A Systematic Review and Meta-analysis of Cohort Studies. *Ann Intern Med* 2019; 171: 703.

52   Astrup A, Hjorth MF. Low-Fat or Low Carb for Weight Loss? It Depends on Your Glucose Metabolism. *EBioMedicine* 2017; 22: 20–21.

53   Hession M, Rolland C, Kulkarni U, Wise A, Broom J. Systematic review of randomized controlled trials of low-carbohydrate vs. low-fat/low-calorie diets in the management of obesity and its comorbidities. *Obes Rev Off J Int Assoc Study Obes* 2009; 10: 36–50.

54   Champagne CM, Broyles ST, Moran LD, Cash KC, Levy EJ, Lin P-H et al. Dietary intakes associated with successful weight loss and maintenance during the Weight Loss Maintenance Trial. *J Am Diet Assoc* 2011; 111: 1826–1835.

55   Astrup A, Grunwald GK, Melanson EL, Saris WH, Hill JO. The role of low-fat diets in body weight control: a meta-analysis of ad libitum dietary intervention studies. *Int J Obes Relat Metab Disord J Int Assoc Study Obes* 2000; 24: 1545–1552.

56   Egan B. Protein intake for athletes and active adults: Current concepts and controversies. *Nutr Bull* 2016; 41: 202–213.

57   Antonio J, Ellerbroek A, Silver T, Orris S, Scheiner M, Gonzalez A et al. A high protein diet (3.4 g/kg/d) combined with a heavy resistance training program improves body composition in healthy trained men and women – a follow-up investigation. *J Int Soc Sports Nutr* 2015; 12. Available from: doi:10.1186/s12970-015-0100-0.

58   Stokes T, Hector AJ, Morton RW, McGlory C, Phillips SM. Recent Perspectives Regarding the Role of Dietary Protein for the Promotion of Muscle Hypertrophy with Resistance Exercise Training. *Nutrients* 2018; 10: 180.

59   Bray GA, Smith SR, de Jonge L, Xie H, Rood J, Martin CK et al. Effect of dietary protein content on weight gain, energy expenditure, and body composition during overeating: a randomized controlled trial. *JAMA* 2012; 307: 47–55.

60   Kassis A, Godin J-P, Moille SE, Nielsen-Moennoz C, Groulx K, Oguey-Araymon S et al. Effects of protein quantity and type on diet induced thermogenesis in overweight adults: A randomized controlled trial. *Clin Nutr Edinb Scotl* 2019; 38: 1570–1580.

61   Hall KD, Ayuketah A, Brychta R, Cai H, Cassimatis T, Chen KY et al. Ultra-processed diets cause excess calorie intake and weight gain: A one-month inpatient randomized controlled trial of ad libitum food intake. *Cell Metab* 2019. Available from: doi:10.31232/osf.io/w3zh2.

62   Merriam-Webster. *Definition of diet.* Available from: https://www.merriam-webster.com/dictionary/diet (accessed 5 Feb 2020).

63   Blomain ES, Dirhan DA, Valentino MA, Kim GW, Waldman SA. Mechanisms of Weight Regain following Weight Loss. *ISRN Obes* 2013; 2013. Available from: doi:10.1155/2013/210524.

64   Trexler ET, Smith-Ryan AE, Norton LE. Metabolic adaptation to weight loss: implications for the athlete. *J Int Soc Sports Nutr* 2014; 11: 7.

65   Klem ML, Wing RR, McGuire MT, Seagle HM, Hill JO. A descriptive study of individuals successful at long-term maintenance of substantial weight loss. *Am J Clin Nutr* 1997; 66: 239–246.

66   Feller S, Müller A, Mayr A, Engeli S, Hilbert A, de Zwaan M. What distinguishes weight loss maintainers of the German Weight Control Registry from the general population? *Obes Silver Spring Md* 2015; 23: 1112–1118.

67   Karfopoulou E, Brikou D, Mamalaki E, Bersimis F, Anastasiou CA, Hill JO et al. Dietary patterns in weight loss maintenance: results from the MedWeight study. *Eur J Nutr* 2017; 56: 991–1002.

68   Soini S, Mustajoki P, Eriksson JG. Weight loss methods and changes in eating habits among successful weight losers. *Ann Med* 2016; 48: 76–82.

69   Oostenbach LH, Slits E, Robinson E, Sacks G. Systematic review of the impact of nutrition claims related to fat, sugar and energy content on food choices and energy intake. *BMC Public Health* 2019; 19. Available from: doi:10.1186/s12889-019-7622-3.

70   Helms E, Prnjak K, Linardon J. Towards a Sustainable Nutrition Paradigm in Physique Sport: A Narrative Review. *Sports* 2019; 7: 172.

71   Van Dyke N, Drinkwater EJ. Relationships between intuitive eating and health indicators: literature review. *Public Health Nutr* 2014; 17: 1757–1766.

72   Ingels JS, Misra R, Stewart J, Lucke-Wold B, Shawley-Brzoska S. The Effect of Adherence to Dietary Tracking on Weight Loss: Using HLM to Model Weight Loss over Time. *J Diabetes Res 2017*; 2017. Available from: doi:10.1155/2017/6951495.

73   Jorge R, Santos I, Teixeira VH, Teixeira PJ. Does diet strictness level during weekends and holiday periods influence 1-year follow-up weight loss maintenance? Evidence from the Portuguese Weight Control Registry. *Nutr J* 2019; 18. Available from: doi:10.1186/s12937-019-0430-x.

74   Gibson AA, Sainsbury A. Strategies to Improve Adherence to Dietary Weight Loss Interventions in Research and Real-World Settings. *Behav Sci* 2017; 7: 44.

75   Dansinger ML, Gleason JA, Griffith JL, Selker HP, Schaefer EJ. Comparison of the Atkins, Ornish, Weight Watchers, and Zone Diets for Weight Loss and Heart Disease Risk Reduction: A Randomized Trial. *JAMA* 2005; 293: 43–53.

76   Phelan S, Wadden TA. Combining behavioral and pharmacological treatments for obesity. *Obes Res* 2002; 10: 560–574.

77   Wadden TA, Berkowitz RI, Sarwer DB, Prus-Wisniewski R, Steinberg C. Benefits of Lifestyle Modification in the Pharmacologic Treatment of Obesity: A Randomized Trial. *Arch Intern Med* 2001; 161: 218–227.

78   Wadden TA, Berkowitz RI, Womble LG, Sarwer DB, Phelan S, Cato RK et al. Randomized trial of lifestyle modification and pharmacotherapy for obesity. *N Engl J Med* 2005; 353: 2111–2120.

79   Burke LE, Wang J, Sevick MA. Self-monitoring in weight loss: a systematic review of the literature. *J Am Diet Assoc* 2011; 111: 92–102.

80   Andy Morgan. *Macro Counting 101: The Comprehensive, No-Nonsense Guide*. 2014. Available from: https://rippedbody.com/how-to-count-macros/ (accessed 5 Feb 2020).

7. The hierarchy of nutrition

Want to ride a bike? Take the stabilisers off before you start buying lycra one suits and carbon fibre bike frames. Don't overlook the basics before trying to change the specifics.

Hierarchy of food intake for body composition:

1. *Total daily calorie intake*
2. *Protein intake*
3. *Fat and carbohydrate intake*
4. *Supplements*

(Assuming adequate sleep and micronutrition, and minimal life stress).

Work out the number of calories you need. Then work out how much protein you need. Then work out the minimum amount of fat you need, plus any additional fat according to personal preference. The remaining calories to meet your total calorie needs can then be allocated to carbohydrates. This may sound like a single diet, but this framework actually encompasses any diet. Your total calorie intake will vary depending on your goal, your protein intake will vary based on your goal, and your fat and carbohydrate will vary based on your goal and what you enjoy eating.

There are many aspects of diets that can influence body composition. But, some are more important than others in terms of the influence they can have. How can we gauge which factors we need to focus on first? Think about *riding a bike*. Riding a more aerodynamic bike, using a more streamlined body position and wearing a tight lycra suit can reduce drag, improve performance and result in better time trial times. These are important factors for elite and trained cyclists who can achieve high speeds for long periods of time. Shaving a few seconds off a time-trial time can make the difference between first and second place. But, an untrained cyclist cannot generate enough speed for long enough for the effects of drag to be meaningful. Any benefit of a more aerodynamic bike and new lycra is insignificant and minimal at best for the beginner. The untrained cyclist is better off focussing on improving their aerobic capacity and cycling performance. Getting out on a bike and riding with effort and sufficient volume and frequency will do more for performance more than anything else. Even if a certain factor can make a difference, understanding whether it will have a *meaningful* difference relative to other factors is important. As with cycling, dietary factors form a hierarchy of importance. We can understand what we should put the majority of our focus on by considering these factors as a hierarchy, starting with the most important factors working down to the least important factors for body composition. The hierarchy assumes that other lifestyle factors are met. This includes adequate sleep, good overall nutrition (no macronutrient or micronutrient deficiencies) and general life stress is not excessive. These factors can significantly influence changes in body composition[1,2].

1. Total daily calorie intake

To lose weight, consume fewer calories than you expend[3]. To gain weight (i.e. muscle mass), consume more calories than you expend*.

Muscles can grow in a deficit, but this is sub-optimal – the nuances of growing muscle in different people such as untrained beginners and those with high body fat levels was discussed in chapter 6[3].

Calculating the calorie intake necessary for your goal will be discussed next in this chapter.

2. Protein intake

Protein intake influences how much weight gained or lost is from muscle or fat.

As an absolute minimum to prevent deficiencies in a sedentary person, 0.8g/kg of body weight of protein per day is required[4]. Participating in any form of exercise will increase this minimum up to 1.2g/kg of body weight. When looking to optimise body composition, protein intakes should be increased above this.

Weight loss: as a complete beginner with higher body fat levels, aim for 1.6g/kg of body weight per day of protein. Increase intake up to 1.8-2.7g/kg of body weight or 2.3–3.1 g/kg of lean mass per day* as you become leaner and with resistance training experience[3,5,6].

Lean mass as opposed to body weight. This is obviously difficult to identify for the average person and the simplified measure relative to body weight may be easiest for most. For lean mass, a simple rule of thumb is to take your body weight, estimate your rough body fat percentage (e.g. 15%, 20%, 25%), and take this away from your body weight. Then use this adjusted value.

Muscle growth (weight gain): aim for a total protein intake of 1.6g/kg of body weight per day. With training experience, intakes up to 2.2g/kg of body weight per day have been suggested.

3a.   Fat intake

A minimum of 0.5g/kg of body weight per day, or 15-20% of total calorie intake regardless of body composition goals[5,6].

3b.   Carbohydrate intake

The remainder of your calories to reach your target daily calorie intake should be from carbohydrate[5].

4.   Supplementation

The least important factor in the hierarchy. The clue is in the name, supplements are not essential. Supplements are discussed in chapter 25.

There are very few supplements with proven benefits to performance or body composition[5]:

- Protein.
- Creatine monohydrate.
- Caffeine.
- Beta-alanine.
- HMB.
- Citrulline malate.

Before even considering supplements, make sure points 1 to 3 are in place. Then, decide which of the proven supplements support your body composition goals. If achieving protein intake (point 2) is difficult, a protein supplement may be beneficial.

Evidence-based nutrition for body composition

Evidence-based recommendations for how to structure a diet based on the body composition goals of an individual have been developed by a range of authorities and researchers, including the *International Society of Sports Nutrition* (ISSN)[3].

Studies on nutrition and weight change utilise a wide range of research study designs, including interventional randomised controlled trials and observational studies. A large number of systematic reviews and meta-analyses exist, meaning the knowledge of the effects of different diets is fairly well understood, but not conclusive. With regards to weight loss, the vast majority of studies are on overweight and obese people. In normal weight people, the majority of research so far has been in young untrained males. What may work well in young untrained males may not work so well for young females or those with training experience, and possibly even less so for older females. However, it is likely that the outcomes will be at least relatively similar, and this is the best we currently have in terms of evidence. Increasingly more studies are being conducted in females and with those with training experience, which are included in this book[3].

Below is a condensed summary regarding diet and weight change[5,6].

> *When in a calorie deficit, ensuring weight loss is gradual by consuming only slightly less than your maintenance calorie intake and not drastically reducing calorie consumption will help to ensure muscle mass is maintained. The body will break down proportionately more muscle than fat with a larger deficit compared to a smaller deficit. This effect is heightened as your body fat levels drop.*

> *A larger calorie deficit can be used if you are of a higher body fat percentage. A higher body fat percentage would be 20 to 25% or more for males, and 30 to 35% or more for females.*

> *The size of the calorie surplus and the training experience of the individual can affect the magnitude of muscle gain (e.g. the largest muscle gains are in untrained beginners with a relatively large surplus, and the smallest muscle gains are in experienced trainers with a small surplus). However, the size of the calorie surplus will also dictate how much extra body fat will be gained during this period.*

> *There are many diet strategies (e.g. low carbohydrate, low fat, ketogenic), all of which can similarly improve body composition. In other words, choose the dietary style which suits your lifestyle, not because there may be some health benefit or other benefit to one diet over the others, because there isn't.*

> *One of the main factors determining long term diet success is adherence. A well-designed plan still needs to be conducted for success. This is where it becomes important to make dietary choices that you can stick to in the long term.*

Calculating your total daily calorie intake and your initial daily calorie intake required to meet your goals

Track your food intake for a few days when your weight has been stable for a period of time, or use a rough calculator. Once calorie intake has been initially set, adjust as necessary by monitoring changes. The key is monitoring and adjusting.

Even the most accurate scientific methods of calculating energy requirements to maintain body weight are only accurate to within 5% of the true value[7]. And as mentioned in chapter 5, total daily energy expenditure can vary day to day due to changes in exercise and non-exercise activity thermogenesis (you just move around more on some days than others). Therefore, using a rough calorie estimator is sufficient to gauge a ballpark figure of your energy needs, to then adjust energy intake over time with monitoring.

The average 70kg person would need 1500 calories if they did absolutely nothing and sat on the sofa all day (their basal metabolic rate). However, most people will be active through non-exercise activity thermogenesis during the day (even without realising it), such as walking to work, climbing stairs or doing housework. Therefore, the calories we need during the day will be higher, but usually only by a few hundred calories. Adding in exercise activity thermogenesis and the fact energy is used to obtain the energy in food (TEF) will bump this number up further. Of course, a smaller person or larger person would need less and more calories respectively, and the amount of energy expended as exercise and non-exercise activity thermogenesis will vary considerably between people. These differences in energy expenditure can be roughly accounted for with calorie estimation.

There are two simple methods to estimate your calorie intake:

- Track food intake.
- Use a calorie calculator.

Track food intake

Track food intake during a period of weight maintenance. If you keep a stable weight for an extended length of time (over several days), it means that your calorie intake is similar to your energy expenditure (calories in and calories out are roughly the same). Keeping a record of the calories in the food you eat during this period and finding the average daily calorie intake can give a pretty good idea about your energy expenditure. This method however is lengthy and requires a lot of effort, especially if you have never tracked calorie intake before. Significant daily variations in food intake and activity can make this difficult to measure. Your day-to-day activities need to be fairly consistent for several days so that total daily energy expenditure does not vary too much.

Calorie calculator

Probably the easiest way to estimate your energy needs is to use an approximate calorie calculator. These calculators will never be exact. But, given the day to day variability in energy intake and expenditure, they are accurate enough as a starting point for your plan.

Several calculators exist that each take slightly different approaches to estimating energy expenditure. Commonly used calculators which can be quite accurate include the *Harris-Benedict* and *Cunningham* equations[8,9]. The Cunningham equation requires knowledge of fat-free mass to be known, which for our purposes can really only be estimated and adds unneeded complexity. The Harris-Benedict equation has since been updated by the *Mifflin and St Jeor* calculator[10,11]. The *Dietary Reference Intakes* method is a nice straightforward method to calculate your daily energy needs, and is the calculator outlined below[6,12]. With the Dietary Reference Intakes method, your basal metabolic rate is multiplied by a *scaling factor* based on how active you are, to calculate your maintenance calorie intake (which will equal your total daily energy expenditure when your weight is stable).

To calculate your total daily energy expenditure with the formula below, you will need your:

- Age in years.
- Weight in kilograms.
- Height in metres.

You will also need to estimate your *daily physical activity levels*. This is different to how much exercise you do per day. Activity levels depends on how much you are on your feet, moving and not being sat down all day, which includes your activity at work and at home. A 20 minute high intensity sprint session does not constitute a high physical activity level, but a labour intensive job such as bricklaying does. Determine which of the three categories below best describes your *physical activity level* (PAL):

- **Sedentary to low activity level.** You spend most of your day sat at a desk with minimal walking, no exercise and recreational time spent not moving (such as watching TV, reading, or sitting down).
- **Moderate activity to high activity level.** You do not have a very physically strenuous job but participate in exercise regularly or your recreational time is spent doing physical activities, or active travel to work (evening gym session, running, cycling).
- **Very high activity level.** You have a job that is very active (such as a labourer) or you spend all day walking or performing physical exercise for several hours per day (such as a 4 hour run or 50 mile bike ride)[13].

Most people with an office job who exercise most days of the week will fall in the moderate to high activity level category.

We will use your physical activity level to scale your basal metabolic rate to match the extra calories burnt during the day to generate your estimated total daily energy expenditure, accounting for EAT and NEAT. Of course, this is an approximate measure. It should be used to get an *approximate* idea of your calorie needs, not exactly.

The *National Institute of Diabetes and Digestive and Kidney Diseases* (NIDDK) has developed a body weight planner; their model can be used by inputting your age, gender, height and weight to estimate your total daily energy expenditure, to find the calorie intake you need to result in a given weight change. Use this calculator for informative purposes only[14].

Males

If you are male, use your age, weight, height and physical activity level to find your *estimated energy requirement* (EER) (which is your total daily energy expenditure when your body weight is maintained). This is your maintenance calorie intake[12].

Estimated energy requirement for men aged 19 and over (in kcal):

$$EER = 662 - (9.53 \times age) + PA \times (15.91 \times weight + 539.6 \times height)[12]$$

Where PA is the physical activity coefficient[12]:

PA = 1.00 if PAL is estimated to be sedentary.
PA = 1.12 if PAL is estimated to be low active.
PA = 1.27 if PAL is estimated to be moderate active.
PA = 1.45 if PAL is estimated to be very active.

So, for a male weighing 80kg, 1.75m tall, aged 30, who is sedentary (PA = 1.00), then:

EER = 662 − (9.53 x 30) + 1 x (15.91 x 80 + 539.6 x 1.75)
EER = 2593.2kcal ~ 2600 kcal

Females

If you are female, use your age, weight, height and physical activity level to find your *estimated energy requirement* (EER) (which is your total daily energy expenditure when your body weight is maintained). This is your maintenance calorie intake[12].

Estimated energy requirement for women aged 19 and over (in kcal):

$$EER = 354 - (6.91 \times age) + PA \times (9.36 \times weight + 726 \times height)[12]$$

Where PA is the physical activity coefficient[12]:
PA = 1.00 if PAL is estimated to be sedentary.
PA = 1.12 if PAL is estimated to be low active.
PA = 1.27 if PAL is estimated to be moderate active.
PA = 1.45 if PAL is estimated to be very active.

So, for a female weighing 60kg, 1.55m tall, aged 22, who is active (PA = 1.27), then:

EER = 354 − (6.91 × 22) + 1.27 × (9.36 × 60 + 726 × 1.55)
EER = 2344 kcal ~ 2350 kcal

Calorie intake for weight change

Now that you know your approximate maintenance calorie intake, you can now work out the calorie intake to match your goals, experience and preferences.

Weight loss: calorie deficit

Reduce calories below your calculated total daily energy expenditure.

The more body fat you have, the larger your calorie deficit can be with the majority of weight loss derived from fat stores, not muscle mass. The leaner you are and the leaner you become, a smaller calorie deficit is desirable because this helps to maximise the weight lost as fat whilst preserving muscle mass[3,5,15]. Resistance training and optimal protein intake should feature in any plan of fat loss or being in a caloric deficit to preserve muscle mass[16].

A smaller calorie deficit (the difference between your total daily energy expenditure and your energy intake) is beneficial to maximise the proportion of weight lost as fat and minimise weight lost as muscle[17,18]. A systematic review of mostly observational studies has shown that the amount of weight lost as fat decreases when using larger calorie deficits. This is apparent across a wide range of body mass indices (weight ÷ height squared)[19]. In other words, more weight is being lost from fat-free mass such as muscle, with bigger calorie deficits[20,21]. For example, a randomised study into weight loss in athletes (although not necessarily *'normal'* individuals, they are healthy and lean) showed more optimal outcomes in body composition (preservation of muscle mass and greater fat loss) when losing weight at a slower rate (0.7% of body weight per week) versus a faster rate (1.0% of body weight per week)[22].

Weight loss at 0.5kg per week rather than 1kg per week has also been suggested in normal weight women[23]. Under medical supervision, large calorie deficits can result in successful weight loss predominantly from fat mass, but in individuals with much higher body fat percentages (such as those who are obese)[24]. The risk of weight loss from muscle for a given calorie deficit increases as body fat levels decrease[3,17,19,24].

How much fat you have and how quickly you try to lose weight (the size of your calorie deficit) will influence the ratio of *fat mass:muscle mass* you lose[25]. Higher fat mass:muscle mass weight loss is preferable because this means you are losing more fat, and less muscle[17].

- Higher fat mass:muscle mass weight loss can occur with higher body fat percentages and/or smaller calorie deficits.
- Lower fat mass:muscle mass weight loss can occur with lower body fat percentages and/or larger calorie deficits.

As a rough measure, a 3500kcal deficit is required to drop 1lb (0.45kg) of body weight as fat mass[26]. This measure is a large oversimplification, and more complex models have been developed to calculate changes in weight loss with changes in energy intake[27]. So, for simplicity, to *initially* drop 1 pound per week, be in a 500kcal deficit per day (7 days x 500 = 3500kcal weekly deficit)[7]. This rate of weight loss will *not* continue indefinitely, due to the reductions in total daily energy expenditure with weight loss that have been discussed. Considering the rough nature of calculating our energy needs, this is good enough to provide a starting point with which to begin our weight loss goals, before adjusting with time as our total daily energy expenditure decreases with weight loss.

Because males and females carry different levels of body fat, the optimal rate of weight loss is sex specific[3,5,28]. There is not enough data to recommend specific optimal rates of weight loss based on gender and body fat percentage, but general ranges of weight loss can be suggested.

Target percentage reduction in body weight per week based on starting body fat percentage and gender:

Males:

1. *Below 10% body fat: lose weight at a rate of 0.25-0.5% per week.*
2. *Between 10-20% body fat: lose weight at a rate of 0.5-1% per week.*
3. *Over 20% body fat: lose weight at a rate of 1-2% per week.*

Females:

1. **Below 20% *body fat*: *lose weight at a rate of 0.25-0.5% per week.***
2. **Between 20-30% *body fat*: *lose weight at a rate of 0.5-1% per week.***
3. **Over 30% *body fat*: *lose weight at a rate of 1-2% per week.***

You do not need to know your exact body fat level, just a rough estimate. This is difficult to accurately measure without complex technology such as a *dual-energy x-ray absorptiometry* (DEXA) scan or training in using skinfold callipers. You could use a *bioelectrical impedance analysis* (BIA) scanner, which you may find in your local gym[29]. With a BIA scanner, you stand on a metal platform, which can estimate your body fat percentage based on electrical resistances in the body. These can be highly variable (influenced by hydration status, food intake, body length, body cross sectional area, age, sex, ethnicity, ambient temperature, muscle mass and prior activity), but a single initial reading will suffice in giving you a ball park figure of your starting body fat level as a healthy, young, hydrated individual[3]. Another simple method to roughly gauge your body fat level is by visual inspection. Below 10% bodyfat in males and 20%

body fat in females, you will have some level of visible abdominal musculature. Between 10-20% body fat in males and 20-30% body fat in females, at the lower end you will have visible abs. At the higher end, you will not have any visible abs. Over 20% body fat in males and over 30% body fat in females, you will not have any visible abs. Clearly this is highly subjective, especially as body fat distribution varies. Gauging your body fat level is only needed to provide a rough estimate as to the size of your calorie deficit. If in doubt as to your body fat percentage, aim for a *slower* rate of weight loss.

At lower ends of each body fat range, aim for the lower end of the weight loss per week range (i.e. as a female with 20% body fat, aim for 0.5% body weight loss per week. As a female with 30% body fat, aim nearer 1% body weight loss per week).

Example: male

So, for our male dietary reference intakes example above who has a total daily energy expenditure of around 2600 kcal, he has estimated his body fat percentage to be around 15%. Therefore, he is aiming to lose 0.75% body weight per week. His body weight is 80kg, which would equate to 80 x 0.0075 = 0.6kg weight loss per week. Assuming a deficit of 3500kcal is required to burn 0.45kg of fat, then a weekly deficit of 4667kcal is required. Across the week, this would mean a daily deficit of 667kcal. Therefore, our male should have an initial calorie intake of 2600 – 667 = 1933kcal. Given the approximate nature of measurements, a ballpark figure around 1900-2000kcal is suitable as a starting point.

An important point to note here is that this male is sedentary. If he then decided at the same time as trying to lose weight that he would also participate in exercise, then his estimated total daily energy expenditure calculation would increase. Unless this was accounted for, this would mean the actual deficit is much larger than the calculated deficit.

Example: female

So, for our female in the dietary reference intakes example above who has a total daily energy expenditure of around 2350kcal, she has estimated her body fat percentage is around 25%. Therefore, she is aiming to lose 1% body weight per week. Her body weight is 60kg, which would equate to 60 x 0.001 = 0.6kg weight loss per week. Assuming a deficit of 3500kcal is required to burn 0.45kg of fat, then a weekly deficit of 4667kcal is required. Across the week, this would mean a daily deficit of 667kcal. Therefore, our female should have an initial calorie intake of 2350 – 667 = 1683kcal. Given the approximate nature of measurements, a ballpark figure around 1650-1750kcal is suitable.

An important point to note here is that this female is active. If she then stopped performing exercise or her activity levels dropped, such that she moved less during the day (perhaps a new job or commuting to work by car instead of bike), then her estimated total daily energy expenditure calculation would decrease. Unless this was accounted for, this would therefore mean the actual deficit is much smaller than the calculated deficit.

The body will adapt to underfeeding and total daily energy expenditure will decrease. Any initial calorie deficit will slowly become smaller as weight is lost and adaptive mechanisms kick in. To maintain the same rate of weight loss over time, you would need to slowly reduce your calorie intake over time[7].

Any initial reduction in calories is a starting point. From here, you should *monitor* changes (such as body weight and visual changes) and *adjust* after allowing time (at least a few weeks) for any meaningful changes in weight to occur. Create an initial calorie deficit and then monitor and adjust as the deficit becomes smaller over time (by assessing the rate of weight loss), to maintain the same rate of weight loss[30]. The rate of weight loss should not be the only factor considered. Also think about:

- **General levels of fatigue and energy**. You are unlikely to feel very energetic during calorie restriction, but significantly elevated lethargy and slow recovery may indicate the deficit is too large.
- **Training performance.** If your ability to train is significantly impaired, it may indicate the deficit is too large.
- Also, consider the optimal amount of **training volume** to preserve muscle mass without excessive fatigue and recovery during calorie restriction (discussed in chapter 19).

After a few weeks, assess progress and determine the next step:

- Weight loss is within the optimal range for your estimated body fat percentage; maintain current calorie intake.
- Weight loss is too fast, visibly losing muscle mass, feeling excessively tired, and poor performance in training; increase calorie intake.
- Weight loss is too slow (which is not necessarily an issue) or no weight change; reduce calorie intake.

Further changes in calorie intake should be small, increasing or decreasing by around 100-200kcal before further assessment, after allowing time for any changes to occur. Over the course of a weight loss period, small, frequent changes in intake will result in a '*stepwise*' appearance of your calorie intake, and a roughly linear change in your weight (see graph below)[30].

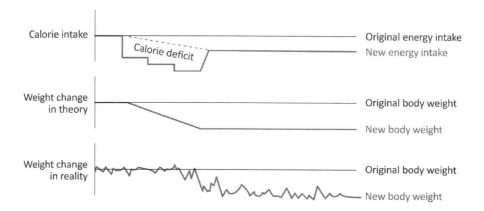

Calorie intake will not fall linearly during a period of weight loss. It will have a stepwise appearance as energy intake is adjusted by 100-200kcal after monitoring for several weeks. Similarly, weight loss does not occur in a linear fashion in real life. A conscious approach can allow for long-term weight change to be monitored, despite short-term fluctuations.

Weight gain for muscle mass: calorie surplus

Add calories to your total daily energy expenditure.

An optimal diet for increasing muscle mass is in a calorie surplus. Calorie deficits are sub-optimal (but possible) for muscle growth[3]. The ability to build muscle mass in a calorie deficit is more likely in untrained individuals with higher body fat levels, than a trained individual with lower body fat levels[31]. Smaller surpluses are more suitable with resistance training experience where the ability to grow muscle is reduced compared to untrained beginners. Larger surpluses increase the possibility of additional fat gain. Resistance training and optimal protein intake (at least 1.6g/kg of body weight per day) should underpin any plan of muscle gain or being in a caloric surplus[16].

From a health perspective, a calorie surplus will result in some increase in fat mass. Ensuring a suitable but not excessive surplus will prevent avoidable increases in fat mass. Consult a medical professional such as your GP before beginning a muscle building plan.

In individuals with little to no resistance training experience (beginners), it is possible to gain meaningful amounts of muscle with a sub-optimal diet whilst training (i.e. not necessarily be in a calorie surplus, or with sub-optimal protein intake). However, this also results in sub-optimal muscle growth[3]. A caloric surplus can augment protein synthesis and the response to a resistance training programme[25]. A period of replete energy provides a more optimal environment for the accretion of lean mass. The research behind specific calorie surpluses and muscle growth (with a resistance training programme) is limited. A calorie surplus alone does not facilitate improvements in body composition. Although muscle mass can increase when in a surplus and without training, this is relatively small compared to the amount of fat mass added[32]. A resistance training programme is necessary as the primary stimulus for muscle growth[31].

The size of the calorie surplus depends on the individual. When in a surplus, excess energy will be stored as muscle mass and fat mass. A bigger calorie surplus will result in a higher fat mass:muscle mass weight gain[32]. The relative proportions of fat gain and muscle gain (*fat mass:muscle mass* weight gain) can be influenced by several factors. Given that increases in fat mass can influence health, minimising increases in fat mass should be carefully considered. In the scenario outlined in this book, any increases in fat mass would occur within an already healthy individual at a normal body fat level, such that marginal increases in fat mass coupled with increases in muscle mass would have a negligible influence on health outcomes. *Consult a medical professional such as your GP if you have concerns.*

Your training experience will influence your potential to build muscle (whether you are new to resistance training, have some experience, or lots of experience). Untrained individuals have a greater potential for muscle growth than trained individuals. In untrained individuals, larger calorie surpluses can result in greater increases in muscle mass and relatively smaller increases in fat mass compared to trained individuals. Larger surpluses in trained individuals result in greater fat mass accumulation, but with only marginal increases in muscle mass compared to smaller surpluses[3,32]. In trained people, the limited ability to build muscle means larger surpluses result in additional fat mass and little extra muscle mass[32]. Complete beginners can consume larger surpluses which may be more optimal, facilitating larger increases in muscle mass with less weight gained as fat. As a more experienced trainer, a smaller surplus may be more optimal because of the limited potential to increase muscle mass. With experience it becomes harder to gain muscle and larger calorie surpluses result in more fat storage with little extra muscle growth[32].

Body fat percentage also influences muscle growth. For the same calorie surplus, higher body fat levels result in a higher fat mass:muscle mass weight gain[7,17,24]. Increased levels of fat mass can augment increases in muscle protein synthesis following resistance exercise and protein ingestion[15,33]. People who are leaner gain a greater proportion of weight as muscle mass when in a given calorie surplus[17,24].

The energy cost of building muscle mass is currently *unknown*. The rationale behind the size of the calorie surplus for muscle gain is a result of the theoretical minimum energy requirements of the constituents of any additional muscle tissue (muscle consists of 75% water, 20% protein and 5% other molecules), meaning 1 kilogram of muscle contains around 1200kcal of energy content[31]. However, energy will also be needed to build new muscle, and there is also a need to take into account metabolic adaptation (an increase in energy expenditure) from the relative increase in calorie intake[7]. We do not actually know how much energy is required to build muscle. Similarly, metabolic adaptation is highly variable between people. There is *no* conclusive or mutually agreed estimate for the energy cost of adding 1kg of muscle mass[31].

A very small surplus can be sub-optimal to promote any meaningful increases in muscle mass. A very large surplus will promote excessive and unnecessary fat gain and minimal additional muscle growth. A small to moderate surplus is a trade-off between ensuring sufficient muscle growth and limiting excessive increases in fat mass. With training experience, the upper optimum limit of energy intake for muscle growth is smaller and closer to maintenance intake, than for a beginner[32]. For a very in-depth theoretical read of how to gain muscle in a calorie surplus and whether to have a very large surplus, moderate surplus, or very small surplus, then I recommend reading the publicly available article *'How to bulk without getting fat'* by Andy Morgan[34].

As a starting point, a moderate daily calorie surplus of 100-500kcal can result in muscle growth whilst minimising excess fat gain. Choose a larger surplus as a beginner if excess fat gain is not of concern and muscle gain is a priority. Choose a smaller surplus as an experienced lifter, if excess fat gain is of concern or the possibility of not maximising muscle growth is not of concern. This will depend on personal preference as to the amount of additional fat you are happy to carry. A larger surplus may be achievable with a more intuitive, untracked intake of calories. A smaller surplus may require a greater element of tracking energy intake.

There are different ways to classify training experience. One rule is on duration, and another is on rate of muscle growth:

- o **Beginner:** 0-6 months of resistance training experience. Highest potential rate of muscle growth.
- o **Intermediate:** 6 months - 2 years of resistance training experience. Moderate potential rate of muscle growth.
- o **Advanced:** >2 years of resistance training experience. Lowest potential rate of muscle growth.

Being *'resistance trained'* (i.e. not a beginner) has been defined as having at least 6 months of resistance training experience[35].

Similarly to weight loss, there is not enough data to recommend specific optimal rates of weight gain based on body fat percentage and training experience, but general ranges of weight gain can be suggested.

Target percentage increase in body weight per month based on training experience:

1. ***Beginner: 1-2% increase in body weight per month. Add 500-1000kcals per day onto your calculated energy expenditure.***
2. ***Intermediate: 0.25-0.5% increase in body weight per month. Add 200-500kcals per day onto your calculated energy expenditure.***
3. ***Experienced: 0.25% increase in body weight per month. Add 100-200kcals per day onto your calculated energy expenditure[32].***

Example: male

So, for our male dietary reference intakes example above who has a total daily energy expenditure of around 2600kcal, he has estimated his training experience is at a beginner level. Therefore, he is aiming to gain 1-2% body weight per month. His starting body weight is 80kg, which would equate to 80 x 1-2 = 0.8-1.6kg weight gain per month. This would need roughly a daily surplus of 500-1000kcal. Therefore, our male should have an initial calorie intake of 2600 + 500-1000 = 3100-3600kcal as a starting point.

An important point to note here is that this dietary reference intake is based on a male who is sedentary. The inclusion of resistance exercise to build muscle means his estimated total daily energy expenditure calculation would increase. This can be achieved by using a higher physical activity coefficient (PA) in the dietary reference intake equation. Unless this was accounted for, this would mean the actual surplus is smaller than the calculated surplus.

Example: female

So, for our female in the dietary reference intakes example above who has a total daily energy expenditure of around 2350kcal, she has estimated her training experience is advanced. Therefore, she is aiming to gain 0.25% body weight per month. Her starting body weight is 60kg, which would equate to 60 x 0.25 = 0.15kg weight gain per month. This would need roughly a daily surplus of 100-200kcal. Therefore, our female should have an initial calorie intake of 2350 + 100-200 = 2450-2550kcal as a starting point.

The female is already performing resistance exercise, so there should be little change to her total daily energy expenditure calculation. An important point to note here is that this female is active. If she then stopped performing exercise or her activity levels dropped, such that she moved less during the day (perhaps a new job or commuting to work by car instead of bike), then her estimated total daily energy expenditure calculation would decrease. Unless this was accounted for, this would therefore mean the actual surplus is much bigger than calculated.

How much muscle can I expect to build?

Data from meta-analyses show that over the course of 12 weeks, young healthy males can add *on average* 1.6kg of lean mass whilst participating in a resistance training programme and consuming sufficient protein[36-38]. Individuals in these studies trained on average, 3 times per week.

Unsurprisingly, there will be variation from these averages and the ability to build muscle differs greatly. With experience, the anticipated rates of muscle growth decrease and therefore the necessary size of the calorie surplus decreases. For a given individual, the surplus will decrease in size with experience, to prevent excess fat gain. However, between people, some experienced trainers might require larger surpluses than some untrained beginners. Whether your required surplus is larger or smaller will be identified following adjustments from the initial calorie increase from your estimated total daily energy expenditure. This can also be as a result of the uncertainty behind the size of the surplus needed to build muscle.

The initial addition of calories is a starting point, and are only approximate additions for each category. From here, you should *monitor* changes and *adjust* after giving time (at least a few weeks) for any meaningful changes in weight to occur.

The rate of weight gain should not be the only factor considered. Also think about:

- **General levels of fatigue and energy.** Slower recovery and fatigue may indicate the surplus is too small or training volume is excessive (training for muscle growth is discussed from chapter 16 onwards).
- **Training performance**. It is expected that your training should progressively increase over time with muscle growth. A lack of progression may indicate the surplus is too small or there is a training related issue (chapter 18).

- Also, consider the optimal amount of **training volume** to build muscle mass, such as whether your volume is insufficient or excessive (chapter 19).

After a few weeks, assess progress and determine the next step:

- Weight gain is within the range optimal for your training experience; maintain current calorie intake.
- Gaining weight but too much as fat (weight gain is too fast, visibly increasing fat mass); reduce calorie intake.
- Weight gain is too slow or no weight change; increase calorie intake.

Further changes in calorie intake should be small, around 100-200kcal at a time, before further assessment after allowing time for any changes to occur.

There is a lack of evidence to suggest whether it is beneficial to only be in a calorie surplus on training days and at calorie maintenance on rest or recovery days, to increase muscle mass whilst preventing unnecessary increases in fat mass. This is known as *calorie cycling*, but is usually implemented by varying carbohydrate intake, and hence is also known as *carbohydrate cycling*[31]. Varying carbohydrate intake to meet training demands is discussed in chapters 8 and 24. Similarly, there is also a lack of evidence to suggest if this is detrimental for body composition compared to a constant calorie surplus across the week, as muscle growth will also be occurring on rest or recovery days. Therefore, whether you choose to remain in a surplus on rest days or not is down to personal preference. Daily variation in energy intake of course requires more effort, conscious thought and adjustment. And, there is not necessarily any benefit in doing so. The main overriding principle is adherence. Therefore, unless you want to vary calorie intake between training and rest days and you think you can adhere to such a plan, don't bother and focus on a consistent daily calorie intake to generate the required calorie surplus. If you do choose to calorie cycle, bear in mind that resistance training will expend energy (exercise activity thermogenesis). Therefore, this additional expenditure would also be no longer present on the rest day, and so calories may need to be reduced anyway to maintain the same size calorie surplus if no other exercise is performed.

Adjustment over time: other considerations for weight gain and weight loss

Besides the scale, there are other valuable methods of tracking weight change, which includes:

- Regular **tape measure readings** at select locations (e.g. hip, waist, thigh and chest)
- **Visual perceptions.** Do you look and feel more muscular or leaner? Are your clothes feeling looser or tighter?
- **Energy levels.** How do you feel? Are you making progress without becoming too fatigued?

No tool is perfectly accurate. The more tools you use to track change, the better the overall picture you will have to assess if change has occurred. The use of several tools also means a more conscious approach to changing body composition.

Self-weighing

Knowing how to correctly and accurately measure your body weight can be one tool you use to track changes. There is strong evidence from systematic reviews, meta-analyses and individual studies to show that self-weighing is associated with weight loss during weight loss interventions, with no evidence of adverse effects[39-46]. Self-weighing can aid adherence to energy intake and energy expenditure targets[47]. Even so, self-weighing should not be used in isolation to dictate how successful your weight change is. Tools such as visual perceptions, mood and energy levels should also be considered. When in a calorie deficit, weight loss is not a nice linear scale where you drop 0.1kg a day, every day, until the end of your weight loss period. Instead, your weight will *fluctuate* on a daily basis; sometimes not changing for several days before dropping say, 0.5kg in one day, or sometimes possibly even increasing (see graph on page 128). Weight can fluctuate for numerous reasons, including changes in water retention, food intake or with the time of day when you weigh yourself. Therefore, aim to weigh yourself at a consistent time, first thing in the morning. Being more consistent with weighing leads to better weight loss results, because infrequent weighing accentuates these small fluctuations in weight, and makes it harder to judge if you are on track. Aim to weigh yourself more frequently than less frequently, more than once per week, but not necessarily every day.

One final consideration as you progress through a body composition plan is that daily protein intake may also need to change as a result of you becoming lighter during a caloric deficit or heavier during a calorie surplus. This does not need to be adjusted on a daily or weekly basis, but over the course of months it can be useful to readjust protein intake to your new body weight (in a calorie surplus) or estimated fat-free mass (in a calorie deficit).

Where should I start?

There may be more productive goals for positive body composition outcomes, based on body fat percentage and resistance training experience. As an untrained individual or beginner, consider:

- As a female with >30% body fat or a male with >20% body fat: focus on a calorie deficit, muscle growth can still occur. Reducing fat mass would be more of a priority.
- As a female with <15% body fat or a male with <10% body fat: focus on a calorie surplus, fat stores are already low. Increasing muscle mass would be more of a priority.
- As a female with 15-30% body fat or a male with 10-20% body fat: choose based on the main goal you want to achieve (muscle gain or fat loss).

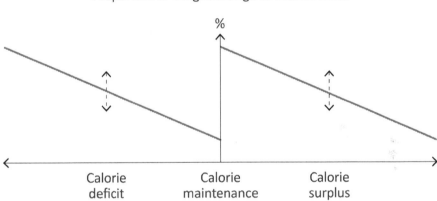

Proportion of weight change as muscle mass

The ratio of fat mass:muscle mass gained or lost is influenced by the size of the calorie deficit or calorie surplus. The smaller the calorie deficit, the less weight that is lost as muscle. The smaller the calorie deficit, the less weight that is gained as fat. With training experience, larger deviations from calorie maintenance will have a greater influence on the ratio of fat mass:muscle mass gained or lost compared to an untrained beginner (indicated by the dashed arrows).

Summary

Certain elements of a diet are more important for body composition than others. Energy balance is the most important element.

Fat intake should be kept above a minimum to prevent health complications. Beyond this, fat and carbohydrate intake should be primarily based on personal preference.

Weight change occurs through changes in fat-free mass and fat mass. Research has identified the relative amounts of energy and protein that can promote successful and more ideal changes in body composition. This will be influenced by current body fat levels, gender and training experience.

For a more conscious approach to weight change, the energy needs for the goal of interest can be estimated to provide a starting point, before consciously monitoring changes and making adjustments over time.

Measures that can be tracked to assess changes in body composition can include body weight, changes in visual appearance, energy levels, training performance and tape measure readings.

References

1   Bartholomew JB, Stults-Kolehmainen MA, Elrod CC, Todd JS. Strength gains after resistance training: the effect of stressful, negative life events. *J Strength Cond Res* 2008; 22: 1215–1221.

2   Nedeltcheva AV, Kilkus JM, Imperial J, Schoeller DA, Penev PD. Insufficient sleep undermines dietary efforts to reduce adiposity. *Ann Intern Med* 2010; 153: 435–441.

3   Aragon AA, Schoenfeld BJ, Wildman R, Kleiner S, VanDusseldorp T, Taylor L et al. International society of sports nutrition position stand: diets and body composition. *J Int Soc Sports Nutr* 2017; 14. Available from: doi:10.1186/s12970-017-0174-y.

4   Rand WM, Pellett PL, Young VR. Meta-analysis of nitrogen balance studies for estimating protein requirements in healthy adults. *Am J Clin Nutr* 2003; 77: 109–127.

5   Helms ER, Aragon AA, Fitschen PJ. Evidence-based recommendations for natural bodybuilding contest preparation: nutrition and supplementation. *J Int Soc Sports Nutr* 2014; 11: 20.

6   American Dietetic Association, Dieticians of Canada, American College of Sports Medicine, Rodriguez NR, Di Marco NM, Langley S. American College

of Sports Medicine position stand. Nutrition and Athletic Performance. *Med Sci Sports Exerc* 2009; 41: 709–731.

7   Hall KD. Modeling metabolic adaptations and energy regulation in humans. *Annu Rev Nutr* 2012; 32: 35–54.

8   Cunningham JJ. A reanalysis of the factors influencing basal metabolic rate in normal adults. *Am J Clin Nutr* 1980; 33: 2372–2374.

9   Harris JA, Benedict FG. A Biometric Study of Human Basal Metabolism. *Proc Natl Acad Sci U S A* 1918; 4: 370–373.

10   Frankenfield D, Roth-Yousey L, Compher C. Comparison of Predictive Equations for Resting Metabolic Rate in Healthy Nonobese and Obese Adults: A Systematic Review. *J Am Diet Assoc* 2005; 105: 775–789.

11   Mifflin MD, St Jeor ST, Hill LA, Scott BJ, Daugherty SA, Koh YO. A new predictive equation for resting energy expenditure in healthy individuals. *Am J Clin Nutr* 1990; 51: 241–247.

12   Trumbo P, Schlicker S, Yates AA, Poos M. Dietary Reference Intakes for Energy, Carbohydrate, Fiber, Fat, Fatty Acids, Cholesterol, Protein and Amino Acids. *J Am Diet Assoc* 2002; 102: 1621–1630.

13   World Health Organisation (WHO). *Human energy requirements.* Available   from: https://www.who.int/nutrition/publications/nutrientrequirements/9251052123/en/ (accessed 5 Feb 2020).

14   National Institute of Diabetes and Digestive and Kidney Diseases (NIDDK). *About the Body Weight Planner.* Available from: https://www.niddk.nih.gov/health-information/weight-management/body-weight-planner (accessed 5 Feb 2020).

15   Trommelen J, Betz MW, van Loon LJC. The Muscle Protein Synthetic Response to Meal Ingestion Following Resistance-Type Exercise. *Sports Med Auckl NZ* 2019; 49: 185–197.

16   Stokes T, Hector AJ, Morton RW, McGlory C, Phillips SM. Recent Perspectives Regarding the Role of Dietary Protein for the Promotion of Muscle Hypertrophy with Resistance Exercise Training. *Nutrients* 2018; 10: 180.

17   Hall KD. Body fat and fat-free mass inter-relationships: Forbes's theory revisited. *Br J Nutr* 2007; 97: 1059–1063.

18   Helms ER, Zinn C, Rowlands DS, Brown SR. A systematic review of dietary protein during caloric restriction in resistance trained lean athletes: a case for higher intakes. *Int J Sport Nutr Exerc Metab* 2014; 24: 127–138.

19   Chaston TB, Dixon JB, O'Brien PE. Changes in fat-free mass during significant weight loss: a systematic review. *Int J Obes* 2007; 31: 743–750.

20   Hector AJ, Phillips SM. Protein Recommendations for Weight Loss in Elite Athletes: A Focus on Body Composition and Performance. *Int J Sport Nutr Exerc Metab* 2018; 28: 170–177.

21   Odysseos C, Avraamidou M. Weight Management for Athletes: Important Things to be Considered. *Arab J Nutr Exerc AJNE* 2016; 1: 155–170.

22   Garthe I, Raastad T, Refsnes PE, Koivisto A, Sundgot-Borgen J. Effect of two different weight-loss rates on body composition and strength and power-

related performance in elite athletes. *Int J Sport Nutr Exerc Metab* 2011; 21: 97–104.

23   Mero AA, Huovinen H, Matintupa O, Hulmi JJ, Puurtinen R, Hohtari H et al. Moderate energy restriction with high protein diet results in healthier outcome in women. *J Int Soc Sports Nutr* 2010; 7: 4.

24   Forbes GB. Body fat content influences the body composition response to nutrition and exercise. *Ann N Y Acad Sci* 2000; 904: 359–365.

25   Lambert CP, Frank LL, Evans WJ. Macronutrient considerations for the sport of bodybuilding. *Sports Med Auckl NZ* 2004; 34: 317–327.

26   Hall KD. What is the Required Energy Deficit per unit Weight Loss? *Int J Obes* 2008; 32: 573–576.

27   Hall KD, Heymsfield SB, Kemnitz JW, Klein S, Schoeller DA, Speakman JR. Energy balance and its components: implications for body weight regulation. *Am J Clin Nutr* 2012; 95: 989–994.

28   Chappell AJ, Simper T, Helms E. Nutritional strategies of British professional and amateur natural bodybuilders during competition preparation. *J Int Soc Sports Nutr* 2019; 16: 35.

29   Dehghan M, Merchant AT. Is bioelectrical impedance accurate for use in large epidemiological studies? *Nutr J* 2008; 7: 26.

30   Trexler ET, Smith-Ryan AE, Norton LE. Metabolic adaptation to weight loss: implications for the athlete. *J Int Soc Sports Nutr* 2014; 11: 7.

31   Slater GJ, Dieter BP, Marsh DJ, Helms ER, Shaw G, Iraki J. Is an Energy Surplus Required to Maximize Skeletal Muscle Hypertrophy Associated With Resistance Training. *Front Nutr* 2019; 6. Available from: doi:10.3389/fnut.2019.00131.

32   Iraki J, Fitschen P, Espinar S, Helms E. Nutrition Recommendations for Bodybuilders in the Off-Season: A Narrative Review. *Sports* 2019; 7: 154.

33   Beals JW, Burd NA, Moore DR, van Vliet S. Obesity Alters the Muscle Protein Synthetic Response to Nutrition and Exercise. *Front Nutr* 2019; 6. Available from: doi:10.3389/fnut.2019.00087.

34   Morgan A. *How to Adjust Your Diet to Successfully Bulk Without Getting Fat.* 2015. Available from: https://rippedbody.com/how-to-bulk/ (accessed 5 Feb 2020).

35   Nunes JP, Grgic J, Cunha PM, Ribeiro AS, Schoenfeld BJ, Salles BF de et al. What influence does resistance exercise order have on muscular strength gains and muscle hypertrophy? A systematic review and meta-analysis. *Eur J Sport Sci* 2020; 0: 1–22.

36   Morton RW, Murphy KT, McKellar SR, Schoenfeld BJ, Henselmans M, Helms E et al. A systematic review, meta-analysis and meta-regression of the effect of protein supplementation on resistance training-induced gains in muscle mass and strength in healthy adults. *Br J Sports Med* 2018; 52: 376–384.

37   Cermak NM, Res PT, de Groot LC, Saris WH, van Loon LJ. Protein supplementation augments the adaptive response of skeletal muscle to resistance-type exercise training: a meta-analysis. *Am J Clin Nutr* 2012; 96: 1454–1464.

38   Jakubowski JS, Wong EPT, Nunes EA, Noguchi KS, Vandeweerd JK, Murphy KT et al. Equivalent Hypertrophy and Strength Gains in β-Hydroxy-β-Methylbutyrate- or Leucine-supplemented Men. *Med Sci Sports Exerc* 2019; 51: 65–74.

39   Gorin AA, Gokee LaRose J, Espeland MA, Tate DF, Jelalian E, Robichaud E et al. Eating pathology and psychological outcomes in young adults in self-regulation interventions using daily self-weighing. *Health Psychol* 2019; 38: 143–150.

40   LaRose JG, Fava JL, Steeves EA, Hecht J, Wing RR, Raynor HA. Daily self-weighing within a lifestyle intervention: impact on disordered eating symptoms. *Health Psychol Off J Div Health Psychol Am Psychol Assoc* 2014; 33: 297–300.

41   Shieh C, Knisely MR, Clark D, Carpenter JS. Self-weighing in weight management interventions: A systematic review of literature. *Obes Res Clin Pract* 2016; 10: 493–519.

42   Zheng Y, Klem ML, Sereika SM, Danford CA, Ewing LJ, Burke LE. Self-weighing in weight management: a systematic literature review. *Obes Silver Spring Md* 2015; 23: 256–265.

43   Benn Y, Webb TL, Chang BPI, Harkin B. What is the psychological impact of self-weighing? A meta-analysis. *Health Psychol Rev* 2016; 10: 187–203.

44   Wilkinson L, Pacanowski CR, Levitsky D. Three-Year Follow-Up of Participants from a Self-Weighing Randomized Controlled Trial. *J Obes* 2017; 2017. Available from: doi:10.1155/2017/4956326.

45   Zheng Y, Burke LE, Danford CA, Ewing LJ, Terry MA, Sereika SM. Patterns of self-weighing behavior and weight change in a weight loss trial. *Int J Obes* 2016; 40: 1392–1396.

46   Rosenbaum DL, Espel HM, Butryn ML, Zhang F, Lowe MR. Daily self-weighing and weight gain prevention: a longitudinal study of college-aged women. *J Behav Med* 2017; 40: 846–853.

47   Zheng Y, Sereika SM, Ewing LJ, Danford CA, Terry MA, Burke LE. Association between Self-Weighing and Percent Weight Change: Mediation Effects of Adherence to Energy Intake and Expenditure Goals. *J Acad Nutr Diet* 2016; 116: 660–666.

8. Diets

An incredibly wide range of diets can result in successful changes in body composition, provided the basic underlying principles are followed for the goal of interest.

A healthy balanced diet for optimising body composition does not require excluding any food group or particular food from your diet. Instead, it is about choosing low energy density, high nutrient density foods *most* of the time, whilst still allowing enjoyment of high energy density, low nutrient density foods *some* of the time. A good habit is to refrain from referring to foods as *'unhealthy'* or *'healthy'*, *'bad'* or *'good'*. Such associations can set up bad relationships with food. Any food can be consumed in moderation or occasionally as part of a healthy balanced diet (discussed in chapter 12). Similarly, any food can be included in a poor diet. Eating an apple each day within the context of a poor diet is *still* a poor diet.

Different dietary styles can be used to achieve the *same* body composition goals. No single diet strategy will suit everyone. Consider what each diet strategy entails and see how they fit in with your current lifestyle. Some will be more appealing than others and these will be the strategies that you find easiest to adhere to. The diet you find most successful will depend on your lifestyle preferences and is therefore your decision. Diet styles are not mutually exclusive. Diets that manipulate timing, food source and macronutrient content, can be combined. Intermittent fasting could be utilised with a low fat omnivorous diet or a low fat vegetarian diet. However, some combinations may be more difficult to practically implement, such as a low carbohydrate vegetarian diet (as most fruit, grains, legumes and vegetables contain at least some carbohydrates, and probably too much to adhere to a low carbohydrate diet).

Dietary styles can be considered as one of three broad categories[1]:

1. Manipulation of **macronutrients**.
2. Manipulation of **food groups and food sources**.
3. Manipulation of **food timing**.

Manipulation of macronutrients

High protein diet	25% or more of total calories or consuming more than 1.2g/kg of body weight of protein per day.
Low carbohydrate diet	50-150g or less of carbohydrates per day.
Ketogenic diet	Very low proportion of carbohydrates (no more than 5-10% of total energy, or 50g per day), alongside a very high proportion of fats (85%), and some protein (10%).
Low fat diet	Fat intake makes up less than 35% of total calories. A very low fat intake would be around 10-20% of total calories.
Very low calorie diet	500 calories per day.

Adapted from Thom and Lean, 2017[2].

Manipulation of food groups and food sources

Vegan	Exclusion of animal products.
Vegetarian	Exclusion of meat products including fish.
Pescatarian	Exclusion of meat products, but inclusion of fish.
Plant-based diet	Predominantly plant-based whole foods, but animal products can also be consumed in moderation.
Geographically associated diets:	
Mediterranean-style diet	Rich in plant-based foods (fruit, vegetables, legumes, nuts, cereals), fish, olive oil and low in processed meats[3].
Western diet	High in protein, saturated fat, refined grains, sugar and low in fruit and vegetables[4].

Manipulation of food timing

Intermittent fasting	Where periods of prolonged fasting are split up with periods of food intake. This can be on a daily or weekly basis.
Intermittent fasting across the day: time-restricted feeding	Timing restrictions placed on food intake to say, an 8 hour feeding window.
Intermittent fasting across the week: whole-day fasting and alternate-day fasting	Days of low calorie intake (fasted) interspersed with days of calorie intake at or near maintenance calorie intake.
Continuous energy restriction (CER)	A daily calorie deficit with no restrictions placed on food timing.
Intermittent energy restriction (IER)	Another way of saying intermittent fasting. A calorie deficit with restrictions placed on food timing at certain points of the day or week.
Intermittent energy restriction: refeed	During a calorie deficit, a short-term increase in calorie intake (usually carbohydrate), e.g. 5 days in a calorie deficit and 1-2 days at calorie maintenance, before returning to the deficit.
Intermittent energy restriction: diet break	Longer periods of increased calorie intake during a calorie deficit, e.g. 4 weeks in a calorie deficit and 1-2 weeks at calorie maintenance, before returning to the deficit.

Manipulation of macronutrients[5]

Different diets can manipulate the three main macronutrients, protein, carbohydrate and fat. We can look at the research of diets with different distributions of these macronutrients to see how varying them influences body composition outcomes for fat loss or muscle growth. There have been many studies looking at manipulating macronutrients and weight change. As such, high quality meta-analyses exist. Like most nutrition research, the majority of which is in sedentary and/or overweight people.

Eating too much or too little is the primary cause of weight change. Diets that vary carbohydrate content will inevitably mean fat and/or protein intake will also vary as a result, if calorie intake is maintained. Similarly, diets varying fat content will alter carbohydrate and/or protein intake.

A *high protein diet* is generally considered to be where 25% or more of total calories are from protein, or when consuming more than 1.2g/kg of body weight of protein per day.

A *low fat diet* is where fat intake makes up 20-35% of total calories[5]. Note that this level of fat intake is not below the recommended minimum intake for health (discussed in chapter 6). A very low fat intake would be around 10-20% of total calorie intake. A *high fat diet* is usually a consequence of adhering to a low carbohydrate diet, where fat makes up more than 45% of total calories. However, there is no agreed proportion of fat intake to classify a high fat diet[6].

There are many diets that primarily alter carbohydrate content. However, they can all fit within 4 broad categories. Definitions vary, but a common framework is:

- **High carbohydrate diet** (more than 45% of daily calories from carbohydrate). Usually a consequence of adhering to a low fat diet.
- **Moderate carbohydrate diet** (between 25–45% of daily calories from carbohydrate). This is the range recommended by most national dietary guidelines.
- **Low carbohydrate diet** (below 25% of daily calories, less than 600kcal or less than <150g carbohydrate).
- Very low carbohydrate diet / **ketogenic diet** (less than 50g of carbohydrate per day or <10% of daily calories of a 2000 kcal/day diet)[7].

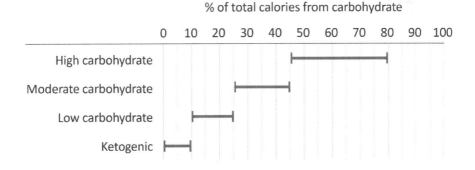

The relative proportion of carbohydrates within different diets.

High protein diets

High protein diets are safe in people with no pre-existing health problems (such as kidney problems).

Many of the benefits associated with other diets are actually the result of a higher protein intake from compensating for restricted fat or carbohydrate intake, rather than from those diets themselves.

When calories are equated, high protein diets result in the same amount of weight loss as other diets. But, diets higher in protein result in more of that weight lost as fat, and less of that weight lost as muscle, compared to a lower protein diet.

The minimum recommended protein intake is designed to prevent deficiencies. Active (regardless of the type of exercise) individuals need more protein than the recommended minimum protein intake. Higher protein intakes preserve muscle mass during a calorie deficit. Higher than the recommended minimum levels of protein intake per day maximise muscle protein synthesis and muscle growth.

Protein is *essential*. Even if you do not eat what would be considered typical protein-rich foods (such as meat, dairy, fish or plant-based sources such as legumes and nuts), your diet will contain protein. Low to moderate protein content can be found in cereals, bread, pasta and some vegetables. Very low protein diets are not recommended for health reasons. *Any* diet should contain as an absolute minimum, 0.8g/kg of body weight per day to prevent muscle loss[8]. For a young female weighing 50kg, this would equate to 40g throughout the day. This minimum value is often misinterpreted as being what is considered optimal[9]. In fact, it has been argued that it is still too low as a minimum for a range of populations, including the young and the old[10].

When making changes to a diet for weight loss, protein is rarely considered. Decreasing foods containing fat or carbohydrate seem to be the first choice for many. However, when making changes to build muscle, pretty much everyone associates protein with muscle building. Increasing protein intake is often so much of a focus when trying to build muscle, that intakes may be greater than what is considered optimum and to the detriment of consuming 'enough' fat or carbohydrate. In the context of weight loss or weight gain, does altering the amount of protein in the diet have any significant influence on body composition outcomes?

A high protein diet is typically considered to be where protein accounts for 25% or more of total calories or consuming more than 1.2g/kg of body weight of protein per day. At this point it is important to note that high protein intakes, and even very high protein intakes (over 4g/kg of body weight per day) have been shown to be *safe* in healthy individuals. See chapter 9 for a detailed discussion on the safety of high protein diets[11,12].

When daily protein intake is increased from lower (0.8-1.2g/kg of body weight per day) to higher intakes (>1.2g/kg of body weight per day), there are notable changes. The effect of increasing dietary protein intake results in several potentially advantageous alterations[1]:

- Promotion of muscle growth and muscle maintenance.
- Increased satiety.
- Greater thermic effect of food than fat or carbohydrate.

Combined, these can result in the generation of a calorie deficit and the preservation of muscle mass whilst in a calorie deficit. Similarly, higher protein diets result in greater increases in muscle mass when in a calorie surplus[9]. Whether different protein sources influence energy expenditure, satiety and fat loss differently, is unknown. But, the current evidence suggests any difference is minor or not meaningful[13].

Higher protein intakes promote greater improvements in body composition than lower protein intakes. The majority of meta-analyses assessing protein intake find that higher protein intakes result in a reduction in body mass, a reduction in fat mass, and preservation of muscle mass whilst in a caloric deficit[5]. However, when total calories are equated, high protein diets result in the *same* amount of weight loss as other diets[1]. Weight change is dictated by the size of the calorie deficit, but the *origin* of this weight change differs. The importance of protein intake for body composition will be discussed in more detail in chapter 9.

Protein intake has important implications for optimising body composition, hence why high protein diets have been discussed first. In order to accurately assess the relative efficacy of other diets (such as low carbohydrate or low fat diets), protein intakes need to be equated due to the influence protein can have on body composition.

Are low carbohydrate diets or low fat diets best for weight loss?

You can lose fat with a very wide range of carbohydrate or fat intakes.

You can gain muscle with a very wide range of carbohydrate or fat intakes.

Relative energy balance determines whether you lose or gain weight. For the same energy deficit or energy surplus, it does not matter whether you eat a high carbohydrate diet, low carbohydrate diet, high fat diet or low fat diet. The weight lost or gained will be the same.

Below is a condensed summary of low carbohydrate and low fat diets. The points outlined in the table will be discussed, as well as the role of carbohydrate and fat for weight loss and muscle gain.

Low fat diets	Low carbohydrate diets
There are no superior benefits to low fat diets compared to any other diet strategy for weight loss.	There are no superior benefits to low carbohydrate diets compared to any other diet strategy for weight loss.
When total calories and protein are equated, weight loss is the same between low fat diets and any other diet.	When total calories and protein are equated, weight loss is the same between low carbohydrate diets and any other diet.
Low fat diets can promote muscle growth if sufficient carbohydrates are consumed, which is the primary fuel source for resistance training workouts.	Low carbohydrate diets can promote muscle growth, provided carbohydrate intake is sufficient to fuel resistance training workouts. Very severely restricted carbohydrate intake may impair anaerobic performance and therefore muscle growth.
Opt for a low fat diet if you would rather prioritise carbohydrate.	Opt for a low carbohydrate diet if you do not mind eating fewer carbohydrates and would rather prioritise fat.
There is no advantage or disadvantage to consuming fewer fats (i.e. a low fat diet) compared to consuming more fats (i.e. a high fat diet) for body composition, when calories are equated for weight loss.	For weight loss, there does not appear to be an advantage or disadvantage to consuming fewer or severely restricting carbohydrates (i.e. a low carbohydrate diet or ketogenic diet) compared to consuming adequate carbohydrates (i.e. a moderate or high carbohydrate diet) for body composition, when calories and protein are equated.

Daily fat intake should be set to personal preference, but kept above a minimum of 0.5/kg/day for health, or at least 15% of daily calories.	Daily carbohydrate intake should be set to personal preference.

Adapted from: Aragon et al., 2017[5].

Unlike protein or fat, there is no lower limit as to how many carbohydrates we must consume. Some individuals think that because of this, we do not need and should not eat carbohydrates. They argue that they are the cause weight gain. On the other hand, some people think fat is the cause of weight gain and therefore fat should be kept to the absolute minimum.

It is proposed that *low fat, high carbohydrate diets* supposedly promote weight loss because eating fat will cause all that fat to be stored, meaning that by limiting fat intake, it is possible to limit fat storage. Another suggestion is that fats are the most energy dense macronutrient at 9kcal per gram (carbohydrates and protein are around 4kcal per gram). Therefore, gram-for-gram, by reducing fat intake this will supposedly have the largest effect on total calorie intake. This is true, but it does not mean that *any* fat intake is stored as fat. It also ignores dietary food choices (i.e. the sources of fat intake).

On the other hand, others have proposed that *low fat, high carbohydrate diets* promote weight gain because eating carbohydrates stimulates insulin release into the blood. It is proposed that by limiting carbohydrate intake (i.e. *high fat, low carbohydrate diets)* it is possible to limit fat storage. This is supposedly superior to *low fat, high carbohydrate diets,* because it results in lower levels of insulin. Insulin promotes the movement of blood sugar (glucose) into muscles, liver and fat cells, to be used and stored. Insulin prevents the release and use of fat from fat cells, promoting fat storage[14]. Therefore, lower insulin levels *supposedly* allow fat stores to be utilised and burnt[1].

However, others then counterargue that these *low carbohydrate, high fat diets* actually promote weight gain because the high fat intake is stored as fat (and hence proposing *low fat, high carbohydrate diets* as mentioned before). Clearly, people have argued both for and against reducing fat or carbohydrate intake to induce weight loss.

These propositions are largely incorrect, because the arguments used consider energy regulation on too short a timescale.

Whether fat is stored or used depends on the rate of fat storage and fat oxidation (fat burning) across longer durations of time.

In a low fat, high carbohydrate diet, more carbohydrates are used as energy to fuel cells. This means there is *less fat oxidation* (the amount of fat used by cells for energy). But also, *less fat* is stored because less fat is being consumed.

In a high fat, low carbohydrate diet, *more fat oxidation* occurs because fat is now the main energy source available, and there are fewer carbohydrates available as energy to fuel cells. But also, *more fat* is stored because more fat is being consumed.

Any diet results in some level of fat oxidation and some level of fat storage. A high fat, low carbohydrate diet will involve greater fat storage and fat oxidation. A low fat, high carbohydrate diet will involve lower fat storage and lower fat oxidation.

Whilst consuming a high fat, low carbohydrate diet or a low fat, high carbohydrate diet, whether weight is stored or gained is the *difference* between *fat oxidation* and *fat storage*. In both, if you equate calories and equate protein, there is no difference in weight change between diets[15,16]. Regardless of the amount of carbohydrate or fat you consume, any weight loss is associated with the size and duration of the calorie deficit, not with the restriction of carbohydrates or fat[1,17]. In both scenarios, fat oxidation will be greater than fat storage when in a calorie deficit (i.e. weight loss). Fat oxidation will be lower than fat storage when in a calorie surplus (i.e. weight gain). A meta-analysis of 32 controlled feeding studies where calories and protein were matched, showed that low fat or low carbohydrate diets are equivalent for weight loss[18]. Controlled feeding studies are where participants are provided with their food. This means they eat exactly what the study intends to give them. People are usually very bad at recording food intake by themselves, which makes these studies more reliable than studies where participants self-report food intake[5,18]. Another meta-analysis of 59 studies (48 of which being randomised controlled trials) also found no difference in weight loss in obese or overweight people from *any* type of low carbohydrate or low fat diet[19]. Adherence to a low carbohydrate diet results in similar changes in body composition as adhering to any other diet that generates a similar sized calorie deficit. Numerous studies show that when calories are matched, weight loss is similar regardless of whether carbohydrate intake is relatively high or low[2].

The concept that carbohydrates and fats are 'bad' and need to be excluded from the diet for weight loss to occur is unfounded. If you consumed a low carbohydrate diet and consumed a lot of protein and fat such that you were in a calorie surplus, you'd still gain weight. You can lose weight eating lots of sugar, so long as you're in a calorie deficit[20]. Similarly, diets high in fat still result in weight loss when in a calorie deficit[7]. A prime example is the *ketogenic diet*, which will be discussed later in this chapter.

The success of these diets often results from the *restriction* of foods. Limiting the intake of a macronutrient limits food choice. Limiting either fat or carbohydrate often leads to an increase in protein intake, which then results in the beneficial effects noted from high protein diets[21]. Increasing protein intakes can explain the differential improvements in body composition seen between diet groups in studies where protein is not matched. Any apparent superior success of a low carbohydrate weight loss diet is often due to the higher protein intake as a result of restricting carbohydrate, rather than the effect of low carbohydrate intake itself.

"Lowered carbohydrate intake per se has no effect on decrease in BW [body weight] and BF% [body fat percentage] during energy restriction, while daily elevated absolute protein intake of 1·1 vs. 0·7 g/kg BW promotes BW loss while reducing BF%."
Westerterp-Plantenga et al., 2012[21].

Restricting fat intakes typically means opting for lower energy density foods. Low fat diets can result in increased consumption of fruit and vegetables (being mostly higher in carbohydrate and lower in fat) which can aid satiety and promote a reduction in calorie intake. This may provide a means to enter a caloric deficit whilst remaining satiated[18].

Returning to the football match analogy from chapter 4, for a team to win a match they must score more goals than the opposition. Supporters of low fat or low carbohydrate diets for weight loss would say that having more possession than the opposition, or more corners during the match is what results in winning matches. Indeed, having more possession than the opposition or having more corners during the match means it is *more likely* that a team will score more goals and therefore win. But, it does not mean they *will* win. A team can win a match with very little possession and no corners during a match. Similarly, a team can have all the possession and many corners, and still lose. With diets, you can have carbohydrates and fats at varying levels of intake. At any relative variation there can be weight gain, maintenance or loss. High intakes of fat or carbohydrate can still result in weight loss if energy expenditure is greater than energy intake. Weight change is dependent on relative energy intake (goals scored vs goals conceded) not dietary constituents (match possession or corners). You can still lose a match even if you score 4 goals, if the other team scores 5.

If you want to read more about the low carbohydrate versus low fat diet debate, Layne Norton has written an excellent publicly available summary, *'Science, stories and side-stepping'*[22], including whether carbohydrates and insulin drive weight gain and not energy balance (spoiler: they do not)[14]. The carbohydrate/fat debate is mainly focussed from the perspective of weight loss and weight gain from fat. In the interest of optimising body composition, it is important to consider these two macronutrients from the perspective of muscle growth as well.

There appears to be no difference in overfeeding with a high carbohydrate or a high fat diet on weight gain[10].

In the same manner as calorie restriction for weight loss, current evidence suggests that weight gain is dictated by the size of the calorie surplus, not the fat or carbohydrate content of the diet. However, the evidence is far more limited[10].

Carbohydrate for muscle growth

Research assessing the effect of dietary carbohydrate on hypertrophy alongside a resistance training programme is very limited. There is low quality evidence to suggest a need for a specific amount of carbohydrate to maximise muscle growth, but moderate quality evidence to suggest there is a minimum quantity of carbohydrate per day needed to support resistance training sessions. Assuming resistance training is the only exercise being performed, the minimum quantity appears to be quite low.

Resistance training primarily uses carbohydrate stores to fuel activity. Therefore, consuming at least a low to moderate amount of carbohydrates (i.e. not severely restricting carbohydrate intake to below 10% of daily calories) may benefit a goal of increasing muscle mass, by fuelling training performance. Carbohydrate intake may vary depending on the volume of training being performed (higher carbohydrate intake when performing higher volumes, lower carbohydrate intake when performing lower volumes). It appears that high intensity performance is impaired when carbohydrate intake is too low[5].

Carbohydrates are not essential to human life, however for the majority of people they are found in highly palatable foods. They are the primary fuel source of energy during high intensity exercise. Similar to low carbohydrate and low fat diets, when in a calorie surplus, there appears to be no difference between overfeeding on high carbohydrate or high fat diets when protein and calories are equated[10].

Research on the importance of carbohydrate intake for endurance exercise performance is very well documented. There is also good evidence to support a role of carbohydrates for strength and power performance, with reduced carbohydrate intake impairing anaerobic performance[23]. The evidence base for muscle growth outcomes with different carbohydrate intakes however, is limited.

There are only a handful of research studies assessing carbohydrate intake and resistance training. These studies are also short in duration and assess exercise performance, not muscle growth[24]. Many research authorities including the American College of Sports Medicine (ACSM) and the International Society of Sports Nutrition (ISSN) do not specifically state carbohydrate intake for resistance training in their nutrition guidelines[24-26]. As such, recommendations for resistance training (and muscle growth) have arisen from endurance exercise recommendations and expert opinion. There are currently *no* specific carbohydrate recommendations for resistance training beyond ensuring at least a minimum intake through a typical diet (i.e. moderate carbohydrate intake)[25]. However as will be discussed, the minimum carbohydrate intake for optimal resistance training and muscle growth may be well below a moderate carbohydrate intake. It is important to note that unless you opt for a diet low in carbohydrate, the discussion of whether you are consuming adequate carbohydrate is unlikely to be of any concern if you are only resistance training without performing any aerobic exercise. The need for additional carbohydrate with aerobic exercise is discussed in chapter 24.

Extrapolating the effects of different carbohydrate intakes on endurance exercise performance to resistance training is of limited value. The way that muscles use energy to fuel endurance exercise or resistance training is different[23]. Performance demands are also different. Endurance training recommendations are based on optimising performance. Resistance training recommendations need to be based on optimising muscle growth. Higher carbohydrate intakes are beneficial for endurance exercise performance, but this does not necessarily mean higher carbohydrate intakes are beneficial for resistance training performance and hypertrophy.

The minimum amount of carbohydrate required will vary hugely between individuals, depending on how much exercise is performed and how intense that exercise is. The argument that additional carbohydrate intake itself helps promote muscle growth is also invalid. Variable carbohydrate intakes do *not* influence net protein balance when sufficient protein is consumed. *Muscle protein synthesis* needs to be higher than *muscle protein breakdown* to build muscle (a positive net protein balance). With an adequate resistance training programme and sufficient protein intake, additional carbohydrate intake does not further facilitate increases in net protein balance to promote muscle growth[24,27,28]. Any benefit of additional carbohydrate would be from consuming the extra calories to ensure a caloric surplus. Therefore, it is clear that high carbohydrate intakes are not more beneficial than moderate or low carbohydrate intakes for muscle growth, when calories are equated[27]. However, is a severely restricted carbohydrate intake detrimental to performance and therefore muscle growth?

It has been proposed that very low carbohydrate intakes may impair muscle growth. However, long-term evidence directly comparing the effect of low carbohydrate intakes to moderate or high carbohydrate intakes on muscle growth are lacking[27]. The reasoning is therefore primarily from indirect and lower quality evidence. The theoretical rationale is that resistance training for muscle growth primarily uses carbohydrates, so a lack of carbohydrate supposedly means you cannot train well. Indeed, high intensity exercise primarily uses muscle glycogen stores to fuel exercise[29]. The consensus from peer-reviewed literature is that low carbohydrate, high fat diets will impair anaerobic performance[23]. However, many studies assess anaerobic performance using whole-body, high intensity interval strategies, rather than typical resistance training protocols. Studies show that high fat, low carbohydrate diets increase fat oxidation and reduce the rate that muscle glycogen stores are used for energy during exercise[23]. An increase in fat use is suggested to limit the amount of work performed during intense resistance exercise (energy use during exercise is discussed in detail in chapter 16). This mechanistic evidence plus the few studies showing a reduction in high intensity performance with low carbohydrate diets have been used to suggest that severe carbohydrate restriction may be sub-optimal for resistance training performance and hypertrophy[5,23]. Adequate training performance is important, and sub-optimal performance may impair muscle growth. But, where the minimum required carbohydrate intake cut-off lies, is inconclusive. Some studies have shown resistance training performance has not been impaired with lower intakes[23]. However, these studies are generally of a short duration across a few days. Whether this is sufficient time for any effect of a low carbohydrate diet (e.g. to deplete muscle glycogen stores) to be meaningful is unclear[30]. As such, severely restricted carbohydrate intake will likely have *some* negative effect, but defining this cut-off is far from conclusive.

"More research, however, is necessary to determine a carbohydrate consumption threshold to support hypertrophy in resistance training athletes." **Vargas et al., 2018[31].**

We could *estimate* where this minimum threshold may lie by considering how much energy is used in a resistance training session, and therefore how much carbohydrate we may need to consume before the next session to ensure adequate performance. The total energy content of muscle glycogen and liver glycogen stores represents only 2000-3000kcal in the average person, with the majority in muscles (80-85%)[27,32]. Fat cannot be converted into carbohydrate. Therefore, if glycogen stores are completely depleted, we would theoretically need to consume that amount carbohydrate to ensure glycogen stores are replete for the next session. However, other energy sources can be converted into carbohydrate to replenish glycogen stores[33-35] and, a typical resistance training session will only deplete up to 30-40% of the glycogen stores in the muscle trained. Even the most taxing of resistance training sessions will not completely deplete the glycogen stores from a muscle[27]. Bear in mind that the total glycogen stores of 2000-3000kcal are the total glycogen stores of *all* muscles and the liver, not just the glycogen stores in an *individual* muscle. This means that when *exclusively* performing resistance training (and not performing any aerobic exercise), the minimum amount of carbohydrate required to ensure replete muscle glycogen stores is quite low. Indeed, the fact that glycogen stores are not fully depleted after resistance training indicates that glycogen stores do not necessarily need to be maximised for a typical resistance training session. Muscle glycogen stores begin to be replenished after being depleted from exercise, even without post-exercise food intake[36]. Post-workout carbohydrate consumption does increase the rate of glycogen replenishment. But even with varied carbohydrate intakes, muscle glycogen stores are similarly replenished 24 hours after muscle glycogen-depleting exercise[37]. Inadequate glycogen store replenishment may only be an issue when training the same muscle with a very high frequency (more than once per day), but this would only apply to highly demanding endurance exercise and not to people resistance training a few times per week[24]. Considering that a specific muscle may only be trained a maximum of 2 or 3 times per week for muscle growth, it is probable that low intakes of carbohydrate are sufficient, when resistance training without any concurrent aerobic exercise.

A range of authors recommend moderate carbohydrate intakes between 4-7g/kg of body weight per day to optimise performance and to avoid inadvertently dropping below the minimum threshold[27]. Some researchers have drawn attention to the fact that the theoretical minimum carbohydrate threshold may *vary* with exercise volume. As such, they suggest that when following a diet lower in carbohydrate, it may be beneficial to increase carbohydrate intake to match the exercise demands for that day[23].

"When workouts involve high-intensity/volume/quality/technique, the day's eating patterns should provide high CHO [carbohydrate] availability. When workouts involve exercise of lower intensity/quality, it is less important to follow patterns that achieve high CHO availability."
Burke, 2015[23].

In other words, when there is a resistance training period or training session that is of higher volume, then additional carbohydrates may be of benefit. When there is a period of lower volume training, then a lower intake of carbohydrates may result in no performance impairment.

The amount of carbohydrates you consume daily can therefore scale with[27]:

- The **volume** (intensity of **load** and **duration)** of a resistance training workout (chapter 19).
- The intensity of **effort** of a workout (chapter 19).

- The **volume** of any endurance exercise you perform (chapter 24).
- Your **personal preference** to consume carbohydrate.

The considerations above will be more important if you follow a very low carbohydrate diet, but most people do not. Chapter 24 discusses the additional carbohydrate needs when also performing aerobic exercise. Provided you consume adequate carbohydrate during the day that is sufficient to fuel resistance training workouts, any level of carbohydrate should allow for similar muscle growth when protein and calories are equated. Severely restricted carbohydrate intakes may limit high volume training. However, even with very low carbohydrate intakes, performance decrements can be minimised by consuming the limited daily carbohydrate intake prior to exercise, so that it can be utilised during exercise[27].

It may be beneficial to avoid severely low carbohydrate intakes during periods of high volume training, or to consume any limited dietary carbohydrates before a workout to allow for their utilisation. For most people, severe carbohydrate restriction is unlikely to be an issue.

Fat for muscle growth

Different daily fat intakes do not appear to influence muscle growth. Daily fat intake should be kept above a minimum of 0.5g/kg of body weight per day for health reasons, or at least 15-20% of daily calories.

There is limited evidence comparing different fat intakes on muscle growth. The effect of modifying fat intake will be less important than ensuring a calorie surplus and sufficient protein intake alongside a structured resistance training plan. Resistance training primarily uses carbohydrate stores to fuel activity. Therefore, consuming fewer fats (i.e. a low fat diet) compared to consuming higher fats (i.e. a high fat diet) to allow for adequate carbohydrate intake (i.e. a moderate to high carbohydrate diet) may benefit a goal of increasing muscle mass to fuel high volume training. However, as a more energy dense macronutrient (9 kcal/gram) compared to protein or carbohydrate (4kcal/gram), it may be beneficial to consume additional fat to ensure a caloric surplus is present. Conversely, if excess weight gain is a problem, then limiting energy dense, high fat foods may aid adherence to a smaller calorie surplus.

Weight gain occurs when you consume a surplus of calories. When in a calorie surplus, the relative proportions of weight gained as fat (adipose tissue) or as lean muscle mass, can be affected by the type of fat consumed.

Anaerobic resistance training primarily uses muscle glycogen to fuel performance. The role of fat intake for anaerobic exercise performance is fairly limited. Significantly limiting fat intake for long periods of time can be sub-optimal for muscle growth, because fats are required to build hormones, including testosterone[15,38]. Reducing fat intake from 40% to 20% of total calorie intake results in a reduction in testosterone in the blood[29,39]. Testosterone is an important hormone promoting muscle growth*. However, this is complicated by other factors including the types of fats consumed (e.g. saturated or polyunsaturated fats). And indeed, the long-term significance of this on muscle growth has not been studied[29,39]. The fact that an individual aiming to build muscle should be in a calorie surplus may also mitigate any hormonal changes, as being in an extended period of calorie restriction with resulting low levels of body fat may have a much larger influence on reducing testosterone than any alteration in fat intake[39]. Even so, during weight loss studies, muscle loss is not greater with a low fat diet compared to a higher fat diet[39]. Therefore, a range of fat intakes are likely to be suitable for muscle growth, but very low fat intakes (i.e. below 15% of total calories) should be avoided for health reasons and to minimise any potential reductions in circulating testosterone[40,41].

* Note that acute post-workout changes in hormones such as testosterone do not appear to be relevant for muscle growth[42].

However, as fat is the most energy dense macronutrient (9 kcal/gram) compared to protein or carbohydrate (4kcal/gram), it may be beneficial to consume additional fat to ensure a caloric surplus is present, if sufficient energy intake is an issue for you.

Overfeeding with different types of fat

Weight gained as fat mass (adipose tissue) or as lean muscle mass in a calorie surplus can be affected by the type of fat consumed. This is only relevant when you are in a calorie surplus.

A double-blind (neither the people in the study nor the researchers conducting the study know who is in which study group) randomised controlled trial showed that if you take two groups of normal weight individuals and make them consume a calorie surplus that is equal between groups, they both gain the same amount of weight[43,44]. Nothing new here. Except, one group were fed muffins rich in *saturated fatty acids* (SFA), and the other group were fed muffins rich in *polyunsaturated fatty acids* (PUFA) (see chapter 6 regarding types of fats). The group consuming the saturated fatty acid muffins gained relatively more weight as fat than the group eating polyunsaturated fatty acid muffins. The ratio of lean mass:fat mass weight gain was 1:1 in the polyunsaturated fatty acid group, and 1:4 in the saturated fatty acid group. There were no other differences between the two groups (such as total calorie intake, total weight gain or macronutrient proportions in the diet) except for the fatty acid proportions. However, the participants were *not* participating in any resistance exercise. Again, this does not mean that saturated fat makes you fat or makes you fatter. The driving factor for the weight gain was the calorie surplus. If no surplus was present, there would have been no weight gain. The importance is that when in a calorie surplus, the relative proportions of different fats in the diet may affect how weight is gained[10,45]. The conclusions of this study for now regarding implications for optimising body composition whilst in a caloric surplus can only be made for the sources of saturated fatty acids (palm oil) and polyunsaturated fatty acids (sunflower oil) used in the study, *without* resistance training. Perhaps if participants performed resistance exercise, the effect would be different. More research is needed before recommendations of types of fat can be made for muscle growth.

Ketogenic diets

A ketogenic diet is a form of low carbohydrate diet, consisting of a high fat intake (85%) and low protein (10%) and carbohydrate (5%) intake.

The current evidence base shows that when total calories and protein intake are equated, a ketogenic diet does not lead to greater fat loss compared to non-ketogenic diets. A ketogenic diet is just as effective.

There is debate as to whether ketogenic diets can promote similar levels of muscle growth as higher carbohydrate diets, because carbohydrate is the primary fuel source for resistance training workouts.

It is appearing increasingly likely that the high levels of fat intake in ketogenic diets are unlikely to have adverse health consequences. However, ketogenic diets can limit dietary fibre intake and exclude many plant-based food groups.

Ketogenic diets may help to suppress appetite.

Only opt for a ketogenic diet if you do not mind eating very little carbohydrate.

In a ketogenic diet, the body switches its preferred fuel source from carbohydrates, to fats and *ketone bodies*. Ketone bodies are made by the liver and are another energy source that can used under certain circumstances. This occurs by a process called *ketosis*, where fat stores in the body are transported to the liver and converted into ketone bodies. The body can enter ketosis when calorie intake is very low (i.e. starvation), when carbohydrate intake is very low, or after exhaustive exercise (very long duration endurance exercise)[46]. These ketones are then used by the body for energy. Ketone bodies provide 7kcal per gram of ketone. A ketogenic diet is defined by the level of circulating ketones in the blood. This is achieved by consuming a very low proportion of carbohydrates (no more than 5-10% of total energy, or <50g), alongside a very high proportion of fats (60-80%), and moderate protein (15-35%)[5,31]. A ketogenic diet induces ketosis due to its low carbohydrate content. Protein levels can be relatively low in ketogenic diets without significant muscle loss because ketones are *protein sparing* (during starvation, their protein sparing effects help to minimise muscle wasting)[46]. Ketogenic diets have been used clinically to treat medical conditions, such as epilepsy[47,48].

* Physiological or nutritional ketosis as described above is distinct and different from the potentially fatal ketoacidosis that can occur in type 1 diabetes mellitus, which is the result of very low blood sugar (glucose) levels, resulting in excessive circulating ketones that leads to blood becoming very acidic.

Ketogenic diets may suppress appetite

One potential benefit of the ketogenic diet is that it may *suppress* appetite. When people go on a ketogenic diet and eat freely (ad libitum), such that they are not restricted on how much they can eat, weight loss can occur. This appears to be due to a *reduction* in energy consumption upon entering ketosis. The majority of the evidence showing an effect of ketogenic diets on appetite is anecdotal[49]. The mechanisms by which a ketogenic diet may reduce appetite is also still inconclusive[49].

A systematic review and meta-analysis of 12 studies showed ketogenic diets led to a reduction in appetite and a greater feeling of being satiated, despite being in a calorie deficit. Usually it would be expected that appetite would increase, and feelings of satiety would decrease during calorie restriction[50]. Appetite suppression may be through increased consumption of protein whilst on the ketogenic diet, as a result of restricting carbohydrate. Higher protein intakes can suppress appetite (discussed in chapter 9). But, the suppressive effect in ketosis appears to be separate from any protein-induced appetite suppression that may also occur[5]. This may aid individuals looking to achieve a calorie deficit (the primary mechanism for weight loss) but may make the ability to achieve a calorie surplus (for goals aimed at increasing muscle mass) more difficult by reducing the drive to consume food[21,51,52]. Appetite suppression may be limited in its utility due to the restriction of carbohydrate and lower intake of fibre, meaning foods high in fat which can be of a higher energy density are more likely to be consumed.

The ketogenic diet involves severe restriction of one macronutrient (carbohydrate) and high intakes of another (fat). This impacts on *food choice*. The majority of ketogenic diet studies are short-term in humans or animals, meaning very little is known about their long-term effects[53]. As discussed later in chapter 12 regarding dietary fat, high fat ketogenic diets may influence circulating levels of lipids, such as LDL-cholesterol (*bad* cholesterol) in the blood[1,52]. But, the influence of ketogenic diets and dietary fat in general on health is inconclusive, with some evidence that such diets may benefit cardiovascular disease risk factors[53]. As such, the effect on cardiovascular disease is inconclusive[1,54]. Another consideration of ketogenic diets is that by limiting carbohydrate intake, this results in all but no consumption of fruit, grains, vegetables and fibre. These are important for daily micronutrition and long-term health. The long-term consequences of ketogenic diets are inconclusive and largely unknown. Therefore, this should be considered before adopting a ketogenic diet. If you are unsure, consult your GP for advice.

Ketogenic diet for weight loss

There does not appear to be an advantage or disadvantage to a ketogenic diet compared to a diet containing adequate carbohydrates (i.e. moderate to high carbohydrate diets) for body composition, when calories and protein are equated for weight loss.

The theoretical rationale is that ketogenic diets can lead to greater fat loss because the body is now burning more fat compared to a non-ketogenic diet. This is a similar concept as to why people thought (and still think) high fat diets would lead to greater fat loss than low fat diets (greater fat oxidation) and is incorrect for the same reason (there is also greater fat storage). Another theory is that because ketones offer a unique metabolic state where they prevent using protein and carbohydrate for energy, they could also aid weight loss[46]. Ketogenic diets do indeed display a higher level of fat oxidation (using fat for energy). However, the majority of this is from using (oxidising) the fat that is consumed as part of the ketogenic diet (similar to high fat diets). So, this would be expected given what is being eaten. Carbohydrate oxidation is simultaneously very low because there is low carbohydrate content in the diet. Regardless, weight loss is still determined by relative calorie intake. Similar to other low carbohydrate diets, the effects on body composition can be *confounded* due to the effect of higher protein intakes when limiting other macronutrients[55]. All studies to date (except one[56]) show that when total calorie and protein intake is equated, there is *no advantage* to a ketogenic diet over other diets[5,51,55,57-60]. And, the largest meta-analysis of controlled feeding studies to date found no influence of different fat or carbohydrate intakes on weight loss[18].

If you can live with restricted carbohydrate intake, the appetite suppressing effect of a ketogenic diet may support reduced calorie intake and the generation of a calorie deficit for weight loss[31].

Ketogenic diet for building muscle mass

Research assessing ketogenic diets and hypertrophy with a resistance training programme is very limited.

Ketogenic diets involve severely restricting carbohydrate intake. This may limit high intensity and high volume training. It may be beneficial to consume the limited carbohydrates in a ketogenic diet during the pre-workout period to allow for their utilisation during the resistance training session.

Resistance training primarily uses carbohydrate stores to fuel activity. Consuming at least a low to moderate amount of carbohydrates (i.e. not severely restricting carbohydrate intake to below 10% of daily calories) may benefit a goal of increasing muscle mass by fuelling training performance. The evidence base is still fairly small. However, it appears that high intensity performance is impaired when carbohydrate intake is severely low[5].

Studies assessing ketogenic diets and a resistance training programme on muscle growth are very limited[27]. One study in young males found a ketogenic diet resulted in comparable muscle growth after 8 weeks when calorie and protein intakes were matched to a control diet, alongside a resistance training programme[27]. However, both groups also lost fat mass[27]. A recent randomised controlled trial compared a hypercaloric (a calorie surplus) ketogenic diet to a non-ketogenic diet in young males alongside an 8 week resistance training programme, with protein intakes equated. The ketogenic diet group consumed <10% of daily calories from carbohydrate. The non-ketogenic group consumed 55% of daily calories from carbohydrate. They found that the ketogenic diet did not increase muscle mass. Only the non-ketogenic diet group significantly gained weight (as muscle mass)[31]. Both the ketogenic and non-ketogenic groups lost weight as fat mass. But importantly, this was only significant in the ketogenic diet group. The study aimed for participants to be in a calorie surplus, but the study did not monitor whether participants were *actually* in a calorie surplus. After questioning participants about their lifestyles and activity levels, a diet plan was created that would put them in a surplus. How closely participants followed this plan or whether the plan was accurate may have affected results. The lack of controlling participant diets is a limitation of the study (like many other dietary studies). The researchers found greater weight loss on the ketogenic diet, despite a high protein intake (2g/kg of body weight per day), but *no increase* in muscle mass during the 8 week resistance training programme. It seems probable that the ketogenic group were probably *not* in a surplus, whereas the non-ketogenic group were. The ketogenic group were possibly in a calorie deficit, and the higher protein intake helped to maintain muscle mass. The appetite suppressing effect of ketogenic diets and the higher protein intake may explain why they consumed less energy[27,50]. The participants were familiar with resistance training and not complete beginners, meaning ensuring a calorie surplus would be more important to promote muscle growth. Another interventional controlled study on resistance trained participants over 12 weeks found fat loss occurred with a ketogenic diet compared to a control diet (the participants' usual diet)[27,52]. Although both groups maintained similar levels of muscle mass, there was a *trend* for muscle loss in the legs of ketogenic diet participants[52]. Upon following to the ketogenic diet, participants significantly *decreased* their calorie intake from 2499 to 1948 kcal per day. However, only 4 out of 7 ketogenic diet participants completed the food logs, and the study did not record the energy intake of the control group. So, it is unknown if the control group were in a calorie surplus or not[52]. Again, participants on ketogenic diets were unlikely to have been in a calorie surplus as they were advised to eat at free will, and as a result, their energy intake decreased (i.e. calorie intake was not equated)[52]. This reduction in intake again may have been due to the appetite suppressing effects of the diet.

Studies to date therefore show the ketogenic diet results in *less* muscle growth than a diet with moderate carbohydrate intake. But, often calories and/or protein have *not* been equated[45]. As such, there is currently a lack of high quality research assessing muscle growth with a ketogenic diet in a calorie surplus, and therefore whether it can be an effective diet for hypertrophy is unclear. Given the importance of ensuring a caloric surplus, this limits any recommendations that can be made from these studies regarding ketogenic diets and muscle growth. It would be short-sighted to conclude ketogenic diets are inferior. More studies are needed that address these study design flaws. However, one benefit is that the studies may suggest that a ketogenic diet limits the ability to consume a daily surplus and promotes generation of a spontaneous caloric deficit, promoting fat loss and preserving muscle mass[31,48].

"Regarding to LBM [lean body mass], an adequate carbohydrate intake (non-ketogenic or conventional dietary approach), in conjunction with a caloric surplus and a higher protein intake, might be the most viable option for inducing muscle hypertrophy after RT [resistance training]."
Vargas et al., 2018[31].

There are theoretical reasons why a ketogenic diet may be sub-optimal for muscle growth. Such as, a lack of carbohydrate intake to ensure adequate energy for a resistance training session, or the appetite suppressing effects which may make it more difficult to consume a caloric surplus. A ketogenic diet can reduce muscle glycogen stores, which are important for anaerobic performance[51].

Recommendations for a ketogenic diet would be similar to a non-ketogenic diet with a low carbohydrate intake. With all things equal, if you like carbohydrates it would probably be best to not opt for a ketogenic diet for a muscle building plan. Considering the evidence showing the benefit of carbohydrates on anaerobic performance, if you were to utilise a ketogenic diet then consider consuming your limited carbohydrate intake prior to your workout. There is variability regarding how quickly a carbohydrate meal can be turned into glycogen in the muscle and liver following eating, but on average it takes around 4 hours. So, consuming your carbohydrates a few hours before training may be optimal. Also, it is likely that any additional exercise performed during a ketogenic diet (such as high volume resistance training workouts, or aerobic exercise) may excessively deplete glycogen stores. The increase in exercise activity thermogenesis, combined with the potential effects of the ketogenic diet on calorie intake may further impair the ability to generate a calorie surplus. Again, there is limited data on this.

If you opt for a ketogenic diet, then the same basic principles for building muscle will apply; ensure you are in a calorie surplus, ensure you consume sufficient amounts of protein, and participate in a resistance training programme[31].

Ketogenic diet: summary

Given there is no superior benefit to a ketogenic diet, it should not be adopted if carbohydrates are an enjoyable part of your diet. From a practical viewpoint, a ketogenic diet is only suitable for a handful of individuals who are happy to pretty much completely omit carbohydrates from their diet. Most people would struggle to adhere to this. That being said, for those who enjoy such a diet and can adhere to it, it can be just as successful for weight loss outcomes as any other diet. Whether it can result in similar muscle growth compared to other diets remains to be seen with more research.

(Very) low calorie diet

Unless you have a lot of additional fat mass, avoid large calorie deficits.

Best utilised in very overweight, obese individuals, and should be avoided in the healthy population.

The diet does work well in very overweight, obese individuals, reducing feelings of hunger and appetite. Sustainable weight loss can be achieved without leading to eating disorders. Aggressive dieting in obese people can work in the long term under clinical supervision.

Very low calorie diets are not suitable for those slightly overweight or lean because it will just lead to significant losses in muscle mass.

Very low calorie diets contain considerably fewer calories than an individual's daily maintenance calorie intake. This means that there is a large calorie deficit, and therefore a fast rate of weight loss. Very low calorie diets (VLCD) typically contain 500kcal per day and are often in liquid form, containing all required nutrients. *Low calorie diets (LCD)* are typically around 1000kcal per day.

The purpose of a VLCD or LCD is to induce *rapid weight loss*, which is achieved by a *large calorie deficit*. The issue with this is that although there is rapid weight loss, a significant proportion of this weight loss comes from muscle being broken down, not just additional fat loss. The risk of excessive muscle loss is greater in leaner individuals. However, with very high body fat levels, the risk of muscle loss in a caloric deficit is reduced. The large health benefit from significantly reducing fat mass outweighs the small detrimental effect from marginal losses in muscle mass. As such, VLCDs and LCDs can be useful in obese individuals. Larger calorie deficits have been shown to lead to greater long-term weight loss to reach a moderate body fat level in obese people[61]. Furthermore, a randomised controlled trial in untrained and obese individuals showed that resistance training can help to limit the loss of muscle mass during a LCD[62].

Even so, VLCD and LCDs are not ideal diets for those who are already relatively lean and healthy, because it will significantly increase the proportion of muscle loss relative to fat loss (see chapter 7 regarding calorie deficits and the ratio of fat loss:muscle loss). VLCDs are clinically prescribed to obese or overweight individuals by a doctor. Even so, they are not routinely used[63]. There are other lifestyle and dietary interventions that a doctor may prescribe to obese individuals instead that use methods already discussed in chapter 6. This includes creating a calorie deficit by planning food intake (a tracked approach) or choosing low energy density, high nutrient density foods to create a calorie deficit from reduced calorie intake (an intuitive approach)[64].

VLCDs and LCDs are severe forms of energy restriction and should *not* be considered a long-term dietary strategy for healthy individuals. Even when used clinically in obese individuals, they are used in the short-term under the close supervision of healthcare professionals[63]. Common adverse events can include susceptibility to colds, fatigue and dizziness. For an obese, untrained individual, a short term VLCD or LCD *may* be suitable under medical supervision[65]. For non-obese healthy individuals, VLCD and LCDs carry more detrimental effects than beneficial effects. Unless a doctor prescribes you a VLCD or LCD, it would be best to avoid using such a strategy.

Manipulation of food groups and food sources

Vegan, vegetarian and pescatarian diets

The majority of research on vegan and vegetarian diets is from observational data and focusses on their health effects. Limited high quality data exists comparing vegan and vegetarian diets to other diets for fat loss and muscle gain[66,67].

Vegan or vegetarian diets can be used in conjunction with any diet strategy that manipulates macronutrients as discussed above (e.g. low fat, low carbohydrate or high protein) or diet that manipulates timing as discussed later. Therefore, from a theoretical perspective and expert opinion, vegan and vegetarian diets can be effective tools for fat loss and muscle gain, provided the nutritional principles that apply to any other diet are followed.

Opt for a vegan or vegetarian diet for ethical or environmental reasons, not health reasons.

Vegetarian diets can vary depending on the specific foods excluded, but generally exclude meat, and include dairy and eggs[68]. *Pescatarian* diets exclude meat, but include fish[69]. In a *vegan* diet, all animal-based foods are excluded such as meat, fish, dairy and eggs. This is also extended to products containing animal-based sources[70]. Compared to meat-eaters, observational studies have shown that vegan diets tend to have higher intakes of fibre, vitamins B_1, C and E and phytonutrients, and generally consume fewer calories, saturated fat and cholesterol. Vegan diets also tend to have lower intakes of omega-3 fatty acids, vitamin D, zinc, calcium and vitamin B_{12}. Vegetarian and pescatarian diets have intermediate nutrient intakes compared to omnivorous and vegan diets[69].

Currently, *no* conclusive evidence supports the complete exclusion of animal-based foods from a diet to further improve health outcomes. *No* conclusive evidence supports even completely excluding red and processed meat intake, where the recommendation is to limit intake. When comparing vegetarians, vegans or pescatarians (who are health conscious) with *health conscious* omnivores, there is no influence of vegetarianism on all-cause mortality[71]. Most studies comparing vegan or vegetarian diets with meat-eating diets focus on excessive consumption of red and processed meat, and do not consider the influence of white meats (chicken or turkey), fish, eggs or dairy. Systematic reviews and meta-analyses of observational studies show that consumption of white meats, fish, eggs and dairy are associated with improved health outcomes and a reduction in all-cause mortality, and consumption is not associated with poorer health[72–89]. Health authorities *do not recommend* excluding animal-based foods from a diet. Instead, authorities recommend limiting processed meat intake, and moderating red meat intake[90,91]. Many of the benefits associated with vegan and vegetarian diets are the result of increasing *whole, plant-based food* intake (e.g. fruit, cereals and legumes) and behavioural and lifestyle changes (e.g. greater exercise levels, not smoking or drinking alcohol), rather than as a result of completely eliminating animal-based food sources[70]. In the same way that low carbohydrate or low fat diets may restrict food choice, the exclusion of certain foods in vegan and vegetarian diets can result in nutritional deficiencies and health implications[26]. But, these can be avoided with careful dietary planning and supplementation. Macronutrient and micronutrient deficiencies are the result of a poorly designed vegan or vegetarian diet, rather than as a result of the diet itself[69,70].

For a complete overview of potential deficiencies in vegan and vegetarian diets, read the '*Position paper on vegetarian diets from the working group of the Italian Society of Human Nutrition*'[68] or '*Vegan diets: practical advice for athletes and exercisers*' by David Rogerson[66]. If you are considering excluding animal-based food sources such as in a vegan, vegetarian or pescatarian diet, speak to your GP first for health advice.

Some of the main potential deficiencies include:

Protein

Protein consumption is generally lower in non meat-eaters than in meat-eaters[66]. Plant-protein sources are incomplete, meaning compared to diets containing animal sources, vegan and vegetarian diets require relatively higher protein intakes and varied protein sources across the day, due to the lower protein quality (chapter 9 will discuss protein intake and types of protein sources)[66,68]. The issue of incomplete protein sources can be resolved by consuming a range of plant-based protein sources. This results in a complete intake of *essential amino acids*. High protein plant-based sources include seeds, nuts and legumes. A plant-based protein supplement such as soy protein can be beneficial to meet daily protein needs without additional calories from fat and carbohydrate. Vegetarians can utilise eggs and dairy sources which are high in protein, and pescatarians can make use of high protein fish sources.

Polyunsaturated fatty acids (PUFAs)

Common sources of polyunsaturated fatty acids are eggs and fish; therefore, intakes can be low in vegans and vegetarians[70].
Seaweed is a good plant-based source of polyunsaturated fatty acids, and animal-free supplements are available.

Micronutrients

The following micronutrients are primarily obtained from animal-based sources, and therefore intake may be low in diets restricting animal foods[26,66,70].

- Vitamin B_{12}
- Vitamin D
- Iron
- Zinc
- Calcium

Vegan, vegetarian and pescatarian diets for body composition goals

For success with a vegan, vegetarian or pescatarian diet for body composition goals, follow the same evidence-based recommendations as for any other diet.

Studies of vegetarian diets show they are neither superior nor inferior to other diets for aerobic exercise, anaerobic exercise, or strength performance[68]. However, there are *no* randomised controlled studies comparing vegan or vegetarian diets to omnivorous diets and muscle growth. Studies of vegan and vegetarian diets and body composition are very limited[26,66]. Most of the recommendations for vegan and vegetarian diets and body composition rely on indirect research, which is then extrapolated to vegan and vegetarian diets. More research is needed, but considering the recent rise in their popularity, it is likely there will be many studies in the future. However, consensus is that there does not appear to be any reason why it is not perfectly possible to meet either weight loss or muscle gain goals whilst on a vegan or vegetarian diet, provided the key principles for fat loss or muscle gain are adhered to and any diet-specific nutritional deficiencies are covered[66].

Vegan, vegetarian and pescatarian diets for fat loss

Current evidence suggests that when calories are equated, a vegan, vegetarian or pescatarian diet does not lead to greater fat loss compared to any other diet, but is just as effective.

In the usual sense of a vegan or vegetarian diet, the availability of low energy density, high nutrient density foods (i.e. a diet consisting primarily of *whole, plant-based food sources* such as fruit, nuts, grains, legumes and vegetables) may make it easier to achieve a calorie deficit and remain satiated, due to the large food volume[66]. However, with modern food development, overfeeding is still possible in a vegan or vegetarian diet with the availability of plant-derived high energy density and low nutrient density foods (i.e. vegan and vegetarian ultra-processed foods such as crisps or sweets).

Possibly the most difficult issue with a vegetarian or vegan diet would be ensuring a calorie deficit whilst still consuming sufficient protein[66]. Considering the higher protein requirements in a calorie deficit for trained individuals (1.8-2.7g/kg of body weight or 2.3–3.1 g/kg of lean mass per day), and the need for relatively higher intakes due to incomplete protein sources, it may be difficult to consume enough protein to meet daily needs to prevent muscle loss without consuming extra carbohydrates and/or fats. Unlike lean meat, poultry or fish, plant-based protein sources often contain carbohydrates or fats at relatively similar quantities to its protein content; high protein plant-based sources often contain protein:carbohydrate/fat at a 1:1 ratio. Therefore, it can be difficult to consume sufficient protein without consuming additional calories. In such cases, a plant-based protein supplement such as soy protein can be beneficial to meet daily protein needs without additional calories from fat and carbohydrate.

Vegan, vegetarian or pescatarian diet for muscle growth

In theory, provided calories are equated and sufficient protein is consumed, a vegan, vegetarian or pescatarian diet should not be superior or inferior for muscle growth compared to any other diet, but be just as effective.

In contrast to fat loss, the availability of low energy density, high nutrient density foods (i.e. whole-food plant-based sources) may make it harder to achieve a calorie surplus, especially with high training volumes (and therefore a higher total daily energy expenditure)[66,68]. However, overfeeding is still possible in a vegan or vegetarian diet with the availability of high energy density and low nutrient density foods (i.e. ultra-processed foods such as sweets). But, the nutrient content of food sources should be taken into consideration and not just the calorie content alone (see chapter 12). If food volume is an issue, then to ensure a calorie surplus it may be beneficial to opt for an increased proportion of fat intake. Fat is more calorie dense. Fat rich plant foods can have a higher energy density, such as nuts and oils. This may help to ensure adequate energy and nutrient intake[66].

Similar to fat loss, the greater need for protein may be difficult due to the lower energy density of whole, plant-based foods. Again, a plant-based protein supplement such as soy protein can be beneficial to meet daily protein needs without additional food volume.

Many plant-based foods (e.g. fruits, cereals and vegetables for example) contain large quantities of carbohydrate. Therefore, inadequate carbohydrate intake for anaerobic performance is unlikely to be an issue[66].

(Whole food) plant-based diet

The contents of a plant-based diet can vary greatly. A *whole food, plant-based* diet refers to the consumption of unprocessed, minimally processed or processed foods such as fruits, vegetables, nuts, plant oils, grains, pulses and legumes, with a focus on limiting intakes of ultra-processed foods. A *plant-based* diet however, can also be *low* in whole food, plant-based sources such as fruits, vegetables, nuts and legumes, and be *high* in ultra-processed foods. Furthermore, a plant-based diet does *not* mean a diet free from animal-based foods. The concepts of plant-based and animal-based diets are a continuum from vegan (plants only) diets, through omnivorous (plants and animals) diets, to carnivorous (animals only) diets[92]. Vegan and vegetarian diets *are* plant-based, but a plant-based diet does *not* have to be vegan or vegetarian. It has similar dietary emphases to the *Mediterranean diet*[3].

"A plant-based diet is based on foods derived from plants, including vegetables, wholegrains, legumes, nuts, seeds and fruits, with few or no animal products." **British Dietetic Association**[93].

A plant-based diet is very similar to vegan and vegetarian diets, except for the possible addition of low to moderate intakes of animal food sources. Similarly, evidence regarding plant-based diets and muscle growth or fat loss is incredibly limited. But again, there does not appear to be any reason why it is not perfectly possible to meet either weight loss or muscle gain goals whilst on a plant-based diet, provided the key principles for fat loss or muscle gain are adhered to, and any diet-specific nutritional deficiencies covered.

The addition of low to moderate animal food sources provides a wider selection of dietary protein sources. Therefore, issues with protein intake in vegan and vegetarian diets can be mitigated in plant-based diets containing animal food sources.

Fad Diets

No evidence supports the use of fad diets, such as detoxes or juice cleanses for improving body composition or health.

Any benefit of a fad diet is simply because it puts you in a calorie deficit, which is likely outweighed by the detrimental effects of the extreme caloric and nutritional restrictions they involve[94].

The majority of fad diets have little to no scientific backing. They are predominantly based on anecdotal evidence, incorrect science (*pseudoscience*), and media influencing. A major issue with fad diets is that they often involve extreme dietary measures such as the exclusion of major food groups, which can result in very low calorie intakes[95]. More importantly, this can lead to severe nutritional deficiencies[94]. Such diets are not representative of peoples' habitual diets, and therefore they often fail in achieving long-term weight loss maintenance because there is no long-term behavioural or lifestyle change (see chapter 6).

Fad diets include:

- Detox diets.
- Juice cleanses.
- Tea detoxes.
- Diets excluding complete food groups or macronutrients (avoiding sugar, fruit, gluten, grains etc.).
- Alkali diets.

Juicing and detoxification diets

The concept behind a *detox* diet is that toxins build up in the body. These toxins then need to be eliminated in order to maintain and promote improved health. They are also used as a means to induce weight loss[96]. A detox is *not* necessary to remove waste products from the body. In normal people, toxins do not build up and specific diets are not needed to remove such toxins. The body has its own detoxification systems to remove toxins in the form of the liver and kidneys. The skin, gut and lungs also have important roles in eliminating substances[96]. Alcohol is a toxin (see chapter 13 regarding alcohol and body composition). The liver does an excellent job in metabolising alcohol and slowly clearing it from the body[96]. A *'toxin'* is also a very vague term. Water can be toxic when consumed in great excess.

- *No* randomised controlled trials have assessed the effectiveness of detox diets in humans for health or body composition[96].
- There is *very limited* high-quality research into juice or detox diets. Current studies have major limitations due to methodological issues generating high risks of bias (e.g. a lack of blinding or control groups), and the majority of evidence is from case studies or expert opinion[96].
- Juice and detox diets involve extreme limitation of calorie intake and extreme limitation of food groups. For example, such diets will likely fail to meet the minimum dietary recommendations for fat, protein and some micronutrients. This can result in severe nutrient deficiencies, fatigue and lethargy. There are numerous case reports of severe nutritional deficiencies and overdoses with such diets[94].
- Some of the apparent weight loss from such diets is the result of consuming liquids, not eating much food, loss of faecal matter and less food volume. All of which can reduce the amount of content in the digestive system, making an individual feel *'lighter'* and *'thinner'*, and make the stomach look flatter[94].
- Juice and detox diets are used as *drastic short-term interventions* (a few days to a couple of weeks). The return to the habitual diet then means any apparent weight lost is regained, and the possibility of gaining additional weight[94].
- Such diets are not sustainable for long periods of time.

There are nutritional components of foods that possess detoxifying qualities that can be obtained by consuming a typical, varied dietary pattern. Even so, there is still no evidence to suggest that detoxification is necessary. This also does not provide evidence that a diet wholly focussed on detoxification is necessary nor superior[96].

"At present, there is no compelling evidence to support the use of detox diets for weight management or toxin elimination. Considering the financial costs to consumers, unsubstantiated claims and potential health risks of detox products, they should be discouraged by health professionals and subject to independent regulatory review and monitoring."
Klein and Kiat, 2014[96].

Summary

When calorie intake and protein intake are equated, all diets are equally effective for weight change.

Individuals find that some diets work better than other diets because they are easier to adhere to. Dietary adherence is associated with more successful weight change.

Dietary styles can manipulate macronutrient content, manipulate food groups, or manipulate food timing. Dietary styles can be combined and are not mutually exclusive.

The dietary style of choice should largely be dictated by personal preference.

References

1   Freire R. Scientific evidence of diets for weight loss: Different macronutrient composition, intermittent fasting, and popular diets. *Nutrition* 2020; 69: 110549.

2   Thom G, Lean M. Is There an Optimal Diet for Weight Management and Metabolic Health? *Gastroenterology* 2017; 152: 1739–1751.

3   Davis C, Bryan J, Hodgson J, Murphy K. Definition of the Mediterranean Diet: A Literature Review. *Nutrients* 2015; 7: 9139–9153.

4   Statovci D, Aguilera M, MacSharry J, Melgar S. The Impact of Western Diet and Nutrients on the Microbiota and Immune Response at Mucosal Interfaces. *Front Immunol* 2017; 8. Available from: doi:10.3389/fimmu.2017.00838.

5   Aragon AA, Schoenfeld BJ, Wildman R, Kleiner S, VanDusseldorp T, Taylor L et al. International society of sports nutrition position stand: diets and body composition. *J Int Soc Sports Nutr* 2017; 14. Available from: doi:10.1186/s12970-017-0174-y.

6   Zinn C, Rush A, Johnson R. Assessing the nutrient intake of a low-carbohydrate, high-fat (LCHF) diet: a hypothetical case study design. *BMJ Open* 2018; 8. Available from: doi:10.1136/bmjopen-2017-018846.

7   Noakes TD, Windt J. Evidence that supports the prescription of low-carbohydrate high-fat diets: a narrative review. *Br J Sports Med* 2017; 51: 133–139.

8   Rand WM, Pellett PL, Young VR. Meta-analysis of nitrogen balance studies for estimating protein requirements in healthy adults. *Am J Clin Nutr* 2003; 77: 109–127.

9   Carbone JW, Pasiakos SM. Dietary Protein and Muscle Mass: Translating Science to Application and Health Benefit. *Nutrients* 2019; 11. Available from: doi:10.3390/nu11051136.

10   Leaf A, Antonio J. The Effects of Overfeeding on Body Composition: The Role of Macronutrient Composition – A Narrative Review. *Int J Exerc Sci* 2017; 10(8): 1275-1296.

11   Antonio J, Ellerbroek A, Silver T, Vargas L, Tamayo A, Buehn R et al. A High Protein Diet Has No Harmful Effects: A One-Year Crossover Study in Resistance-Trained Males. *J Nutr Metab* 2016. Available from: doi:10.1155/2016/9104792.

12   Antonio J, Ellerbroek A, Silver T, Vargas L, Peacock C. The effects of a high protein diet on indices of health and body composition – a crossover trial in resistance-trained men. *J Int Soc Sports Nutr* 2016; 13. Available from: doi:10.1186/s12970-016-0114-2.

13   Johnstone A. Safety and efficacy of high-protein diets for weight loss. *Proc Nutr Soc* 2012; 71: 339–49.

14   Hall KD. A review of the carbohydrate-insulin model of obesity. *Eur J Clin Nutr* 2017; 71: 323–326.

15   Gardner CD, Trepanowski JF, Gobbo LCD, Hauser ME, Rigdon J, Ioannidis JPA et al. Effect of low-fat VS low-carbohydrate diet on 12-month weight loss in overweight adults and the association with genotype pattern or insulin secretion the DIETFITS randomized clinical trial. *J Am Med Assoc* 2018; 319: 667–679.

16   Lammert O, Grunnet N, Faber P, Bjørnsbo KS, Dich J, Larsen LO et al. Effects of isoenergetic overfeeding of either carbohydrate or fat in young men. *Br J Nutr* 2000; 84: 233–245.

17   Astrup A, Meinert Larsen T, Harper A. Atkins and other low-carbohydrate diets: hoax or an effective tool for weight loss? *Lancet Lond Engl* 2004; 364: 897–899.

18   Hall KD, Guo J. Obesity Energetics: Body Weight Regulation and the Effects of Diet Composition. *Gastroenterology* 2017; 152: 1718-1727.e3.

19   Johnston BC, Kanters S, Bandayrel K, Wu P, Naji F, Siemieniuk RA et al. Comparison of weight loss among named diet programs in overweight and obese adults: a meta-analysis. *JAMA* 2014; 312: 923–933.

20   Surwit RS, Feinglos MN, McCaskill CC, Clay SL, Babyak MA, Brownlow BS et al. Metabolic and behavioral effects of a high-sucrose diet during weight loss. *Am J Clin Nutr* 1997; 65: 908–915.

21   Westerterp-Plantenga MS, Lemmens SG, Westerterp KR. Dietary protein – its role in satiety, energetics, weight loss and health. *Br J Nutr* 2012; 108: S105–S112.

22   Norton L. *Science, Stories, and Side-Stepping: The Stephan Guyenet vs. Gary Taubes Debate.* 2019. Available from: https://www.biolayne.com/articles/research/science-stories-and-side-stepping-the-stephan-guyenet-vs-gary-taubes-debate/ (accessed 5 Feb 2020).

23   Burke LM. Re-Examining High-Fat Diets for Sports Performance: Did We Call the 'Nail in the Coffin' Too Soon? *Sports Med Auckl NZ* 2015; 45 Suppl 1: S33-49.

24   Escobar KA, VanDusseldorp TA, Kerksick CM. Carbohydrate intake and resistance-based exercise: are current recommendations reflective of actual need? *Br J Nutr* 2016; 116: 2053–2065.

25   Kerksick CM, Wilborn CD, Roberts MD, Smith-Ryan A, Kleiner SM, Jäger R et al. ISSN exercise & sports nutrition review update: research & recommendations. *J Int Soc Sports Nutr* 2018; 15. Available from: doi:10.1186/s12970-018-0242-y.

26   Thomas DT, Erdman KA, Burke LM. Position of the Academy of Nutrition and Dietetics, Dietitians of Canada, and the American College of Sports Medicine: Nutrition and Athletic Performance. *J Acad Nutr Diet* 2016; 116: 501–528.

27   Cholewa JM, Newmire DE, Zanchi NE. Carbohydrate restriction: Friend or foe of resistance-based exercise performance? *Nutrition* 2019; 60: 136–146.

28   Kerksick C, Arent S, Schoenfeld B, Stout J, Campbell B, Wilborn C et al. International society of sports nutrition position stand: Nutrient timing. *J Int Soc Sports Nutr* 2017; 14: 33.

29   Lambert CP, Frank LL, Evans WJ. Macronutrient considerations for the sport of bodybuilding. *Sports Med Auckl NZ* 2004; 34: 317–327.

30   Slater G, Phillips SM. Nutrition guidelines for strength sports: sprinting, weightlifting, throwing events, and bodybuilding. *J Sports Sci* 2011; 29 Suppl 1: S67-77.

31   Vargas S, Romance R, Petro JL, Bonilla DA, Galancho I, Espinar S et al. Efficacy of ketogenic diet on body composition during resistance training in trained men: a randomized controlled trial. *J Int Soc Sports Nutr* 2018; 15. Available from: doi:10.1186/s12970-018-0236-9.

32   Murray B, Rosenbloom C. Fundamentals of glycogen metabolism for coaches and athletes. *Nutr Rev* 2018; 76: 243–259.

33   Franz MJ. Protein: Metabolism and Effect on Blood Glucose Levels. *Diabetes Educ* 1997; 23: 643–651.

34   Roberts BM, Helms ER, Trexler ET, Fitschen PJ. Nutritional Recommendations for Physique Athletes. *J Hum Kin* 2020; 71(1): 79-108 Available from: doi:http://dx.doi.org/10.2478/hukin-2019-0096.

35   Volek JS, Freidenreich DJ, Saenz C, Kunces LJ, Creighton BC, Bartley JM et al. Metabolic characteristics of keto-adapted ultra-endurance runners. *Metab - Clin Exp* 2016; 65: 100–110.

36   Robergs RA, Pearson DR, Costill DL, Fink WJ, Pascoe DD, Benedict MA et al. Muscle glycogenolysis during differing intensities of weight-resistance exercise. *J Appl Physiol Bethesda* 1991; 70: 1700–1706.

37   Aragon AA, Schoenfeld BJ. Nutrient timing revisited: is there a post-exercise anabolic window? *J Int Soc Sports Nutr* 2013; 10: 5.

38   Dorgan JF, Judd JT, Longcope C, Brown C, Schatzkin A, Clevidence BA et al. Effects of dietary fat and fiber on plasma and urine androgens and estrogens in men: a controlled feeding study. *Am J Clin Nutr* 1996; 64: 850–855.

39   Helms ER, Aragon AA, Fitschen PJ. Evidence-based recommendations for natural bodybuilding contest preparation: nutrition and supplementation. *J Int Soc Sports Nutr* 2014; 11: 20.

40   Hämäläinen EK, Adlercreutz H, Puska P, Pietinen P. Decrease of serum total and free testosterone during a low-fat high-fibre diet. *J Steroid Biochem* 1983; 18: 369–370.

41   Volek JS, Kraemer WJ, Bush JA, Incledon T, Boetes M. Testosterone and cortisol in relationship to dietary nutrients and resistance exercise. *J Appl Physiol Bethesda* 1997; 82: 49–54.

42   Schoenfeld BJ. Postexercise hypertrophic adaptations: a reexamination of the hormone hypothesis and its applicability to resistance training program design. *J Strength Cond Res* 2013; 27: 1720–1730.

43   Iggman D, Rosqvist F, Larsson A, Arnlöv J, Beckman L, Rudling M et al. Role of dietary fats in modulating cardiometabolic risk during moderate weight gain: a randomized double-blind overfeeding trial (LIPOGAIN study). *J Am Heart Assoc* 2014; 3: e001095.

44   Rosqvist F, Iggman D, Kullberg J, Cedernaes J, Johansson H-E, Larsson A et al. Overfeeding Polyunsaturated and Saturated Fat Causes Distinct Effects on Liver and Visceral Fat Accumulation in Humans. *Diabetes* 2014; 63: 2356–2368.

45   Slater GJ, Dieter BP, Marsh DJ, Helms ER, Shaw G, Iraki J. Is an Energy Surplus Required to Maximize Skeletal Muscle Hypertrophy Associated With Resistance Training. *Front Nutr* 2019; 6. Available from: doi:10.3389/fnut.2019.00131.

46   Dearlove DJ, Faull OK, Clarke K. Context is key: exogenous ketosis and athletic performance. *Curr Opin Physiol* 2019; 10: 81–89.

47   Sharma S, Jain P. The ketogenic diet and other dietary treatments for refractory epilepsy in children. *Ann Indian Acad Neurol* 2014; 17: 253–258.

48   Paoli A, Cancellara P, Pompei P, Moro T. Ketogenic Diet and Skeletal Muscle Hypertrophy: A Frenemy Relationship? *J Hum Kinet* 2019; 68: 233–247.

49   Paoli A, Bosco G, Camporesi EM, Mangar D. Ketosis, ketogenic diet and food intake control: a complex relationship. *Front Psychol* 2015; 6. Available from: doi:10.3389/fpsyg.2015.00027.

50   Gibson AA, Seimon RV, Lee CMY, Ayre J, Franklin J, Markovic TP et al. Do ketogenic diets really suppress appetite? A systematic review and meta-analysis. *Obes Rev Off J Int Assoc Study Obes* 2015; 16: 64–76.

51   Greene DA, Varley BJ, Hartwig TB, Chapman P, Rigney M. A Low-Carbohydrate Ketogenic Diet Reduces Body Mass Without Compromising Performance in Powerlifting and Olympic Weightlifting Athletes. *J Strength Cond Res* 2018; 32: 3373–3382.

52   Kephart WC, Pledge CD, Roberson PA, Mumford PW, Romero MA, Mobley CB et al. The Three-Month Effects of a Ketogenic Diet on Body Composition, Blood Parameters, and Performance Metrics in CrossFit Trainees: A Pilot Study. *Sports* 2018; 6. Available from: doi:10.3390/sports6010001.

53   Kosinski C, Jornayvaz FR. Effects of Ketogenic Diets on Cardiovascular Risk Factors: Evidence from Animal and Human Studies. *Nutrients* 2017; 9. Available from: doi:10.3390/nu9050517.

54   Liu AG, Ford NA, Hu FB, Zelman KM, Mozaffarian D, Kris-Etherton PM. A healthy approach to dietary fats: understanding the science and taking action to reduce consumer confusion. *Nutr J* 2017; 16. Available from: doi:10.1186/s12937-017-0271-4.

55   Soenen S, Bonomi AG, Lemmens SGT, Scholte J, Thijssen MAMA, van Berkum F et al. Relatively high-protein or 'low-carb' energy-restricted diets for body weight loss and body weight maintenance? *Physiol Behav* 2012; 107: 374–380.

56   Wilson JM, Lowery RP, Roberts MD, Sharp MH, Joy JM, Shields KA et al. The Effects of Ketogenic Dieting on Body Composition, Strength, Power, and Hormonal Profiles in Resistance Training Males. *J Strength Cond Res* 2017. Available from: doi:10.1519/JSC.0000000000001935.

57   Hall KD, Chen KY, Guo J, Lam YY, Leibel RL, Mayer LE et al. Energy expenditure and body composition changes after an isocaloric ketogenic diet in overweight and obese men. *Am J Clin Nutr* 2016; 104: 324–333.

58   Johnston CS, Tjonn SL, Swan PD, White A, Hutchins H, Sears B. Ketogenic low-carbohydrate diets have no metabolic advantage over nonketogenic low-carbohydrate diets. *Am J Clin Nutr* 2006; 83: 1055–1061.

59   Stimson RH, Johnstone AM, Homer NZM, Wake DJ, Morton NM, Andrew R et al. Dietary Macronutrient Content Alters Cortisol Metabolism Independently of Body Weight Changes in Obese Men. *J Clin Endocrinol Metab* 2007; 92: 4480–4484.

60   Veum VL, Laupsa-Borge J, Eng Ø, Rostrup E, Larsen TH, Nordrehaug JE et al. Visceral adiposity and metabolic syndrome after very high–fat and low-fat isocaloric diets: a randomized controlled trial. *Am J Clin Nutr* 2017; 105: 85–99.

61   Nackers LM, Ross KM, Perri MG. The association between rate of initial weight loss and long-term success in obesity treatment: does slow and steady win the race? *Int J Behav Med* 2010; 17: 161–167.

62   Bryner RW, Ullrich IH, Sauers J, Donley D, Hornsby G, Kolar M et al. Effects of resistance vs. aerobic training combined with an 800 calorie liquid diet on lean body mass and resting metabolic rate. *J Am Coll Nutr* 1999; 18: 115–121.

63   National Institute for Health and Care Excellence (NICE). *NCG. Very-low-calorie diets.* 2014 Available from: https://www.ncbi.nlm.nih.gov/books/NBK311324/ (accessed 6 Feb 2020).

64   Jensen MD, Ryan DH, Apovian CM, Ard JD, Comuzzie AG, Donato KA et al. 2013 AHA/ACC/TOS Guideline for the Management of Overweight and Obesity in Adults. *Circulation* 2014; 129: S102–S138.

65   Tsai AG, Wadden TA. The Evolution of Very-Low-Calorie Diets: An Update and Meta-analysis. *Obesity* 2006; 14: 1283–1293.

66   Rogerson D. Vegan diets: practical advice for athletes and exercisers. *J Int Soc Sports Nutr* 2017; 14. Available from: doi:10.1186/s12970-017-0192-9.

67   Le LT, Sabaté J. Beyond Meatless, the Health Effects of Vegan Diets: Findings from the Adventist Cohorts. *Nutrients* 2014; 6: 2131–2147.

68   Agnoli C, Baroni L, Bertini I, Ciappellano S, Fabbri A, Papa M et al. Position paper on vegetarian diets from the working group of the Italian Society of Human Nutrition. *Nutr Metab Cardiovasc Dis* 2017; 27: 1037–1052.

69   Davey GK, Spencer EA, Appleby PN, Allen NE, Knox KH, Key TJ. EPIC–Oxford:lifestyle characteristics and nutrient intakes in a cohort of 33 883 meat-eaters and 31 546 non meat-eaters in the UK. *Public Health Nutr* 2003; 6: 259–268.

70   Craig WJ. Health effects of vegan diets. *Am J Clin Nutr* 2009; 89: 1627S-1633S.

71   Appleby PN, Crowe FL, Bradbury KE, Travis RC, Key TJ. Mortality in vegetarians and comparable nonvegetarians in the United Kingdom. *Am J Clin Nutr* 2016; 103: 218–230.

72   Daniel CR, Cross AJ, Graubard BI, Hollenbeck AR, Park Y, Sinha R. Prospective Investigation of Poultry and Fish Intake in Relation to Cancer Risk. *Cancer Prev Res (Phila Pa)* 2011; 4: 1903–1911.

73   Kim K, Hyeon J, Lee SA, Kwon SO, Lee H, Keum N et al. Role of Total, Red, Processed, and White Meat Consumption in Stroke Incidence and Mortality: A Systematic Review and Meta-Analysis of Prospective Cohort Studies. *J Am Heart Assoc* 2017; 6. Available from: doi:10.1161/JAHA.117.005983.

74   Deng C, Lu Q, Gong B, Li L, Chang L, Fu L et al. Stroke and food groups: an overview of systematic reviews and meta-analyses. *Public Health Nutr* 2017. Available from: doi:10.1017/S1368980017003093.

75   Mishali M, Prizant-Passal S, Avrech T, Shoenfeld Y. Association between dairy intake and the risk of contracting type 2 diabetes and cardiovascular diseases: a systematic review and meta-analysis with subgroup analysis of men versus women. *Nutr Rev* 2019. Available from: doi:10.1093/nutrit/nuz006.

76   Keum N, Lee DH, Marchand N, Oh H, Liu H, Aune D et al. Egg intake and cancers of the breast, ovary and prostate: a dose-response meta-analysis of prospective observational studies. *Br J Nutr* 2015; 114: 1099–1107.

77   Alexander DD, Miller PE, Vargas AJ, Weed DL, Cohen SS. Meta-analysis of Egg Consumption and Risk of Coronary Heart Disease and Stroke. *J Am Coll Nutr* 2016. Available from: doi:10.1080/07315724.2016.1152928.

78   Lu W, Chen H, Niu Y, Wu H, Xia D, Wu Y. Dairy products intake and cancer mortality risk: a meta-analysis of 11 population-based cohort studies. *Nutr J* 2016; 15. Available from: doi:10.1186/s12937-016-0210-9.

79   Guo J, Astrup A, Lovegrove JA, Gijsbers L, Givens DI, Soedamah-Muthu SS. Milk and dairy consumption and risk of cardiovascular diseases and all-cause mortality: dose-response meta-analysis of prospective cohort studies. *Eur J Epidemiol* 2017; 32: 269–287.

80   Qin L-Q, Xu J-Y, Han S-F, Zhang Z-L, Zhao Y-Y, Szeto IM. Dairy consumption and risk of cardiovascular disease: an updated meta-analysis of prospective cohort studies. *Asia Pac J Clin Nutr* 2015; 24: 90–100.

81   Goede J de, Soedamah-Muthu SS, Pan AX, Gijsbers L, Geleijnse JM. Dairy Consumption and Risk of Stroke: A Systematic Review and Updated Dose–

Response Meta-Analysis of Prospective Cohort Studies. *Journal of the American Heart Association* 2016. Available from: doi:10.1161/JAHA.115.002787.

82   Zhang Z, Chen G-C, Qin Z-Z, Tong X, Li D-P, Qin L-Q. Poultry and Fish Consumption in Relation to Total Cancer Mortality: A Meta-Analysis of Prospective Studies. *Nutr Cancer* 2018; 70: 204–212.

83   Larsson SC, Orsini N. Fish consumption and the risk of stroke: a dose-response meta-analysis. *Stroke* 2011; 42: 3621–3623.

84   Xun P, Qin B, Song Y, Nakamura Y, Kurth T, Yaemsiri S et al. Fish consumption and risk of stroke and its subtypes: accumulative evidence from a meta-analysis of prospective cohort studies. *Eur J Clin Nutr* 2012; 66: 1199–1207.

85   Zhao W, Tang H, Yang X, Luo X, Wang X, Shao C et al. Fish Consumption and Stroke Risk: A Meta-Analysis of Prospective Cohort Studies. *J Stroke Cerebrovasc Dis Off J Natl Stroke Assoc* 2019; 28: 604–611.

86   He K, Song Y, Daviglus ML, Liu K, Van Horn L, Dyer AR et al. Fish consumption and incidence of stroke: a meta-analysis of cohort studies. *Stroke* 2004; 35: 1538–1542.

87   Mente A, de Koning L, Shannon HS, Anand SS. A systematic review of the evidence supporting a causal link between dietary factors and coronary heart disease. *Arch Intern Med* 2009; 169: 659–669.

88   Lippi G, Mattiuzzi C, Cervellin G. Meat consumption and cancer risk: a critical review of published meta-analyses. *Crit Rev Oncol Hematol* 2016; 97: 1–14.

89   Bernstein AM, Pan A, Rexrode KM, Stampfer MJ, Hu FB, Mozaffarian D et al. Dietary protein sources and the risk of stroke in men and women. *Stroke* 2012. Available from: doi:10.1161/STROKEAHA.111.633404.

90   World Cancer Research Fund. *Limit red and processed meat*. 2018. Available from: https://www.wcrf.org/dietandcancer/recommendations/limit-red-processed-meat (accessed 6 Feb 2020).

91   NHS. *Red meat and the risk of bowel cancer*. 2018. Available from: https://www.nhs.uk/live-well/eat-well/red-meat-and-the-risk-of-bowel-cancer/ (accessed 6 Feb 2020).

92   Medawar E, Huhn S, Villringer A, Veronica Witte A. The effects of plant-based diets on the body and the brain: a systematic review. *Transl Psychiatry* 2019; 9. Available from: doi:10.1038/s41398-019-0552-0.

93   *BDA.   Plant-based   diet.*   Available   from: https://www.bda.uk.com/resource/plant-based-diet.html (accessed 6 Feb 2020).

94   Obert J, Pearlman M, Obert L, Chapin S. Popular Weight Loss Strategies: a Review of Four Weight Loss Techniques. *Curr Gastroenterol Rep* 2017; 19: 61.

95   Roberts DC. Quick weight loss: sorting fad from fact. *Med J Aust* 2001; 175: 637–640.

96   Klein AV, Kiat H. Detox diets for toxin elimination and weight management: a critical review of the evidence. *J Hum Nutr Diet Off J Br Diet Assoc* 2015; 28: 675–686.

9. Advanced nutrition: protein intake for specific goals

Intuitive and tracked approaches to energy intake are not two dietary options, but a *continuum*. A more intuitive approach to dieting is a great strategy for long-term weight maintenance and works for most people. However, when you have specific body composition goals which require a short-term shift in energy intake, then the calories you need can be calculated for this period. Whether you can meet and/or adhere to these numbers may require being more conscious about energy intake during the period of time you intend to achieve your specific goal. This becomes more important when for example, trying to be in a calorie deficit that maximises fat loss, minimises muscle loss, and allows you to train and perform at your best.

A complete approach to calculating your macronutrient needs:

- Calculate your **total daily calorie needs** for your goal (fat loss or muscle gain). Calculate your current calorie expenditure. Calculate the relative size of your calorie surplus or deficit (chapter 7).
- Calculate **how much protein** you need depending on your goals; a minimum of 1.6g/kg of body weight for muscle growth or fat loss, increasing to 1.8-2.7g/kg of body weight or 2.3–3.1 g/kg of lean mass per day if you are trained and in a calorie deficit for fat loss.
- Calculate **how much fat** you need (as a minimum 15-20% of total calories or 0.5g/kg of body weight per day), and then consider adding additional fats above this based on personal preference, keeping within the calculated daily calorie intake for your goal.
- Fill the remainder of your calorie needs with **carbohydrates** depending on your preference of carbohydrates over fats, the volume, duration and intensity of any exercise you perform and your body composition goal.

Protein intake

Total daily protein intake is by far the most important protein-related factor for optimising body composition. Factors such as protein timing, protein source and protein quality are all secondary to this.

The main daily focus should be on consuming your daily protein target.

For muscle growth, 1.6g/kg of body weight per day should be consumed as a minimum. Once this is met, consider splitting this intake evenly across multiple meals in doses that maximally stimulate muscle protein synthesis at each meal (a minimum of 20g).

For preserving muscle mass in a deficit, 1.6g/kg of body weight per day is sufficient for untrained individuals with higher body fat percentages to preserve muscle mass and promote fat loss. Increasing intake to 1.8-2.7g/kg of body weight or 2.3-3.1 g/kg of lean mass per day (depending on body fat percentage) may be more beneficial for leaner, resistance trained individuals.

Whether protein timing, rate of protein digestion (fast vs slow) and types of protein have a significant impact on muscle growth or preservation of muscle mass once total daily protein intake is achieved appears to be small in untrained individuals. Whether these factors are more important in trained individuals remains to be seen with more research. Addressing these factors is a matter of adherence and whether you consider them important enough to be implemented in your diet.

A position stand by the International Society of Sports Nutrition (ISSN) has been conducted on protein consumption and exercise, which is freely available to the public[1]. Similar recommendations to the ISSN have been made in other reviews[2].

Resistance training and ingesting protein both stimulate muscle protein synthesis. Consuming protein before or after resistance training can increase the muscle protein building response above that of resistance training alone. However, when consuming adequate daily protein, protein timing around a workout is relatively unimportant.

The benefits of protein consumption on muscle protein synthesis can occur from pre or post-workout consumption. Timing choice is largely down to personal preference.

High protein intakes (>3g/kg of body weight per day) show no adverse health effects in healthy individuals.

Protein doses should be ideally spread throughout the day in 3 to 6 hour intervals to maintain elevated levels of muscle protein synthesis. This is more important for muscle growth, and less important for fat loss.

0.25g/kg of body weight or around 20-40g of protein per meal is recommended for muscle growth as this quantity maximises muscle protein synthesis with each meal. Recommendations vary depending on age and if you have just trained. This is less important than total protein intake.

Rapidly digesting proteins most effectively elevate muscle protein synthesis. This is less important than total protein intake.

Individuals should aim to consume complete sources of protein (complete sources contain all the amino acids needed to build protein). Consuming a range of incomplete proteins (as may occur in a vegan or vegetarian diet) is suitable. But, due to the lower protein quality, total daily protein intakes need to be greater and varied protein sources are needed when consuming only incomplete protein sources. A slightly greater intake of a range of incomplete protein sources is equivalent to a slightly lower intake of complete protein sources for stimulating muscle protein synthesis and muscle growth.

If needed, individuals can use protein supplements as a convenient source to meet daily protein needs, which have been shown to be completely safe. When daily protein intake is sufficient, protein supplements provide no further benefit on body composition.

Consuming slow-digesting protein such as casein before sleep can elevate overnight muscle protein synthesis. This is less important than total protein intake.

Before we discuss the potential nuances of protein intake, it is important to state that ensuring adequate total protein intake for your intended goal supersedes *any* specific niche of protein intake in terms of muscle growth, such as timing[2]. Once this is achieved, the relative importance of secondary variables such as timing, quality and content of protein intake can then be discussed, as they become more relevant.

Even though the timing, dosage and source of protein supplements can affect acute changes in muscle protein synthesis, the effect of these differences does not necessarily affect muscle growth when total daily protein needs are met[2]. Consuming adequate daily protein through food sources or protein supplements should be the primary focus[3].

The recommended protein intakes for the general population are much lower than position stand recommendations for people that participate in any form of exercise[1]. General protein recommendations for the average person not doing any form of exercise (i.e. sedentary) is around 0.8g/kg of body weight per day[4]. This recommendation is the *minimum* amount of protein to keep the body ticking over and to prevent health problems. This is to avoid nutritional deficiency and is *not* considered to be the optimum intake[5]. As soon as you start doing any form of exercise (which includes aerobic exercise, not just resistance training) protein requirements increase. Higher protein intakes optimise exercise performance and body composition. Higher protein intake is not just to keep the body ticking over, but also to maximise muscle recovery and growth, and optimise fat loss in a calorie deficit[6].

The brick wall analogy

Imagine a *brick wall*. We can keep building a brick wall higher and higher by adding new bricks on top, and we can make it wider by adding new bricks to the sides. However, we can only keep on building the wall so long as the bricks already in place are stable and in good condition. Imagine the bricks at the bottom are old and starting to deteriorate. If we keep adding bricks on top, there will become a point where these weak, old bricks will give way, and the wall will fall. Clearly, the solution is to take out any weak, old bricks and place strong, new bricks in their place to allow us to keep building the wall or at least to make sure that the wall does not deteriorate over time. The *balance* between adding and removing bricks determines whether the wall gets bigger, stays the same or gets smaller.

Muscles are like the brick wall. Proteins are continually being broken down and rebuilt in our muscles. This has an important role in making sure that old, defective protein is removed and replaced with functioning proteins. The *balance* between breaking down and building up determines whether we are gaining, maintaining, or losing muscle.

Net protein balance (NPB) is the difference between *muscle protein synthesis* (MPS) and *muscle protein breakdown* (MPB); i.e. the balance between adding new protein and taking away old protein.

Net protein balance = muscle protein synthesis – muscle protein breakdown

NPB = MPS - MPB

Muscles are in a constant flux between positive net protein balance (building muscle) and negative net protein balance (losing muscle). Muscles will fluctuate between the two depending on stimuli that promote changes in muscle protein synthesis and muscle protein breakdown across the day and week. The balance between muscle protein breakdown and muscle protein synthesis determines net protein balance at a given instant. The long-term net protein balance will determine whether there is muscle growth, maintenance or loss. Many factors can promote, augment or suppress muscle protein synthesis and muscle protein breakdown. Notably, *nutrient status* (how much you have eaten, what you have just eaten, or whether you have eaten at all) and *exercise*, including aerobic and anaerobic training can augment muscle protein synthesis and muscle protein breakdown.

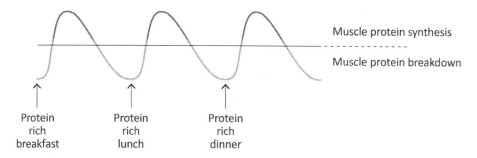

Net protein balance is important during both weight loss and weight gain. The aim of a weight loss plan is to decrease *fat mass*, not *muscle mass*. If net protein balance becomes negative, muscle size will decrease as we will lose muscle, not fat. The aim of a weight gain plan is to increase *muscle mass*, not *fat mass*. If net protein balance is not sufficiently positive, the additional energy from the calorie surplus will be stored as fat, rather than directed towards the energy demands of building muscle. Therefore, during weight loss and weight gain we want net protein balance to remain positive for as long as possible. Strategies that maintain elevated muscle protein synthesis are of importance for optimising body composition.

Muscle protein synthesis can be stimulated by *resistance training* and *protein consumption*. However, resistance training also stimulates muscle protein breakdown. In the absence of nutrition, this results in muscle loss. Therefore, adequate intake and protein consumption are important for muscle growth[7]. This chapter will look at protein consumption to optimise weight loss or weight gain. The training chapters will cover resistance training and its effect on muscle protein synthesis.

Day-to-day elevations in muscle protein synthesis should be the primary protein-related focus, which is achieved by consuming adequate daily protein. Resistance training elevates muscle protein synthesis for 1 to 2 days after a workout. Consuming sufficient protein in this extended window is important for muscle growth.

The acute rise in muscle protein synthesis immediately after a resistance training session does *not* appear to correlate with muscle growth[8,9]. This is seen in untrained individuals when a workout generates large amounts of muscle damage, such as a novel workout (note that most research is on untrained individuals performing novel resistance training workouts). The immediate resistance-training induced increase in muscle protein synthesis does not correlate with long-term muscle hypertrophy, most likely because this acute increase also incorporates increases in muscle protein synthesis due to muscle damage, which does not contribute to muscle growth and instead is directed to repairing damaged muscle[10]. Once an individual has been on a training programme for a few weeks, the extent of muscle damage appears to attenuate. Resistance training-induced increases in muscle protein synthesis are lower several weeks into a training programme than at the beginning of the programme, suggesting that elevations in muscle protein synthesis become *'refined'*. Levels of muscle protein synthesis on a longer scale of days rather than on an acute scale of minutes to hours after a workout then start to correlate with hypertrophy[11]. Hypertrophy therefore appears to be the result of multiple rises in muscle protein synthesis across the day, after controlling for elevations in muscle protein synthesis due to *exercise-induced muscle damage*. One study looked at the levels of muscle protein synthesis and muscle damage after a resistance training workout over the course of a 10-week training programme. They found that muscle protein synthesis only correlated with long-term muscle growth once the initial elevation in muscle damage from the first sessions was attenuated[10]. Muscle protein synthesis was measured over a period of 48 hours after the resistance training session, not acutely after the workout.

Day to day elevations in muscle protein synthesis (once the initial muscle damage from a new training programme has attenuated) correlates with muscle hypertrophy[9]. Increasing muscle protein synthesis is important, but no single increase in muscle protein synthesis across the day is more important than overall daily elevations in muscle protein synthesis. Sufficient overall increases in daily muscle protein synthesis should be the focus[9,10].

Similarly, consumption of protein after a workout acutely elevates markers of muscle growth and increases muscle protein synthesis, above the elevated levels seen from resistance training alone[12]. However, this acute increase does *not* correlate well with long-term hypertrophy, at least in novel sessions or in untrained individuals. As noted by multiple authors, post-workout elevations in muscle protein synthesis appears to be insignificant in the context of adequate daily protein intake[9,12,13].

"While the positive effects of the protein or amino acid ingestion on muscle hypertrophy signalling can often be clear when studied acutely after each exercise, especially when the study was performed in a fasting state, the long-term positive effects may not be as robust with normal daily high protein consumption."
Hulmi et al., 2009[13].

Following a resistance training session, the trained muscle is more sensitive to protein consumption and the elevation in amino acids in the blood (from consuming protein) for at least 24 and up to 48 hours afterwards, not just for a few minutes or hours after. Therefore, total daily protein intake will have a greater influence on long term hypertrophy regardless of any immediate protein-mediated post-workout increase in muscle protein synthesis. As discussed later in chapter 10, immediate pre-workout or post-workout protein or carbohydrate consumption is fairy irrelevant for muscle growth in the content of sufficient daily protein and adequate carbohydrate intake. Indeed, muscle protein synthesis measured over the course of several weeks rather than on an acute post-exercise scale, within the context of a prolonged resistance training programme, appears to predict increases in muscle mass[11].

"Resistance physical exercise increases muscle tissue sensitivity to AA [amino acids] for up to 24 hours post-exercise, regardless of whether protein is consumed prior to, during or 1 to 3 hours post-workout. The major factor is evenly spread protein intake throughout the day, according to individual recommendations. Incremental induction of an anabolic state by repeated resistance physical exercise and diet is what boosts skeletal muscle remodelling and hypertrophy."
de Sousa Santos and Nascimento, 2019[9].

As important as protein-induced elevations in muscle protein synthesis are, single, acute elevations are much less important than day-to-day elevations in muscle protein synthesis. Therefore, the post-workout rise in muscle protein synthesis is not as important as once thought. *It is not a single resistance training session, nor a single protein-rich meal, but the long-term and consistent application of a resistance training programme coupled with adequate nutrition that results in muscle growth*[10,12]. Imagine a marathon. It doesn't matter if you run the last mile really fast, if the other 25 were slow, your time will be slow. It is much more effective to be consistent over each mile. A big dose of post-workout protein is less important than several well-sized doses across the day.

When at caloric maintenance without resistance training, muscle protein synthesis and muscle protein breakdown are usually *balanced* over the course of the day. To build significant muscle, muscle cells need to be stimulated primarily by resistance training and then with sufficient calorie intake and protein consumption. Resistance training can increase muscle protein synthesis and stimulate muscle growth. By consuming protein around your weight lifting session, you can increase muscle protein synthesis further. However, this acute effect appears to be fairly redundant when total protein intake is optimised[3]. So long as the protein source is sufficient to maximise muscle protein synthesis (which is usually a minimum 20g serving), it doesn't matter if you have this a couple of hours before your gym session, or a couple of hours after.

Protein for weight loss

How much protein do I need when in a calorie deficit or losing weight?

For preserving muscle mass in a deficit, 1.6g/kg of body weight per day is sufficient for untrained individuals with higher body fat percentages to preserve muscle mass and promote fat loss. Increasing protein intake up to 1.8-2.7g/kg of body weight or 2.3–3.1g/kg of lean mass per day may be beneficial to preserve muscle mass and promote fat loss in resistance trained individuals, but the evidence is limited.

There have been a good number of studies assessing weight loss with varying amounts of protein intake, but mainly in untrained people with higher body fat percentages. The effect of different protein intakes on trained individuals is less well researched.

When in a calorie deficit, weight loss comes from both fat and muscle mass, not just fat. Two individuals could both have a starting weight of 75kg. Over 10 weeks they could both lose 5kg of body weight whilst on a calorie deficit, which is a reasonable 0.5-1% of body weight loss per week. However, depending on certain factors, one person could lose mainly fat (e.g. 4.5kg or 90% of weight lost as fat mass and the remainder as muscle mass), and the other could lose significantly more muscle and less fat (e.g. 2kg or 40% of weight lost as fat mass, but also a

3kg or 60% drop in muscle mass). Clearly, the former individual has had the more successful weight loss (a more optimal change in body composition).

1.6g/kg of body weight of protein should be consumed throughout the day to minimise muscle loss whilst in a caloric deficit, and may need to be higher during a period of energy restriction[14]. Energy restriction results in a reduction in muscle protein synthesis, and therefore a more negative net protein balance. Higher protein intakes can offset this reduction in muscle protein synthesis. A systematic review demonstrated that with resistance training experience or in athletes, higher protein intakes appear to be more beneficial in preserving muscle mass. Intakes around 1.8-2.7g/kg of body weight or 2.3-3.1g/kg of lean mass per day have been recommended by researchers[14-17]. Studies using higher protein intakes during a calorie deficit result in the same weight loss, but with greater fat loss and less muscle loss, when calories are equated. This will scale with the size of the calorie deficit, and the body fat percentage of the individual[16]. Scaling protein intake to fat-free (lean) mass has been proposed to prevent underestimating protein intake in lean individuals, and overestimating protein intake in individuals with higher body fat levels. Previous researchers have recommended 1.8-2.7g/kg of body weight per day, which does not account for body composition[14,17]. The lower ends of the 2.3-3.1g/kg range may be sufficient for a resistance trained individual with a higher body fat percentage and smaller calorie deficit. For a resistance trained individual with a lower body fat percentage and a larger calorie deficit, the higher end of the range may be necessary[15]. The exact amount an individual may need currently cannot be assessed beyond these ranges. Scaling protein intake to fat-free mass is of course more complicated (how to roughly gauge your fat-free mass was discussed in chapter 7). The simpler 1.8-2.7g/kg of body weight measure is likely to be the more practical, useable form of the two recommendations for most people.

However, other authors have argued that protein intakes may not need to be so high in trained individuals[18]. Where you exactly set your protein intake will be largely down to personal preference. It is clear that intakes of 1.6g/kg of body weight are more beneficial than lower intakes, but the benefit from further increasing protein intake requires further study. Increasing protein intake above this appears to be more beneficial with training experience, at lower body fat percentages, and with larger calorie deficits. There appears to be no detrimental effect to consuming a slightly higher protein intake. As a means to 'cover all bases', higher intakes above 1.6g/kg of body weight can be considered to maximise any theoretical benefit, but possibly to the detriment of limiting fat or carbohydrate intake.

Losses in muscle mass during a calorie deficit are largely driven by reductions in muscle protein synthesis, not increases in muscle protein breakdown.

It can be tempting to think that if we are losing muscle during a calorie deficit then there must be a greater rate of muscle protein breakdown to result in a reduction in muscle mass. However, this does not appear to be the case.

Studies assessing variations in protein intake during a calorie deficit show muscle protein breakdown is pretty constant regardless of protein intake or training status during a calorie deficit[19,20]. There is some evidence for muscle protein breakdown to increase in lean individuals[17]. But, muscle protein breakdown is unlikely to increase significantly, because it is an energy costly process. It is unlikely any energy costly processes will increase during a period when energy availability is already limited, especially when considering the general adaptive response to *reduced* calorie intake is to *reduce* energy expenditure (chapter 5)[20]. Using our brick wall analogy, when in a calorie deficit there is a relatively constant level of taking out old bricks, but a reduced rate of adding new bricks. In other words, rather than using more energy to remove more bricks, less energy is used by adding fewer bricks.

Diet and exercise have a large influence on muscle protein synthesis. Studies have shown that having higher protein intakes during a calorie deficit can attenuate the calorie deficit-induced reduction in muscle protein synthesis[20]. This helps to preserve muscle mass, meaning a greater proportion of weight loss is derived from fat mass. Meta-analyses have demonstrated this to be true in normal weight people[21,22]. A systematic review has shown this to also be true in people with resistance training experience[16]. This does *not* mean you lose *more* weight. If you had two diets with the same size calorie deficit, but one diet provided protein intake at 0.8g/kg/day and the other at 2g/kg/day, you would lose the *same* amount of weight. But, the higher protein diet would lead to more weight lost as fat than muscle, compared to the lower protein diet.

The main factors that affect the ratio of *fat loss:muscle loss* during a calorie deficit include:

1. The **size of the calorie deficit**; proportionally more muscle is lost with a larger calorie deficit (when energy intake is far less than total daily energy expenditure).
2. The **body fat percentage** of the individual; higher body fat percentages will lose relatively less muscle mass compared to lower body fat percentages for a given calorie deficit.
3. **Daily protein intake**; greater protein intakes appear to preserve lean muscle mass better than low protein intakes during a calorie deficit (to an extent).
4. **Resistance training**; resistance training compared to no resistance training results in significantly greater preservation of muscle mass.
5. Other factors such as insufficient **sleep**, chronic **stress** and **nutritional deficiencies** will also result in greater muscle loss.

Use the points above as a *checklist* against your own plan to ensure you are not unknowingly losing unnecessary amounts of muscle during a calorie deficit. See chapter 7 to estimate the size of the calorie deficit you should aim for depending on your approximate body fat levels and gender.

How to increase protein intake in a calorie deficit

How would you go about shifting your diet to higher protein whilst *simultaneously* decreasing energy intake? Any dietary changes need to be sustainable and ones you can adhere to. There are two points to consider. How and with what foods are you going to *increase* protein intake, and how and with what foods are you going to ensure a *reduction* in daily calorie intake to ensure a calorie deficit?

If you were to enter a calorie deficit and increase protein intake, your fat and carbohydrate intakes are going to have to decrease. This may be aided by the appetite suppressing effects of protein (discussed later on in this chapter). Should you reduce both? Or primarily one? And if only one, which one? Although we are discussing macronutrients, the reality is that this would be achieved by reducing the quantity of food and/or drink you consume. You therefore need to consider through which elements of your diet you will achieve a reduction in energy intake. There's no right or wrong answer, just what suits you and your goals. The role of carbohydrate and fat intake during a calorie deficit have been discussed in chapter 8. You should consider:

- We *need* fats in our diet, therefore you should not reduce fat intake below the minimum recommendation of 0.5 g/kg of body weight per day (or 15-20% of total calorie intake)[16].
- Carbohydrates are not essential, but they are the primary fuel source for high intensity exercise. If you take part in resistance training and/or you need to ensure adequate exercise performance, then you may want to ensure carbohydrate intake is not severely restricted. A key part of preserving muscle in a calorie deficit is the stimulus of resistance training, ensuring that your training sessions are productive and that you do not lose strength or performance. Therefore, it may be beneficial to maintain carbohydrate intake and reduce fat intake to meet daily needs[16]. However, the extent to which you do this will be highly individualised.
- Your food choices. Protein, carbohydrate and fat are consumed within foods, not in isolation. Consider the foods in your overall dietary pattern, including your relative intake of *whole, plant-based foods* (e.g. fruit and vegetable intake) and *ultra-processed foods* (e.g. chocolate and chips). Consider how much you enjoy eating certain foods in your diet. Foods could be switched for alternatives that provide similar levels of satiety,

but with a lower energy content. Lower energy intake can be achieved by *replacing* higher energy density food choices with lower energy density food choices, or by reducing the energy density of your meals, rather than by reducing food volume. Chapter 12 will discuss food energy densities and their influence on energy intake. This should also give you a good idea of where you could reduce your calorie intake. If your fat intake is already low, trying to further reduce fat intake would not be ideal.

- Fat is more energy dense. Carbohydrate may provide greater satiety per calorie which may help to reduce appetite during the deficit, but this is highly dependent on your specific food choices.

You could achieve a higher protein intake with a more intuitive approach. You could as a one off, see how much protein you roughly consume per day. Say it is around 0.8g/kg of body weight per day. You could then just double your protein portions (provided your protein sources contain minimal fat or carbohydrate), or by having protein snacks in between meals, or adding 50% to the size of your protein portions at meals. Of course, this leaves room for significant error. Keeping a rough track, or exact track on protein intake may be easier for you.

Of note, professional muscle building athletes use a high protein, high carbohydrate and low fat strategy. Both carbohydrates and fats are dropped to preserve protein intake, as calories are gradually reduced to maintain the same rate of weight loss[23].

How often should I consume protein during the day whilst in a calorie deficit?

Spreading protein intake across the day is less important for reducing fat mass and preserving muscle mass during a calorie deficit.

Focus on total daily calorie and protein intake and eat protein-rich meals when they suit you.

Long-term studies show that the timing of protein and carbohydrate around a workout and having more frequent protein-rich meals does *not* result in greater fat loss and muscle preservation, when daily protein and carbohydrate intakes are sufficient[24]. Notably, most timing studies do not equate protein. Therefore, if the non-timing group has a sub-optimal intake, it could just be that the daily *absolute* increase in protein results in better outcomes, not the *timing* of the additional dose[24]. If there were to be any theoretical benefit to spreading protein intake across the day when losing weight, it is likely to be in trained individuals at lower body fat percentages. But, this is currently unproven due to a lack of research on the topic[24]. Although meal frequency is less important during a calorie deficit provided protein intake is sufficient, it is unlikely that you would consume protein across fewer than 3 meals per day. While unstudied, consuming all of your daily protein in one single meal would likely be sub-optimal for muscle preservation in a calorie deficit from the sub-optimal elevation in muscle protein synthesis across the day. However, such a feeding pattern is very uncommon. So, the general consensus is that any theoretical benefit of timing is probably already achieved with typical meal patterns, when considering elevations in muscle protein synthesis after a mixed meal lasts around 3-6 hours[17].

"The functional impact of differences in meal frequency at moderate ranges (e.g., 3–6 meals per day containing a minimum of 20 g protein each) are likely to be negligible in the context of a sound training program and properly targeted total daily micronutrition."
Helms et al., 2014[24].

Protein for muscle growth

How much protein do I need for building muscle?

Consume 1.6g of protein per kg of body weight per day (g/kg/day) when consuming complete protein sources (e.g. animal-based proteins).

Increase consumption to 1.8g/kg/day when consuming primarily incomplete protein sources (e.g. plant-based proteins within a vegan or vegetarian diet).

The minimum daily protein recommendation for sedentary individuals is 0.8g/kg/day[4].

When overfeeding (a calorie surplus), higher protein intakes result in improved outcomes in body composition, with proportionally more weight gain as muscle and less as fat [25]. However, this relationship does not continue indefinitely. There is a *limit* to the benefit of increasing protein intake during a calorie surplus. In people who do *not* resistance train, this benefit appears to increase up to 1.2-1.3g/kg/day. However, to optimise muscle growth *with* resistance training, this intake increases to 1.6g/kg/day[26]. The most recent and largest systematic review and meta-analysis on protein supplementation for muscle growth to date was of 49 randomised controlled trials[3]. The analysis found that protein supplementation does indeed result in greater increases in fat-free mass when daily protein intakes are low. A benefit of additional protein consumption to changes in fat-free mass is evident until daily protein consumption reaches 1.62g/kg/day. In other words, protein intake above 1.6g/kg/day does not result in further improvements in body composition. Similar daily intakes in other studies have been shown to promote muscle growth and is currently considered to be the optimum daily intake for muscle growth[24].

In resistance trained individuals, is there a limit as to how much additional protein is beneficial for muscle growth?

From the current evidence, the consensus is that 1.6g/kg/day is sufficient to optimise muscle growth in a surplus. However, the confidence interval in this estimate may mean that a slightly higher intake may be beneficial, up to 2.2g/kg/day. Also, most research is on untrained individuals. Some researchers have speculated a possible role of protein intakes greater than 1.6g/kg/day for muscle growth in trained individuals, but this is inconclusive.

If eating more protein results in more muscle growth for the same calorie surplus, what happens if we just keep eating more protein? More muscle? Unfortunately not. There appears to be a dose-response relationship between daily protein intake and muscle growth, up to a certain intake. Above which, protein intake has no additional benefit (i.e. a plateau)[3]. Meta-analyses demonstrate increased muscle mass when increasing protein intake up to 1.6g/kg/day; consuming greater amounts per day does not translate into further increases in muscle size. But, meta-analyses and other studies consider protein intake in individuals with a wide range of characteristics, including a large number of untrained individuals. Furthermore, the *confidence interval* (the range of values between which the true optimal protein intake probably lies, see chapter 4) in the most recent meta-analysis on protein intake varied from 1.0 to 2.2g/kg/day[2]. Therefore, some researchers have suggested that trained individuals looking to maximise daily muscle protein synthesis may opt for the upper limits of the confidence interval[3]. And as always, the response to protein intake will vary between individuals, such that some individuals may need slightly more, and some slightly less protein per day.

For very experienced resistance trained individuals, some researchers have suggested that even higher protein intakes during a caloric surplus may promote greater improvements in body composition, but not necessarily greater muscle growth[15]. Such suggestions are based on a few studies with limitations and expert opinion, meaning the strength of the recommendation to do so is weak.

One study by Antonio et al. demonstrated that feeding resistance trained people with 4.4g of protein per kg of body weight per day (g/kg/day) did *not* result in greater improvements in body composition compared to resistance trained individuals consuming 1.8g/kg/day[27]. In this study, participants continued their typical training regime. In another study by Antonio et al., they compared

2.3g/kg/day and 3.4g/kg/day in resistance trained men and women[28]. However in this study, the training programme of participants was changed. They were given a new heavy resistance training programme. The addition of a heavy programme led to improved outcomes in body composition in the higher protein group. Both groups gained similar levels of fat-free mass, but the 3.4g/kg/day group lost more fat mass than the 2.3g/kg/day group. This is somewhat complicated by the fact that the 3.4g/kg/day group also consumed more calories than the 2.3g/kg/day group. Although interesting, given the recovery demands of the new programme, the difference could be explained by the different energy intakes and other factors such as hydration, sleep quality, compliance to training or the accuracy of participants self-reporting their food intake[28]. It is probable that whether higher protein intakes are beneficial will depend on the demands of the training being performed and training experience. In a double-blind study (neither the researchers nor participants knew who received which intervention), researchers gave army soldiers either whey protein supplements or energy-matched carbohydrate supplements. Both drinks added 580kcal to the daily calorie intakes of the soldiers[29]. After 8 weeks of intensive army training, greater improvements in body composition were found in those consuming the whey protein supplement. Both groups maintained weight and both similarly increased muscle mass. But, a greater reduction in fat mass was seen in the whey protein group. It cannot be overlooked that due to the greater fat loss, participants consuming whey protein may have been in a caloric deficit. Both groups initially consumed around 1.6g/kg/day. During the study, the whey protein group consumed 2.8g/kg/day and the carbohydrate group consumed 1.6g/kg/day. Participants were beginning an initial entry training programme for the army, which is physically demanding and likely involving high levels of muscle damage[29]. Therefore, higher protein intakes may be more beneficial when training demands are greater. Trained individuals require a greater *training volume* than untrained people to promote muscle growth (chapter 19). The additional training volume may explain the beneficial effects of higher protein intakes than 1.6g/kg/day seen in some studies of trained individuals.

Theoretically, protein *may* need to be higher in trained individuals, to counterbalance a potential increase in muscle protein breakdown with a greater increase in muscle protein synthesis[30]. In contrast, other researchers have argued *against* a need for higher intakes because of the limited evidence showing a benefit. Some studies have demonstrated that trained individuals become more efficient with using protein, such that protein requirements might be lower in trained individuals[30].

Higher protein intakes have been shown to be safe. As a trained individual, consume at least 1.6g/kg of body weight per day, possibly up to 2.2g/kg of body weight per day or higher depending on personal choice[2,15,25]. Even if trained individuals are more efficient with protein, there is little benefit to reducing intake (i.e. it would not result in greater muscle growth) below 1.6g/kg/day, when compared to the greater risk of a sub-optimal protein intake. Given the possible, but inconclusive evidence suggesting benefit to higher intakes, further consumption should be down to personal preference. There appears to be little negative implications to a marginal increase. When considering total daily energy intake, increasing protein intakes above 1.6g/kg of body weight per day may limit fat and/or carbohydrate intake.

You can't just eat unlimited protein in a calorie surplus; it can be stored as fat if you overeat. However, overfeeding on protein appears to differ from fat or carbohydrate overfeeding.

Eating too much of any macronutrient (fat, carbohydrate or protein) such that you enter a calorie surplus, will lead to weight gain. Protein is energy. Eating large amounts of protein can induce fat storage in a calorie surplus. A biochemical pathway of protein being converted to fat in humans exists[31]. In the same way that fat can be oxidised (burnt to be used as energy), eating more protein can also allow for surplus protein to be used for energy, with an increase in protein oxidation[32]. The thought is that the higher thermic effect of protein reduces how much protein is stored as fat. However, weight gain is the result of a calorie surplus, and weight will still be gained because any fat or carbohydrate that is consumed can be readily stored. Increasing protein intake can promote increases in fat-free mass during a surplus unlike overfeeding on carbohydrate or fat[15]. But, metabolic ward studies show overfeeding on protein can still increase fat mass as a result of the extra energy[33,34]. Some studies show that calorie surpluses as a result of higher protein intakes do not lead to increases in fat mass. However, these studies are limited because dietary intakes are *not* tightly controlled or accurately calculated in these studies, as they are in metabolic ward studies. Therefore, calorie surpluses were most likely not present, possibly due to compensatory mechanisms (such as from protein-induced satiety and changes in exercise and non-exercise activity thermogenesis or adaptive thermogenesis)[35]. Differences between participants' dietary reporting and their *actual* energy expenditure may also account for this difference. Self-reporting of energy intake is often significantly less than peoples' true energy intake[36].

How much protein do I need per meal to build muscle?

The quantity needed will vary depending on your age, weight and if you have just trained. But for young adults, 0.25-0.50g/kg/meal or around 20-40g will result in maximal stimulation of muscle protein synthesis.

A review of the evidence by two evidence-based fitness experts (Brad Schoenfeld and Alan Aragon) suggest that you should calculate your daily protein needs (e.g. 1.6g/kg of body weight per day) and split this between how many meals you habitually consume, rather than worrying specifically about eating too much protein at each meal[26].

A single acute rise in muscle protein synthesis does *not* relate to muscle growth. But, it is the continual elevation of muscle protein synthesis following meals containing protein that chronically elevates muscle protein synthesis, which *does* relate to muscle growth. Each meal is as important as the one before and the one after in elevating muscle protein synthesis, and no meal is more important. Therefore, whenever we have a meal we want to maximally stimulate muscle protein synthesis for muscle growth, to ensure a more positive net protein balance across the day. We can assess this by getting people to eat different amounts of protein and measure rates of muscle protein synthesis. Muscle protein synthesis appears to increase in a dose-dependent manner when consuming up to 20g of protein[11]. Consuming less than 20g of protein, such as 10g, is insufficient to maximally stimulate muscle protein synthesis, or stimulate muscle protein synthesis significantly above no protein intake at all[37,38]. To maximise muscle protein synthesis, some studies show peak muscle protein synthesis occurs after consuming 20g of protein; others show even greater muscle protein synthesis with quantities up to 40g, but studies do not find increased muscle protein synthesis above 40g of protein[11]. 20g will result in a near-maximal increase in muscle protein synthesis. Consuming up to 40g can increase muscle protein synthesis by a further 10-20%[11]. Achieving maximal muscle protein synthesis is commonly referred to in the literature as the *'muscle full'* effect. Muscle protein synthesis peaks around 30 minutes after a sufficient *fast-digesting* protein dose and is elevated for several hours, before returning back to baseline levels[39]. The larger the dose, the longer the duration of elevated muscle protein synthesis. There appears to be a *'refractory period'*, whereby additional protein consumption does not further elevate muscle protein synthesis, even though muscle protein synthesis will start to decline[40]. Several hours after the initial protein dose, muscle protein synthesis can once again be elevated. Typical meal patterns of 3-4 meals per day seems to best elevate muscle protein synthesis across the day[41].

The context in which the protein is ingested will affect digestion and absorption, but this does not necessarily influence muscle protein synthesis. Most studies assess fast digesting proteins in isolation, which is not necessarily the same as consuming protein within a mixed meal of food containing carbohydrates and fats. Therefore, the changes in muscle protein synthesis from consuming isolated protein in research studies may differ to the changes in muscle protein synthesis from consuming a mixed meal in real-life. For example, consuming minced meat results in a faster rise in amino acid levels in the blood than consuming the same amount of protein as a steak, but with no effect on rates of muscle protein synthesis[42]. Consuming protein from whole eggs compared to an equivalent amount of protein from egg white results in greater muscle protein synthesis after a resistance training session[43]. This occurred even though the egg whites caused a more rapid rise in blood amino acid levels and in particular *leucine*, an important amino acid for muscle protein synthesis[43]. The food matrix itself and the other nutritional content with the protein may augment changes in muscle protein synthesis[39]. And again, most studies assessing muscle protein synthesis after a mixed meal simply add rapidly digesting carbohydrates to protein drinks. The limited evidence suggests a mixed meal would have the effect of slowing the rate of digestion and absorption of protein, such that the protein source in the meal resembles a slow digesting protein[11].

Consuming more than 40g of protein in a single meal does not result in this protein not being digested and absorbed, or 'wasted'. The protein is absorbed. But, it does not further benefit muscle protein synthesis.

Doses higher than 40g per meal are not *'wasted'*. The amino acids in the protein will still be absorbed in the gut and be utilised for building and repairing, or used as energy. In other words, if you eat a large amount of protein in one meal (such as half a chicken), your gut would still digest and absorb the protein content. Muscle protein synthesis would be maximally stimulated. Some of the energy would be lost from the thermic effect of protein. The additional amino acids will be oxidised (used as energy). If in a caloric surplus, fat storage can result through conversion of protein or carbohydrate to fat or direct storage of consumed fat[34]. Doses greater than around 20-40g do not lead to further increases in muscle protein synthesis, but consumed protein is still used in some manner.

*Protein doses above 40g reduce mu*scle *protein breakdown, but this is not necessarily beneficial.*

Studies show that consuming larger doses of protein above 40g does not further increase muscle protein synthesis but can reduce muscle protein breakdown, generating a more positive net protein balance[42,44]. However, these studies measure *whole-body breakdown* (which includes protein breakdown in tissues besides muscle, such as protein breakdown in the gut). Many other cells and tissues continually undergo breakdown and synthesis, not just muscles. This may not be related to the protein breakdown that occurs in muscles, which accounts for around 25% of whole-body muscle protein breakdown[2]. However as discussed in the brick wall analogy, it is likely that muscle breakdown has an important role in the remodelling and repair of muscle[2]. Whether reducing breakdown has any benefit on body composition is not understood. Low quality evidence actually suggests muscle protein breakdown is required for maintaining proper muscle function[2]. There is currently no evidence to suggest a benefit to muscle growth by suppressing muscle protein breakdown. Therefore, it makes sense to just focus on maximising muscle protein synthesis and not to focus on minimising muscle protein breakdown[32]. Jorn Trommellen is an academic who has just completed his PhD researching the effects of protein consumption. He has summarised nicely using the brick wall analogy why focussing on muscle protein synthesis and not on muscle protein breakdown is probably best. Muscle protein breakdown serves as a useful tool to remove weak, old protein[11]. If we have a very large amount of protein and suppress muscle protein breakdown, it may mean that some of these weak, old proteins remain in the muscle. Much like keeping weak, old bricks in the wall, this may lead to issues in the future. Again, the aim should be daily total protein intake. An occasional large amount of protein in a meal to ensure total daily protein intake is achieved is unlikely to have any negative consequences. But, only consuming 1 or 2 very high-protein meals is probably sub-optimal for elevating muscle protein synthesis across the day.

To optimise muscle protein synthesis across the day, consume at least 20g of protein at each meal, but ideally not much greater than 40g. Occasional large protein doses greater than 40g should not be of concern, however.

How often should I consume protein during the day?

Any typical meal frequency of 3-6 meals per day with snacks is perfectly suitable for maintaining elevated muscle protein synthesis across the day, with protein at each meal.

Frequency is largely irrelevant when total daily protein intake is sufficient. However, this is does not mean that one single protein-rich meal is as effective as several meals; these conclusions are from studies where participants have more than one or two protein feedings per day. For muscle growth we want to maximally stimulate muscle protein synthesis across the day. This rise in muscle protein synthesis after a protein-rich meal usually lasts 3-6 hours. Therefore, we can maximise daily muscle protein synthesis by splitting our total daily protein intake throughout the day in 3 to 6-hour intervals to maintain elevated levels of muscle protein synthesis, which is achieved with any 'typical' meal frequency. This is beneficial for increasing muscle mass. To increase the ability to adhere to the diet, consume protein in as few meals as feasibly possible.

Spreading protein throughout the day to maintain elevated levels of muscle protein synthesis is more important during a phase aimed at muscle growth. During a caloric deficit, protein frequency appears to be less important when the goal is fat loss and muscle preservation, where the focus should be to just consume a sufficient total daily protein intake.

Calorie intake is the dietary priority for muscle growth. Relative to this, nutrient timing is secondary and much less important. However, studies assessing daily protein intake have discovered interesting findings. It appears that spreading protein intake out across the day leads to greater muscle protein synthesis and a more positive net protein balance over 24 hours, compared to having *all* protein in one meal, or *unevenly* distributing protein across meals. For example, consuming 75g of protein as 10g, 15g and 50g at three different meals across the day does not maintain muscle protein synthesis as effectively as 3 equal doses of 25g[41,45]. Net protein balance is the difference between muscle protein synthesis and breakdown. If there is greater muscle protein synthesis from spreading protein intake across the day, then there will be relatively greater muscle protein synthesis than breakdown, and therefore a relatively higher net protein balance. With our brick wall analogy, this will result in more bricks being added than taken away, meaning our brick wall gets bigger, and likewise, our muscles get bigger. This achieves a more positive net protein balance without necessarily reducing muscle protein breakdown, which may be important for remodelling and repair[2]. If you haven't eaten any protein all day and you are aiming to consume 1.6g/kg/day, then you would be better off consuming your protein needs in one or two meals, rather than having a much lower protein intake to avoid eating it all in large amounts. Again, the underlying key is to consume enough protein in the first place. Similarly, there isn't a need to, nor is it more beneficial to try and split your daily protein requirements across as many meals as possible with 20g of protein[41].

Nearer 20g, or nearer 40g of protein per meal?

This should largely be dictated by: 1.6g/kg of your body weight in protein divided by the number of meals you consume per day. For 3-6 meals per day, this equates to 0.25-0.50g protein per kg of body weight per meal.

Preference for more frequent, smaller meals = nearer 20g.

Preference for less frequent, larger meals = nearer 40g.

Choice of protein source (complete vs incomplete protein) will also influence the quantity of protein per meal. Larger quantities of incomplete proteins are required to maximise muscle protein synthesis compared to complete proteins.

Whether you opt for the lower or higher end of 20-40g will depend on your calculated total protein intake and how many meals (and any snacks) you wish to have throughout the day. This should simply be dictated by dividing your total protein intake by the number of meals you eat per day. Fewer meals per day, larger quantities of protein per meal. More meals per day, smaller quantities of protein per meal. For example, let's say you are aiming to build muscle, so your total daily protein intake is 1.6g/kg of body weight per day. You like to eat 3 meals per day (breakfast, lunch and dinner) with snacks mid-morning and mid-afternoon. If you were 70kg, this would mean splitting 112g (70 × 1.6) across the day. Splitting this across your 3 meals would mean consuming 35-40g of protein per meal (112 ÷ 3), which is at the upper end of the range. However, you could also split the 112g across the 3 meals and 2 snacks (115 ÷ 5 = 22-25g). Both options are perfectly fine and valid choices[46]. Your meals before and after a workout could contain a higher amount of protein (e.g. 3 × 20g, and 2 × 25-30g several hours before and after a workout).

The literature base on this is still fairly small. Whether a minor increase in spreading protein across *more* than 3 meals leads to any meaningful increases in muscle mass is unclear, but appears unlikely. Less frequent meals will mean larger doses. When consumed in the context of a mixed meal, 3 meals can be sufficient to maximise muscle protein synthesis across the day, as mixed meals can delay protein digestion and absorption compared to protein consumed in isolation[2]. Long term studies are needed as most studies have focussed on the effects of fast-acting protein sources in isolation (e.g. a whey protein drink), and not mixed-meals (consuming protein with carbohydrates and fats from food sources, such as a roast dinner). The main focus is on consuming sufficient daily protein. Then, focus on spreading your protein across sufficiently large and even doses throughout the day. For some that might be 5 to 6 meals or snacks. Similarly, for some this might be achieved with 3 meals.

When should I consume protein around a workout?

The benefits to consuming protein on muscle protein synthesis can occur for several hours pre- or post-workout. Timing is largely down to personal preference. When consuming adequate daily protein, protein timing around a workout is relatively unimportant for muscle growth. Protein can be consumed within a 4 to 6 hour window of the training session. The effect of protein timing is not as important as consuming sufficient protein during the day.

A recent systematic review and meta-analysis of 49 studies showed that when total protein intake is sufficient, the timing of protein intake around a workout is *meaningless* for muscle growth[3]. In other words, timing protein immediately before or after a workout can increase muscle mass and strength when protein intake is sub-optimal, but consuming sufficient protein (1.6g/kg of body weight per day) eradicates the need to consume protein within an hour of a workout. Any differences in hypertrophy are the result of differences in total protein intake[7]. However, considering the role of protein around a workout in further increasing muscle protein synthesis, it would make sense to not completely avoid protein consumption for several hours before or after a workout if it is feasible to do so[26]. Immediate protein intake may not be necessary, but delaying protein intake would not be more beneficial either. If you have the opportunity to consume protein close to a workout, then by all means do so. Of course, if you struggle to consume enough protein daily then by all means consume it as and when you can. A more important factor is just ensuring you are able to consume it, by considering your lifestyle pattern. It is completely fine if that requires consumption very close to your workout. There is no problem with protein consumption near to a workout, there is just unlikely to be any benefit.

If you are meeting your daily protein needs, then don't panic about immediate pre- and post-workout protein. This can be useful to know, if for certain reasons you are unable to consume a meal before or after training, safe in the knowledge that a slightly later meal will not be detrimental.

Chapter 10 covers nutrient timing in more detail.

Are high protein diets (>3 g/kg/day) safe?

Very high protein intakes as great as 4.4g/kg/day have been shown to have no adverse health effects for a range of health markers in healthy individuals. In other words, it's not going to cause any problems if you're a healthy person with no existing problems.

The protein intakes recommended for muscle gain and weight loss are far below the highest intakes shown to still be safe in studies. Even though they are safe, little evidence suggests such high protein intakes (>3.3g/kg/day) are necessary for fat loss or muscle gain.

Any essential nutrient can become toxic at excessively high levels[47]. Water is essential, but overload can be fatal[48]. Minerals such as potassium and sodium are essential, but excess intakes can also be lethal[49]. Therefore, the question isn't whether excessive protein intake may be detrimental, but how high can protein intake be without causing adverse effects? It is important to note that there is *no* universal agreement as to what constitutes a *high protein diet* in the research literature[50]. Typically, high protein intake is considered as 1.2g/kg/day. But, many researchers may consider 1.2g/kg/day to be low, and 3g/kg/day or more as high.

All current literature to date assessing protein intake and health have found *no evidence* of high protein intakes being unsafe or causing any adverse problems in *healthy* people[50,51]. High protein intakes potentially cause problems, but *only* in people with *pre-existing* health problems, such as those with kidney disease[1].

One study found no harmful effects after 12 months on a high protein diet of 2.5-3.3g/kg of body weight per day[52]. Another study found no harmful effects of a high protein diet of 2.6-3.3g/kg of body weight per day after 4 months[53]. Other studies have reported no side effects of high (>3.0g/kg of body weight per day) intakes in healthy individuals[27,47].

Safe upper limits have been determined to be 3.5g/kg of body weight per day for adults[47]. This limit exists because studies have not fully assessed safety at intakes greater than 3.5g/kg/day, meaning recommendations cannot be made for higher intakes, rather than because higher intakes are unsafe.

High protein diets do *not* appear to have a harmful effect on a number of health measures[51]:

- **Cardiovascular health.** Higher protein diets are at worst equivocal to low protein diets, and at best superior to low protein diets for cardiovascular health[47,50]. A meta-analysis of whey protein supplementation on blood lipids demonstrated no effect on blood cholesterol levels[54].
- **Liver function.** The current evidence does not show a risk of high protein intake on kidney function in healthy people[47].
- **Kidney function**. The current evidence does not show a risk of high protein intake on kidney function in healthy people[47].
- **Bone health[55].** A systematic review and meta-analysis of randomised controlled trials assessing protein intake and bone mineral density demonstrated that increased protein intakes positively influence bone health[47,50,56].
- **Sleep.** Short-term studies show no effect of protein intake on sleep quantity or quality[55].

"Multiple review articles indicate that no controlled scientific evidence exists indicating that increased intakes of protein pose any health risks in healthy, exercising individuals. Statements by large regulatory bodies have also indicated that concerns about one's health secondary to ingesting high amounts of protein are unfounded. A series of controlled investigations spanning up to one year in duration utilizing protein intakes of up to 2.5–3.3 g/kg/day in healthy resistance-trained individuals consistently indicate that increased intakes of protein exert no harmful effect on blood lipids or markers of kidney and liver function."
Jäger et al., 2017[1].

Another point to remember is the influence of high protein diets on weight loss. As pointed out by Alexandra Johnstone, a leading researcher on diets from the University of Aberdeen, the health benefits from weight loss would *outweigh* any theoretical (and as yet unproven) risk of high protein diets[50].

High protein diets are associated with animal-based food consumption. However, a large oversight is that a high protein diet can also be achieved on a *plant-based diet*[46]. Such a diet would provide the additional benefit of increased fibre and phytonutrient consumption[46]. The health effects of high protein itself, the effects of different high-protein food sources, and any other physical or dietary changes (e.g. weight gain or loss from a calorie surplus or deficit) need to be controlled for in future studies.

Nevertheless, there is little evidence to support utilising very high protein intakes for body composition. For muscle growth, intake should be in the range of 1.6g/kg, possibly up to 2.2g/kg. For fat loss in a caloric deficit, a minimum of 1.6g/kg in untrained people, increasing to 1.8-2.7g/kg of body weight or 2.3–3.1 g/kg of lean mass per day for trained people. The high intakes recommended during a calorie deficit are still well below intakes that have been studied. Even so, calorie deficits are not long-term phases; higher protein intakes are only used for a relatively short period (e.g. weeks to months) during weight loss.

Very high protein diets are safe, but there isn't any strong evidence to support using them.

Which protein sources should I consume?

Broadly, proteins can be classed on their amino acid content (complete, incomplete), digestibility (fast digesting, slow digesting) and bioavailability. These factors determine the 'quality' of a protein source. Animal-based protein sources are generally of a higher quality than plant-based protein sources. Different proteins have slightly different effects on the body.

Complete sources contain all the essential amino acids. Examples include meat, dairy (whey and casein), fish, soy and eggs. Incomplete sources are missing some or contain low amounts of the essential amino acids. Examples include beans, peas, oats, legumes and nuts. Most plant-based protein sources are incomplete.

For the same quantity, incomplete proteins do not stimulate muscle protein synthesis to the same degree as complete proteins. Consume a larger portion of incomplete protein to ensure maximal muscle protein synthesis. Increase daily protein intake from 1.6g/kg to

1.8g/kg of body weight per day for muscle growth if you primarily eat incomplete proteins, such as in vegan or vegetarian diets. Aim to consume a range of incomplete proteins across the day to prevent amino acid deficiencies.

Most studies assessing protein intake and muscle protein synthesis are acute, lab-based studies of protein intake in isolation which may not reflect long-term, real-world habitual protein intakes from whole foods.

No evidence suggests that once differences in protein sources are considered by adjusting daily protein intake, that any protein source (e.g. animal- vs plant-based, complete vs incomplete, fast vs slow) is superior or more beneficial for fat loss or muscle growth.

Not all protein sources are equal in terms of their effects on the body[2]. Protein sources may contain sufficient quantities of all 9 essential amino acids (a *complete protein*), or contain all 9, but with an inadequate balance, or missing one or more of the 9 essential amino acids (an *incomplete protein*)[32]. Combining incomplete protein sources can provide all the essential amino acids needed to avoid deficiency. Incomplete proteins are seen as lower quality protein sources, because for the same quantity they do not stimulate muscle protein synthesis to the same extent as a complete protein[2].

Complete proteins include:

Casein and whey (milk), poultry, meat (beef, pork, lamb), fish, eggs and soy[57].

Incomplete proteins include:

Most plant protein sources: beans, peas, legumes, nuts and pulses[57].

There are differences beyond this distinction that affects how well a protein stimulates muscle protein synthesis. This includes the quantity of *branched-chain amino acids* (and in particular the amino acid *leucine*), the *digestibility* of the protein source (fast digesting proteins result in a rapid rise in amino acids in the blood, which quickly elevates muscle protein synthesis compared to slow digesting proteins) and the *bioavailability* of the amino acids in the protein, which all affect the rate and extent to which a protein source stimulates muscle protein synthesis[58]. Protein quality can be quantified using the *protein digestibility-corrected amino acid score (PDCAAS)* or the *digestibility indispensable amino acid (DIAA)* score[46,57,59].

Animal based proteins are complete, with high digestibility and bioavailability. Plant-based proteins are generally incomplete with lower digestibility and bioavailability[58]. Milk, egg, whey, casein and beef protein have the highest possible PDCAA score at 1.0. Soy protein has a score of 0.91, pea of 0.67 and oats of 0.57[46].

Whey protein is a high-quality protein. It has a high branched-chain amino acid (BCAA) content, is rapidly digested and contains readily bioavailable amino acids. This means it can rapidly and effectively stimulate muscle protein synthesis[2]. Soy is also complete and is one of the few plant-based complete protein sources[2]. It has a lower BCAA content than whey and fewer bioavailable amino acids[7]. In particular, soy has half the amount of the amino acid leucine compared to whey. Leucine is an important amino acid involved in stimulating muscle protein synthesis*. Maximal muscle protein synthesis is achieved at a certain quantity of leucine within a protein source, and has been termed the 'leucine threshold'[7,39]. Maximal muscle protein synthesis also requires other essential amino acids (EAAs) to be present[2]. To maximally stimulate muscle protein synthesis, a protein source needs to contain a minimum amount of leucine. Because protein sources vary in leucine content, this means the quantity of protein needed to maximally stimulate muscle protein synthesis varies between sources. Plant-based sources typically contain lower quantities of leucine compared to animal-based sources. The threshold to maximise muscle protein synthesis is probably around 2g of leucine at each protein-rich meal, but this can be influenced by age and whether you have just trained. So, this should be considered a minimum[7,46]. You don't need to start checking protein sources for their leucine content. The leucine threshold concept was developed through studies of isolated protein sources, and may not even be relevant to protein intake from mixed meals[39]. Just ensure a meal has at least 20-40g of protein, which would ensure leucine intake is above 2g. For an incomplete protein, aim for the higher end of this range to ensure maximal muscle protein synthesis with each meal to ensure the leucine threshold is met. The lower end of this range is sufficient for maximal muscle protein synthesis when consuming animal-based protein sources.

The result of this means that a diet primarily consisting of protein from incomplete protein sources will require a slightly higher daily protein intake that is above 1.6g/kg of body weight per day. A minimum of *1.8g/kg of body weight per day* is advised to maximally stimulate muscle protein synthesis when consuming incomplete protein sources[2]. For example, studies assessing muscle protein synthesis after ingesting the same quantity of soy or whey protein (25g) show greater muscle protein synthesis after whey consumption[7]. Some studies find greater muscle growth with whey compared to soy protein supplementation (i.e. complete vs incomplete protein). However, this appears to be due to the habitually low protein intakes in participants[7]. At much higher doses of whey, soy or rice protein (>40g), muscle protein synthesis is maximally stimulated in all conditions and no difference exists between groups in terms of muscle growth. Participants in these studies were on high protein diets. Therefore, any differences in protein source quality were attenuated as total daily protein needs were optimised[7,60–62]. It should be noted that these studies supplement with an animal- or plant-based protein source, rather than compare animal- or plant-based diets[58]. No long-term controlled study to date has assessed diets containing *only* complete or incomplete protein (i.e. animal-based compared to plant-based protein sources) and muscle growth. Observational studies show that higher protein intakes result in greater muscle mass. Plant-based diets generally result in less muscle growth, however often this is due to lower protein intakes with plant-based diets. At comparable intakes from animal- or plant-based sources, muscle growth tends to be lower in plant-based diets. But, when plant-based protein intakes are greater, muscle growth appears similar[58].

Again, the primary concern should be achieving a sufficient total daily protein intake. As such, when total protein intake is *adjusted* for protein quality, animal and plant-based protein sources are *equivalent* for body composition outcomes. The choice of protein source should therefore be down to personal preference.

The role of leucine has led to some confusion, with branched-chain amino acid (BCAA) supplementation being perceived to be beneficial to promote muscle protein synthesis (see chapter 25 regarding BCAA supplementation). BCAA supplementation has been shown to result in greater muscle protein synthesis after a workout. But, usually this is compared to a placebo of water, no calories or a carbohydrate control. When compared to a complete protein source such as whey protein, BCAA supplementation provides no benefit, even when adding additional BCAA to an optimal dose of whey protein. BCAAs and in particular leucine, stimulate muscle protein synthesis. However, their effect becomes limited in the presence (or lack of) other amino acids. Therefore, complete protein sources result in greater anabolic responses[2]. Evidence shows no superior benefit to BCAA supplementation on muscle growth compared to whole protein sources[9,63]. Therefore, the focus on protein consumption should be on whole protein sources that are complete, or incomplete but at larger doses.

If you primarily consume plant-based proteins and consume on the lower end of current recommendations (at or lower than 1.6g/kg/day)[64], then it may be wise to consume a greater quantity and range of plant-based protein sources or consider consuming animal-based sources. Increase consumption to at least 1.8g/kg of body weight per day to factor in the lower quality of plant-based incomplete protein sources. It is not necessary to consume a range of incomplete sources at each meal, just a range of incomplete sources across the day to ensure adequate daily essential amino acid intake. If you are vegan or vegetarian, you may wish to consider a plant-based protein supplement to achieve this. So as long as you do not limit yourself to eating only one incomplete protein source, amino acid deficiency should not an issue.

Fast vs slow digesting proteins

Fast digesting proteins result in faster elevations in amino acid (the building blocks of protein) levels in the blood after consumption than slower digesting proteins[32,39,58]. Consuming other macronutrients with protein as a mixed meal will also affect the rate of absorption from the gut, slowing the response[39]. Rapidly digesting protein consumed by itself (such as whey protein in a drink) would logically be absorbed much faster than protein consumed in a solid meal alongside carbohydrates and fats, which will slow down the absorption rate. It may be that rapidly digesting proteins are more likely to be oxidised (used for energy) than protein consumed as a meal, so the same amount of protein in a meal may lead to greater use in protein synthesis than oxidation. The practical use of this in real life is still *unknown* (such as whether it influences body composition). However, considering meta-analyses of many different diets utilising a wide range of protein sources (i.e. from fast digesting protein sources in isolation to slow digesting protein sources within a mixed meal) find a consensus of 1.6g/kg of body weight of protein per day, the influence of consuming protein in a mixed meal compared to in isolation is at best a *minor* consideration[50]. Nevertheless, variations between different protein sources may contribute to the wide confidence interval (1.0-2.2g/kg/day) around the 1.6g/kg/day average from the most-recent meta-analysis[3]. More research needs to be done before further recommendations can be made. *No* controlled study to date has compared diets of fast digesting protein and slow digesting protein on muscle growth. For now, focus on meeting total daily protein needs. Ensure that when you eat protein, you consume more than 20g as a minimum to maximise muscle protein synthesis. If consuming plant-based proteins, aim for the upper ranges of daily intakes and per meal intakes. Beyond this, most other factors appear to be rather irrelevant.

Are protein supplements beneficial?

The primary benefit of a protein supplement is to meet your daily protein needs if you struggle to achieve this through conventional food sources. Protein supplements are a completely safe and convenient method of meeting daily protein needs[2]. Beyond this, protein supplementation does not provide benefit. Protein supplementation is effective at lower daily protein intakes. Once an individual is consuming 1.6g of protein per kg of body weight per day (g/kg/day), there is no further advantage to consuming protein supplements for muscle growth[3].

This is discussed in detail in chapter 25.

The most recent and largest systematic review and meta-analysis on protein supplementation for muscle growth to date was of 49 randomised controlled trials[3]. Previous studies and analyses have shown conflicting findings. However, previous studies often did not control for potentially influential variables, such as training experience, daily protein intakes and the age of participants[65]. By considering these factors and conducting more detailed analyses, the new meta-analysis found protein supplementation does indeed result in greater increases in fat-free mass when daily protein intakes are low. A benefit to fat-free mass is evident until daily protein consumption reaches 1.62g/kg/day. Of note, the average pre-supplementation protein intake was 1.4g/kg/day. Therefore, even small additions of supplemental protein of around 35g per day, or 0.2g/kg/day can have significant beneficial effects on strength and fat-free mass[3]. *Protein supplements are just convenient sources of protein.* There is *no* superior benefit of protein supplementation once total daily protein intake has been optimised. The lack of any effect of protein timing, source, dose or post-exercise protein timing once sufficient daily intake is achieved also highlights the *minor* role these factors have on muscle growth relative to total protein intake[3].

If you struggle to consume sufficient protein from whole food sources due to food volume (this may be more of an issue when consuming low energy density foods), then a protein supplement may be beneficial. If you can consume enough from whole food sources, then a protein supplement may not be necessary. Protein supplements can provide an easily accessible, convenient form of protein that may be more suitable for busy lifestyles. When purchased in large volumes, they can also be a *cost-effective* protein source relative to whole food sources.

Consuming slow-digesting protein such as casein before sleep can stimulate overnight muscle protein synthesis.

Pre-sleep protein intake can be an effective way of ensuring *acute* (post-workout or post-meal elevations in muscle protein synthesis) and *chronic* (consuming sufficient daily protein over a period of days and weeks) responses to resistance training for muscle growth are achieved.

If the last meal of the day is several hours before bed, then assuming a good night of sleep is 7-8 hours in duration, it may well be another 12 hours until the next meal is consumed[2]. Such an extended period may result in the body being in a state of net protein breakdown from a decline in muscle protein synthesis.

A body of studies have assessed protein intake prior to sleep. Notably, the consumption of casein protein (a type of protein found in milk) can stimulate overnight muscle protein synthesis. Studies show consuming casein protein after a resistance training session before bed can promote overnight increases in muscle protein synthesis[66]. The gut does function effectively overnight, and any pre-sleep protein is digested and absorbed[67]. Day to day elevations in muscle protein synthesis result in long-term hypertrophy. Theoretically, keeping muscle protein synthesis elevated across the day and overnight may be beneficial for muscle growth in a calorie surplus. Studies have shown that protein consumed before sleep does get incorporated into new muscle tissue during a resistance training programme[67]. This will also be of more importance if you prefer to perform your resistance training in the evenings.

The duration of the overnight period would imply a slow digesting protein such as casein over a fast digesting protein such as whey would best maintain elevated muscle protein synthesis throughout the night. However, faster digesting proteins appear to also elicit a similar overnight response[67]. The main focus should be on a large (e.g. 40g) pre-sleep protein intake to generate a prolonged elevation in muscle protein synthesis, rather than the specific protein in question.

Putting these acute findings back into context, whether these acute overnight changes in muscle protein synthesis have *any* significance in the long-term for muscle growth is not clear. But, there are no detrimental effects and a theoretical benefit from lab-based studies. Pre-sleep protein intake should be considered within the context of whether you are consuming sufficient daily protein, the spacing of your protein across the day, and your personal preference to *'cover all bases'*. If you already consume a large meal containing protein within a couple of hours before bed, the benefit of further consumption of protein before bed may be attenuated. However, if there is a long period of time between your last meal containing protein and bedtime, then perhaps consider a protein-based snack before bed. A dose of 40g is recommended to ensure a longer duration of elevated muscle protein synthesis overnight. As discussed previously, the benefit of additional protein will be when your total daily protein intake is below 1.6g/kg/day. The benefit of pre-sleep protein consumption has largely been when total daily protein intake has not been equated[17]. When protein intake has been equated, there has been no benefit to pre-sleep protein intake[68,69]. If you already consume 1.6g/kg/day, yet have a large pre-sleep window without protein, it may be wiser to consider shifting your current protein consumption pattern, rather than to consume more protein, to *'cover all bases'*[17].

Lab studies versus real life

The majority of studies assessing protein intake and changes in muscle protein synthesis involve isolated protein supplements (e.g. soy, whey or casein), and monitoring their acute effects on the body over a few hours or a day. This is to understand the direct relationship between the protein source and digestion, absorption and elevations in muscle protein synthesis, removing any potential confounding influence of other foods or drinks consumed. However, the majority of food intake is through the consumption of mixed meals. Mixed meals may contain large protein doses (e.g. a large steak or chicken breast) up to 100g. When such large doses are consumed within a food matrix alongside carbohydrates, fats and fibre, this can result in a slower digestion and absorption of protein, but also augment elevations in muscle protein synthesis. This may mean that typical habitual diets result in a steady release of protein and elevation of muscle protein synthesis throughout the day with several mixed meals, rather than an acute sudden rise and fall in muscle protein synthesis[39]. Consuming sufficient daily protein is by far the most important factor for body composition[17].

Is protein more satiating than carbohydrates or fat?

The general consensus is that diets with a higher protein content result in greater satiety, reduced appetite and increased resting energy expenditure. There is evidence from randomised controlled trials, observational studies and mechanistic data to support this theory. However, this effect may be attenuated with further protein intake, and other factors can influence satiety and appetite. This is again limited by the lack of a universal definition of what constitutes a 'high protein diet'.

So far, we have said a calorie is a calorie. This holds true when eating at calorie maintenance, in a surplus or in a deficit; a bigger deficit means more weight loss, and a bigger surplus means more weight gain. The source of calorie intake is less important than total calorie intake for weight change. Whether this difference is achieved with a low carbohydrate or low fat diet does not matter. However, a higher protein diet compared to a lower protein diet allows for relatively more weight to be lost as fat and less as muscle when in an equivalent calorie deficit. A higher protein diet similarly allows for relatively more muscle gain and less fat gain when in an equivalent calorie surplus. There may also be one other benefit to higher protein intakes. There is mounting evidence to suggest that diets with higher protein intakes lead to greater feelings of *satiety* and suppression of *appetite* compared to diets with lower protein intakes.

The current prevailing academic view is that a higher protein intake increases satiety, with studies finding protein to be more satiating than fat or carbohydrate[50]. This has been concluded from a range of observational studies, randomised controlled studies, dietary studies, and also mechanistic evidence in lab studies that demonstrate how this may be possible. Many studies have reported increased satiety with increased protein intakes on acute, daily and long-term scales[32,50,70,71].

For example, one study compared high fat snacks to high protein snacks and found improved appetite and satiety with the high protein snacks[72]. In another study, participants consumed either 15% of their daily calories as protein compared to 30% of their daily calories as protein[73]. The 30% protein group had reduced their food intake when left to eat at free will, which led to weight loss (participants ended up in a daily calorie deficit)[73].

Several mechanisms may result in increased satiety from protein:

- Elevated amino acid levels in the blood.
- Increases in hormones that promote satiety.
- Increased energy expenditure.

These signals are incorporated by the hypothalamus in the brain and will result in a reduction in appetite and increased satiety (chapter 5)[32,50,71].

The effect of protein satiety will depend on several factors, such as[32]:

- **Protein quality**: complete versus incomplete protein and amino acid content.
- **Protein digestibility**: fast versus slow digesting protein.
- **Protein quantity.**
- The **food matrix**. For example, solid versus liquid food and other components of the food source.
- The possible effect of satiety from inducing **ketosis** (see chapter 8 regarding the ketogenic diet) rather than the effect of high protein itself.
- The relative **metabolic inefficiency** of using (oxidising) amino acids compared to glucose (carbohydrate) and fatty acids (fat)[50].
- **Increased energy expenditure** from the thermic effect of food (TEF), *urea* production (a product of breaking down protein) and *gluconeogenesis* (the formation of glucose, a sugar) from protein metabolism[71].

The generation of a sustained negative energy balance can result from elevated plasma amino acid concentrations, the thermic effect of protein and hunger suppression. Ketogenesis can also contribute when simultaneously consuming a low intake of carbohydrates.

A review found that when calorie intake is controlled, higher protein diets appear to provide no advantage to weight loss (i.e. weight loss is dictated by the size of the calorie deficit). However, when people can eat freely (ad libitum), higher protein diets result in greater weight loss[70,71]. Because calorie intake is *not* matched, the increased satiety, reduced appetite and increase in energy expenditure promotes greater calorie restriction[71].

It therefore has been so far concluded that a diet containing higher levels of protein is more satiating, can increase energy expenditure, and promote weight loss. However, there is debate that protein itself is no more satiating than fat or carbohydrate, or at least, only satiating up to a certain daily intake. It is proposed that limitations of the studies mentioned have led to erroneous conclusions.

Although most studies show greater satiety, not every study assessing higher protein diets show greater ratings of satiety[50,71]. A leading evidence-based fitness expert, Menno Henselmans, has proposed a theory to explain the satiating effects seen in protein studies[74]. His theory is that protein is more satiating, but only up to a point, according to the established *protein leverage hypothesis*[75]. The protein leverage hypothesis is a theory that has been developed to try and explain the obesity epidemic[75]. The concept is that there is an appetite to consume protein, until a certain minimum daily intake has been met[76]. Once this minimum intake has been met, the drive is reduced. However, at lower protein intakes, this appetite drive remains[75,76]. In other words, protein suppresses appetite once this minimum intake is met, but there is no further appetite suppressing benefit to greater intakes. Part of this arises from a cross-over study assessing protein intake and satiety that Menno collaborated on. Their study showed that high (2.9g/kg/day) or low protein (1.8g/kg/day) intakes did *not* influence feelings of satiety in resistance trained individuals in a caloric deficit[18]. However, the low protein intake of 1.8g/kg/day used in the study is already well above levels currently consumed by the majority of the population. There was also no detrimental effect of consuming higher protein intakes, and the study was very short, just 7 days[18]. There may indeed be a threshold. If there is, it most likely lies at a much lower intake than 1.8g/kg/day[76]. Indeed, some studies have found protein to be no more satiating than fat or carbohydrate when other factors have been controlled for. The issue is that there are *many* factors that influence satiety, such as:

- Palatability of food.
- The mass of food consumed.
- Energy density.
- The food matrix (what else the protein being consumed with).
- Fibre content.
- Glycaemic index[50].

Unless we control for these factors, it cannot be concluded for sure that protein is inherently the most satiating macronutrient. Is the increased satiety from the lower energy density of high protein food, rather than protein itself being more satiating? This is useful to know because then recommendations can be to either opt for lower energy density foods in general or to opt for foods with greater protein content. When we control for the energy density of food, it seems that the effect of a high protein diet on satiety appears is attenuated[70]. One study made participants consume foods of the *same* energy density, but from *different* energy sources (alcohol, fat, carbohydrate or protein). Ratings of appetite and satiety were similar between all energy sources when energy density was equated, possibly suggesting that protein is not inherently more satiating[77]. In many previous studies that show increased satiety with protein intake, other factors such as the energy density of the food have not been considered. Even though their protein content is low, many plant-based foods such as fruit, vegetables and whole grains can promote greater satiety for a given energy content in part through their lower energy density (see chapter 12 regarding energy and nutrient density).

Focus on meeting your daily calorie needs and meeting your protein requirements to meet your goals. The general consensus is that protein is more satiating than fats or carbohydrates. It may be that this effect is only present up to a certain protein intake, beyond which protein does not further suppress appetite. Even so, the macronutrients you consume are not the whole picture. You need to consider *where* you get them from. It is important to consider not just the macronutrient, but the food source itself. We don't eat protein, carbohydrates and fats by themselves. We eat mixed meals containing foods with a variety of nutrients and with specific properties. If a person transitioned to a diet with higher protein, there may also be a transition from ultra-processed foods to lean protein sources (e.g. meat, chicken, eggs, plant-based protein sources) which may also increase satiety due to the lower energy density of the foods consumed[18].

Summary

A minimum daily intake of protein is required to prevent health complications.

When exercising, this minimum amount increases due to the increased recovery requirements.

Additional protein intake, to a point, can result in more optimal changes in body composition.

Total daily protein intake is the most important protein related variable. Spacing protein across the day can benefit muscle growth.

Other variables such as protein digestibility, protein quality, protein source and timing appear to be minor factors in relation to total daily protein intake for muscle growth or fat loss.

References

1   Jäger R, Kerksick CM, Campbell BI, Cribb PJ, Wells SD, Skwiat TM et al. International Society of Sports Nutrition Position Stand: protein and exercise. *J Int Soc Sports Nutr* 2017; 14: 20.

2   Stokes T, Hector AJ, Morton RW, McGlory C, Phillips SM. Recent Perspectives Regarding the Role of Dietary Protein for the Promotion of Muscle Hypertrophy with Resistance Exercise Training. *Nutrients* 2018; 10: 180.

3   Morton R, Murphy K, McKellar S, Schoenfeld B, Henselmans M, Helms E et al. A systematic review, meta-analysis and meta-regression of the effect of protein supplementation on resistance training-induced gains in muscle mass and strength in healthy adults. *Br J Sports Med* 2017; 52(6): 376-384.

4   Rand WM, Pellett PL, Young VR. Meta-analysis of nitrogen balance studies for estimating protein requirements in healthy adults. *Am J Clin Nutr* 2003; 77: 109–127.

5   World Health Organisation (WHO). *Protein and amino acid requirements in human nutrition.* Available from: http://www.who.int/nutrition/publications/nutrientrequirements/WHO_TRS _935/en/ (accessed 6 Feb 2020).

6   Phillips SM. A Brief Review of Higher Dietary Protein Diets in Weight Loss: A Focus on Athletes. *Sports Med Auckl Nz* 2014; 44: 149–153.

7   Devries MC, Phillips SM. Supplemental Protein in Support of Muscle Mass and Health: Advantage Whey. *J Food Sci* 2015; 80: A8–A15.

8   Mitchell CJ, Churchward-Venne TA, Parise G, Bellamy L, Baker SK, Smith K et al. Acute Post-Exercise Myofibrillar Protein Synthesis Is Not Correlated with Resistance Training-Induced Muscle Hypertrophy in Young Men. *PLoS ONE* 2014; 9. Available from: doi:10.1371/journal.pone.0089431.

9   Santos C de S, Nascimento FEL. Isolated branched-chain amino acid intake and muscle protein synthesis in humans: a biochemical review. *Einstein* 2019; 17(3). Available from: doi:10.31744/einstein_journal/2019RB4898.

10   Damas F, Phillips SM, Libardi CA, Vechin FC, Lixandrão ME, Jannig PR et al. Resistance training-induced changes in integrated myofibrillar protein synthesis are related to hypertrophy only after attenuation of muscle damage. *J Physiol* 2016; 594: 5209–5222.

11   Trommelen J, Betz MW, van Loon LJC. The Muscle Protein Synthetic Response to Meal Ingestion Following Resistance-Type Exercise. *Sports Med Auckl NZ* 2019; 49: 185–197.

12   Reidy PT, Rasmussen BB. Role of Ingested Amino Acids and Protein in the Promotion of Resistance Exercise–Induced Muscle Protein Anabolism. *J Nutr* 2016; 146: 155–183.

13   Hulmi JJ, Tannerstedt J, Selänne H, Kainulainen H, Kovanen V, Mero AA. Resistance exercise with whey protein ingestion affects mTOR signaling pathway and myostatin in men. *J Appl Physiol Bethesda Md* 2009; 106: 1720–1729.

14   Egan B. Protein intake for athletes and active adults: Current concepts and controversies. *Nutr Bull* 2016; 41: 202–213.

15   Ribeiro AS, Nunes JP, Schoenfeld BJ. Should Competitive Bodybuilders Ingest More Protein than Current Evidence-Based Recommendations? *Sports Med Auckl NZ* 2019; 49: 1481–1485.

16   Helms ER, Zinn C, Rowlands DS, Brown SR. A systematic review of dietary protein during caloric restriction in resistance trained lean athletes: a case for higher intakes. *Int J Sport Nutr Exerc Metab* 2014; 24: 127–138.

17   Roberts BM, Helms ER, Trexler ET, Fitschen PJ. Nutritional Recommendations for Physique Athletes. Journal of Human Kinetics 2020; 71(1): 79-108. Available from: doi:http://dx.doi.org/10.2478/hukin-2019-0096.

18   Roberts J, Zinchenko A, Mahbubani K, Johnstone J, Smith L, Merzbach V et al. Satiating Effect of High Protein Diets on Resistance-Trained Subjects in Energy Deficit. *Nutrients* 2018; 11: 56.

19   Carbone JW, Pasiakos SM, Vislocky LM, Anderson JM, Rodriguez NR. Effects of short-term energy deficit on muscle protein breakdown and intramuscular proteolysis in normal-weight young adults. *Appl Physiol Nutr Metab Physiol Appl Nutr Metab* 2014; 39: 960–968.

20   Hector AJ, McGlory C, Damas F, Mazara N, Baker SK, Phillips SM. Pronounced energy restriction with elevated protein intake results in no change in proteolysis and reductions in skeletal muscle protein synthesis that are mitigated by resistance exercise. *FASEB J Off Publ Fed Am Soc Exp Biol* 2018; 32: 265–275.

21   Wycherley TP, Moran LJ, Clifton PM, Noakes M, Brinkworth GD. Effects of energy-restricted high-protein, low-fat compared with standard-protein, low-fat diets: a meta-analysis of randomized controlled trials. *Am J Clin Nutr* 2012; 96: 1281–1298.

22   Krieger JW, Sitren HS, Daniels MJ, Langkamp-Henken B. Effects of variation in protein and carbohydrate intake on body mass and composition during energy restriction: a meta-regression. *Am J Clin Nutr* 2006; 83: 260–274.

23   Chappell AJ, Simper T, Helms E. Nutritional strategies of British professional and amateur natural bodybuilders during competition preparation. *J Int Soc Sports Nutr* 2019; 16: 35.

24   Helms ER, Aragon AA, Fitschen PJ. Evidence-based recommendations for natural bodybuilding contest preparation: nutrition and supplementation. *J Int Soc Sports Nutr* 2014; 11: 20.

25   Leaf A, Antonio J. The Effects of Overfeeding on Body Composition: The Role of Macronutrient Composition – A Narrative Review. *Int J Exerc Sci 2017*; 10(8): 1275-1296.

26   Schoenfeld BJ, Aragon AA. How much protein can the body use in a single meal for muscle-building? Implications for daily protein distribution. *J Int Soc Sports Nutr* 2018; 15: 10.

27   Antonio J, Peacock CA, Ellerbroek A, Fromhoff B, Silver T. The effects of consuming a high protein diet (4.4 g/kg/d) on body composition in resistance-trained individuals. *J Int Soc Sports Nutr* 2014; 11: 19.

28   Antonio J, Ellerbroek A, Silver T, Orris S, Scheiner M, Gonzalez A et al. A high protein diet (3.4 g/kg/d) combined with a heavy resistance training program improves body composition in healthy trained men and women – a follow-up investigation. *J Int Soc Sports Nutr* 2015; 12. Available from: doi:10.1186/s12970-015-0100-0.

29   McAdam JS, McGinnis KD, Beck DT, Haun CT, Romero MA, Mumford PW et al. Effect of Whey Protein Supplementation on Physical Performance and Body Composition in Army Initial Entry Training Soldiers. *Nutrients* 2018; 10. Available from: doi:10.3390/nu10091248.

30   Phillips SM. Protein requirements and supplementation in strength sports. *Nutr Burbank Los Angel Cty Calif* 2004; 20: 689–695.

31   Charidemou E, Ashmore T, Li X, McNally BD, West JA, Liggi S et al. A randomized 3-way crossover study indicates that high-protein feeding induces de novo lipogenesis in healthy humans. *JCI Insight* 2019; 4. Available from: doi:10.1172/jci.insight.124819.

32   Westerterp-Plantenga MS, Lemmens SG, Westerterp KR. Dietary protein – its role in satiety, energetics, weight loss and health. *Br J Nutr* 2012; 108: S105–S112.

33   Slater GJ, Dieter BP, Marsh DJ, Helms ER, Shaw G, Iraki J. Is an Energy Surplus Required to Maximize Skeletal Muscle Hypertrophy Associated With Resistance Training. *Front Nutr* 2019; 6. Available from: doi:10.3389/fnut.2019.00131.

34   Bray GA, Smith SR, de Jonge L, Xie H, Rood J, Martin CK et al. Effect of dietary protein content on weight gain, energy expenditure, and body composition during overeating: a randomized controlled trial. *JAMA* 2012; 307: 47–55.

35   Campbell B, Aguilar D, Conlin L, Vargas A, Schoenfeld B, Corson A et al. Effects of High vs. Low Protein Intake on Body Composition and Maximal Strength in Aspiring Female Physique Athletes Engaging in an 8-Week Resistance Training Program. *Int J Sport Nutr Exerc Metab* 2018; 28: 1–21.

36   Macdiarmid J, Blundell J. Assessing dietary intake: Who, what and why of under-reporting. *Nutr Res Rev* 1998; 11: 231–253.

37   Macnaughton LS, Wardle SL, Witard OC, McGlory C, Hamilton DL, Jeromson S et al. The response of muscle protein synthesis following whole-body resistance exercise is greater following 40 g than 20 g of ingested whey protein. *Physiol Rep* 2016; 4. Available from: doi:10.14814/phy2.12893.

38   Witard OC, Jackman SR, Breen L, Smith K, Selby A, Tipton KD. Myofibrillar muscle protein synthesis rates subsequent to a meal in response to increasing doses of whey protein at rest and after resistance exercise. *Am J Clin Nutr* 2014; 99: 86–95.

39   van Vliet S, Beals JW, Martinez IG, Skinner SK, Burd NA. Achieving Optimal Post-Exercise Muscle Protein Remodeling in Physically Active Adults

through Whole Food Consumption. *Nutrients* 2018; 10. Available from: doi:10.3390/nu10020224.

40   West DWD, Burd NA, Coffey VG, Baker SK, Burke LM, Hawley JA et al. Rapid aminoacidemia enhances myofibrillar protein synthesis and anabolic intramuscular signaling responses after resistance exercise. *Am J Clin Nutr* 2011; 94: 795–803.

41   Areta JL, Burke LM, Ross ML, Camera DM, West DWD, Broad EM et al. Timing and distribution of protein ingestion during prolonged recovery from resistance exercise alters myofibrillar protein synthesis. *J Physiol* 2013; 591: 2319–2331.

42   Pennings B, Groen BBL, van Dijk J-W, de Lange A, Kiskini A, Kuklinski M et al. Minced beef is more rapidly digested and absorbed than beef steak, resulting in greater postprandial protein retention in older men. *Am J Clin Nutr* 2013; 98: 121–128.

43   van Vliet S, Shy EL, Abou Sawan S, Beals JW, West DW, Skinner SK et al. Consumption of whole eggs promotes greater stimulation of postexercise muscle protein synthesis than consumption of isonitrogenous amounts of egg whites in young men. *Am J Clin Nutr* 2017; 106: 1401–1412.

44   Kim I-Y, Schutzler S, Schrader A, Spencer HJ, Azhar G, Ferrando AA et al. The anabolic response to a meal containing different amounts of protein is not limited by the maximal stimulation of protein synthesis in healthy young adults. *Am J Physiol - Endocrinol Metab* 2016; 310: E73–E80.

45   Mamerow MM, Mettler JA, English KL, Casperson SL, Arentson-Lantz E, Sheffield-Moore M et al. Dietary protein distribution positively influences 24-h muscle protein synthesis in healthy adults. *J Nutr* 2014; 144: 876–880.

46   Lonnie M, Hooker E, Brunstrom JM, Corfe BM, Green MA, Watson AW et al. Protein for Life: Review of Optimal Protein Intake, Sustainable Dietary Sources and the Effect on Appetite in Ageing Adults. *Nutrients* 2018; 10. Available from: doi:10.3390/nu10030360.

47   Wu G. Dietary protein intake and human health. *Food Funct* 2016; 7: 1251–1265.

48   Farrell DJ, Bower L. Fatal water intoxication. *J Clin Pathol* 2003; 56: 803–804.

49   Campbell NRC, Train EJ. A Systematic Review of Fatalities Related to Acute Ingestion of Salt. A Need for Warning Labels? *Nutrients* 2017; 9. Available from: doi:10.3390/nu9070648.

50   Johnstone A. Safety and efficacy of high-protein diets for weight loss. *Proc Nutr Soc* 2012; 71: 339–49.

51   Carbone JW, Pasiakos SM. Dietary Protein and Muscle Mass: Translating Science to Application and Health Benefit. *Nutrients* 2019; 11. Available from: doi:10.3390/nu11051136.

52   Antonio J, Ellerbroek A, Silver T, Vargas L, Tamayo A, Buehn R et al. A High Protein Diet Has No Harmful Effects: A One-Year Crossover Study in Resistance-Trained Males. *J Nutr Metab*; 2016. Available from: doi:10.1155/2016/9104792.

53   Antonio J, Ellerbroek A, Silver T, Vargas L, Peacock C. The effects of a high protein diet on indices of health and body composition – a crossover trial in resistance-trained men. *J Int Soc Sports Nutr* 2016; 13. Available from: doi:10.1186/s12970-016-0114-2.

54   Zhang J-W, Tong X, Wan Z, Wang Y, Qin L-Q, Szeto IMY. Effect of whey protein on blood lipid profiles: a meta-analysis of randomized controlled trials. *Eur J Clin Nutr* 2016; 70: 879–885.

55   Proceedings of the Fifteenth International Society of Sports Nutrition (ISSN) Conference and Expo. *J Int Soc Sports Nutr* 2018; 15: 1-37. Available from: https://jissn.biomedcentral.com/articles/10.1186/s12970-018-0256-5 (accessed 6 Feb 2020).

56   Darling AL, Millward DJ, Torgerson DJ, Hewitt CE, Lanham-New SA. Dietary protein and bone health: a systematic review and meta-analysis. *Am J Clin Nutr* 2009; 90: 1674–1692.

57   Hoffman JR, Falvo MJ. Protein – Which is Best? *J Sports Sci Med* 2004; 3: 118–130.

58   Berrazaga I, Micard V, Gueugneau M, Walrand S. The Role of the Anabolic Properties of Plant- versus Animal-Based Protein Sources in Supporting Muscle Mass Maintenance: A Critical Review. *Nutrients* 2019; 11. Available from: doi:10.3390/nu11081825.

59   Schaafsma G. Advantages and limitations of the protein digestibility-corrected amino acid score (PDCAAS) as a method for evaluating protein quality in human diets. *Br J Nutr* 2012; 108 Suppl 2: S333-336.

60   Candow DG, Burke NC, Smith-Palmer T, Burke DG. Effect of whey and soy protein supplementation combined with resistance training in young adults. *Int J Sport Nutr Exerc Metab* 2006; 16: 233–244.

61   Joy JM, Lowery RP, Wilson JM, Purpura M, De Souza EO, Wilson SM et al. The effects of 8 weeks of whey or rice protein supplementation on body composition and exercise performance. *Nutr J* 2013; 12: 86.

62   Denysschen CA, Burton HW, Horvath PJ, Leddy JJ, Browne RW. Resistance training with soy vs whey protein supplements in hyperlipidemic males. *J Int Soc Sports Nutr* 2009; 6: 8.

63   Kerksick CM, Wilborn CD, Roberts MD, Smith-Ryan A, Kleiner SM, Jäger R et al. ISSN exercise & sports nutrition review update: research & recommendations. *J Int Soc Sports Nutr* 2018; 15. Available from: doi:10.1186/s12970-018-0242-y.

64   Iraki J, Fitschen P, Espinar S, Helms E. Nutrition Recommendations for Bodybuilders in the Off-Season: A Narrative Review. *Sports* 2019; 7: 154.

65   Cermak NM, Res PT, de Groot LC, Saris WH, van Loon LJ. Protein supplementation augments the adaptive response of skeletal muscle to resistance-type exercise training: a meta-analysis. *Am J Clin Nutr* 2012; 96: 1454–1464.

66   Res PT, Groen B, Pennings B, Beelen M, Wallis GA, Gijsen AP et al. Protein Ingestion before Sleep Improves Postexercise Overnight Recovery. *Med Sci Sports Exerc* 2012; 44: 1560–1569.

67   Trommelen J, van Loon LJC. Pre-Sleep Protein Ingestion to Improve the Skeletal Muscle Adaptive Response to Exercise Training. *Nutrients* 2016; 8. Available from: doi:10.3390/nu8120763.

68   Joy JM, Vogel RM, Shane Broughton K, Kudla U, Kerr NY, Davison JM et al. Daytime and nighttime casein supplements similarly increase muscle size and strength in response to resistance training earlier in the day: a preliminary investigation. *J Int Soc Sports Nutr* 2018; 15: 24.

69   Antonio J, Ellerbroek A, Peacock C, Silver T. Casein Protein Supplementation in Trained Men and Women: Morning versus Evening. *Int J Exerc Sci* 2017; 10: 479–486.

70   Wyness L, Weichselbaum E, O'Connor A, Williams EB, Benelam B, Riley H et al. Red meat in the diet: an update. *Nutr Bull* 2011; 36: 34–77.

71   Halton TL, Hu FB. The effects of high protein diets on thermogenesis, satiety and weight loss: a critical review. *J Am Coll Nutr* 2004; 23: 373–385.

72   Ortinau LC, Hoertel HA, Douglas SM, Leidy HJ. Effects of high-protein vs. high- fat snacks on appetite control, satiety, and eating initiation in healthy women. *Nutr J* 2014; 13. Available from: doi:10.1186/1475-2891-13-97.

73   Weigle DS, Breen PA, Matthys CC, Callahan HS, Meeuws KE, Burden VR et al. A high-protein diet induces sustained reductions in appetite, ad libitum caloric intake, and body weight despite compensatory changes in diurnal plasma leptin and ghrelin concentrations. *Am J Clin Nutr* 2005; 82: 41–48.

74   Henselmans M. *Is protein really more satiating than carbs and fats?* 2018. Available from: https://mennohenselmans.com/protein-is-not-more-satiating-than-carbs-and-fats/ (accessed 7 Feb 2020).

75   Simpson SJ, Raubenheimer D. Obesity: the protein leverage hypothesis. *Obes Rev Off J Int Assoc Study Obes* 2005; 6: 133–142.

76   Bekelman TA, Santamaría-Ulloa C, Dufour DL, Marín-Arias L, Dengo AL. Using the protein leverage hypothesis to understand socioeconomic variation in obesity. *Am J Hum Biol Off J Hum Biol Counc* 2017; 29. Available from: doi:10.1002/ajhb.22953.

77   Raben A, Agerholm-Larsen L, Flint A, Holst JJ, Astrup A. Meals with similar energy densities but rich in protein, fat, carbohydrate, or alcohol have different effects on energy expenditure and substrate metabolism but not on appetite and energy intake. *Am J Clin Nutr* 2003; 77: 91–100.

10. Nutrient Timing

Nutrient timing is irrelevant for body composition when at caloric maintenance. It is far less important than total daily calorie intake for body composition when in a calorie surplus or deficit.

For muscle growth in a caloric surplus, timing protein across the day can maximise muscle protein synthesis to maintain a positive net protein balance.

During a caloric deficit, nutrient timing is largely unimportant for protein, carbohydrates and fats.

Timing of carbohydrate and fat for muscle growth is unimportant beyond consuming sufficient fat for health, and consuming sufficient carbohydrate throughout the day to fuel a resistance training workout. Any aerobic exercise lasting more than 1 hour, or very high volume resistance training may require timing considerations of carbohydrate.

Eating smaller meals rather than larger meals throughout the day does not increase metabolic rate.

The time of day during which food is consumed (e.g. early morning or late at night) does not influence whether weight is gained or lost beyond total energy balance across the day.

Nutrient timing in this context refers to improvements in performance, recovery and body composition by manipulating the timing of calorie and macronutrient consumption throughout the day, relative to training sessions.

There have been significant amounts of research on nutrient timing in performance. However, this has mainly been in trained individuals performing endurance exercise. Studies assessing nutrient timing for body composition are generally acute studies in untrained individuals that do not always measure muscle growth[1]. They also often use both pre- *and* post-workout consumption, which limits the ability to determine the individual effects of pre- and post-workout nutritional interventions[2]. There is a lack of controlled long-term trials that distinctly compare the effects of the timing of nutrients independent of quantity, as protein intake is often not matched. If protein is not equated between groups, having protein before a workout may be beneficial because it increases total daily protein intake, rather than because of the timing of the protein[1].

A position stand has been developed by the International Society of Sports Nutrition (ISSN) on nutrient timing and exercise[2]. However, our focus is of timing on *body composition*. The guidelines here are of timing on *exercise performance*. Most of the recommendations apply to long duration endurance performance, not body composition. Nonetheless, a range other reviews cover aspects of nutrient timing for muscle growth and fat loss[1,3-5].

The timing of protein or carbohydrate consumption is less important than consuming adequate amounts of protein or carbohydrate.

In terms of weight loss or weight gain, the overriding factor is total calorie intake, not the timing of calorie intake. Before considering the timing of nutrients, ensure your total energy intake is aligned with your goals. See chapter 7 for calculating your calorie and macronutrient intakes.

Food before and after training: pre-workout and post-workout nutrition

Consume 20-40g of protein to maximally stimulate muscle protein synthesis, which can be several hours before and/or after a resistance training workout.

Post-workout food intake is dependent on the timing and size of pre-workout food intake and vice versa, not on the timing relative to the resistance training session. A larger pre-workout meal immediately before (<1 hour) a workout mitigates the need for immediate post workout nutrition. A smaller pre-workout meal several hours before a workout will increase the need for post workout nutrition sooner rather than later. A large mixed meal before training can also act as an immediate post-workout meal due to the timing of digestion and absorption[1]. This doesn't mean you can't eat immediately before or after a workout, just that you don't necessarily have to.

Protein and carbohydrate timing prior to a resistance training workout are relatively unimportant provided total daily intakes are met. Factors such as food choice and meal size (food volume and macronutrient quantity) should be considered for the pre-training meal, as this can influence gut comfort during training, which will differ between individuals.

Immediate protein and carbohydrate after a workout are relatively unimportant provided total daily intakes are met. Post-workout food choice and meal size (food volume and macronutrient quantity) will primarily depend on the duration of time since the last meal, and the number of calories that need to be consumed to meet daily calorie needs, which will differ between individuals.

The timing of food during the day (such as what you consume before a workout) should primarily be based around your *personal experience* with certain foods and how they make you *feel*[6]. If certain foods make you feel uncomfortable when exercising then it would be wise to not eat them before a workout, or to not eat too much of them. Hunger may also be a factor. Whether or not you feel hungry during a workout may influence how much food you eat before. You may find a big serving of carbohydrates before training provides a psychological *'placebo' or 'meaningful'* boost to train well, or it leaves you feeling drained and lethargic. Knowledge of carbohydrate availability from a meal before exercise can benefit high-intensity performance[7]. How much or what you eat may also be influenced by the exercises you perform in the workout. Other things to consider in terms of a pre-training meal include having a lower fibre and fat content of the meal to aid *gastric* (stomach) emptying (so that the food you eat before the workout can be used quickly) and to reduce any gut distress. A smaller meal may be more suitable when eating soon before training, whereas a bigger meal may be more comfortable if training is not until several hours later[6]. In order to achieve the same macronutrient intake with a smaller meal, the energy density of the food should be considered. A smaller meal may require opting for more energy dense foods.

The importance of pre- and post-workout protein consumption are interdependent. The timing between the pre- and post-workout meal should ideally not exceed 3-6 hours (a larger mixed meal can elevate muscle protein synthesis for up to 6 hours). Therefore, if you eat a meal 1 hour before training, there is no immediate need for post-workout food. If you eat a meal 5 hours before training, then post-workout food may need to be sooner rather than later after a workout to maintain a positive net protein balance.

The anabolic window: protein and carbohydrate for muscle growth

You don't need to eat immediately after a training session to ensure muscle growth and recovery. Eating a meal containing sufficient protein (with some carbohydrate to meet total daily calorie needs if necessary) within a few hours of training is fine.

The 'anabolic window' around a workout is either non-existent, or very large. The time-frame for consuming protein before or after a workout appears to be as large as 6 hours[4]. The concept of post-workout nutrition for muscle growth has stemmed from endurance performance, where intra- and post-workout protein and carbohydrate intake can provide beneficial effects[3,8]. However, the needs of an endurance athlete in terms of recovery and performance are different to that of someone resistance training for muscle growth. The adaptations that are desired following resistance training (hypertrophy) and endurance training (muscular endurance) are also different[3]. The anabolic effects of a mixed meal (proteins and carbohydrates) usually lasts for at least 3 hours, and up to 6 hours. So, training immediately after a meal does not warrant consuming calories immediately after, and vice versa. There does not appear to be any advantage to consuming protein immediately post-workout or pre-workout when consuming sufficient protein during the day for muscle growth[8]. If you have a sufficient amount of protein (20-40g) within a couple of hours of your gym session, you don't need another dose of protein immediately after your workout. Your next protein dose can be consumed at your next planned meal an hour or two after your session.

Do I need to consume carbohydrates before, during or after resistance training?

Carbohydrate timing around a resistance training session for muscle growth or weight loss is unimportant provided adequate carbohydrates are consumed during the day.

Training completely fasted will not be ideal and can impair performance in high volume sessions. But, having carbohydrates in meals before and after training are sufficient for a typical resistance training workout. Intra-workout carbohydrate is unnecessary for typical resistance training workouts. But again, if you personally prefer to consume food around a training session then by all means do so, especially in an attempt to ensure a caloric surplus.

The role of carbohydrate for muscle growth has been covered in depth in chapter 8.

Consuming carbohydrates around a workout would in *theory* be to the benefit of acute exercise performance, or to maximise chronic anabolic adaptations from the training session. This would be because energy is being provided at a time when energy is needed to fuel exercise or recover from exercise.

Muscle glycogen stores (how carbohydrates are stored in muscles and the liver, and the fuel used during anaerobic resistance training) are replete with an adequate carbohydrate diet of 4-7g of carbohydrate per kg of body weight per day. This is a moderate carbohydrate intake which the majority of the population tends to consume[9]. This level of carbohydrate intake is achieved in most diets except for very low carbohydrate diets or ketogenic diets (i.e. sufficient intake is achieved except when severely restricting carbohydrate intake). Replenishment of carbohydrate stores in muscle is achieved well within 24 hours, and replenishment can occur from other sources of energy besides ingested carbohydrate[10]. When resistance training a maximum of once per day, consideration of carbohydrate timing is unnecessary when daily carbohydrate intake is adequate[5]. Beyond the general recommendations for minimum daily carbohydrate consumption, no further recommendations for acute intakes can be made for resistance training sessions typically lasting around 60-90 minutes[11,12]. As such, the need to immediately consume carbohydrate before a resistance training workout is not needed when daily carbohydrate intake is sufficient[12]. Importantly, training fasted would also not be beneficial. Not training fasted (i.e. fed) would be more ideal. Fasted training also places greater emphasis on the need for immediate post-workout nutrition (see chapter 24 regarding fasted exercise)[1]. At least some carbohydrates should be consumed in the day before a workout. For a morning session, this may well mean intake near to the session. For an evening session, this could be intakes across two or three meals earlier in the day.

Having carbohydrate with your post-workout protein intake does not result in a further increase in muscle protein synthesis[13–15]. A recent study in untrained males assessed the effect of consuming protein alone, carbohydrate alone, or both protein and carbohydrate after resistance training on muscle strength, size, and fat mass. They found that if you have a dose of protein after your workout, having carbohydrate with the protein does not further increase muscle strength, size or fat loss over the course of a 12-week resistance training programme[15].

"Carbohydrate coingestion with protein does not enhance the anabolic effect of protein and does not contribute to a greater hypertrophic potential following resistance exercise."
Stokes et al., 2018[13].

This doesn't mean that you *shouldn't* have carbohydrate with your post-workout protein, just that you don't *need* to if you don't want to.

Although the *'anabolic window'* is much larger than previously thought, it doesn't mean that you cannot eat during this period. If you are trying to be in a calorie surplus this may be irrelevant because you just need to focus on consuming sufficient calories during the day. However, if you find it very easy to overeat or you are trying to lose weight in a calorie deficit, it can be useful to know that you do not need to prioritise energy intake during this period. It means that you don't *need* to have big meals before and after the gym, which limits your food choices for the rest of the day. This is also useful if you have a busy schedule and don't have much time to eat before or after training. The knowledge that you do not need to cram your limited calories immediately before or after your workout allows you to enjoy your food whilst ensuring you get the benefits of the workout. If you find you are bloated or uncomfortable when training on a full stomach, this means you could have something lighter before training, with a larger meal after your workout.

Fats

There are currently no timing recommendations of fat intake for muscle growth or fat loss[2].

There is little to say regarding fat timing and body composition goals. The priority is to simply consume a minimum of 0.5g/kg of body weight per day from a health perspective.

Some experts suggest consuming fewer fats around your resistance training workout and consuming more fats at other times of the day. This is suggested because fat consumption can slow the rate of digestion. Therefore, lower intakes before and after a workout may better allow for protein and carbohydrates to be quickly digested and used[6]. *No* studies have actually compared whether fat timing has any influence on body composition. Given the evidence is theoretical and from expert opinion (i.e. low quality), the recommendation to do this is fairly weak. However, it can be very easy to achieve, and you may find that you consume low fat meals around your workouts anyway as you prioritise protein and possibly carbohydrate consumption.

Meal frequency

Meal frequency should be determined by your own personal preference.

Increasing meal frequency does not significantly increase the thermic effect of food (TEF), total daily energy expenditure (TDEE) or basal metabolic rate (BMR).

For muscle growth, it may be beneficial to have protein consumed in at least 3 meals or snacks across the day to maintain elevated muscle protein synthesis. The research regarding meal frequency for muscle growth during intermittent fasting is still minimal and unclear.

For fat loss, meal frequency is not important. An increased meal frequency does not lead to greater weight loss.

A position stand has been produced by the International Society of Sports Nutrition (ISSN) on meal frequency[16]. The current evidence from interventional studies assessing meal frequency is fairly limited. The main takeaway is that your meal frequency should be largely dictated by personal preference.

If you currently eat all your food in one meal, then this is likely to be sub-optimal. There does appear to be some benefit to spreading protein out across the day in more meals for muscle growth. The frequency of fat or carbohydrate feeding throughout the day is irrelevant for fat loss or muscle gain. However, whether to eat three, four or five meals is down to what suits your lifestyle and which you find easiest to adhere to. Although eating more meals per day does not lead to significant increases in energy expenditure, if you prefer eating 6 to 7 small meals a day rather than a few large meals, then by all means do so as the strategy you use to ensure adherence.

Increasing meal frequency does not increase the thermic effect of food, total daily energy expenditure, or basal metabolic rate (the energy you need to just be alive).

When you eat and digest a meal, you burn energy to use that food, called the thermic effect of food (TEF). Therefore, if you eat more meals, would your metabolic rate be higher? The idea is that eating more frequently *'stokes the metabolic furnace'* and increases metabolism. This has been widely promoted in fitness circles. However, the increase in metabolic rate is *proportional* to the size of the meal consumed. If you usually eat 3 meals and decided to eat 6 instead, your meal size with 6 meals would be half the size of the 3 meals per day plan for calories to remain equivalent. This also means that the increase in metabolic rate after each meal is half that of when consuming 3 meals. The result? The rise in metabolic rate across the day is no different between the two. But what if you eat more over the day with the 6 meals, than with 3? Yes, you would have an increase in metabolic rate from an increase in the thermic effect of food. But, thermic effect of food is a *proportion* (8-15%) of the energy you consume. Therefore, you would consume far more calories than this effect would expend, meaning you end up just eating more calories, which would be gained as weight.

Additionally, higher meal frequencies are associated with greater energy intake and higher body mass index (BMI)[10]. Those consuming a higher frequency of smaller meals also tend to have greater feelings of hunger[10].

Meals per day	Total calories	Calories per meal	Thermic effect of food from a mixed meal	TEF per meal	Total daily TEF	Net calorie intake
3	2400	800	15%	120	360	2040
4	2400	600	15%	90	360	2040
6	2400	400	15%	60	360	2040
3	3000	1000	15%	150	450	2550
4	3000	750	15%	112.5	450	2550
6	3000	500	15%	75	450	2550

The effect of changing meal frequency whilst keeping energy intake constant.

Choose the minimum frequency of meals to meet your goal of weight loss or muscle gain.

Some practical advice from Andy Morgan illustrates an excellent strategy for dietary adherence, which features in his highly detailed *'complete nutrition setup guide'*, which is freely available online[17]. Fewer meals minimises the amount of food preparation and planning you need to do. Simpler plans make it easier to adhere to in the long-term, and the overarching factor with any plan is to ensure adherence[17]. His suggestion is to consume 2 to 4 meals when losing weight because one meal is probably sub-optimal for training and muscle preservation, but more frequent feeding does not show greater benefit for muscle preservation. Similarly, fewer meals allows for larger meal sizes. When building muscle, we know that distributing protein across the day can be beneficial for muscle growth, therefore he suggests having 3 to 4 meals per day. Eating a larger amount of food in 1 or 2 meals will also be difficult to achieve without opting for energy dense food sources. However, with high protein snacks being included as a meal, this can easily be increased to 5 or 6 meals if necessary. Eating more frequently is unlikely to have any negative effects (with protein doses kept above 20-25g per meal) except for the added inconvenience of food preparation and/or planning.

Eat as often as preferred, which may be as infrequently as necessary[17].

Late night eating

Total calorie intake, not calorie timing dictates weight loss or weight gain.

How much and how late you eat should be dictated by your calorie requirements, lifestyle and how it influences your sleep quality and quantity.

Most evidence on the timing of meals is focussed on eating or skipping breakfast, and studies of evening food consumption are mainly observational, which limits conclusions about causality (chapter 4)[18,19]. Studies also do *not* equate calorie intake and are more concerned with how meal timing influences daily energy intake, rather than how an equal number of daily calories eaten at different times of the day affects body composition.

You may have heard of the phrase *'no carbohydrates (or food) after 6pm'*. The thought is that any food eaten late at night is converted into fat as there is no need to use the energy it contains. A recent systematic review and meta-analysis of observational and interventional studies found *no* effect of evening meal size on weight loss during a caloric deficit[20]. Non-significance was found when assessing evening food intake from randomised controlled trials where total daily intake is equated. There is no significant effect of the size of the evening meal on weight loss[20]. Even so, many studies used diet diaries to record calorie intake, which can be inaccurate. As outlined in the nutrient hierarchy, the overriding factor with weight loss or weight gain is the total calorie intake for the day. Therefore, if you need to eat 2500kcal to maintain your body weight but have only eaten 2000kcal by 6pm, then eating another 500kcal in the evening will *not* result in weight gain. On the other hand, if you've already eaten 2500kcal, then another 500kcal will put you in a calorie surplus and therefore you *will* gain weight. And similarly, if you have only eaten 1500kcal by 6pm, then another 500kcal late in the evening will mean you are in a calorie deficit and therefore you *will* lose weight, despite late eating. Even so, on a single occasion this would not result in any meaningful weight change. As an example, intermittent fasting (discussed next) is an effective (but not superior) strategy for weight loss, yet it can involve shifting food intake to later in the day.

The main factor determining when you eat during the day should be *personal preference*, and if building muscle, then spreading protein across the day also in at least 3 or so meals. Whether you have a large meal later in the day is up to you. The potentially beneficial role of consuming protein before sleep was discussed in chapter 9. The only things to consider are that you do not eat too much too late, such that it disrupts your ability to sleep from gut distress.

Summary

Nutrient timing is relatively unimportant compared to energy balance. Spacing protein throughout the day can promote greater muscle growth.

The *'anabolic window'* around a workout is either non-existent, or very large.

With severely low carbohydrate intakes, consuming the limited amount of carbohydrate prior to a resistance training workout may aid performance. Timing is irrelevant at moderate carbohydrate intakes for resistance training.

References

1   Aragon AA, Schoenfeld BJ. Nutrient timing revisited: is there a post-exercise anabolic window? *J Int Soc Sports Nutr* 2013; 10: 5.

2   Kerksick C, Arent S, Schoenfeld B, Stout J, Campbell B, Wilborn C et al. International society of sports nutrition position stand: Nutrient timing. *J Int Soc Sports Nutr* 2017; 14: 33.

3   Escobar KA, VanDusseldorp TA, Kerksick CM. Carbohydrate intake and resistance-based exercise: are current recommendations reflective of actual need? *Br J Nutr* 2016; 116: 2053–2065.

4   Schoenfeld BJ, Aragon AA. Is There a Postworkout Anabolic Window of Opportunity for Nutrient Consumption? Clearing up Controversies. *J Orthop Sports Phys Ther* 2018; 48: 911–914.

5   Helms ER, Aragon AA, Fitschen PJ. Evidence-based recommendations for natural bodybuilding contest preparation: nutrition and supplementation. *J Int Soc Sports Nutr* 2014; 11: 20.

6   American Dietetic Association, Dieticians of Canada, American College of Sports Medicine, Rodriguez NR, Di Marco NM, Langley S. American College of Sports Medicine position stand. Nutrition and Athletic Performance. *Med Sci Sports Exerc* 2009; 41: 709–731.

7   Waterworth SP, Spencer CC, Porter AL, Morton JP. Perception of Carbohydrate Availability Augments High-Intensity Intermittent Exercise Capacity Under Sleep-Low, Train-Low Conditions. *Int J Sport Nutr Exerc Metab* 2020; 30(2): 1–7.

8   Reidy PT, Rasmussen BB. Role of Ingested Amino Acids and Protein in the Promotion of Resistance Exercise–Induced Muscle Protein Anabolism. *J Nutr* 2016; 146: 155–183.

9   Potgieter S. Sport nutrition: A review of the latest guidelines for exercise and sport nutrition from the American College of Sport Nutrition, the

International Olympic Committee and the International Society for Sports Nutrition. *South Afr J Clin Nutr* 2013; 26: 6–16.

10   Roberts BM, Helms ER, Trexler ET, Fitschen PJ. Nutritional Recommendations for Physique Athletes. *Journal of Human Kinetics* 2020; 71(1): 79-108. Available from: doi:http://dx.doi.org/10.2478/hukin-2019-0096.

11   Slater GJ, Dieter BP, Marsh DJ, Helms ER, Shaw G, Iraki J. Is an Energy Surplus Required to Maximize Skeletal Muscle Hypertrophy Associated With Resistance Training. *Front Nutr* 2019; 6. Available from: doi:10.3389/fnut.2019.00131.

12   Kerksick CM, Wilborn CD, Roberts MD, Smith-Ryan A, Kleiner SM, Jäger R et al. ISSN exercise & sports nutrition review update: research & recommendations. *J Int Soc Sports Nutr* 2018; 15. Available from: doi:10.1186/s12970-018-0242-y.

13   Stokes T, Hector AJ, Morton RW, McGlory C, Phillips SM. Recent Perspectives Regarding the Role of Dietary Protein for the Promotion of Muscle Hypertrophy with Resistance Exercise Training. *Nutrients* 2018; 10: 180.

14   Staples AW, Burd NA, West DWD, Currie KD, Atherton PJ, Moore DR et al. Carbohydrate does not augment exercise-induced protein accretion versus protein alone. *Med Sci Sports Exerc* 2011; 43: 1154–1161.

15   Hulmi JJ, Laakso M, Mero AA, Häkkinen K, Ahtiainen JP, Peltonen H. The effects of whey protein with or without carbohydrates on resistance training adaptations. *J Int Soc Sports Nutr* 2015; 12: 48.

16   La Bounty PM, Campbell BI, Wilson J, Galvan E, Berardi J, Kleiner SM et al. International Society of Sports Nutrition position stand: meal frequency. *J Int Soc Sports Nutr* 2011; 8: 4.

17   Morgan A. *The Complete Nutrition Set Up Guide*. Available from: https://rippedbody.com/complete-diet-nutrition-set-up-guide/ (accessed 7 Feb 2020).

18   Paoli A, Tinsley G, Bianco A, Moro T. The Influence of Meal Frequency and Timing on Health in Humans: The Role of Fasting. *Nutrients* 2019; 11: 719.

19   Lopez-Minguez J, Gómez-Abellán P, Garaulet M. Timing of Breakfast, Lunch, and Dinner. Effects on Obesity and Metabolic Risk. *Nutrients* 2019; 11. Available from: doi:10.3390/nu11112624.

20   Fong M, Caterson ID, Madigan CD. Are large dinners associated with excess weight, and does eating a smaller dinner achieve greater weight loss? A systematic review and meta-analysis. *Br J Nutr* 2017; 118: 616–628.

11. Manipulating the timing of energy intake: fasting

Intermittent fasting

There are no conclusive superior benefits to intermittent fasting (IF) compared to continuous energy restriction (CER) for weight loss[1].

You should use intermittent fasting if you would rather eat larger meals and prefer not to eat throughout the day, or you find you are not hungry in the morning. Intermittent fasting will not lead to muscle loss any differently to a calorie equated continuous energy restriction regime. You should not use intermittent fasting if you think it will provide superior body composition and health benefits.

There is limited evidence regarding the influence of intermittent fasting on muscle growth. The positioning of the fast in relation to the training session may influence muscle growth.

Intermittent fasting has risen rapidly in popularity. It has been used by many people who say it has worked *'wonders'* for them. But, what actually is intermittent fasting (IF), and what are its supposed benefits?

Fasting means to be without food. Intermittent fasting means to be without food for periods of time.

Everyone fasts from when they have their last meal of the day to when they have their first meal the following day. This means most people *already* fast for 8-12 hours at a time. The fasting discussed here is where you extend the overnight fast and spend prolonged periods of time without any calorie intake. Intermittent fasting is where periods of prolonged fasting are split up with periods of food intake. Intermittent fasting can be[2]:

- On a **time-period basis** (fasting for a certain number of hours a day). This involves several hours with no food, interspersed with breaks of food intake. The most common form is with a feeding window of 8 hours and a fasting window of 16 hours. This is usually achieved by extending the overnight fast in the morning, then breaking the fast at lunchtime and eating until 8pm, before resuming the fast. This is called *time-restricted feeding* (TRF).

- On a **daily basis** (fasting for a certain number of days per week). The most commonly researched intermittent fasting strategy is *alternate-day fasting* (ADF), where there are alternating days of maintenance calorie intake with days of fasting. Every other day is either at an intake of 500kcal or ad libitum (free to eat at will). Another popular, but less researched format is *whole-day fasting* (WDF), such as the 5-2 diet. Here, the individual spends 2 days during the week fasted (usually not on consecutive days) and 5 days at or near calorie maintenance, or ad libitum. Daily fasting diets can involve very low-calorie intakes (<500kcal) on fasted days, or even completely fasted.

Periods of complete fasting longer than a few days are rarely seen and can have detrimental health effects.

Typical intermittent fasting usually does not involve periods of severe calorie restriction that last longer than 7 days. The forms outlined above are the most commonly used intermittent fasting strategies and the ones that have been studied the most in research. There are many more forms of intermittent fasting that are essentially just slightly different versions of these. Studies show that periods of severe energy restriction in the short or long term are not favourable for athletes, but can be successful in obese populations[3]. This is for the same reasons stated for very low calorie diets in chapter 8, due to large calorie deficits.

Intermittent fasting on a time-restricted basis or daily basis is *safe* for humans and can improve body composition and health[4]. Intermittent fasting is typically associated with weight loss because there are long periods of time without consuming food, which may predispose an individual to consuming fewer calories than their daily needs. During feeding periods, there is usually no compensatory increase in calorie intake to offset the fasted days, resulting in a calorie deficit across the day or week. However, like any other diet, intermittent fasting *can* result in weight gain if calorie consumption during the fed hours exceeds the daily (TRF) or weekly (ADF, WDF) maintenance calorie needs. But to date, there are no human studies comparing different forms of intermittent fasting to one another[5]. And therefore, it is unknown whether one fasting strategy is better than another.

Intermittent fasting for weight loss: continuous energy restriction (CER) versus intermittent energy restriction (IER)

Continuous energy restriction is a more formal term for what we call a typical calorie deficit where you restrict calorie intake but eat at any time of the day. *Intermittent energy restriction* is another way of saying intermittent fasting. You restrict calorie intake only at certain times of the day or week.

Systematic reviews and meta-analyses of intermittent energy restriction show that it is *not* superior to continuous energy restriction for weight loss when calories are equated, showing intermittent energy restriction to be comparable to continuous energy restriction for weight loss[4,6–8]. Current evidence does not show a significant benefit of intermittent fasting compared to other dieting strategies to generate a calorie deficit for improving body composition. Intermittent energy restriction is as effective, but not more effective than continuous energy restriction[1,4,6,9,10].

Intermittent fasting is also just as effective, but not superior to any other form of diet plan for improving health (such as reducing type 2 diabetes or reducing resting blood glucose levels)[8,11]. Intermittent fasting can be a successful strategy for weight loss because by restricting the period of time during which you can eat, it leads to a reduction in daily energy intake. This can result in a calorie deficit and weight loss. It is the calorie deficit leading to weight loss and the weight loss resulting in health improvements, not intermittent fasting *per se*. There is no evidence to suggest that intermittent fasting results in improvements in health outcomes beyond the calorie deficit it generates[2,4,12].

For some, intermittent fasting is a great strategy because it can be much easier to adhere to the calorie restriction. For others, the lengthy periods of fasting can be uncomfortable, resulting in hunger and dissatisfaction. Once again, personal preference should dictate whether it is used or not.

As mentioned before, the timing of protein is less important for body composition when in a calorie deficit for weight loss. Therefore, intermittent energy restriction will not impair muscle preservation provided daily protein intake is sufficient. The size of the calorie deficit induced by intermittent energy restriction is the driving factor for the ratio of fat mass:muscle mass lost (chapter 7). The size of the daily calorie deficit is the sum of both the fasted and fed periods.

Time-restricted feeding typically involves skipping breakfast, with food consumption commencing at midday. Indeed, consuming breakfast is not necessarily superior to skipping breakfast for body composition[13]. This is also a strong example of how the study design can heavily influence the findings and subsequent recommendations (chapter 4). A meta-analysis of *randomised controlled trials* comparing breakfast with no breakfast (time-restricted feeding strategies use a similar concept), found a lower total daily calorie intake and lower body weight with no breakfast[14,15]. On the other hand, a meta-analysis of *observational studies* found breakfast skipping was associated with weight gain[16–18]. Some studies have also found no association of breakfast skipping on weight gain[13]. Observational studies suggest a detrimental effect of no breakfast on health and body weight, but controlled interventions show the opposite[19]. There also appears to be a genetic component associated with breakfast skipping, with a higher body mass index in the genetically associated breakfast skippers[19,20]. The influence of meal timing is likely to be *highly individual* and also based on *personal preference*. Most studies are in the general population, who are not necessarily exercising.

Intermittent fasting for muscle growth

The very limited high-quality evidence suggests it is possible to build muscle and fast during part of the day. It is probably wise to train during the fed period of your day to maximise muscle growth if you choose to do so.

Most intermittent fasting studies are in sedentary, overweight individuals. Fewer studies assess active individuals with a focus on weight loss, and even fewer assess the effect of intermittent fasting on resistance training and muscle growth. Earlier randomised controlled studies suggest either equivocal or sub-optimal results with intermittent fasting compared to continuous feeding[21,22]. However, these studies have significant limitations due to differences between the intermittent fasting groups and the continuous feeding groups being studied. Lower protein intakes or lower total calorie intakes (calories and protein were not equated) in the intermittent fasting groups will impact muscle growth regardless of any timing strategy, and therefore does not provide a fair comparison due to confounding (chapter 4). Unless we control for variables that are known to affect muscle growth, we cannot conclude if intermittent fasting is a suitable alternative to continuous energy intake. As discussed in chapter 9, spacing protein intake throughout the day is beneficial for muscle growth. Is this still possible to achieve whilst intermittently fasting?

Fortunately, a very recent randomised, controlled, double-blinded study (a high-quality study design) by Grant Tinsley has addressed many of these concerns. The study assessed *time-restricted feeding* (TRF; fasting during parts of the day) and equated important dietary variables including total calorie and protein intake[23]. Over the course of 8 weeks, 40 females with resistance training experience (they had several years of experience lifting weights) took part in a resistance training programme and either ate continuously throughout the day or consumed all of their daily energy intake between 12am and 8pm (the TRF group). This aligns with the time-restricted feeding form of intermittent fasting, fasting for 16 hours and eating for 8 hours. Both groups had similar diet compositions, training programmes and optimal protein intakes (1.6g/kg/day). Both groups similarly increased muscle mass and lost similarly small, but significant amounts of body fat. Both groups had similar improvements in muscular performance[23]. It is important to note that the intermittent fasting group completed their resistance training *during* their period of feeding. They did *not* train fasted. They had pre-workout and post-workout nutrition. It may well be that if they had trained in the fasted state, the results may have been inferior to the continuous food intake group. As such, the study suggests that intermittent fasting *can* be a viable strategy for muscle growth and equivalent to continuous feeding when training in a fed state.

The fact that the participants were experienced at resistance training suggests that intermediate or advanced lifters can utilise intermittent fasting as a viable option for building muscle[23].

However, it should be noted that participants in the time-restricted feeding group felt hungrier during the study, more fatigued, and more irritable. A major determinant of body composition change success is adherence to your plan. If time-restricted feeding promotes factors that reduce your ability to adhere, it may limit your success with that strategy.

The study highlights once again how the specifics of a diet (such as the timing) are much less important than the top-level factors such as total calorie intake and protein intake. And, the study provides further evidence showing intermittent fasting to be equivocal to, and not superior to, continuous feeding.

Interestingly, a systematic review and meta-analysis of *Ramadan fasting* in amateur and elite athletes (food intake restricted to the hours of darkness) demonstrated that this form of intermittent fasting generally did not impair aerobic exercise performance or workload, but did affect mean and peak power, and sprint performance[24]. This was only over the course of 1 month, therefore the effects may be greater with longer durations of fasting. Also, this is a very different form of fasting to that used by most people who practice intermittent fasting and may not be directly relevant, especially when considering that some of the studies looking at anaerobic performance found no effect, but only assessed hydration status and not food intake[25,26]. If you exercise in the mornings, consuming a breakfast to fuel your workout may be more preferable (see chapter 24 regarding fasted exercise).

Should I use intermittent fasting?

Try it, if you find it works, great. If you find it doesn't, stop.

One of the leading researchers on intermittent fasting, Grant Tinsley (whose studies have been discussed above) has summed up whether to use intermittent fasting nicely:

"Intermittent fasting may be difficult for certain individuals to follow... since adherence is known to be one of the most critical factors for long-term success with a dietary program, intermittent fasting is probably not a good strategy for those who find it especially difficult. With that said, a number of our participants reported that the intermittent fasting program got substantially easier after they had followed it for several days or weeks."
Grant Tinsley, today.ttu.com[27].

If intermittent fasting sounds good to you, which form of intermittent fasting should you choose? We currently do not know which type of fasting is best, or if they are equally effective[5]. Choose the form: time-restricted feeding (TRF), alternate-day fasting (ADF) or whole-day fasting (WDF), that you think best suits you, or try them all.

As a tool for weight loss, intermittent fasting should be used for as long as is needed for the determined weight loss to continue. Extended periods of calorie restriction are not recommended and can have counteracting effects on weight loss (such as reduced total daily energy expenditure and increased feelings of hunger). Intermittent fasting can be a viable strategy for long-term weight maintenance if it results in satiety, appetite regulation and achieving caloric maintenance. The limited feeding window with intermittent fasting may aid long-term maintenance of weight with a more intuitive approach (chapter 6).

Intermittent energy restriction: diet breaks and refeeds for weight loss

The discussion of intermittent fasting so far has considered forms of intermittent energy restriction involving fasting. However, intermittent energy restriction can also include days to weeks of continuous energy restriction interspersed with days of increased calorie intake. In other words, intermittent energy restriction over longer time scales.

Diet breaks and refeeds can be thought of as calorie cycling between a moderate (<30%) calorie deficit, and a period of calorie maintenance. This differs from traditional intermittent fasting which typically involves periods of severe or extreme (usually >75% up to 100%) periods of calorie restriction, and periods of ad libitum (at free will) feeding.

The evidence is currently inconclusive as to whether diet breaks and refeeds are more beneficial than continuous energy restriction. There is suggestion that they can help to minimise the adverse metabolic and hormonal changes that occur with weight loss. Current recommendations are based largely on theory and expert opinion.

Continuous and intermittent energy restriction are *equivalent* for weight loss. The primary driver is a calorie deficit, and the dietary strategy you choose (low carbohydrate and high fat, high fat and low carbohydrate, or continuous or intermittent energy restriction) is down to personal preference that allows for adherence.

There is very recent research that suggests there may be an advantage to adopting novel forms of intermittent energy restriction (IER). These novel forms are over periods longer than a few days. These periods of energy restriction are broken up with shorter periods of energy intake at calorie maintenance. This is slightly different to intermittent fasting because the periods of energy restriction do *not* involve fasting.

There are two main forms, which are essentially the same but differ in their duration:

- **Refeed;** a shorter and more frequent increase in calories (usually carbohydrate), such as 5 days in a calorie deficit and a 1 to 2 day refeed at caloric maintenance, before returning to the deficit.
- **Diet break**; a longer and less frequent period of increased calorie intake, such as 4 weeks in a calorie deficit and a 1 to 2 week diet break at caloric maintenance, before returning to the deficit.

Most assessments of intermittent energy restriction are in the form of intermittent fasting, and do not consider the longer duration forms of intermittent energy restriction: refeeds or diet breaks. Their utility is in *weight loss*, not muscle gain. As stated above, intermittent fasting has been shown to be equivalent to, and not superior to continuous energy restriction for weight loss (when calories and protein are equated)[4,6,10]. The evidence base for intermittent energy restriction in the form of diet breaks and refeeds in humans is very small. Most evidence is in non-athletes (obese and overweight people). This evidence suggests that intermittent energy restriction in the form of diet breaks and refeeds is as effective as continuous energy restriction for fat loss. Some studies suggest there is a slight benefit to using intermittent energy restriction, resulting in more favourable metabolic and hormonal adaptations to weight loss compared to continuous energy restriction[28,29]. No studies exist for intermittent energy restriction as refeeds or diet breaks in athletes compared to continuous energy restriction. However, refeeds are a strategy that some athletes already adopt during periods of weight loss[28,30]. Athletes using refeeds or diet breaks have been questioned in *qualitative* research studies (a type of research where people are interviewed). Athletes said that by refeeding, it *gave* them more energy for workouts. They '*perceived*' having more muscle glycogen, providing greater mental recovery, and they '*perceived*' having a prevention of further negative effects on total daily energy expenditure (TDEE) from dieting. This is of course, anecdotal. '*Feeling*' something does not mean it *actually* happens. Drawing conclusions should be treated with caution until randomised trials have been conducted.

The theoretical rationale for how refeeds and diet breaks work is that by returning to calorie maintenance, some of the hormones involved in regulating fat storage, appetite and metabolism are altered. It is thought that the break in calorie restriction helps to attenuate any adaptive mechanisms that may make it difficult to lose more weight after being in a period of calorie restriction[28]. In other words, they may make it easier to adhere to further calorie restriction. The *psychological break* from calorie restriction may also be important[29]. Calorie restriction is stressful and having a break may aid adherence. It may also be that what is actually occurring is that the diet break makes the deficit slightly smaller across the week as a whole. We know that larger deficits are less optimal in normal individuals, and smaller deficits promote greater fat-free mass retention. Therefore, a diet break would promote relatively greater fat loss and less muscle loss per calorie in the deficit. Also, from the large amount of evidence we have on weight change and metabolism in healthy people, metabolic rate does not seem to be significantly affected by previous dieting history. Also, you cannot '*damage*' your metabolism (as discussed in chapter 5). This would suggest that you also cannot '*improve*' your metabolism beyond alterations in energy intake. It may well be that intermittent energy restriction *works* by just creating a smaller weekly net deficit and therefore more optimal long-term outcomes. Indeed, to achieve the same amount of weight loss from the same calorie deficit, the total dieting period needs to be *longer* when using intermittent energy restriction, than when using continuous energy restriction. This is because of the periods of time spent at calorie maintenance with intermittent energy restriction. Whether there is a benefit or not, is unknown. Like intermittent fasting, *no* studies have compared different refeed or diet break forms, and therefore whether superior forms exist is unknown[29].

Refeed

In a refeed, there is energy restriction for most of the week followed by 1 or 2 days at caloric maintenance. The literature on refeeds is slim. However, such a strategy is popular amongst fitness individuals, using the more extreme concept of '*cheat meals*' (eating high energy density, low nutrient density foods such as pizza or burgers to excess, once per week)[29].

Bill Campbell's lab at the University of South Florida are working on the effects of refeeds in healthy and resistance trained individuals. His lab has performed two studies which have been presented at a recent ISSN conference. The full study design is yet to be published, which limits the ability to critique the study[31]. The first was a randomised controlled pilot study in 2018[31]. 8 resistance trained males and one female were randomly split to have a calorie restricted diet with a refeed (3 participants) or a control continuous energy restriction diet (5 participants) alongside a resistance training programme. Calorie intake was equated such that participants consumed 25% fewer calories than their daily baseline calorie intake. The refeed group consumed more carbohydrates 2 days per week, and were calorie restricted for 5 days per week. The control continuous energy restriction diet group were in a calorie deficit 7 days per week. After 7 weeks, both groups significantly reduced body weight from the start of the study. Both groups achieved equivalent weight loss.

Subsequently, the lab performed a larger randomised controlled study with 14 resistance trained males and 13 resistance trained females[31]. The study design was identical to the pilot study above except for more participants (this means that smaller differences between groups can be identified). This time, the study assessed more variables. After 7 weeks, both groups:

- Significantly reduced **body weight.**
- Significantly reduced **resting metabolic rate** (similar to basal metabolic rate), as expected from weight loss.
- Significantly reduced **fat mass** and **body fat percentage.**
- Significantly reduced **muscle mass.**

However, the refeed group lost slightly less muscle mass than the continuous energy restriction group. The study found that the refeed group also had a slightly smaller reduction in basal metabolic rate (in this case resting metabolic rate, but similar enough; see chapter 5) compared to the continuous energy restriction group[31]. The difference however, was small (a reduction of 40kcal/day compared to a reduction of 78kcal/day). Considering the effects of adaptive thermogenesis, exercise and non-exercise activity thermogenesis on total daily energy expenditure, is this of meaningful significance? Did the preservation of more fat-free mass mean basal metabolic rate was preserved? Or did the preservation of basal metabolic rate from a smaller weekly deficit mean fat-free mass was preserved? Indeed, the control diet lost more weight overall, which would suggest a larger caloric deficit over the dieting period, which may explain these differences[31]. This limited, but well designed study suggests there could be a benefit to refeeds during a calorie deficit. More studies are needed to confirm such findings and to consider the mechanism in more detail.

A novel observational study by Jorge et al. from the *Portuguese Weight Control Registry* looked at how strict people were with their diets on weekends and holidays compared to weekdays, and whether they regained weight during long periods of weight loss maintenance. The study reveals some interesting and relevant findings to the concept of refeeds[32]. Of the 108 individuals studied, those who were less strict on weekends were less likely to regain weight, and no difference was seen with strictness during holidays. This is not too dissimilar from the concept of refeeds as conducted by Bill Campbell's lab. The concepts are similar in that 5 days are spent being *'more strict'* with calorie intake, with 2 days being *'less strict'*. However, one difference is that refeeds are used to *lose* weight, and this study looked at the ability to *maintain* weight (and not add weight).

Others have suggested that 1 to 2 days at calorie maintenance may be too short of a break from a calorie deficit to reverse some of the negative effects of dieting. Thus, the suggestion is that longer periods of additional calories in the form of a diet break may provide a better outcome for body composition.

Diet break

In a diet break, there is a calorie deficit for several weeks before eating at calorie maintenance or above for a week or so, rather than fasting at certain times of the day or on certain days of the week. The specific length of time in a deficit and time on a diet break has not been standardised, nor have different lengths of diet breaks been compared[29]. The main evidence so far is from the MATADOR (*Minimising Adaptive Thermogenesis And Deactivating Obesity Rebound*) randomised controlled trial in obese males[33]. The study found greater fat loss with a diet break compared to the continuous energy restricted diet, but with similar muscle mass retention[33]. Similar findings were seen in overweight and obese females[34]. Of course, how applicable these studies in obese individuals are to healthy individuals performing exercise is limited. Studies have *not* been conducted in individuals of a healthy weight. Unsurprisingly, there are also studies that show no significant benefit over continuous energy restriction[28]. Diet breaks are therefore an interesting research topic for the future.

Jackson Peos, an Australian researcher at the University of Western Australia is conducting a randomised, controlled, single-blinded study (participants do not know which group they are in, but the researchers do)[10]. The key difference is that this study is in healthy athletes. Therefore, this study will be more applicable to the readers of this book. The study will compare a diet break (4 x 3 week blocks of intermittent energy restriction (IER) interspersed with 1 week at calorie maintenance) with a single 12 week block of continuous energy restriction.

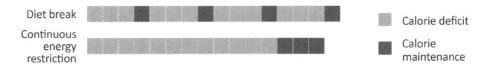

Diet break — Continuous energy restriction

Calorie deficit — Calorie maintenance

The 'Intermittent versus Continuous Energy restriction Compared in an Athlete Population' (ICECAP) study design[10]. One group will be in a continuous calorie deficit for 12 weeks. The other group will be in a calorie deficit for 3 weeks, before having 1 week at calorie maintenance. The diet break group will then return to the calorie deficit and repeat the cycle 4 times, such that they will be in a calorie deficit for a total of 12 weeks. Calorie deficits will be equated between the two groups.

The calorie deficit will be moderate, such that both groups will have a target weight loss of 0.7% of their starting body weight per week. Unlike typical intermittent fasting diets, this period of intermittent energy restriction will last longer than a week[10]. The results will provide important information to guide evidence-based recommendations for using diet breaks to influence body composition.

Expert recommendations for implementing a diet break

A theoretical guide to intermittent energy restriction for dieting has been published by Jackson Peos[28]. The evidence-based recommendations currently are of low quality, relying on studies in obese individuals, theoretical concepts and expert opinion. Many of the recommendations cover the main principles for any other diet, including avoiding rapid weight loss, consuming sufficient protein intake, and performing resistance exercise[28].

The main specific recommendation for a refeed or a diet break is that additional energy intake from carbohydrate consumption may be more beneficial than increasing protein and fat[28]. It may also be beneficial to time higher volume training sessions or periods during these diet breaks or refeeds, to facilitate greater performance and recovery needs[28].

Do diet breaks and refeeds improve adherence? Or do they make it harder because it causes you to break the new habits you are forming? For some, it may reinforce the mindset that you can return to 'normal', which may break the new habits that have been made. As discussed in chapters 5 and 7, when you lose weight your metabolism will be lower. Therefore, your new maintenance energy intake is lower than before, meaning a return to your 'normal' lifestyle may result in weight gain. For others, it may allow you to adhere better by giving a break from the stress of a calorie deficit. Responses to breaks and the *reasoning* behind them are important. Future studies will not only need to look at the body composition changes, but also any psychological or perceived changes with intermittent compared to continuous energy restriction. Other areas to be addressed include how you should implement the break; should you increase calorie intake back to an estimated calorie maintenance, or eat ad libitum (eat as much as you want)? Do diet breaks impair the ability to create sustainable lifestyle changes? These two contrasting views may both be possible, depending on the individual. Two evidence-based fitness experts have given their opinions on utilising a diet break. As noted in chapter 4, expert opinion is a lower quality form of evidence, but there is a paucity of research on the topic, and therefore their insights are useful.

Jackson Peos (an academic researching diet breaks) recommends that a diet break should be 7-14 days in length. Food sources should be kept roughly the same and calorie intake should be increased by increasing portion sizes. Diet breaks should return calories to predicted maintenance, erring on the side of caution (i.e. a calorie surplus), because there tends to not be much benefit from a diet break if the individual is still in a deficit. There is weak evidence to allocate additional calories to carbohydrate, which is primarily a theoretical consideration. Based on the current research, the diet break should be implemented every 2-3 weeks. In real-life, possibly every 4-8 weeks may be more suitable[28,35].

Menno Henselmans recommends that for a diet break you should ask yourself, '*why do you think you need a break?*'; is it because of issues with adherence? What is it that you are doing now that is so unsustainable or stressful that you need a break? It will be just as unsustainable after. Even though a caloric deficit should not be maintained in the long term, it should be similar to your habitual maintenance diet. If you choose to take a diet break, then keep food choices as similar as possible, without any focus on increasing any particular macronutrient (i.e. just increase portion sizes). Menno suggests there is never a theoretical need, but they can used when the time seems right[35].

Anecdotally, refeeds and diet breaks are commonly used in individuals dieting, but there is a lack of solid evidence for their efficacy. Experts have suggested they may be beneficial, but more high quality evidence is needed[28,29]. Therefore, use them if you find it easier when dieting or if it helps you to be compliant to the weight loss plan. But, whether they are actually beneficial remains to be seen. They may have use as a mental and psychological break from calorie restriction and the stress involved. But they may also affect adherence and break any habits that have formed during the weight loss process.

Summary

When calorie and protein intake are equated, intermittent fasting and continuous eating regimes are equivocal for weight change outcomes.

The decision to use intermittent fasting should be down to personal preference.

Restricting food intake to certain periods of the day or week can help adhere to a calorie restricted diet.

Diet breaks and refeeds may be useful tools to minimise the adverse effects of periods of calorie restriction. However, the evidence is limited at this stage.

References

1   Aragon AA, Schoenfeld BJ, Wildman R, Kleiner S, VanDusseldorp T, Taylor L et al. International society of sports nutrition position stand: diets and body composition. *J Int Soc Sports Nutr* 2017; 14. Available from: doi:10.1186/s12970-017-0174-y.

2   Tinsley GM, La Bounty PM. Effects of intermittent fasting on body composition and clinical health markers in humans. *Nutr Rev* 2015; 73: 661–674.

3   Casazza K, Fontaine KR, Astrup A, Birch LL, Brown AW, Bohan Brown MM et al. Myths, Presumptions, and Facts about Obesity. *N Engl J Med* 2013; 368: 446–454.

4   Seimon RV, Roekenes JA, Zibellini J, Zhu B, Gibson AA, Hills AP et al. Do intermittent diets provide physiological benefits over continuous diets for weight loss? A systematic review of clinical trials. *Mol Cell Endocrinol* 2015; 418: 153–172.

5   Obert J, Pearlman M, Obert L, Chapin S. Popular Weight Loss Strategies: a Review of Four Weight Loss Techniques. *Curr Gastroenterol Rep* 2017; 19: 61.

6   Davis CS, Clarke RE, Coulter SN, Rounsefell KN, Walker RE, Rauch CE et al. Intermittent energy restriction and weight loss: a systematic review. *Eur J Clin Nutr* 2016; 70: 292–299.

7   Harris L, Hamilton S, Azevedo LB, Olajide J, De Brún C, Waller G et al. Intermittent fasting interventions for treatment of overweight and obesity in adults: a systematic review and meta-analysis. *JBI Database Syst Rev Implement Rep* 2018; 16: 507–547.

8   Headland M, Clifton PM, Carter S, Keogh JB. Weight-Loss Outcomes: A Systematic Review and Meta-Analysis of Intermittent Energy Restriction Trials

Lasting a Minimum of 6 Months. *Nutrients* 2016; 8. Available from: doi:10.3390/nu8060354.

9   Schübel R, Nattenmüller J, Sookthai D, Nonnenmacher T, Graf ME, Riedl L et al. Effects of intermittent and continuous calorie restriction on body weight and metabolism over 50 wk: a randomized controlled trial. *Am J Clin Nutr* 2018; 108: 933–945.

10   Peos JJ, Helms ER, Fournier PA, Sainsbury A. Continuous versus intermittent moderate energy restriction for increased fat mass loss and fat free mass retention in adult athletes: protocol for a randomised controlled trial—the ICECAP trial (Intermittent versus Continuous Energy restriction Compared in an Athlete Population). *BMJ Open Sport Exerc Med* 2018; 4. Available from: doi:10.1136/bmjsem-2018-000423.

11   de Cabo R, Mattson MP. Effects of Intermittent Fasting on Health, Aging, and Disease. *N Engl J Med* 2019; 381: 2541–2551.

12   Trepanowski JF, Canale RE, Marshall KE, Kabir MM, Bloomer RJ. Impact of caloric and dietary restriction regimens on markers of health and longevity in humans and animals: a summary of available findings. *Nutr J* 2011; 10: 107.

13   Zhang L, Cordeiro LS, Liu J, Ma Y. The Association between Breakfast Skipping and Body Weight, Nutrient Intake, and Metabolic Measures among Participants with Metabolic Syndrome. *Nutrients* 2017; 9. Available from: doi:10.3390/nu9040384.

14   Levitsky DA, Pacanowski CR. Effect of skipping breakfast on subsequent energy intake. *Physiol Behav* 2013; 119: 9–16.

15   Sievert K, Hussain SM, Page MJ, Wang Y, Hughes HJ, Malek M et al. Effect of breakfast on weight and energy intake: systematic review and meta-analysis of randomised controlled trials. *BMJ* 2019; 364. Available from: doi:10.1136/bmj.l42.

16   Watanabe Y, Saito I, Henmi I, Yoshimura K, Maruyama K, Yamauchi K et al. Skipping Breakfast is Correlated with Obesity. *J Rural Med JRM* 2014; 9: 51–58.

17   Otaki N, Obayashi K, Saeki K, Kitagawa M, Tone N, Kurumatani N. Relationship between Breakfast Skipping and Obesity among Elderly: Cross-Sectional Analysis of the HEIJO-KYO Study. *J Nutr Health Aging* 2017; 21: 501–504.

18   Horikawa C, Kodama S, Yachi Y, Heianza Y, Hirasawa R, Ibe Y et al. Skipping breakfast and prevalence of overweight and obesity in Asian and Pacific regions: a meta-analysis. *Prev Med* 2011; 53: 260–267.

19   Lopez-Minguez J, Gómez-Abellán P, Garaulet M. Timing of Breakfast, Lunch, and Dinner. Effects on Obesity and Metabolic Risk. *Nutrients* 2019; 11. Available from: doi:10.3390/nu11112624.

20   Dashti HS, Merino J, Lane JM, Song Y, Smith CE, Tanaka T et al. Genome-wide association study of breakfast skipping links clock regulation with food timing. *Am J Clin Nutr* 2019; 110: 473–484.

21   Tinsley GM, Forsse JS, Butler NK, Paoli A, Bane AA, Bounty PML et al. Time-restricted feeding in young men performing resistance training: A randomized controlled trial. *Eur J Sport Sci* 2017; 17: 200–207.

22   Moro T, Tinsley G, Bianco A, Marcolin G, Pacelli QF, Battaglia G et al. Effects of eight weeks of time-restricted feeding (16/8) on basal metabolism, maximal strength, body composition, inflammation, and cardiovascular risk factors in resistance-trained males. *J Transl Med* 2016; 14: 290.

23   Tinsley GM, Moore ML, Graybeal AJ, Paoli A, Kim Y, Gonzales JU et al. Time-restricted feeding plus resistance training in active females: a randomized trial. *Am J Clin Nutr* 2019; 110: 628–640.

24   Abaïdia A-E, Daab W, Bouzid MA. Effects of Ramadan Fasting on Physical Performance: A Systematic Review with Meta-analysis. *Sports Med Auckl NZ* 2020. Available from: doi:10.1007/s40279-020-01257-0.

25   Hoffman JR, Stavsky H, Falk B. The effect of water restriction on anaerobic power and vertical jumping height in basketball players. *Int J Sports Med* 1995; 16: 214–218.

26   Cheuvront SN, Carter RI, Haymes EM, Sawka MN. No Effect of Moderate Hypohydration or Hyperthermia on Anaerobic Exercise Performance. *Med Sci Sports Exerc* 2006; 38: 1093–1097.

27   Young G. *Researcher: Intermittent Fasting Has Benefits, But It's Not For Everyone.* Texas Tech Today. Available from: https://today.ttu.edu/posts/2019/07/Stories/intermittent-fasting-benefits-not-for-everyone (accessed 7 Feb 2020).

28   Peos J, Norton L, Helms E, Galpin A, Fournier P. Intermittent Dieting: Theoretical Considerations for the Athlete. *Sports* 2019; 7: 22.

29   Roberts BM, Helms ER, Trexler ET, Fitschen PJ. Nutritional Recommendations for Physique Athletes. *Journal of Human Kinetics* 2020; 71(1): 79-108. Available from: doi:http://dx.doi.org/10.2478/hukin-2019-0096.

30   Mitchell L, Hackett D, Gifford J, Estermann F, O'Connor H. Do Bodybuilders Use Evidence-Based Nutrition Strategies to Manipulate Physique? *Sports* 2017; 5: 76.

31   Proceedings of the Fifteenth International Society of Sports Nutrition (ISSN) Conference and Expo. *J Int Soc Sports Nutr* 2018; 15: 1-37. Available from: https://jissn.biomedcentral.com/articles/10.1186/s12970-018-0256-5 (accessed 6 Feb 2020).

32   Jorge R, Santos I, Teixeira VH, Teixeira PJ. Does diet strictness level during weekends and holiday periods influence 1-year follow-up weight loss maintenance? Evidence from the Portuguese Weight Control Registry. *Nutr J* 2019; 18. Available from: doi:10.1186/s12937-019-0430-x.

33   Byrne NM, Sainsbury A, King NA, Hills AP, Wood RE. Intermittent energy restriction improves weight loss efficiency in obese men: the MATADOR study. *Int J Obes* 2018; 42: 129–138.

34   Davoodi SH, Ajami M, Ayatollahi SA, Dowlatshahi K, Javedan G, Pazoki-Toroudi HR. Calorie Shifting Diet Versus Calorie Restriction Diet: A Comparative Clinical Trial Study. *Int J Prev Med* 2014; 5: 447–456.

35   Henselmans M. *Should you do diet breaks?* 2019. Available from: https://mennohenselmans.com/diet-break-debate/ (accessed 7 Feb 2020).

12. Food choice and dietary patterns for health

You can eat anything you want, just not everything you want. No food is so good that you must eat it, and no food is so bad that you must avoid it.

No single nutrient is more important than the diet as a whole. Superfoods do not exist; the term is a marketing tool. Foods are not inherently unhealthy or healthy, they just contain different amounts of energy and nutrients within a given volume of food. A diet consisting of only a single food that is considered 'healthy' (e.g. only eating apples) would actually be 'unhealthy' due to nutritional deficiencies. A food can only be 'healthy' in the context of a wide and varied diet. Any food can be considered in this context.

A single food consumed at a given instant will not influence health. But, the repeated consumption over a long period of time of certain foods will relate to better or poorer health outcomes. In other words, the long-term dietary pattern influences health, not specific food choices at a given moment in time.

Any food can be part of an 'unhealthy' diet, any food can be part of a 'healthy' diet.

The discussion so far has centred around macronutrients (protein, carbohydrate and fat) in isolation. However, the reality is that we consume these in the form of food and drink. Foods can vary greatly in terms of their:

- Energy content.
- Nutritional value.
- Palatability.

These are all important considerations when assessing your own diet.

Energy density and nutrient density: a model for understanding food choices for a varied, balanced diet

The concept of specific foods being *'bad' or 'good, 'healthy,* or *'unhealthy'* is outdated and illogical. Dietary habits and choices can influence physical, social and mental health. This can be through the relationships developed with foods, and through the foods consumed themselves. A diet with what would be considered *'healthy'* foods (e.g. fruits and vegetables) could be unhealthy if an individual develops a poor relationship with their diet. Diets can therefore be healthier or unhealthier as a whole. But, any specific food can be in an unhealthy diet, and any food can be in a healthy diet. No food is inherently fattening, nor is any food inherently slimming. Besides allergies, there is no evidence to suggest that any particular food group or food should be completely excluded from a diet for health reasons. If this were the case, we would be able to see an improvement in health outcomes from excluding specific foods, but this has not been conclusively shown. Instead, research finds that *dietary patterns* (the relative proportions of *food groups* that make up the majority of someone's diet) relate with differences in health outcomes. Food groups can be split into plant-based and animal-based food groups, and then further categorised. This list is not definitive, and food groups can be categorised in other ways.

Plant-based food groups:

- Fruit
- Vegetables
- Nuts
- Legumes
- Whole grains
- Refined grains
- Plant oils

- Sugar-sweetened drinks (plant-based beverages)
- Tea and coffee (plant-based beverages)

Animal-based food groups:

- Dairy
- Eggs
- Fish
- Poultry
- Red meat. Mammalian muscle meats such as beef, pork or lamb. Red meat does not include chicken, turkey, duck, rabbit or fish.

- Processed meat. Any meat that has been salted, smoked, cured or been through processing to improve its flavour or allow for its preservation (e.g. hot dogs, sausages, sliced meat, salami, bacon, canned meat). Processed meat is usually red meat, but processed white meat may also be included.

Animal or plant-based food groups:

- Ultra-processed foods. Industrial productions with the addition of ingredients that are not used in home cooking.

Because of this, it is more appropriate to consider foods in terms of their *energy density* and *nutrient density*, and to consider food choices from the perspective of food groups, not from the perspective of specific foods or nutrients.

Energy density

Energy density refers to the number of calories in a food relative to its weight (kcal/gram)[1,2]. Energy dense foods contain more calories within a given amount of food. Some foods provide a lot of calories whilst providing minimal satiety. This can create a scenario whereby it is easier to overfeed and consume calories in excess of your daily calorie needs, and therefore result in weight gain. Similarly, other foods provide fewer calories whilst also providing similar or greater levels of satiety. Consuming these foods can promote a scenario where you are less likely to overconsume before feeling satiated, less likely to be in a caloric surplus, and potentially be in a calorie deficit.

Nutrient density

Nutrient density refers to the quantity of important dietary elements in a food relative to its weight or energy content. This can include vitamins, minerals, fibre and phytonutrients (non-specific chemicals found in plants that are thought to be beneficial to health) and other chemicals. Assessing nutrient density is more complex than assessing energy density[1]. Nutrient density has been calculated in different ways, but often assesses the relative quantity of certain nutrients such as protein, fibre and specific vitamins and minerals against the quantity of other nutrients such as saturated fat and added sugar. Beyond simply calorie intake, consuming sufficient quantities of these nutrients can also influence appetite and satiety, and impact on health.

Energy dense diets have been linked with increased risks of obesity, whereas nutrient dense diets have not[1]. There is an inverse relationship between energy density and nutrient density[1]; *reducing* the energy density *increases* the ratio of nutrient:energy content.

Energy density varies from:

- 0kcal/gram – water.
- 4kcal/gram – carbohydrate and protein.
- 7kcal/gram – alcohol.
- 9kcal/gram – fat.

The relative contributions of each component in a food will dictate its energy density. The main factor influencing the energy density of a food is its water content. Water content increases food volume with *no* additional caloric content. Water content therefore decreases energy density[2]. Similarly, soft drinks have low energy densities due to their water content, which is true for any liquid. But, they are of very low nutrient density and it is easier to overconsume liquids. Fat content will increase energy density[2]. Nuts, seeds and eggs are energy dense due to their fat content, but they are also nutrient dense.

Some examples of food energy densities:

Food	Energy density (kcal/100g)
Milk (whole fat)	61
Meat (beef)	219
Fruit (citrus)	50
Vegetables (lettuce)	17
Vegetables (dark green veg)	31
Fish	182
Eggs	171
Ice-cream	232
Cakes (biscuits, muffins)	334
Soft drinks	39

Food energy densities. From Drewnowski, 2018[1].

Let's take two extreme examples:

1. Fruit

Despite common belief that fruits are high in sugar, fruits actually have a low energy density.

Pretty much all sources of fruit count towards your '*5 a day*', including fresh, frozen, tinned, dried varieties and fruit juice.

Observational studies show an inverse relationship between consuming fruit and body weight and body fat levels[2-5].

Fruits are:

- Low energy density and high nutrient density.
- A good source of vitamins and minerals.
- A source of dietary fibre (chapter 6).
- Contain a large amount of water[2].
- Associated with improved health.

2. Ultra-processed foods

Most ultra-processed foods such as cakes, crisps and chocolate are high energy density and low nutrient density.

Ultra-processed foods are:

- High energy density and low nutrient density.
- A poor source of vitamins and minerals.
- A poor source of dietary fibre
- Contain a small amount of water.
- Associated with poorer health.

The energy density within food groups will vary with the specific food tested. The table below provides a rough guide.

Energy Density (kcal/g)	Example
<0.6	Most fruit and non-starchy vegetables.
0.6-1.5	Whole grains, legumes, lean meats, dairy.
1.6-3.9	Refined grains (e.g. white breads, rice) cheese, higher fat meats.
4.0-4.9	Ultra-processed foods (e.g. fried foods, sweets, cookies).

Energy density classifications. From Rolls, 2018[6,7].

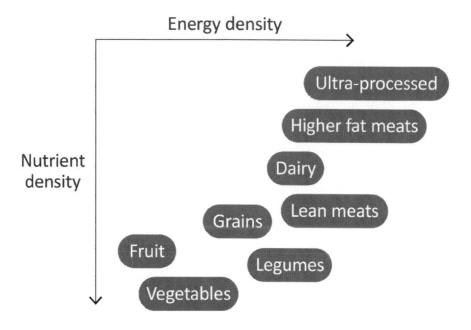

The energy and nutrient density graph. All foods and food groups are located in some region of the graph.

There is a common misconception that fruits contain large amounts of sugar. Therefore, some have suggested that fruit intake should be limited or even excluded to prevent excess sugar and calorie intake. However, fruits actually have a low energy density compared to other foods which are considered high in sugar content. Gram for gram, strawberries contain *1/10th* the sugar content and *5.8%* of the energy content of chocolate (see table below). This is partially because of the additional water content of strawberries, and the additional fat content of chocolate[2]. It should be pointed out that naturally occurring sugars such as those found in fruits are *not* included in the government dietary guidelines to reduce sugar intake (as outlined in chapter 6). In other words, there is *no* recommendation to limit the intake of naturally occurring sugars[8,9].

Per 100g	Cadbury dairy milk chocolate[10]	Strawberries, raw[11]
Energy density (kcal)	534	31
Fat	30	0.17
(of which saturates)	18	0
Carbohydrate	57	7.6
(of which sugars)	56	5.3
Fibre	2.1	1.8

The relative energy and nutrient densities of an ultra-processed food (chocolate) and a fruit (strawberry).

This only considers the energy density of the food. When we consider the nutrient density, fruits also contain a rich mixture of vitamins, minerals, fibre and phytonutrients. Therefore, they have a high nutrient density compared to ultra-processed foods such as chocolate, which contains little nutritional value besides its calorie content. This means that when comparing fruits with other processed high sugar foods, there are multiple contrasts and distinctions between them.

In summary, fruit has a low energy density and high nutrient density, and food such as ultra-processed chocolate has a high energy density and low nutrient density. Their relative position on the graph above highlights the large difference in their densities.

High fibre content makes a food source less energy dense, such as vegetables, fruit and grains[7,11]. As the *World Health Organisation* states, lower energy density foods are generally high in dietary fibre and water, such as fruits, legumes, vegetables and whole grain cereals. Energy dense and micronutrient-poor foods tend to be ultra-processed and contain high quantities of fat and/or sugar and/or salt[12]. Increased consumption of fibre-rich foods is correlated with a lower body mass index, lower body fat percentage and smaller waist circumference[13]. This effect can in part be attributed to the increase in satiety and resulting reduction in caloric intake from consuming less energy dense foods[2]. Decreasing the energy density of food (i.e. by increasing water or fibre content) can reduce daily calorie intake without reducing the total volume of food consumed and without increasing feelings of hunger or generating a lack of feeling full[7,14,15]. As an example, dried fruits are a great source of vitamins, minerals and fibre, and can be very convenient forms of fruit on the go. Because the water content has been removed, dried fruits are more energy dense than whole fruits[2]. For example, whole mango contains 60kcal/100g[16]. Dried mango contains 319kcal/100g[17]. An 80g portion of whole fruit is classed as one of your '5 a day', compared to a 30g portion of dried fruit, which counts as one of your

'5 a day'. This means that the same volume of dried fruit and whole fruit will have different energy and nutrient densities, and this may influence energy intake when eating intuitively[2].

As noted above, the volume of strawberries that could be consumed compared to chocolate is vastly greater for the same energy intake. Food volume is a large factor influencing satiety. People often go on brief periods of excluding ultra-processed foods such as cakes, chips, crisps and chocolate and discover they lose weight. The assumption made is that ultra-processed foods cause weight gain or prevent weight loss due to their fat or sugar content. What is really happening is that these ultra-processed foods provide little satiety and can result in calorie overconsumption. During these periods of ultra-processed food exclusion, these foods are replaced by the consumption of fruit, vegetables or other low energy density foods[2]. Interventional studies show that adding fruit or vegetables to meals can reduce the energy density of meals. Participants that are given meals of a similar palatability but a different energy density consume a similar volume of food. Participants consuming lower energy density meals therefore end up with a *reduction* in energy intake whilst *maintaining* satiety[18]. This reduction in energy intake occurs whether people are aware of the lower energy density or not[2]. Weight loss can be achieved intuitively without tracking, in some people. The maintained food volume promotes satiety alongside the consumption of fewer calories, which can result in the generation of a calorie deficit whilst eating at free will. If sustained, this can result in weight loss. Eventually, adaptive mechanisms will result in slower weight loss before eventual weight maintenance at a lower body weight as energy expenditure matches energy intake. The nutritional value of high fibre and phytonutrient content (non-specific chemicals found in plants that are thought to be beneficial to health) also likely contributes to the effects seen on body weight[2].

The influence of specific nutrients or foods on health: *'superfoods'*

How do you define a superfood? There is no universally accepted definition. Even so, no studies or meta-analyses (studies of studies) show evidence that a single food can significantly improve health outcomes compared to the whole dietary pattern itself. Focus on the overall diet and not on consuming specific foods. Consuming a range of food groups (fruit, vegetables, nuts, seeds etc) is far more important than the specific foods you consume within these groups.

"The current scientific evidence strongly suggests that it is not the consumption of one or two varieties of vegetables and fruit that confer a benefit, but rather the intake of a wide variety of plant foods."
Johnstone, 2012[21].

What is a superfood? Depending on who you ask, it has different meanings:

- A superfood is generally rich in nutrients and good for you.
- A superfood can help to *'prevent'*, *'reduce'* or even *'treat'* specific diseases.
- A superfood contains specific qualities or nutrients that provide health benefits that cannot be obtained elsewhere. For example, if the food source contains a *nutraceutical* (molecules found within foods that have both nutritional and pharmaceutical properties). Unlike macronutrients or micronutrients, nutraceuticals are not necessarily needed for maintenance of the body but may provide additional health benefits[22]. It is possible to test the effects of a nutraceutical with a randomised controlled trial (chapter 4). Examples of nutraceuticals include *carotenoids* and *polyphenols*.

A general definition which most people would probably agree with is:

"Broadly, they [superfoods] refer to foodstuffs and dietary supplements that are thought to contain a particularly beneficial set or sets of health-promoting properties (often in the form of vitamins and minerals contained in the foods themselves) and are believed to fight or prevent degenerative disease. Properties of foods like antioxidants, polyphenols, phytochemicals, and enzymes are highlighted as particularly health promoting."
Sikka, 2019[23].

Why has the concept of superfoods become so prevalent in recent years?

This comes down to a range of factors. One explanation is the search for a *'magic pill'*, something that can be taken with an instant benefit. In the hunt for such, there has been a rise in studies looking for specific foods that may benefit health. If one exists, wouldn't it be great if we can bottle it up or make it into a pill and sell it for lots of money? Also, when studies produce possible positive findings, the media has poorly interpreted and mis-reported such studies (which is not helped at times by overly optimistic researchers). A *'superfood'* newspaper headline grabs the attention of a reader much more than *'eat a range of nutritious foods'*. The vast *majority* of studies on superfoods or nutraceuticals are in cells or in animals in the lab, with very few studies in humans (see chapter 4 regarding research and study design)[24]. Any study that is not conducted within humans is immediately limited in its applicability. The interpretations of these studies are often too simplistic or flawed[22]. Studies may examine an extract, or a particular nutrient from the food in question, which is given at an incredibly high dose to a lab animal or cell. The study may then find improvements in a *proxy* outcome for an actual health outcome. For example, a biological marker which *correlates* with the actual disease of interest. These results are then *wrongly* interpreted as saying that the particular food that the extract originated from can prevent or reduce a particular disease. Extracts or components of foods are not eaten in isolation, but within a food matrix (i.e. a chemical of interest in a fruit is consumed as part of the fruit, not by itself)[25]. On the face of it, this research may appear applicable to humans. But, the evidence is actually completely different in terms of the population studied (animals versus humans), the intervention (a high dose of an isolated nutrient versus the nutrient within a food) and the outcome (a proxy marker versus an actual health outcome). This ultimately leads to a widespread belief about certain foods having certain health properties, which hasn't really been proven at all.

Even when studies assess humans, usually they are observational studies, which are lower quality forms of evidence[26]. Observational dietary studies are essentially in-depth questionnaires where researchers ask people about their dietary and lifestyle habits and measure health outcomes such as body weight, blood pressure or mortality. This can be at a single point in time or by studying people for many years. Researchers can then see how dietary and lifestyle habits associate with these health outcomes. These studies can only show correlations, *not* causations. They are limited by confounding variables.

When trying to assess whether a particular food is beneficial for health in a human association study, it is hard to separate it from the other variables (such as other foods consumed, lifestyle, socio-economic factors and other factors that can affect health) that are associated with increased consumption of that food. For example, eating apples is associated with improved health outcomes[27]. However, the actual effect is probably smaller than we think, because people who eat apples generally eat more fruit and vegetables than people who do not eat apples, and are more likely to be health conscious, perform exercise and not smoke. We can adjust the data for these confounding factors, but this can only be achieved to a certain extent. Statistical adjustment never fully removes confounding. Similarly, some people can have very healthy lifestyles and never eat apples, possibly because apples do not feature regularly in their culture or lifestyle, or simply because they do not like them and prefer to eat other fruits. The influence of the overall lifestyle will mask the relatively small effect of apple consumption. We know apples are a low energy density and high nutrient density food with beneficial outcomes for health. But, whether actually eating an apple every day compared to just consuming *any* other fruit has a significantly greater effect, is unlikely. And if there was, it would not be meaningful in a real-life context. Consider, if consuming 5 portions of fruit or vegetables a day added years onto life expectancy compared to no fruit or vegetable consumption, then if eating a specific fruit or vegetable (e.g. an apple) within those 5 portions had an effect on life expectancy, it might add just a few seconds or minutes onto life expectancy.

Foods are not drugs, it is not possible to isolate the effects of a specific food within the context of the whole dietary pattern.

To show a superfood (or any food) provides superior (or particular) health benefits, you would need to conduct a randomised controlled trial. But, testing food is far more complex and difficult than testing a drug, due to the complex nature of food intake and dietary patterns[26,28]. Changing *one* aspect of a diet results in changes in *other* aspects of a diet. Therefore, differences between groups may be due to changes in the *other* aspects, and not in the *one* you are interested in. This is part of the reason why nutrition recommendations are based on lower quality forms of evidence, such as observational studies and short-term randomised controlled trials that assess indirect markers of long-term health[29]. Ideally, you would conduct many randomised controlled trials and analyse the results in a meta-analysis. Randomised controlled trials have been conducted on a range of supposed superfoods on health. However, studies are limited due to the inherently difficult nature of trying to assess how a superfood or nutraceutical can influence health within a complex dietary pattern. For example, how to blind participants, how to equate calorie intake, and what is the trial food being compared to[28]? Removing or adding food from a diet results in a change to the rest of the diet, making it difficult to isolate the effect of the food itself, from the effect of the other changes that have occurred in the diet[26].

As discussed before, the perceived benefit of a low fat or low carbohydrate diet on body composition is often the result of a subsequent increase in protein intake. Randomised controlled trials of diets also suffer the same fate as more basic studies, being short in duration and using proxy measures of health (e.g. insulin sensitivity or blood pressure) rather than hard clinical endpoints (e.g. mortality)[28]. This means that most evidence regarding diets and important health outcomes are from observational evidence, not interventional evidence. Similarly, if they have a wide range of effects, which health outcomes should be measured? The more we measure, the greater the risk of generating a significant finding by chance; flip a coin enough times and eventually you will land five heads in a row.

"Systematic reviews of randomized controlled trials (RCTs) of nutrition interventions have inherent methodologic constraints. For example, RCTs of dietary interventions cannot be controlled with true placebos, but rather with certain constraints on nutrient compositions, food groups, or dietary patterns. Other limitations include lack of double blinding, poor compliance and adherence, crossover bias, and high dropout rates. Thus, in the field of nutritional epidemiology, in which RCTs are constrained, well-designed prospective cohort studies can provide important evidence."
Schwingshackl et al., 2016[30].

In reality, studies and meta-analyses (studies of studies) repeatedly demonstrate that food groups or dietary patterns, *rather* than specific foods, are strongly related to health outcomes. If particular nutrients or nutraceuticals are found to have a health benefit, the nutrient can usually be found in a *broad range* of foods. For example, *polyphenols* have been linked to a range of health benefits including protective effects against cardiovascular disease and type 2 diabetes. Polyphenols are found in a wide range of plant-based foods such as fruits and vegetables, tea, coffee and other food sources[31]. *Nitrates* also have increasing evidence for a benefit in health and performance (discussed in chapter 25), but are also found in many dark leafy greens (e.g. spinach and beetroot), water and some animal-based foods[32]. Hence, it is consuming *any* food within a certain food group, and not consuming specific foods within that food group, that is important[22]. There may well be particular foods or nutraceuticals that have particular health benefits, but for now there is no conclusive evidence to support any claims or to make any specific recommendations[22]. And, given most populations have overall dietary patterns that are not associated with good health, focussing on specific foods is missing the woods for the trees.

"You will have gathered by now that there's no real evidence that superfoods exist, if by that we mean a single food or compound that will keep us healthy, stop illness in its tracks or save our life. When it comes to keeping healthy, it's best not to concentrate on any one food in the hope it will work miracles. Current advice is to eat a balanced diet with a range of foods, to ensure you get enough of the nutrients your body needs."
NHS, 2011[33].

The *European Union* (EU) has a register for nutrition and health claims[34]. A product in the EU can only state a claim if it meets the criteria set by the register. Many of these claims are not of superior benefits, but simply '*product X is needed for normal growth and development*'. In other words, the dietary requirement of most specific foods or chemicals is to simply ensure you are not deficient in it.

Fat intake and health

Recommendations for fat intake can be understood from the perspective of food groups and dietary patterns.

Total fat intake in the diet does not appear to be linked to poor health outcomes. But, high intakes of certain types of fat may increase the risk of poor health. There is conflicting opinion on whether saturated fat intake should be reduced, and if it should be replaced with polyunsaturated fat or monounsaturated fat. Current evidence points towards replacing saturated fat with unsaturated fat to improve health. If so, such a change can be achieved by increasing plant-based food consumption and moderating ultra-processed food consumption without having to consider the types of fats consumed. Regardless, the overconsumption of fat (in generating a calorie surplus and weight gain) would have greater health effects than the moderate consumption of different proportions of fat.

The role of dietary fats and health is still hotly debated (for types of fats and fat food sources, see chapter 6)[35,36]. The main link between fat intake and health is via their effects on cardiovascular disease. Cardiovascular disease is the largest cause of death worldwide, accounting for a third of global deaths. *Strokes* and *heart attacks* are the most common cardiovascular events.

This is only a brief mention of an important but controversial topic, as it relates to the discussion of food choice. High total fat intake does *not* appear to be linked to poor health outcomes[29,37]. A *Cochrane** systematic review of randomised controlled trials found no effect of reducing total fat intake on the risk of a cardiovascular event[38]. There was also no effect of changes in dietary fat intake on all-cause mortality and mortality from cardiovascular disease[38]. But, the *types* of fat within the diet may have some influence on health[36]. If there is a benefit to manipulating fat intake, it appears to be by *modifying* the types of fats consumed, rather than by *reducing* the quantity of fat consumed[38]. High saturated fat diets can lead to higher cholesterol levels in the blood[39]. Higher cholesterol (and in particular LDL-cholesterol) is a major risk factor for heart disease[40,41]. The relationship is slightly more complicated than this, because it also depends on the size of the cholesterol particle and other factors[29]. Short-term (a few weeks) trials show that replacing saturated fat with other unsaturated fats can lower the cholesterol levels in the blood[39,42]. The effect is greater when replacing saturated fats with polyunsaturated fats. One 19 week trial found a reduction in blood LDL-cholesterol levels with low saturated fat intake (6%) and higher unsaturated fat intake (21-31%), with no change in body weight[43]. Notably, all diets contained a low to moderate intake of animal-based food sources. But, replacing saturated fat with other fats or carbohydrates can alter the levels of other lipids in the blood, such as *'good'* HDL-cholesterol and *triglycerides* (a type of fat)[29]. This may have a *confounding* influence on any changes in 'bad' LDL-cholesterol[29].

* Cochrane systematic reviews have the aim of minimising bias, with a team of select experts to produce as reliable findings as possible.

Despite the effect of increased saturated fatty acid consumption on cholesterol levels, increased saturated fatty acid consumption does not appear to be associated with increases in other cardiovascular risk factors, such as inflammation, blood pressure or blood vessel function.

Some studies find that high levels of saturated fat intake increases the risk of heart disease[44]. But, evidence of increased heart disease and mortality with increased saturated fatty acid consumption is not conclusive, with weak associations from prospective observational cohort studies[37,45–47]. Systematic reviews and meta-analyses of observational cohort studies and randomised controlled trials find minimal evidence to suggest that saturated fat increases the risk heart disease[35,48–50]. Cochrane systematic reviews of randomised controlled trials found no effect of increasing polyunsaturated fat, omega-3 (the main form of polyunsaturated fat found in oily fish) or omega-6 (the main form of polyunsaturated fats in vegetable oils, nuts and seeds) intake in *isolation* on reducing cardiovascular disease or all-cause mortality[51–53]. Furthermore, meta-analyses of prospective cohort studies shows no benefit of increasing monounsaturated fat intake to reduce the risk of stroke and heart disease[50,54,55].

But, some have argued that the over-adjustment of blood lipid (i.e. cholesterol) levels in observational studies has reduced the size of the actual effect seen from having a high saturated fat intake in randomised controlled trials. Indeed, it appears that the effect of saturated fat intake and intake of other fatty acids and heart disease is influenced by the *source* of the saturated fat, and what the dietary saturated fat is *replaced* with, rather than the effect of increasing or decreasing saturated or unsaturated fat in *isolation*. Increasing unsaturated fat intake may inadvertently result in an increase in saturated fat intake, and decreasing saturated fat intake may inadvertently result in a decrease in unsaturated fat intake[56]. This could explain the lack of any significant effect on heart disease in cohort studies and randomised controlled trials from trying to change only saturated or unsaturated fat intake. In other words, the *relative* proportions of saturated and unsaturated fat intake relate to increased or decreased health risk, rather than the *absolute* proportions. Randomised controlled trials of reducing total fat intake from reducing saturated and unsaturated fat intake tend to find little to no benefit on reducing the risk of heart disease[56]. Low fat diets do *not* reduce the risk of heart disease compared to high fat diets[57]. Reducing dietary saturated fat intake isn't inherently beneficial, because it *depends* on what it is replaced with[35,56,58,59]. Cochrane systematic reviews of randomised controlled trials find that replacing saturated fat intake, in particular by replacing saturated fat with polyunsaturated fat reduces the risk of a cardiovascular event by 10%, but does not necessarily reduce all-cause mortality or mortality from cardiovascular disease (i.e. replacement reduces the risk of a stroke or heart attack, but does not necessarily reduce the risk of death)[38,42,56]. The reduced risk of a cardiovascular event was in proportion with the reduction in total cholesterol levels. Lowering non-HDL cholesterol (cholesterol other than the *'good'* cholesterol) is important to reduce the risk of cardiovascular disease[40]. Depending on what saturated fat is replaced with, influences the changes in total cholesterol, *'bad'* LDL-cholesterol and *'good'* HDL-cholesterol, which appears to influence the size of the effect on cardiovascular disease[56]. There is a tendency for greater benefit with greater replacement of saturated fat intake with unsaturated fat intake. Other observational studies find that diets with a larger proportion of polyunsaturated fats to saturated fats are associated with improved health outcomes[48,58]. Interestingly, one randomised controlled trial found a 50-70% reduced risk of heart disease after 46 months with a *Mediterranean-style* diet with lower saturated fat (8%) and higher unsaturated fat (18%), *without* any change to blood cholesterol levels[60]. The diet contained a low to moderate intake of animal-based foods (fish, dairy, poultry, eggs and little red meat)[60]. It is likely that fats will also influence health through mechanisms besides just cholesterol levels, such as affecting blood pressure, blood sugar (glucose), inflammation and importantly, body weight[37].

Replacing saturated fats with unsaturated fats may improve the cholesterol profile in the blood, lowering the risk of a cardiovascular event (e.g. a stroke or a heart attack)[42,59]. Large *observational cohort* studies have assessed the effect of replacing saturated fat with *other* sources of fat or carbohydrate[47,48]. One study assessed the risk of fat intake and *heart disease,* while another study assessed fat intake and the association with *mortality.* Replacement of 5% of total energy intake from saturated fatty acids with 5% of total energy intake from plant-based monounsaturated fats, polyunsaturated fats or starchy carbohydrates from whole grains was associated with a reduced risk of heart disease[48]. And, replacement of 5% of total energy intake from saturated fatty acids with 5% of total energy intake from monounsaturated fats was associated with 13% lower mortality, and replacement with polyunsaturated fats was associated with 27% lower mortality[47]. The greatest benefit on heart disease and mortality is seen with replacing saturated fat with polyunsaturated fat (increasing the ratio of polyunsaturated fat to saturated fat in the diet). However, replacement of 5% of total energy intake from saturated fatty acids with 5% of total energy intake from refined starches and sugars or trans fats was *not* associated with a change in heart disease risk[48]. In fact, the benefit on heart disease does not just occur from replacing saturated fat with unsaturated fat. Replacing carbohydrates from refined starches and sugars with carbohydrates from whole grains, or with polyunsaturated fats, is also associated with a reduced risk of heart disease[48]. Studies of *randomised controlled trials* demonstrate similar findings. A systematic review and meta-analysis of randomised controlled trials assessed the effect of replacing saturated fat with polyunsaturated fat[48]. Again, replacement of 5% of total energy intake from saturated fatty acids with 5% of total energy intake from polyunsaturated fats was associated with a 10% reduction in heart disease risk[48]. Similar findings have been reported in a review[42].

Total fat intake does not appear to influence the risk of heart disease, but replacing saturated fat with unsaturated fat appears to have a beneficial effect in reducing the risk of heart disease.

"The effect of a specific fatty acid depends strongly on the source of calories with which it is compared. Little or no cardiovascular benefits were seen when

SFA [saturated fats] is replaced by total carbohydrate, but a significant reduction in CVD [cardiovascular disease] risk is achieved when SFA is replaced by MUFA [monounsaturated fats] and/or PUFA [polyunsaturated fats]."
Wang and Hu, 2017[56].

Different foods contain different relative quantities of these different *forms* of fat and carbohydrate. As such, any benefit in reducing saturated fat intake and increasing unsaturated fat intake can be related to the dietary pattern as a whole and to the food sources of fats, rather than considering the type of fat itself in isolation[35,48]. Even so, there is conflict amongst scientists about the direct role of saturated fat and heart disease. This is because replacing saturated fat with whole grain carbohydrates does not confer as great a benefit as unsaturated fats and, replacing saturated fat with refined carbohydrates or trans fats does not change, or even increases the risk of heart disease[37,47,56]. Meaning, replacement of saturated fat with other foods is *not* inherently better for cardiovascular health.

"When all these lines of evidence are considered, the role of saturated fat in CHD [coronary heart disease] is controversial, including among the writing group of the present manuscript. Some scientists believe that reduction in saturated fat must continue to be prioritized, based on its LDL-raising effects and causality for CVD [cardiovascular disease], on the benefits of replacing saturated fat with PUFA [polyunsaturated fat], and on concerns that in the absence of recommendations to limit saturated fat, ingredients high in saturated fat (e.g., palm oil) could be added to foods. Other scientists believe that heterogeneous effects of saturated fat on blood lipids and lipoproteins, of different individual saturated fatty acids, and of saturated fat from different food sources raises questions on the biologic and practical relevance of any focus on saturated fat, and that food-based recommendations are both more biologically sound and more practical."
Liu et al., 2017[35].

Some experts and health organisations recommend reducing saturated fat intake and increasing unsaturated fat intake (in particular, polyunsaturated fat)[40,47,56,61,62]. The *extent* to which saturated fats should be decreased, and unsaturated fats increased, is *inconclusive*. Many authorities suggest keeping saturated fat below 10% of total calorie intake[39]. However, some authorities no longer recommend limiting saturated fat intake[35,63].

Dietary patterns associated with improved heart health (e.g. Mediterranean-style diet) typically contain saturated fat below 10%, and unsaturated fat intake around 20-30% of total calorie intake[37]. As discussed in chapter 6, the primary sources of saturated fats include animal fats such as red meat and butters. Major sources of polyunsaturated fat include oily fish, nuts and seeds. Olive oil is a major source of monounsaturated fat[56]. Dairy and meats both contain saturated and monounsaturated fat. UK dietary recommendations are *not* to reduce total fat intake, but to *alter* the sources of dietary fats: reducing saturated fat intake, and increasing the intake of monounsaturated and polyunsaturated fats[59,64]. Therefore, increasing the relative dietary intake of polyunsaturated fat to saturated fat can be achieved simply by consuming more whole plant-based foods, and consuming fewer ultra-processed foods[65]. Organisations are now starting to recommend changes at the level of food choices and dietary patterns to meet the recommended intakes of specific types of fat[36,66,67].

It is also important to remember that saturated fat intake is typically high with excessive meat consumption and use of animal fat spreads. However, many meats are low in saturated fat, and some animal-based sources are rich in unsaturated fats. Poultry, turkey, and lean cuts of meat are low in saturated fat. Oily fish are low in saturated fat, and high in polyunsaturated fat. A higher polyunsaturated:saturated fat ratio can also be achieved with moderate animal-based food consumption by consideration of the animal-based food groups that are consumed. The *Joint British Societies'* (including the *British Heart Foundation, Heart UK* and the *British Cardiovascular Society*) recommend keeping saturated fat below 10% of total daily calories by consuming lean meats and low fat dairy[62]. Even so, the dietary pattern may be even more important, as saturated fat from dairy has been associated with a reduced cardiovascular disease risk, and saturated fat from meat associated with an increased cardiovascular disease risk[68]. Meaning, the *same* types of fat from *different* food sources may have *different* effects[29]. Dietary fat recommendations can be achieved by considering food groups alone[29], and does not require the exclusion of animal-based food sources[43].

Even so, the primary concern regarding fat intake should be overall energy consumption and the avoidance of overconsumption. Overconsumption will result in weight gain and adverse health effects from obesity related complications (e.g. diabetes)[69].

"Indeed, excess consumption of calories has greater effects on weight and energy balance than the amount and type of fat consumed."
Liu et al., 2017[35].

The *greatest* risk of cardiovascular disease arises from excess body weight, being overweight or obese, and from high blood pressure[68].

Unprocessed vs processed vs ultra-processed foods

Just because a food is processed, does not mean it is of high energy and low nutrient density (consider tinned or frozen fruit and vegetables, which have been processed). Cooking food is a form of processing. Unless you only eat raw food, you consume processed food.

Foods can be classified on their level of processing[1]:

1. **Unprocessed** or **minimally processed** foods. Drying, crushing, roasting, boiling, fresh, frozen: vegetables, fruits, legumes, meat, fish, eggs and milk.
2. **Processed** culinary ingredients. Foods that are added to other foods (oils, butter, vinegar, sugar, salt).
3. **Simple processed** foods. The addition of fats, sugar or salt to minimally processed foods (cheese, ham).
4. **Ultra-processed** foods. Industrial productions with the addition of ingredients that are not used in home cooking. There is added salt, sugar and fat, and use of additives, flavourings and sweeteners. This does actually mean that many foods such as bread, pasta or cereals are classed as ultra-processed. It also includes sweets, meat products (sausages), pastries, soft drinks, cakes, chocolate and crisps amongst others.

An important and recent area of interest is the difference between ultra-processed foods and other processed foods. Ultra-processed foods:

"typically contain little or no whole foods, are ready-to-consume or heat up, and are fatty, salty or sugary and depleted in dietary fibre, protein, various micronutrients and other bioactive compounds."
Monteiro et al., 2018[70].

A recent, randomised controlled cross-over trial compared the calorie intake from an ultra-processed diet to an unprocessed diet (a cross-over study design is where participants receive both interventions, in this case the ultra-processed and unprocessed diets). The study was performed in a metabolic ward, meaning energy intake and expenditure could be very closely measured. The study let people eat freely on each diet for 2 weeks[71]. One diet contained only ultra-processed foods, and the other contained only unprocessed food. Participants were provided with meals. Unprocessed and ultra-processed meals were matched for calories, energy density, macronutrients, sugar, sodium and fibre content[71]. After eating one of the diets for 2 weeks, consuming as much or as little as they desired, participants consumed the other diet for 2 weeks. They found that the ultra-processed diet resulted in eating 508 more calories than the unprocessed diet as a result of eating more fat and carbohydrate, but not protein. Weight change was very closely related to energy intake. A diet of purely ultra-processed foods resulted in overfeeding, a calorie surplus, and subsequent energy storage and weight gain. The study was not designed to identify the cause behind different energy intakes in the diets. Despite wide claims that processed foods are less than ideal, food processing serves a vital purpose in global food sustainability and can preserve the nutritional value of food (such as tinned and frozen fruit and vegetables). The energy and nutrient density framework allows for food processing to be factored into the effect of consuming a food. High energy, low nutrient density foods are not inherently fattening, but they can increase the likelihood of energy overconsumption and therefore weight gain.

"Diets are more likely to meet food guidance recommendations if nutrient-dense foods, either processed or not, are selected."
Weaver et al., 2014[72].

The differentiation between unprocessed foods being *'healthy'* and processed foods being *'unhealthy'* is an incorrect generalisation. The effect of processing (canning or freezing) fruit and vegetables does not impact on their nutritional quality[73]. Drying out fruit and vegetables would have the effect of increasing the energy density. But this also extends its shelf life. The nutritional quality of food will vary with cooking, processing, storage and geographical location. For example, soil quality can influence the mineral content within a plant.

The type of processing used to produce the fruit juice will influence its energy and nutrient density. 100% fruit juice (which includes fruit juice from concentrate) when commercially blended, loses some of its nutrient content because it is filtered, which removes all or most of the fibre content[74]. Blending without removing any fibre will maintain the nutrient and energy content. Removing the skin also lowers some of the micronutrient content found in the fruit. This will *increase* its energy density and decrease its nutrient density. However, the density is also affected by how much water is added to the fruit juice, and whether the juice is fortified with vitamins and minerals. Blending breaks down the cell walls of the fruit, which releases the sugar and other energy bound within the fruit cells. This can make it easier for the gut to digest and absorb the content within the fruit, which can increase the amount and rate at which energy is obtained. Supermarket fruit smoothies can often contain *added* sugar (distinct to the naturally occurring sugars within the fruit). Fruit smoothies that are blended from whole fruits with little content removed retain similar energy and nutrient characteristics. Current limited evidence from systematic reviews and meta-analyses show *no* associations of moderate 100% fruit juice consumption (which includes fruit juice from concentrate) with long-term health problems[74].

When eating intuitively for weight maintenance or weight loss, one habit-based rule to utilise could be the *80:20 split*. 80% of the time, choose whole food sources such as lean meats, fish, vegetables, fruits, whole grains and plant oils, whether processed or not. Such food sources are *typically* lower energy density and higher nutrient density. For the other 20%, consume any ultra-processed foods or other foods of personal preference such as cakes, chips or sweets. These food sources are *typically* higher energy density and lower nutrient density. You could have a 90:10, or even a 95:5 split depending on your appetite and preference for high energy density, low nutrient density foods. The foods that suppress appetite and provide satiety for one individual can differ completely to the foods that suppress appetite and provide satiety for another individual. As you increase the split, such as a ratio of 60:40, or 50:50, there will be a shift towards consuming more calories, and consuming fewer nutrients.

The key is not exclusion, but moderation, and not following someone else's diet, but discovering your own.

Summary

Food densities are not discrete, but a continuum from a low to high density of nutrient and energy content. *All* foods and food groups can be a part of a diet designed for optimising body composition and better health outcomes. The importance is in the relative proportions of the food groups. Dietary recommendations from health organisations can be summarised as being *'additive'* or *'subtractive'*; consume more of X, or less of Y[29].

The *Mediterranean-style* diet is one of the most well researched dietary patterns to date. Adherence to a Mediterranean-style diet is associated with improved health outcomes and reduced cardiovascular disease risk[28]. In fact, it is proposed as a dietary pattern to support general improved health and to reduce the risk of disease[75]. There is a strong emphasis on the consumption of fruits, vegetables, whole grains, nuts, plant oils and oily fish. The Mediterranean diet still contains red meat, alcohol and dairy, but in moderation[75]. Ultra-processed foods such as pastries and cakes are *not* excluded, but consumed in low amounts. The diet typically contains a relatively high amount of fat, but a greater proportion of polyunsaturated fat to saturated fat. Even one of the healthiest dietary patterns studied to date does not exclude food groups nor animal-based food sources, and contains large amounts of fat and naturally occurring sugar[76].

Moderate portions of energy dense, low nutrient density food can be part of any healthy lifestyle that can simultaneously allow for achievement of body composition goals. However, in order to achieve the discussed key points for a particular goal, it is likely that daily food choices will need to be derived mainly from the middle to the bottom left regions of the graph, and fewer choices from the top right region.

The energy density and nutrient density model is essentially another way of saying that a dietary pattern (diet):

- consisting predominantly of plant-based food sources (fruit, vegetables, legumes, whole grains, plant oils, nuts),
- with low to moderate intake of animal-based sources (lean meats, dairy, eggs, fish and poultry),
- whilst not excluding any food groups (except for allergies or ethical/environmental concerns),
- but avoiding excessive (i.e. limiting) consumption of ultra-processed foods,

aligns with most health outcomes and with most health authority dietary recommendations[35,76,77]. Dietary variation by consuming foods from a range of food sources ensures complete nutritional adequacy[76].

The energy density of a diet should be considered when assessing your diet for weight loss or weight gain. Diets lower in energy density promote a reduction in calorie intake whilst remaining satiated, which would benefit a calorie restricted plan. But, a diet lower in energy density may hinder the ability to increase calorie intake to a surplus to optimise muscle growth, especially with a more intuitive approach to energy intake. The nutrient density also needs to be considered in the same manner, which is important for health and to ensure training adaptations. Nutrient rich foods tend to have a lower energy density, nutrient poor foods tend to have a higher energy density.

"It is important to note that the overall quality of one's diet, combined with the types and quantity of food, have more impact on health than any single nutrient such as saturated fat."
Heart and Stroke[63].

References

1 Drewnowski A. Nutrient density: addressing the challenge of obesity. *Br J Nutr* 2018; 120: S8–S14.

2 Rolls BJ, Ello-Martin JA, Tohill BC. What Can Intervention Studies Tell Us about the Relationship between Fruit and Vegetable Consumption and Weight Management? *Nutr Rev* 2004; 62: 1–17.

3 Pem D, Jeewon R. Fruit and Vegetable Intake: Benefits and Progress of Nutrition Education Interventions- Narrative Review Article. *Iran J Public Health* 2015; 44: 1309–1321.

4 Yu ZM, DeClercq V, Cui Y, Forbes C, Grandy S, Keats M et al. Fruit and vegetable intake and body adiposity among populations in Eastern Canada: the

Atlantic Partnership for Tomorrow's Health Study. *BMJ Open* 2018; 8. Available from: doi:10.1136/bmjopen-2017-018060.

5   Nour M, Lutze SA, Grech A, Allman-Farinelli M. The Relationship between Vegetable Intake and Weight Outcomes: A Systematic Review of Cohort Studies. *Nutrients* 2018; 10. Available from: doi:10.3390/nu10111626.

6   Foreyt JP. The Ultimate Volumetrics Diet: Smart, Simple, Science-Based Strategies for Losing Weight and Keeping It Off. *Am J Clin Nutr* 2012; 96: 681–682.

7   Rolls BJ. Dietary energy density: Applying behavioural science to weight management. *Nutr Bull* 2017; 42: 246–253.

8   GOV.UK. *NDNS: results from years 7 and 8 (combined)*. Available from: https://www.gov.uk/government/statistics/ndns-results-from-years-7-and-8-combined (accessed 5 Feb 2020).

9   GOV.UK. *NDNS: results from Years 1 to 4 (combined)*. Available from: https://www.gov.uk/government/statistics/national-diet-and-nutrition-survey-results-from-years-1-to-4-combined-of-the-rolling-programme-for-2008-and-2009-to-2011-and-2012 (accessed 5 Feb 2020).

10   Cadbury. *Cadbury Dairy Milk*. Available from: http://www.cadbury.co.uk/products/cadbury-dairy-milk-11294 (accessed 7 Feb 2020).

11   FoodData Central. *Strawberries, raw*. Available from: https://fdc.nal.usda.gov/fdc-app.html#/food-details/327699/nutrients (accessed 7 Feb 2020).

12   World Health Organisation. *NCDs. Diet, nutrition and the prevention of chronic diseases - Report of the joint WHO/FAO expert consultation*. Available from: http://www.who.int/ncds/prevention/technical-report-series-916/en/ (accessed 7 Feb 2020).

13   Gibson R, Eriksen R, Chambers E, Gao H, Aresu M, Heard A et al. Intakes and Food Sources of Dietary Fibre and Their Associations with Measures of Body Composition and Inflammation in UK Adults: Cross-Sectional Analysis of the Airwave Health Monitoring Study. *Nutrients* 2019; 11. Available from: doi:10.3390/nu11081839.

14   Blatt AD, Roe LS, Rolls BJ. Hidden vegetables: an effective strategy to reduce energy intake and increase vegetable intake in adults. *Am J Clin Nutr* 2011; 93: 756–763.

15   Rouhani MH, Surkan PJ, Azadbakht L. The effect of preload/meal energy density on energy intake in a subsequent meal: A systematic review and meta-analysis. *Eat Behav* 2017; 26: 6–15.

16   FoodData Central. *Mangos, raw*. Available from: https://fdc.nal.usda.gov/fdc-app.html#/food-details/169910/nutrients (accessed 7 Feb 2020).

17   FoodData Central. *Mango, dried*. Available from: https://fdc.nal.usda.gov/fdc-app.html#/food-details/341488/nutrients (accessed 7 Feb 2020).

18   Bell EA, Castellanos VH, Pelkman CL, Thorwart ML, Rolls BJ. Energy density of foods affects energy intake in normal-weight women. *Am J Clin Nutr* 1998; 67: 412–420.

19   Smajis S, Gajdošík M, Pfleger L, Traussnigg S, Kienbacher C, Halilbasic E et al. Metabolic effects of a prolonged, very-high-dose dietary fructose challenge in healthy subjects. *Am J Clin Nutr* 2020; 111: 369–377.

20   Vos MB, Kimmons JE, Gillespie C, Welsh J, Blanck HM. Dietary fructose consumption among US children and adults: the Third National Health and Nutrition Examination Survey. *Medscape J Med* 2008; 10: 160.

21   Johnstone A. Safety and efficacy of high-protein diets for weight loss. *Proc Nutr Soc* 2012; 71: 339–49.

22   McClements DJ. *Nutraceuticals: Superfoods or Superfads? In: Future Foods.* SpringerLink; 2019. Available from: https://link.springer.com/chapter/10.1007/978-3-030-12995-8_6 (accessed 4 Feb 2020).

23   Sikka T. The contradictions of a superfood consumerism in a postfeminist, neoliberal world. *Food Cult Soc* 2019; 22: 354–375.

24   Tomé-Carneiro J, Visioli F. Polyphenol-based nutraceuticals for the prevention and treatment of cardiovascular disease: Review of human evidence. *Phytomedicine* 2016; 23: 1145–1174.

25   Mie A, Andersen HR, Gunnarsson S, Kahl J, Kesse-Guyot E, Rembiałkowska E et al. Human health implications of organic food and organic agriculture: a comprehensive review. *Environ Health Glob Access Sci Source* 2017; 16: 111.

26   Johnston BC, Seivenpiper JL, Vernooij RWM, de Souza RJ, Jenkins DJA, Zeraatkar D et al. The Philosophy of Evidence-Based Principles and Practice in Nutrition. *Mayo Clin Proc Innov Qual Outcomes* 2019; 3: 189–199.

27   O'Neil CE, Nicklas TA, Fulgoni VL. Consumption of apples is associated with a better diet quality and reduced risk of obesity in children: National Health and Nutrition Examination Survey (NHANES) 2003–2010. *Nutr J* 2015; 14. Available from: doi:10.1186/s12937-015-0040-1.

28   Jacobs DR, Tapsell LC. Food synergy: the key to a healthy diet. *Proc Nutr Soc* 2013; 72: 200–206.

29   Forouhi NG, Krauss RM, Taubes G, Willett W. Dietary fat and cardiometabolic health: evidence, controversies, and consensus for guidance. *The BMJ* 2018; 361. Available from: doi:10.1136/bmj.k2139.

30   Schwingshackl L, Knüppel S, Schwedhelm C, Hoffmann G, Missbach B, Stelmach-Mardas M et al. Perspective: NutriGrade: A Scoring System to Assess and Judge the Meta-Evidence of Randomized Controlled Trials and Cohort Studies in Nutrition Research. *Adv Nutr* 2016; 7: 994–1004.

31   Williamson G. The role of polyphenols in modern nutrition. *Nutr Bull* 2017; 42: 226–235.

32   Ma L, Hu L, Feng X, Wang S. Nitrate and Nitrite in Health and Disease. *Aging Dis* 2018; 9: 938–945.

33   NHS. *Miracle foods: a special report.* 2017. Available from: https://www.nhs.uk/news/food-and-diet/miracle-foods-a-special-report/ (accessed 7 Feb 2020).

34   European Commission. *EU Register of Nutrition and Health Claims.* Available   from: https://ec.europa.eu/food/safety/labelling_nutrition/claims/register/public/? event=register.home&CFID=533127&CFTOKEN=b25fc8446fd1391f-3139661B-0ADE-FD50-E617EC7B575FCDE0 (accessed 7 Feb 2020).

35   Liu AG, Ford NA, Hu FB, Zelman KM, Mozaffarian D, Kris-Etherton PM. A healthy approach to dietary fats: understanding the science and taking action to reduce consumer confusion. *Nutr J* 2017; 16. Available from: doi:10.1186/s12937-017-0271-4.

36   Nettleton JA, Brouwer IA, Geleijnse JM, Hornstra G. Saturated Fat Consumption and Risk of Coronary Heart Disease and Ischemic Stroke: A Science Update. *Ann Nutr Metab* 2017; 70: 26–33.

37   Billingsley HE, Carbone S, Lavie CJ. Dietary Fats and Chronic Noncommunicable Diseases. *Nutrients* 2018; 10. Available from: doi:10.3390/nu10101385.

38   Hooper L, Summerbell CD, Thompson R, Sills D, Roberts FG, Moore HJ et al. Reduced or modified dietary fat for preventing cardiovascular disease. *Cochrane Database Syst Rev* 2012. Available from: doi:10.1002/14651858.CD002137.pub3.

39   Mensink RP, World Health Organisation. *Effects of saturated fatty acids on serum lipids and lipoproteins: a systematic review and regression analysis.* World Health Organization, 2016. Available from: https://apps.who.int/iris/handle/10665/246104 (accessed 29 Feb 2020).

40   Jacobson TA, Ito MK, Maki KC, Orringer CE, Bays HE, Jones PH et al. National lipid association recommendations for patient-centered management of dyslipidemia: part 1--full report. *J Clin Lipidol* 2015; 9: 129–169.

41   Marmot MG, Syme SL, Kagan A, Kato H, Cohen JB, Belsky J. Epidemiologic studies of coronary heart disease and stroke in Japanese men living in Japan, Hawaii and California: prevalence of coronary and hypertensive heart disease and associated risk factors. *Am J Epidemiol* 1975; 102: 514–525.

42   Hooper L, Martin N, Abdelhamid A, Davey Smith G. Reduction in saturated fat intake for cardiovascular disease. *Cochrane Database Syst Rev* 2015; 6: CD011737.

43   Swain JF, McCarron PB, Hamilton EF, Sacks FM, Appel LJ. Characteristics of the Diet Patterns Tested in the Optimal Macronutrient Intake Trial to Prevent Heart Disease (OmniHeart): Options for a Heart-Healthy Diet. *J Am Diet Assoc* 2008; 108: 257–265.

44   Kromhout D, Menotti A, Bloemberg B, Aravanis C, Blackburn H, Buzina R et al. Dietary saturated and trans fatty acids and cholesterol and 25-year mortality from coronary heart disease: the Seven Countries Study. *Prev Med* 1995; 24: 308–315.

45   Hu FB, Stampfer MJ, Manson JE, Rimm E, Colditz GA, Rosner BA et al. Dietary fat intake and the risk of coronary heart disease in women. *N Engl J Med* 1997; 337: 1491–1499.

46   Oh K, Hu FB, Manson JE, Stampfer MJ, Willett WC. Dietary fat intake and risk of coronary heart disease in women: 20 years of follow-up of the nurses' health study. *Am J Epidemiol* 2005; 161: 672–679.

47   Wang DD, Li Y, Chiuve SE, Stampfer MJ, Manson JE, Rimm EB et al. Association of Specific Dietary Fats With Total and Cause-Specific Mortality. *JAMA Intern Med* 2016; 176: 1134–1145.

48   Li Y, Hruby A, Bernstein AM, Ley SH, Wang DD, Chiuve SE et al. Saturated Fat as Compared With Unsaturated Fats and Sources of Carbohydrates in Relation to Risk of Coronary Heart Disease: A Prospective Cohort Study. *J Am Coll Cardiol* 2015; 66: 1538–1548.

49   Siri-Tarino PW, Sun Q, Hu FB, Krauss RM. Meta-analysis of prospective cohort studies evaluating the association of saturated fat with cardiovascular disease. *Am J Clin Nutr* 2010; 91: 535–546.

50   Chowdhury R, Warnakula S, Kunutsor S, Crowe F, Ward HA, Johnson L et al. Association of dietary, circulating, and supplement fatty acids with coronary risk: a systematic review and meta-analysis. *Ann Intern Med* 2014; 160: 398–406.

51   Abdelhamid AS, Martin N, Bridges C, Brainard JS, Wang X, Brown TJ et al. Polyunsaturated fatty acids for the primary and secondary prevention of cardiovascular disease. *Cochrane Database Syst Rev* 2018. Available from: doi:10.1002/14651858.CD012345.pub3.

52   Hooper L, Al-Khudairy L, Abdelhamid AS, Rees K, Brainard JS, Brown TJ et al. Omega-6 fats for the primary and secondary prevention of cardiovascular disease. *Cochrane Database Syst Rev* 2018. Available from: doi:10.1002/14651858.CD011094.pub4.

53   Abdelhamid AS, Brown TJ, Brainard JS, Biswas P, Thorpe GC, Moore HJ et al. Omega-3 fatty acids for the primary and secondary prevention of cardiovascular disease. *Cochrane Database Syst Rev* 2018. Available from: doi:10.1002/14651858.CD003177.pub4.

54   Cheng P, Wang J, Shao W. Monounsaturated Fatty Acid Intake and Stroke Risk: A Meta-analysis of Prospective Cohort Studies. *J Stroke Cerebrovasc Dis Off J Natl Stroke Assoc* 2016; 25: 1326–1334.

55   Schwingshackl L, Hoffmann G. Monounsaturated fatty acids, olive oil and health status: a systematic review and meta-analysis of cohort studies. *Lipids Health Dis* 2014; 13. Available from: doi:10.1186/1476-511X-13-154.

56   Wang DD, Hu FB. Dietary Fat and Risk of Cardiovascular Disease: Recent Controversies and Advances. *Annu Rev Nutr* 2017; 37: 423–446.

57   Howard BV, Van Horn L, Hsia J, Manson JE, Stefanick ML, Wassertheil-Smoller S et al. Low-fat dietary pattern and risk of cardiovascular disease: the Women's Health Initiative Randomized Controlled Dietary Modification Trial. *JAMA* 2006; 295: 655–666.

58   Jakobsen MU, O'Reilly EJ, Heitmann BL, Pereira MA, Bälter K, Fraser GE et al. Major types of dietary fat and risk of coronary heart disease: a pooled analysis of 11 cohort studies. *Am J Clin Nutr* 2009; 89: 1425–1432.

59   Siri-Tarino PW, Chiu S, Bergeron N, Krauss RM. Saturated Fats Versus Polyunsaturated Fats Versus Carbohydrates for Cardiovascular Disease Prevention and Treatment. *Annu Rev Nutr* 2015; 35: 517–543.

60   Kris-Etherton P, Eckel RH, Howard BV, St Jeor S, Bazzarre TL, Nutrition Committee Population Science Committee and Clinical Science Committee of the American Heart Association. AHA Science Advisory: Lyon Diet Heart Study. Benefits of a Mediterranean-style, National Cholesterol Education Program/American Heart Association Step I Dietary Pattern on Cardiovascular Disease. *Circulation* 2001; 103: 1823–1825.

61   Sacks FM, Lichtenstein AH, Wu JHY, Appel LJ, Creager MA, Kris-Etherton PM et al. Dietary Fats and Cardiovascular Disease: A Presidential Advisory From the American Heart Association. *Circulation* 2017; 136: e1–e23.

62   JBS3 Board. Joint British Societies' consensus recommendations for the prevention of cardiovascular disease (JBS3). *Heart Br Card Soc* 2014; 100 Suppl 2: ii1–ii67.

63   Heart & Stroke. *Position Statement: Saturated Fat, Heart Disease and Stroke*. Available from: https://www.heartandstroke.ca/-/media/pdf-files/canada/2017-position-statements/saturatedfat-ps-eng.ashx (accessed 5 Mar 2020).

64   GOV.UK. *Saturated fats and health: SACN report*. Available from: https://www.gov.uk/government/publications/saturated-fats-and-health-sacn-report (accessed 29 Feb 2020).

65   Martínez-González MA, Sánchez-Tainta A, Corella D, Salas-Salvadó J, Ros E, Arós F et al. A provegetarian food pattern and reduction in total mortality in the Prevención con Dieta Mediterránea (PREDIMED) study. *Am J Clin Nutr* 2014; 100: 320S-328S.

66   Kromhout D, Spaaij CJK, de Goede J, Weggemans RM. The 2015 Dutch food-based dietary guidelines. *Eur J Clin Nutr* 2016; 70: 869–878.

67   Becker W, Lyhne N, Pedersen AN, Aro A, Fogelholm M, Phorsdottir I et al. Nordic Nutrition Recommendations 2004 - integrating nutrition and physical activity. *Scand J Nutr* 2004; 48: 178–187.

68   Siri-Tarino P, Krauss R. Diet, lipids, and cardiovascular disease. *Curr Opin Lipidol* 2016; 27: 323–328.

69   Hooper L, Abdelhamid A, Bunn D, Brown T, Summerbell CD, Skeaff CM. Effects of total fat intake on body weight. *Cochrane Database Syst Rev* 2015. Available from: doi:10.1002/14651858.CD011834.

70   Monteiro CA, Cannon G, Moubarac J-C, Levy RB, Louzada MLC, Jaime PC. The UN Decade of Nutrition, the NOVA food classification and the trouble with ultra-processing. *Public Health Nutr* 2018; 21: 5–17.

71   Hall KD, Ayuketah A, Brychta R, Cai H, Cassimatis T, Chen KY et al. Ultra-processed diets cause excess calorie intake and weight gain: A one-month

inpatient randomized controlled trial of ad libitum food intake. *Cell Metab* 2019. Available from: doi:10.31232/osf.io/w3zh2.

72   Weaver CM, Dwyer J, Fulgoni VL, King JC, Leveille GA, MacDonald RS et al. Processed foods: contributions to nutrition. *Am J Clin Nutr* 2014; 99: 1525–1542.

73   Rickman JC, Barrett DM, Bruhn CM. Nutritional comparison of fresh, frozen and canned fruits and vegetables. Part 1. Vitamins C and B and phenolic compounds. *J Sci Food Agric* 2007; 87: 930–944.

74   Auerbach BJ, Dibey S, Vallila-Buchman P, Kratz M, Krieger J. Review of 100% Fruit Juice and Chronic Health Conditions: Implications for Sugar-Sweetened Beverage Policy. *Adv Nutr* 2018; 9: 78–85.

75   Freire R. Scientific evidence of diets for weight loss: Different macronutrient composition, intermittent fasting, and popular diets. *Nutrition* 2020; 69: 110549.

76   Valavanidis A. Dietary Supplements: Beneficial to Human Health or Just Peace of Mind? A Critical Review on the Issue of Benefit/Risk of Dietary Supplements. *Pharmakeftiki* 2016; 28: 60–83.

77   Arnett DK, Blumenthal RS, Albert MA, Buroker AB, Goldberger ZD, Hahn EJ et al. 2019 ACC/AHA Guideline on the Primary Prevention of Cardiovascular Disease: A Report of the American College of Cardiology/American Heart Association Task Force on Clinical Practice Guidelines. *J Am Coll Cardiol* 2019; 74: e177–e232.

13. Alcohol

Alcohol is toxic and contains calories. It can affect fat loss and muscle gain. It is metabolised as a priority when simultaneously ingested with protein, fat or carbohydrate, because of its toxicity. Alcoholic drinks are high energy density (compared to other drinks), and low nutrient density.

You can lose weight and consume alcohol. Similarly, you can gain muscle mass and drink alcohol. The effect will be dependent on the frequency and quantity you drink, as well as your calorie intake from food sources.

The more serious your goals are, the more likely you will need to monitor and consider restricting your alcohol intake, which will also depend on how much and how often you consume alcohol.

Alcohol is toxic and calorie dense at around 7 kcal per gram, however it does have a fairly high thermic effect (the energy required to access the energy in food or drink) at around 20%[1], which is comparable to that of a mixed meal. Drinking alcohol means consuming calories. There are *no* calorie-free alcoholic drinks. Therefore, alcohol consumption *can* impact on muscle growth and weight loss. The simplistic approach would be to just tell everyone to be tee-total. However, the evidence-based approach would be to consider that alcohol is a core part of many peoples' lifestyles. Cutting out alcohol is not a long-term strategy for well-being or happiness for many individuals. The question therefore is, '*how much* and *how often* can I drink whilst still achieving any body composition goals?'. In other words, does my preferred level of drinking have an effect on my body composition? The evidence-based approach to alcohol intake for body composition will depend heavily on personal preference, by considering how much and how often you like drinking and how serious your body composition goals are. If you have one or two drinks infrequently and are pretty relaxed about any body composition goals, there probably is no issue at all. If you '*binge drink*' multiple times per week but also want to build a lot of muscle and have low levels of fat mass, then a trade-off will probably need to be made.

To the best of my knowledge, there is only *one* short to moderate term study in healthy individuals, trained or untrained, on the effects of alcohol consumption on muscle growth or weight loss[2]. No long-term study has compared a group of people drinking alcohol with another group not drinking alcohol and the effect on body composition. Unfortunately, whether a big night on the town will significantly affect muscle growth after training chest and arms isn't high on the priority list for many research organisations. The majority of human research (which is quite limited) into alcohol consumption and body composition is in chronic excessive daily alcohol consumption (i.e. research on those with *alcohol use disorders* (AUD)), or the acute effects after a single drink or several drinks[3]. Research on people with AUDs is not representative of, nor generalisable to healthy individuals who may have a casual drink during the week, due to many confounding factors (mis-users of alcohol are more likely to smoke and perform other detrimental activities to health) and co-existing health issues (such as liver disease). Due to the ethical issues in giving people a toxin (alcohol), evidence is currently limited to acute or short-term trials of alcohol consumption or evidence from observational studies, expert opinion and lab evidence. The majority of evidence comes from studies where animals (e.g. rodents) are given alcohol to assess its effects on health and body composition. The amounts of alcohol used in rodent studies is equivalent to very high daily chronic alcohol consumption in humans, and therefore is also of limited use in this discussion[3]. Therefore, guidance on alcohol usually utilises lower quality forms of evidence and makes strong use of expert and coaching opinion.

There are no hard and fast rules with alcohol consumption. It is *not* possible to say that having X drinks or drinking more than Y times per week will impair weight loss or muscle growth. The effect of alcohol on body composition is *dose-responsive* and *frequency* dependent. The more you drink and the more frequently you drink, the larger the effects will be. Do you need to be tee-total? No. Can you drink as much as you want, whenever you want? No. The judgement of how much and how often you drink alcohol simply comes down to how much it forms part of your social life, and how serious your body composition goals are. At calorie maintenance or with no goals, frequent moderate drinking is unlikely to be an issue because the aim is just to maintain current condition. As you become leaner, or as you intend to build muscle, the effects become more important. A casual glass every other week will essentially have no effect. A few heavy nights per week will indeed have an effect.

Some important points about alcohol:

- Alcohol contains calories (7kcal per gram of alcohol)[4].
- Different alcoholic drinks contain additional calories from fats or carbohydrates (in particular, sugar). For the same alcohol content, two different drinks (e.g. a shot of spirit and a glass of wine) will contain the same number of calories from alcohol, but will contain different

amounts of additional calories from other macronutrients (see table below).

- Alcohol does not get stored as fat. It is utilised as energy because it is toxic and so the body aims to clear it from the body. Because of this, it has a high thermic effect of food.
- Because of this toxicity, alcohol is preferentially used for energy, meaning any fat, carbohydrate or protein will be directed towards fat storage until the alcohol in the body has been cleared[5].
- Therefore, alcohol can indirectly result in weight gain. Whether there is weight gain is again ultimately dependent on whether alcohol consumption results in a calorie surplus. Consuming alcohol whilst remaining in a calorie deficit will not result in weight gain.
- Alcohol disrupts sleep. Not just quantity, but quality. Even if you sleep for 7-9 hours, the quality of that sleep is reduced. Alcohol can therefore disrupt recovery and alter muscle protein synthesis. In a calorie deficit, alcohol consumption can promote muscle breakdown. The more you drink, the greater the effect.

The type of alcoholic drink or whether you mix alcoholic drinks does not influence how hungover you are (technically called *veisalgia*).

The only determinant of *hangover* magnitude is how high your blood alcohol levels reach and therefore how much alcohol you drink. A randomised controlled trial compared consuming beer then wine, wine then beer, beer only, or wine only and found no difference between the extent of hangovers when reaching the same blood alcohol levels (as measured by breath testing)[6]. The extent of a hangover will of course vary between individuals, depending on the ability to metabolise alcohol and clear it from the system, which is influenced by genetics and whether someone frequently drinks alcohol[6].

There are also no hangover cures[6].

In fact, the actual process of how alcohol consumption results in hangover symptoms is not really understood at all. If you want to reduce your morning hangover, reduce how high your blood alcohol levels reach the night before (discussed below).

There is only one controlled study to date assessing alcohol intake alongside an exercise programme for changes in body composition (suitably named the BEER-HIIT study)[2]. The good news? Frequent beer or equivalent alcohol consumption did not affect body composition outcomes.

As the most relevant study to date, it is important to discuss the study design and results. The BEER-HIIT study involved 72 adults (bigger than most studies on alcohol in healthy humans) and was partially randomised[2]. Getting someone drunk is pretty hard to conceal, so the study was not blinded. Participants had the choice of whether to be involved in training, and whether to drink alcohol or not. Those choosing alcohol were randomly assigned to consume 1 standard 330ml beer or vodka in sparkling water. Those not choosing alcohol were assigned to receive an alcohol-free beer or sparkling water. Men drank one drink at lunch and one drink at dinner. Women had one drink at dinner only. Those choosing training performed high intensity interval training (HIIT) twice per week, for 10 weeks. 40-65 minutes of high intensity interval training was performed per week. High intensity interval training sessions involved a range of weight-bearing exercises including squats, deadlifts, push ups and burpees at high intensities of effort (a rating of perceived exertion* > 8) with moderate intensity intervals (rating of perceived exertion = 6).

The rating of perceived exertion (RPE) as a marker of intensity of effort is discussed on in chapter 19.

After 10 weeks? Those who performed high intensity interval training significantly increased lean mass and decreased fat mass compared to those who did not train. The effect of alcohol consumption had *no* differential effect on body composition. The *same* change in body composition occurred in those who trained and drank a beer or vodka, compared to those who drank water or alcohol-free beer. Body mass did not change between any group, because the training groups gained muscle and lost fat (termed 'body recomposition'). Similar findings have been seen in overweight and obese individuals. Consuming 10% of calories from white wine or 10% of calories from grape juice on a calorie restricted and calorie equated diet resulted in the same amount of weight loss over 3 months[7].

The role of high intensity interval training on muscle growth and fat loss is discussed in chapter 24. The participants were not currently taking part in any exercise programme. Therefore, the high intensities and novelty of high intensity interval training may well have acted as a stimulus to increase muscle mass. One limitation of the study is that we do not know the diets of participants. Protein intake influences body composition when in a calorie surplus or deficit. The training groups significantly lost fat mass and significantly gained muscle. Concomitant muscle gain and fat loss is usually only seen in complete beginners. It cannot be assumed that participants were in a caloric deficit. They may have been at caloric maintenance or even in a surplus. A surplus despite increased exercise activity thermogenesis and therefore increased total daily energy expenditure from the high intensity interval training sessions could be explained by the additional calorie content of alcoholic drinks and alcohol-free beers. However, the fact that similar changes occurred in the group drinking water suggests that this cannot explain the results entirely.

Considering the low frequency of training and the lack of tracking of any measure of diet, this study would be most applicable to those who train infrequently and utilise a more intuitive approach to calorie intake. Participants were not on any training programme and their training history was unknown. The effect of high intensity interval training in promoting muscle growth can be seen in untrained individuals, but not in trained individuals. Further increases in high intensity interval training-mediated muscle growth may be attenuated after the initial training novelty. Whether differences in body composition may arise in durations longer than 10 weeks cannot be confirmed. But as the first study of its kind, it does a great job in suggesting that moderate alcohol consumption does not appear to significantly influence body composition in untrained males and females when high intensity interval training twice per week.

The table below outlines the calorie content of popular drinks. Note that the examples are a guide. Different wines, beers or ciders will vary in calorie and alcohol content.

Drink	Volume (ml)	Alcohol content (g)	Calories (kcal)	Alcohol calories (kcal)	Other calories (kcal)	Kcal/g of alcohol
Vodka	25	7.8	54	54	0	7
Gin	25	7.5	52	52	0	7
Whisky	25	7.8	54	54	0	7
White wine (10%)	250	24.7	196	172.9	23.1	7.9
Red wine (10%)	250	26.5	212	185	36	8
Lager (5.1%)	568 (1 pint)	22.7	240	158.9	81.1	10.6
Beer (5%)	568 (1 pint)	22.2	244	154	90	11
Cider (4.5%)	568 (1 pint)	20.2	256	141.4	114.6	12.7

Energy content of different alcoholic drinks. Data from MyFitnessPal and calorieking[8-10].

Lowest calorie content per unit of alcohol:

- Spirits
- Dry wines

Highest calorie content per unit of alcohol:

- Beers, ales, lagers
- Sugar-sweetened mixers
- Alcopops

Alcohol consumption and decreasing fat mass

You can drink alcohol and lose weight. The more alcohol you drink and the more frequent you drink it, the more difficult it would be to lose weight. Alcohol contains calories. Therefore, across the day when drinking alcohol, this additional calorie intake needs to be taken into account otherwise you may not be in a calorie deficit, and possibly even spill into a calorie surplus. A few drinks once a week is very feasible with weight loss. Heavy drinking sessions multiple times per week, less so.

Alcohol contains calories, but with *no* nutritional value. It has a high energy density (compared to other liquids) and a low nutrient density. Liquids are much easier to consume than whole food sources and can be less satiating. We also need to consider the additional calories in alcoholic drinks. Mixers, beers and wines for example contain additional calories besides just the alcohol, usually as carbohydrate. Whether you lose weight depends on whether you are in a calorie deficit. So, you can still lose weight and drink alcohol provided you consider the additional calories you drink. If you consumed 500kcal worth of drinks in an evening (which, depending on the drink, may be 2-4 drinks), then to ensure the same calorie deficit you would need to drop 500kcal from your usual energy intake. Occasionally this is fine. But as this becomes more frequent it limits your ability to consume foods that may aid satiety, and the ability to obtain sufficient nutrition from food to prevent deficiencies.

A systematic review and meta-analysis shows that when people consume alcohol, they tend to not compensate for the additional calories by reducing their calorie intake elsewhere[4]. Alcohol intake may also promote food intake by promoting appetite[11], and through the effects of alcohol on reducing inhibitions, making post-alcohol food consumption of highly palatable foods more likely (i.e. the post-night out kebab).

An important consideration is, what do you do when you drink alcohol? For many, this involves visiting bars and clubs, and often a stint on the dancefloor. Weight change is the result of differences between energy intake and expenditure. If energy intake is increasing from alcohol, then one strategy may be to increase energy expenditure, rather than to decrease energy intake from food. The amount of exercise activity thermogenesis you participate in on a night out will affect your overall energy balance. Hitting the dancefloor and cutting some shapes may help to minimise any excess calorie intake by increasing exercise activity thermogenesis and therefore total daily energy expenditure.

Alcohol consumption and increasing muscle mass

Alcohol consumption can result in an acute reduction in a range of muscle building related markers after a resistance training workout. No long-term studies have directly assessed the effect alcohol intake on muscle growth. It is probable that the more alcohol consumed and the more frequently it is consumed, the greater the effect.

The current evidence does *not* allow for quantification of how much alcohol will result in a certain impairment of muscle growth. For a detailed non-peer reviewed article on the mechanistic literature on the topic, read Menno Henselmans' freely available article[12]. Many of the studies cited in the article assess chronic alcoholics, rodents and acute alcohol consumption. Indeed, going by lab-based work on cells and rodent models of alcohol intake and exercise, binge-drinking alcohol immediately after resistance training will likely limit long-term improvements in muscle growth[13].

But what about *human* studies? The limited pool of acute studies looking at alcohol consumption after a workout show:

- The effect on testosterone (important for muscle growth) is dose-dependent. At lower levels of alcohol consumption some studies have found circulating testosterone (in the blood) to increase post-workout following alcohol consumption (potentially from reduced uptake by muscle)[14,15]. But at higher levels of alcohol consumption, circulating testosterone is acutely reduced[16,17].
- A reduction in post-workout markers of muscle protein synthesis[18-20]. However, most studies assessing post-workout muscle protein synthesis have participants drink large amounts of alcohol *immediately* after the training session, and they only assess the effect after a single training session in isolation[18,19].
- As will be discussed in the training chapters, a resistance training workout will reduce the ability of the trained muscle to produce force in the following days, whilst damage is being repaired. Does alcohol further reduce this reduction in force? Impaired recovery from a workout and greater impaired performance in the days following a muscle damaging workout has been documented[21,22]. However, most studies assessing the effects of alcohol on subsequent force production show no effect[20]. It may well be that the effect on recovery depends on how damaging the

278

workout is. Highly damaging workouts result in greater decrements in performance compared to less damaging workouts with post-workout alcohol consumption[23,24].

- Interestingly, the effects of alcohol consumption in women appears to be attenuated compared to men. Increases in testosterone and/or oestrogen and no change in markers of muscle protein synthesis have been noted[18], and there appears to be less of an effect on muscle recovery[23,25].

However, despite notable changes in some biomarkers, a non-systematic review of acute alcohol ingestion post-workout found little influence of alcohol intake on a range of biological, physical and cognitive markers within 2 to 48 hours after exercise with or without alcohol[3]. Despite some studies showing impaired recovery following alcohol, this review found measures of force, power, soreness or muscle damage were unchanged between groups drinking or not drinking alcohol post-workout. Indeed, the review did find lower acute levels of circulating testosterone and markers of muscle protein synthesis, and higher levels of cortisol (as outlined in chapter 5, cortisol is elevated from stress) which may be more relevant for our muscle building interests. Testosterone is important for muscle growth and chronically elevated cortisol can result in muscle breakdown. But, whether these *acute* alcohol-induced hormonal changes have any long-term effect on body composition is not clear, especially when considering that post-workout acute changes in testosterone and cortisol without alcohol consumption have been shown to not be relevant for muscle growth[3,26]. Of course, the literature base is thin with low participant numbers. These acute changes cannot be considered to be comprehensive.

A randomised cross-over trial found that even though muscle protein synthesis was lower when consuming alcohol and protein (or carbohydrate) post-workout compared to protein alone post workout, it was still significantly elevated above baseline levels (57% increase for alcohol and protein), albeit significantly lower than protein alone (109%)[19]. Of note, not consuming protein post-workout (alcohol and carbohydrate) had the lowest rise in muscle protein synthesis (29%). The practical implications of the findings in acute studies are limited. Reduced markers of muscle protein synthesis in the acute setting when consuming alcohol after a single resistance training session does not necessarily mean that muscle growth is reduced or impaired. As discussed in chapter 9, acute changes in muscle protein synthesis post-workout do not correlate with muscle growth and is not as important as total protein intake or maintaining elevated muscle protein synthesis across the day. Consuming protein post-workout may help mitigate alcohol-induced reductions in muscle protein synthesis. But, how meaningful are these changes for long-term changes in muscle growth? Analogously, lower testosterone and lower levels of markers of muscle protein synthesis are also seen during weight loss phases with calorie restriction. These reductions are chronic, yet muscle growth is still possible in these scenarios, albeit less optimal than with a calorie surplus. Even so, when consuming alcohol once or twice per week, changes in muscle protein synthesis would only occur acutely on those days for several hours. These alcohol-mediated changes are unlikely to be beneficial, but whether they meaningfully reduce muscle growth is unknown[3]. Genetics most likely plays a large role in the individual response to alcohol consumption and muscle growth.

Considering we cannot quantify alcohol consumption and changes in muscle growth, we can instead try to *qualitatively* assess whether a bout of drinking has affected or will affect performance, recovery and muscle building goals. The morning after drinking (whether moderate or as binge drinking), consider:

- How much sleep did you get? Do you feel well rested or slightly fatigued?
- How well recovered do your muscles feel, do you have excessive delayed onset of muscle soreness (DOMS)? Compare this to the typical muscle soreness you experience for a similar workout without alcohol consumption (see chapter 17 regarding muscle damage and DOMS).
- Do you feel as though you could perform a productive workout? Not necessarily hitting personal records, but can train near to failure (see chapter 16 regarding training recommendations).

The more tired you feel, the more achy you are, and the less likely you think you could have a productive workout, the more likely the alcohol you drank had an effect on your muscle building potential. Similarly, the less tired you feel, the less achy you are, and the more likely you could have a productive workout, the more likely the alcohol you drank had minimal effects on your muscle building potential. This is a crude measure, but it provides a useful starting point to determine how much alcohol you can *'get away with'* on a night out without impacting your muscle building potential.

Regardless of how much you drink, some basic strategies can be used to minimise any potential effect of alcohol on your muscle building plan.

- ***The timing of alcohol in relation to training.*** *Maximise* the time between training and drinking alcohol. Train as early in the morning as possible and start drinking as late as possible in the evening.
- ***Have a rest day the day after drinking***. Sleep is likely to be compromised after drinking, which can impair recovery from previous training and worsen subsequent workout performance. Having a rest day means an extra full night of sleep before the next session, which can be much more productive. Other experts suggest having a rest day on the day of your drinking[27]. If your training frequency is 5 or fewer sessions per week, placing your rest days on the day of and day after a large session of drinking may help to optimise the productivity of your

sessions. In other words, reduce your training volume during the part(s) of the week that you drink.

Is it worse (in terms of body composition) to have one or two drinks more frequently (e.g. a few times a week), or one big drinking session less frequently (i.e. a binge drinking session on the weekend)?

It depends.

Moderate drinking is defined as 1 or 2 drinks per day, several times per week. Binge drinking is defined as anything more than 2 drinks in one sitting. Most people reading this book may binge drink at most once or twice per week, and possibly on only 5 or 6 drinks.

Again, the research on such a topic is very limited, but we can make inferences:

Moderate drinking: 1 or 2 drinks per day, several times per week.	Binge drinking: anything more than 2 drinks in one sitting, once per week.
Unlikely to have any effect or only mild effects on muscle growth.	Likely to impair muscle growth.
Unlikely to impair or only mild impair sleep or recovery.	Likely to impair sleep and recovery.
Consideration of the alcohol content will limit daily food energy intake.	Unlikely to be able to consider calories from drinks and therefore unlikely to factor this into food intake.
Unlikely to affect or only mildly affect training the day after.	Likely to affect training from that day and the day after, unlikely to affect training or muscle growth during the rest of the week.
May be significant during a period of weight loss when calories are already limited, by further limiting nutrient intake. Or, the frequent consumption of alcohol without consideration for the additional calories could prevent the generation of a calorie deficit for weight loss. The calorie content of a couple of drinks multiple times per week may be similar to one night of binge drinking. The minor effect of	May be significant during a period of weight loss from an inability to track calorie intake and loss of inhibitions which may promote food consumption leading to a caloric surplus and excess fat gain.

changes to muscle protein synthesis and testosterone may shift protein balance to be more negative and promote more breakdown of muscle mass when in a deficit, considering this may occur multiple times per week.	
May be significant during a period of weight gain for muscle growth. The additional calories during a calorie surplus from alcohol may promote additional fat storage, and the frequent moderate drinking may have a minor, but more chronic suppression of muscle protein synthesis.	May be significant during a period of weight gain where muscle growth will be affected.

How to maximise the effects of alcohol and minimise the effects on body composition

At a crude level, people drink alcohol for a range of reasons, including:

1. To enjoy some drinks and not get too drunk.
2. To enjoy some drinks and maybe get a little tipsy or drunk, but not so much that a hangover is present the following day.
3. To get as drunk as possible, with total disregard for the hangover the following day.

The effects of alcohol (the social effects, whether we get a hangover, and some of the effects relating to body composition) are dependent on the blood alcohol levels that are reached whilst drinking. The effect of alcohol on calorie intake is primarily dependent on the amount of alcohol and types of drinks consumed, and not on blood alcohol levels (besides any cognitive effects resulting in a late night kebab). Several factors influence blood alcohol content. Therefore, whether you aim to get drunk or limit how drunk you get, you can consider the following factors:

- **Rate of alcohol consumption** (i.e. the number of drinks per hour). Drinking at a faster rate will mean that blood alcohol levels will reach a much higher level. Your liver can only metabolise so much alcohol at any given instant. Pacing your drinking will mean that blood alcohol content will not be as high, as alcohol absorption by the gut and alcohol metabolism by the liver will be better matched. The elevation in blood alcohol will depend on the rate of drinking. Downing a beer or some shots will rapidly raise blood alcohol content. Sipping on a beer all afternoon will not elevate blood alcohol much at all.

- **Eating food** before drinking will slow down the rate of alcohol absorption into the blood[28,29]. Avoid eating food and drinking alcohol in close proximity if you want to get drunk. Conversely, to minimise the effects of alcohol (you want to drink alcohol but without the effects of high blood alcohol levels), space your drinks out as much as possible with a big meal before you start drinking and meal(s) during drinking[27]. Food consumption will slow the rate at which you can drink alcohol. But, calorie intake needs to be considered.

There are two ways to factor alcohol into your diet.

Drinking in moderation (2 or fewer drinks per sitting):

- Such as a glass of wine with dinner or an afternoon beer.
- Consider how many drinks you will have or have had and reduce calories from your daily food intake. It is likely best to reduce calories from fat and carbohydrate (without dropping fat below 0.5g/kg of body weight) to spare protein, which is satiating and beneficial for body composition.
- Few drinks display their calorie content. Use the average calorie value in the table above to estimate the calorie content of drinks.

Binge-drinking (more than 2 drinks per sitting):

- Avoid highly fatiguing workouts with high levels of muscle damage near to drinking alcohol. Recovery from highly fatiguing workouts appears to be worse after alcohol consumption than less fatiguing workouts.
- Either train as early as possible in the morning and drink as late as possible to maximise recovery time or have a rest day on the day of drinking.
- Avoid training the day after binge drinking.
- To maximise blood alcohol content, avoid eating food immediately before or during alcohol consumption and drink at a fast rate.
- To minimise blood alcohol content, eat food immediately before or during alcohol consumption and drink at a slow rate.
- Avoid any attempt to track alcohol calories and compensate from food calories, as you will be left with no calories for food and nutrient intake.
- Maintain protein intake.
- Consume fibrous vegetables to aid satiety from food volume.
- Limit fat on the day of drinking as it will be readily stored and helps to reduce calorie intake from food, whilst maintaining satiety from protein and vegetables[27].

- Choose spirits with a calorie free mixer or dry red wines to limit additional calories from alcoholic drinks. Avoid drinks that have extra calories besides alcohol, such as beers, ales, alcopops and sugar-based mixers.
- Try and move more. Increase total daily energy expenditure to try and offset energy intake. Walk during the day or hit the dancefloor on the night out.

Two great resources for alcohol and body composition are Andy Morgan's very useful and simple guide for drinking alcohol and its effects on body composition[30]. Menno Henselmans has written a useful expert opinion guide on binge drinking and how to minimise or maximise the effect of alcohol[27].

References

1   Suter PM, Jéquier E, Schutz Y. Effect of ethanol on energy expenditure. *Am J Physiol* 1994; 266: R1204-1212.

2   Molina-Hidalgo C, De-la-O A, Jurado-Fasoli L, Amaro-Gahete FJ, Castillo MJ. Beer or Ethanol Effects on the Body Composition Response to High-Intensity Interval Training. The BEER-HIIT Study. *Nutrients* 2019; 11. Available from: doi:10.3390/nu11040909.

3   Steiner JL, Lang CH. Dysregulation of skeletal muscle protein metabolism by alcohol. *Am J Physiol - Endocrinol Metab* 2015; 308: E699–E712.

4   Kwok A, Dordevic AL, Paton G, Page MJ, Truby H. Effect of alcohol consumption on food energy intake: a systematic review and meta-analysis. *Br J Nutr* 2019; 121: 481–495.

5   Raben A, Agerholm-Larsen L, Flint A, Holst JJ, Astrup A. Meals with similar energy densities but rich in protein, fat, carbohydrate, or alcohol have different effects on energy expenditure and substrate metabolism but not on appetite and energy intake. *Am J Clin Nutr* 2003; 77: 91–100.

6   Köchling J, Geis B, Wirth S, Hensel KO. Grape or grain but never the twain? A randomized controlled multiarm matched-triplet crossover trial of beer and wine. *Am J Clin Nutr* 2019; 109: 345–352.

7   Flechtner-Mors M, Biesalski HK, Jenkinson CP, Adler G, Ditschuneit HH. Effects of moderate consumption of white wine on weight loss in overweight and obese subjects. *Int J Obes Relat Metab Disord J Int Assoc Study Obes* 2004; 28: 1420–1426.

8   MyFitnessPal. *MyFitnessPal.com.* Available from: https://www.myfitnesspal.com/ (accessed 7 Feb 2020).

9   CalorieKing (United Kingdom). *Food Nutrition Facts and Free Calorie Counter.* Available from: https://www.calorieking.com/gb/en/ (accessed 7 Feb 2020).

10   CalorieKing. *Food Nutrition Facts and Free Calorie Counter.* Available from: https://www.calorieking.com/us/en/ (accessed 7 Feb 2020).

11   Yeomans MR. Short term effects of alcohol on appetite in humans. Effects of context and restrained eating. *Appetite* 2010; 55: 565–573.

12   Henselmans M. *The effects of alcohol on muscle growth.* Available from: https://mennohenselmans.com/the-effects-of-alcohol-on-muscle-growth/ (accessed 7 Feb 2020).

13   Bamji ZD, Haddad GE. Convergence of Theories of Alcohol Administration Postanabolic Stimulation on mTOR Signaling: Lessons for Exercise Regimen. *Alcohol Clin Exp Res* 2015; 39: 787–789.

14   Vingren JL, Hill DW, Buddhadev H, Duplanty A. Postresistance exercise ethanol ingestion and acute testosterone bioavailability. *Med Sci Sports Exerc* 2013; 45: 1825–1832.

15   Sarkola T, Eriksson CJP. Testosterone increases in men after a low dose of alcohol. *Alcohol Clin Exp Res* 2003; 27: 682–685.

16   Mendelson JH, Mello NK, Ellingboe J. Effects of acute alcohol intake on pituitary-gonadal hormones in normal human males. *J Pharmacol Exp Ther* 1977; 202: 676–682.

17   Vatsalya V, Issa JE, Hommer DW, Ramchandani VA. Pharmacodynamic effects of intravenous alcohol on hepatic and gonadal hormones: influence of age and sex. *Alcohol Clin Exp Res* 2012; 36: 207–213.

18   Duplanty AA, Budnar RG, Luk HY, Levitt DE, Hill DW, McFarlin BK et al. Effect of Acute Alcohol Ingestion on Resistance Exercise-Induced mTORC1 Signaling in Human Muscle. *J Strength Cond Res* 2017; 31: 54–61.

19   Parr EB, Camera DM, Areta JL, Burke LM, Phillips SM, Hawley JA et al. Alcohol Ingestion Impairs Maximal Post-Exercise Rates of Myofibrillar Protein Synthesis following a Single Bout of Concurrent Training. *PLOS ONE* 2014; 9: e88384.

20   Lakićević N. The Effects of Alcohol Consumption on Recovery Following Resistance Exercise: A Systematic Review. *J Funct Morphol Kinesiol* 2019; 4: 41.

21   Barnes Matthew J, Mündel T, Stannard SR. The effects of acute alcohol consumption and eccentric muscle damage on neuromuscular function. *Appl Physiol Nutr Metab* 2011; 37: 63–71.

22   Barnes MJ, Mündel T, Stannard SR. Post-exercise alcohol ingestion exacerbates eccentric-exercise induced losses in performance. *Eur J Appl Physiol* 2010; 108: 1009–1014.

23   Levitt D, Luk H-Y, Duplanty A, McFarlin B, Hill D, Vingren J. Effect of alcohol after muscle-damaging resistance exercise on muscular performance recovery and inflammatory capacity in women. *Eur J Appl Physiol* 2017; 117. Available from: doi:10.1007/s00421-017-3606-0.

24   Barnes MJ, Mündel T, Stannard SR. Acute alcohol consumption aggravates the decline in muscle performance following strenuous eccentric exercise. *J Sci Med Sport* 2010; 13: 189–193.

25   McLeay Y, Stannard SR, Mundel T, Foskett A, Barnes M. Effect of Alcohol Consumption on Recovery From Eccentric Exercise Induced Muscle Damage in Females. *Int J Sport Nutr Exerc Metab* 2017; 27: 115–121.

26   Schoenfeld BJ. Postexercise Hypertrophic Adaptations: A Reexamination of the Hormone Hypothesis and Its Applicability to Resistance Training Program Design. *J Strength Cond Res* 2013; 27: 1720–1730.

27   Henselmans M. *The science of binge drinking: 7 Tips to get wasted without wasting your gains.* Available from: https://mennohenselmans.com/science-binge-drinking/ (accessed 7 Feb 2020).

28   Sadler DW, Fox J. Intra-individual and inter-individual variation in breath alcohol pharmacokinetics: The effect of food on absorption. *Sci Justice J Forensic Sci Soc* 2011; 51: 3–9.

29   Jones AW, Jönsson KA, Kechagias S. Effect of high-fat, high-protein, and high-carbohydrate meals on the pharmacokinetics of a small dose of ethanol. *Br J Clin Pharmacol* 1997; 44: 521–526.

30   Morgan A. *A Guide to Alcohol and Fat Loss.* Available from: https://rippedbody.com/alcohol/ (accessed 7 Feb 2020).

14. Non-sugar sweeteners and artificial sweeteners

There is a large body of evidence in humans from meta-analyses of randomised controlled trials and observational studies that non-sugar sweeteners have no adverse health effects in humans and are safe to consume, even in high quantities. They are a useful tool in maintaining satiety, especially during periods of calorie deficits. Whether they are incorporated should be a matter of personal preference.

* The only people who should be concerned with artificial sweetener consumption are those with Phenylketonuria, who cannot consume the sweetener aspartame. This is because aspartame is converted to phenylalanine in the body, which these individuals cannot metabolise (break down), due to a genetic disorder. And don't worry, in the UK it is diagnosed at birth, you'd know if you had it.

Non-sugar sweeteners, more commonly known as artificial sweeteners (however this definition excludes naturally occurring calorie free sweeteners) are increasingly being found in food products and available as separate products that can be added to food. Non-sugar sweeteners are used to replace sugar-based sources of sweetness, allowing for the same enjoyment of sweet foods without the additional calories. Non-sugar sweeteners can be used to replace *added* sugars, which the UK government recommends limiting[1,2]. This can reduce daily calorie intake and therefore support weight loss or maintenance (not because of any particular detrimental effects of sugar itself, but the fact that high sugar consumption often leads to a calorie surplus, weight gain and therefore any health implications that come with weight gain)[3].

The most common sweeteners are:

- Aspartame (an amino acid)
- Sucralose
- Stevia

- Xylitol (often found in chewing gum)
- Sorbitol (often found in chewing gum)
- Acesulfame K
- Saccharin

A systematic review and meta-analysis has been conducted on 56 randomised and non-randomised controlled trials and observational studies regarding sweetener consumption. This review was prepared to inform new *World Health Organisation* (WHO) guidelines on the use of non-sugar sweeteners. A range of health measures were assessed, including[4]:

- Body weight.
- Oral health.
- Energy intake and appetite.
- Diabetes.
- Cancer.
- Cardiovascular disease.
- Mood and behaviour.

The studies in the meta-analysis compared consumption of sweetener against no consumption, and the amount of sweetener consumed. The conclusions were that sweeteners are *safe* for consumption and they have *no* significant effect on health measures[4]. They also concluded that there is *no* evidence to suggest health benefits from their consumption. In other words, sweeteners are pretty *neutral* in terms of their effects[4].

Furthermore, a recent consensus workshop of 17 experts came to similar conclusions:

"The panel agreed that the safety of LCS [low calorie sweeteners] is demonstrated by a substantial body of evidence reviewed by regulatory experts and current levels of consumption, even for high users, are within agreed safety margins."
Ashwell et al., 2020[3].

In fact, there have been many systematic reviews and other reviews on sweetener consumption. Some of these use different search criteria and data collection methods, meaning different studies are included or excluded. They *all* still conclude that artificial sweeteners are *safe* for consumption, including:

- No effect of artificial sweeteners on metabolic health[5].
- No effect of artificially sweetened drinks on chronic kidney disease[6].
- No conclusive trend between artificially sweetened drinks and type 2 diabetes[7].

- A systematic review and meta-analysis of randomised controlled trials showing a reduction in body mass index (BMI) when consuming food and drinks with non-sugar sweeteners, compared to an increase in BMI when consuming food and drinks with sucrose (a type of sugar)[8].
- Another systematic review and meta-analysis of randomised controlled trials found no effect of non-sugar sweeteners on BMI, fat mass or waist circumference[9].
- The *European Food Safety Authority*, an advisory committee for the *European Union* on food safety, have also reported that xylitol, sorbitol and sucralose have been shown to be beneficial to oral health (maintenance of tooth mineralisation)[10].

It should be noted that most reviews highlight the importance of the need for further randomised controlled trials with more participants to make robust recommendations, as there is a lack of high quality research on non-sugar sweeteners[4]. But, the comparatively large body of evidence compared to other diet-related topics suggests no effect from their consumption on many health outcomes.

* Note that *excessive consumption of polyols (e.g. xylitol and sorbitol) can have laxative effects.*

Sucralose and aspartame

The most common non-sugar sweeteners are sucralose and aspartame.

Sucralose

Sucralose is an artificial sweetener that is around 600 times sweeter than regular sugar[11]. It is commonly found in soft drinks, puddings, chewing gum, breakfast cereals and pre-prepared salads[12]. The majority of sucralose is not absorbed by the body and is excreted. Around 10 to 20% enters the blood stream, but leaves the body relatively unchanged in the urine.

The *European Union's Scientific Committee on Food* concluded that sucralose is *safe* for human consumption and is not harmful to the immune system. It also does not cause cancer, create infertility or cause problems during pregnancy. There is also no evidence for any meaningful effects of sucralose on blood glucose (sugar) regulation[12].

The acceptable limit is currently 15mg/kg of body weight per day. A typical sucralose-sweetened diet drink contains 15-30mg of sucralose. Meaning, if you weighed 70kg, the maximum current upper safe limit would be around 35 sucralose-sweetened drinks per day.

Aspartame

Aspartame is a very common sweetener found in many popular drinks. It is an amino acid (a building block of protein) and therefore it does actually contain calories. But, because it is 200 times sweeter than sugar, the quantity used is small. Meaning, the calorie content is *negligible* and essentially zero[13]. Health concerns regarding aspartame first arose in the 1990s following studies into rats. However, after years of human studies and data collection, the consensus from health authorities is that aspartame is *safe* for human consumption and does not cause cancer or brain damage[13]. In fact, like sucralose, the safe upper intake levels for aspartame are quite high:

"An adult weighing 60 kg drinking 12 (330ml) cans of a diet soft drink (containing aspartame at the maximum permitted levels of use), every hour would still have a blood phenylalanine concentration below 6 mg/dl as recommended by current clinical guidelines and that is with no reported health effects."
European Food Safety Authority, 2014[13].

Summary

Non-sugar sweeteners have been demonstrated to be safe. The recommended safe upper limits are far higher than the intakes typically consumed by individuals. As a tool to limit additional sugar consumption, they can be a valuable tool. Whether they are used is down to *personal preference*, but there is no evidence of any detrimental effect from their use.

References

1   GOV.UK. *NDNS: results from Years 1 to 4 (combined)*. Available from: https://www.gov.uk/government/statistics/national-diet-and-nutrition-survey-results-from-years-1-to-4-combined-of-the-rolling-programme-for-2008-and-2009-to-2011-and-2012 (accessed 5 Feb 2020).

2   GOV.UK. *NDNS: results from years 7 and 8 (combined)*. Available from: https://www.gov.uk/government/statistics/ndns-results-from-years-7-and-8-combined (accessed 5 Feb 2020).

3   Ashwell M, Gibson S, Bellisle F, Buttriss J, Drewnowski A, Fantino M et al. Expert consensus on low-calorie sweeteners: facts, research gaps and suggested actions. *Nutr Res Rev* 2020; 13: 1–10.

4   Toews I, Lohner S, Küllenberg de Gaudry D, Sommer H, Meerpohl JJ. Association between intake of non-sugar sweeteners and health outcomes: systematic review and meta-analyses of randomised and non-randomised controlled trials and observational studies. *The BMJ* 2019; 364. Available from: doi:10.1136/bmj.k4718.

5   Brown RJ, de Banate MA, Rother KI. Artificial sweeteners: a systematic review of metabolic effects in youth. *Int J Pediatr Obes IJPO Off J Int Assoc Study Obes* 2010; 5: 305–312.

6   Cheungpasitporn W, Thongprayoon C, O'Corragain OA, Edmonds PJ, Kittanamongkolchai W, Erickson SB. Associations of sugar-sweetened and artificially sweetened soda with chronic kidney disease: a systematic review and meta-analysis. *Nephrol Carlton Vic* 2014; 19: 791–797.

7   Greenwood DC, Threapleton DE, Evans CEL, Cleghorn CL, Nykjaer C, Woodhead C et al. Association between sugar-sweetened and artificially sweetened soft drinks and type 2 diabetes: systematic review and dose-response meta-analysis of prospective studies. *Br J Nutr* 2014; 112: 725–734.

8   Wiebe N, Padwal R, Field C, Marks S, Jacobs R, Tonelli M. A systematic review on the effect of sweeteners on glycemic response and clinically relevant outcomes. *BMC Med* 2011; 9: 123.

9   Azad MB, Abou-Setta AM, Chauhan BF, Rabbani R, Lys J, Copstein L et al. Nonnutritive sweeteners and cardiometabolic health: a systematic review and meta-analysis of randomized controlled trials and prospective cohort studies. *CMAJ Can Med Assoc J J Assoc Medicale* Can 2017; 189: E929–E939.

10   European Food Safety Authority. *Scientific Opinion on the substantiation of health claims related to the sugar replacers xylitol, sorbitol, mannitol, maltitol, lactitol, isomalt, erythritol, D-tagatose, isomaltulose, sucralose and polydextrose and maintenance of tooth mineralisation by decreasing tooth demineralisation (ID 463, 464, 563, 618, 647, 1182, 1591, 2907, 2921, 4300), and reduction of post-prandial glycaemic responses (ID 617, 619, 669, 1590, 1762, 2903, 2908, 2920) pursuant to Article 13(1) of Regulation (EC) No 1924/2006.* Available from: https://efsa.onlinelibrary.wiley.com/doi/epdf/10.2903/j.efsa.2011.2076 (accessed 7 Feb 2020).

11   AlDeeb OAA, Mahgoub H, Foda NH. Sucralose. *Profiles Drug Subst Excip Relat Methodol* 2013; 38: 423–462.

12   The Scientific Committee for Food (European Commission). *Opinion of the Scientific Committee on Food on Sucralose.* Available from: https://documents.pub/document/opinion-of-the-scientific-committee-on-food-on-sucralose.html (accessed 7 Feb 2020).

13   European Food Safety Authority. *EFSA explains the Safety of Aspartame.* Available from: https://www.efsa.europa.eu/en/corporate/pub/factsheetaspartame (accessed 8 Feb 2020).

15. Organic food

Organic foods are not more nutritious than conventional foods.

Organic foods have become very popular recently and are defined as:

"growing crops and raising livestock that avoids synthetic chemicals, hormones, antibiotic agents, genetic engineering, and irradiation." **Forman et al., 2012[1].**

Numerous claims have been made about organic food consumption, compared to *conventional* food consumption (i.e. food not grown *'organically'*). Surveys demonstrate that people purchase organic foods with a greater emphasis on the belief that they are more *nutritious*, rather than because they believe they are better for the *environment*[2]. Despite such claims, the literature on organic food and health outcomes in humans to date, is quite limited[3]. Organic products are more expensive than conventional products[1]. There are no long-term studies that compare people consuming organic food with people consuming conventionally produced food, whilst factoring socioeconomic status[1,4]. Observational studies comparing organic and conventional food intake are limited in their use, because there are many other differences (confounding factors) between organic consumers and non-organic consumers, such as education, income, health awareness, exercise levels and smoking history[3]. People making the decision to consume organic food also make other decisions that influence their health, including an altered overall dietary pattern[3]. Even so, observational studies are very limited to place any causality on organic food and outcomes[3,4].

There is *no* difference between organic or conventional plant and animal foods in terms of their vitamin, mineral or overall nutritional content. This has been demonstrated in a range of meta-analyses[1,3,5]. Some meta-analyses show greater element content in conventional food compared to organic food. For example, elevated iodine and selenium in conventional milk[3]. Some meta-analyses show elevated nutrient content in organic food compared to conventional food. There may be differences in omega-3 fatty acid content in animal-based organic products including milk and meat[6]. A meta-analysis showed an increase in omega-3 fatty acid content in organic meat[7]. As the authors noted, there was very high variability between studies (such as the animals studied, the country or the diets of the animals), which limits the strength of such findings. Indeed, some conventional milks produced in a certain manner have a similar omega-3 content to organically produced milk[1]. However, even if differences do exist (such as in omega-3 content), they are too small to be of *meaningful* consequence within a diet[3]. For example, in a typical diet containing animal products, switching conventional food sources for organic food sources would only increase dietary omega-3 fatty acid intake by 2.5-8% (with dairy) and 2.5-4% (with meat). Meat and dairy are *minor* sources of omega-3 in typical diets[3]. However, this has *not* been formally assessed in a randomised controlled trial. Some research shows no difference between organic and conventional foods and some research shows a difference, but this has *not* been proven to be *meaningful* within the context of the whole diet for health[1,8]. There also appears to be no detrimental effects of organic foods[8]. As such, from a nutritional perspective, the choice of whether to consume organic or conventional foods should be *personal preference*.

"Despite the widespread perception that organically produced foods are more nutritious than conventional alternatives, we did not find robust evidence to support this perception."
Smith-Spangler et al., 2012[4].

"The published literature lacks strong evidence that organic foods are significantly more nutritious than conventional foods. Consumption of organic foods may reduce exposure to pesticide residues and antibiotic-resistant bacteria."
Smith-Spangler et al., 2012[4].

"No clear positive effects on human health have been presented as a result of consuming an organic diet in comparison with a conventional diet."
Haugen et al., 2014[8].

A point to remember is that there are many other factors in the production of food within both organic and conventional farming methods that may influence nutritional quality. For example, the country and geographical location of the farm, soil type, climate, storage methods, length of storage and time of season[1,3].

Despite a lack of nutritional benefit, organic foods have been shown to have a beneficial impact on the environment compared to conventional food production[1]. Organic foods may also reduce exposure to pesticides[8]. Whether this is of any benefit is unknown, because no studies have experimentally examined a causal relationship between pesticide consumption and any health issues with the nervous system[1,8]. Further discussion is beyond the scope of this book.

References

1   Forman J, Silverstein J, Nutrition CO, Health C on E. Organic Foods: Health and Environmental Advantages and Disadvantages. *Pediatrics* 2012; 130: e1406–e1415.

2   Shepherd R, Magnusson M, Sjödén P-O. Determinants of consumer behavior related to organic foods. *Ambio* 2005; 34: 352–359.

3   Mie A, Andersen HR, Gunnarsson S, Kahl J, Kesse-Guyot E, Rembiałkowska E et al. Human health implications of organic food and organic agriculture: a comprehensive review. *Environ Health Glob Access Sci Source* 2017; 16: 111.

4   Smith-Spangler C, Brandeau ML, Hunter GE, Bavinger JC, Pearson M, Eschbach PJ et al. Are Organic Foods Safer or Healthier Than Conventional Alternatives?: A Systematic Review. *Ann Intern Med* 2012; 157: 348.

5   Dangour AD, Lock K, Hayter A, Aikenhead A, Allen E, Uauy R. Nutrition-related health effects of organic foods: a systematic review. *Am J Clin Nutr* 2010; 92: 203–210.

6   Srednicka-Tober D, Barański M, Seal CJ, Sanderson R, Benbrook C, Steinshamn H et al. Higher PUFA and n-3 PUFA, conjugated linoleic acid, α-tocopherol and iron, but lower iodine and selenium concentrations in organic milk: a systematic literature review and meta- and redundancy analyses. *Br J Nutr* 2016; 115: 1043–1060.

7   Srednicka-Tober D, Barański M, Seal C, Sanderson R, Benbrook C, Steinshamn H et al. Composition differences between organic and conventional meat: a systematic literature review and meta-analysis. *Br J Nutr* 2016; 115: 994–1011.

8   Haugen M, Halvorsen R, Iversen PO, Mansoor MA, Meltzer HM, Torjusen H et al. *Comparison of organic and conventional food and food Production. Part III: Human health – an evaluation of human studies, animal models studies and biomarker studies.* Available from: https://vkm.no/download/18.13735ab315cffecbb51386ae/1509703709701/ (accessed 8 Feb 2020)

16. Evidence-based training for optimising body composition

Exercise has an important role in determining body composition. This section will focus on exercise to optimise body composition during a calorie surplus (i.e. to increase muscle mass) and during a calorie deficit (i.e. losing fat mass whilst preserving muscle mass). Both *resistance training* and *aerobic exercise* will be covered.

This book will *not* cover how to *specifically* (i.e. as the primary goal) train for performance. However, elements of performance relevant to muscle building will be discussed, and certain performance aspects *will* improve as a result of training for muscle growth and weight loss. Performance is highly specific to the discipline (e.g. how to be a faster sprinter, be a stronger powerlifter, or be a better tennis player). Influencing body composition can increase or decrease performance, which is highly dependent on the athletic or sporting discipline, or aspect of performance being measured. For example, consider the optimal body weights in different positions of professional rugby players. Not just body composition, but optimal body fat and muscle levels are sport-specific[1]. *Strength* (the ability to produce a force) will be discussed in the context of building muscle. *Absolute strength* (the maximum force that can be produced) is determined by several factors including:

- Biomechanics (how the body moves).
- Genetics.
- Tendon stiffness (what connects muscles to the skeleton).
- Neural adaptations (an ability to recruit all the *muscle fibres* in a muscle, using the right muscles and specifically learning the correct movement).
- Baseline muscle mass.

Improvements in strength from resistance training however, have long been proposed to be the result of[2]:

- Initial neural adaptations from training.
- Subsequent *muscle hypertrophy* (increased muscle mass)[3,4].

It is proposed that at a certain point, neural adaptations are essentially maximised and improvements in strength are the result of increased muscle mass[4]. In other words, beginner improvements in strength may be unrelated to increases in muscle size, but with training experience, increases in strength can be accounted for by increases in muscle mass. However, authors have questioned the relative influence of muscle growth on strength gains as there is actually *no* direct evidence demonstrating this association[2,5]. The rationale is based on *retrospective* analyses showing an association between muscle growth and increases in strength after a period of training[5]. The association between increases in muscle mass and strength from resistance training may just be a *correlation*. Relative increases in muscle size and strength will be influenced by the loads used during training. As will be discussed, light, moderate and heavy weight loads can build muscle, but strength is primarily increased through heavy loads[6]. Correlation does not mean causation. The exact influence of muscle growth or neural adaptations on strength is still inconclusive[2,7]. For further discussion, Greg Nuckols has written an in-depth publicly available article discussing the role of muscle growth on strength, based on the peer-reviewed literature[8].

Although this book focuses on increasing muscle mass, in doing so this will facilitate the ability to be stronger through some similar training principles, albeit not to the extent that a dedicated strength training programme may be able to achieve. Training primarily for muscle mass can improve strength in powerlifting[9,10]. As a beginner, there are large similarities between training for strength and training for hypertrophy. However with experience, training will need to become more specific for the goal in mind, but there will always be some overlap. For a comprehensive overview of strength training I recommend reading '*The Complete Strength Training Guide*' by Greg Nuckols, which is freely available[11].

Exercise

Many books, articles and blogs are readily available on training for specific goals, training for specific sports and how to exercise for general health. Many resources are written from an anecdotal perspective; discussing what worked an *individual,* outlining the key differences between *their* success and failure based on *their* experience. For example, your favourite sportsman or sportswoman may share their favourite workouts and exercises that they '*believe*' are key to their success. You may have followed one of these workouts or training plans, following the instructed exercises, number of reps and rest, and so on. But, what elements of a workout or plan are the key elements that make it effective? Or even, is it any good at all? When your favourite star with chiselled abs or well-defined legs promotes a specific exercise, rep range, or technique as the secret to success, it can be very easy to consider this to be true, without any actual *evidence* to indicate this.

This book will cover what is important, what isn't important and look at what is still unknown about training for muscle growth. This will include how to train to grow muscle and how to design your workout and programme so that you achieve what is needed, but in a framework that suits *your* lifestyle. It is important to clarify what has no benefit or may even be detrimental to your goals. This allows you to focus on what is important. However, there are still things that are not fully understood. It is at these boundaries of our understanding that expert experience and personal preference are important in providing recommendation. This is where you can consider trying things that *'feel'* good or *'seem'* to work, but are not necessarily the focus of your training.

"If physical activity were a drug, we would refer to it as a miracle cure, due to the great many illnesses it can prevent and help treat."
UK Chief Medical Officers' Physical Activity Guidelines, 2019[1].

Exercise is more than just a tool to shape the body. All forms of exercise provide a wealth of health benefits, and this should not be overlooked.

Aerobic exercise

Do you need to perform cardio to lose weight? No. Should you perform cardio to be healthy? Yes.

However you may call it, *aerobic, cardiovascular* or *endurance* exercise, is where the body uses oxygen during physical activity. It is well ingrained in society as being beneficial for health and for improving physical performance. Take for example, someone who has cardiovascular problems, such as a *heart attack*. One of the first treatments that a doctor will recommend is a supervised exercise programme. Quite literally, getting patients with cardiovascular disease to work with a physiotherapist or cardiac rehabilitation nurse to improve their cardiovascular endurance. For instance, to increase the distance they can walk.

For some it can be easy to view aerobic exercise solely as a tool to burn calories. But, there are numerous benefits including improved cardiovascular function and improved brain function. There are many general health benefits that *no* drug, pill, or expensive *'detox'* could provide. Aerobic exercise is seen as the primary mechanism for increasing cardiorespiratory fitness, which can be quantified with measures such as VO_2max (the maximum rate at which you can breathe in and use oxygen)[12].

Despite popular belief, aerobic exercise does *not* increase lung function or lung capacity in healthy people[13]. Oxygen delivery and carbon dioxide removal from exercising muscles is limited by the ability of the heart and blood vessels to deliver and remove them, not the ability of the lungs to deliver and remove them. An elite long-distance athlete may have lungs that are a limiting factor because their cardiovascular system is so efficient, or someone with lung disease because their lung capacity is limited, but this is very much in the minority.

The role of aerobic exercise on body composition and how you may wish to implement it, is discussed in chapter 24.

Resistance training

Adults of all ages should resistance train for long-term health, regardless of any body composition goals.

Resistance training is defined as:

"a form of periodic exercise whereby external weights provide progressive overload to skeletal muscles in order to make them stronger and often result in hypertrophy."
Phillips and Winett, 2010[14].

Resistance training covers a range of disciplines including *powerlifting* and *weightlifting*, and can be used to improve muscle strength, endurance, power or hypertrophy, depending on the specifics of the training. It is usually seen only as a tool to increase muscle size, strength or power. But, resistance training in itself provides a wide range of health benefits as well as using significant amounts of energy during the exercise session. Each type of resistance training can produce specific adaptations. Any individual looking to be healthier and fitter regardless of whether body composition is a goal, should consider incorporating resistance training into their lifestyle[15]. In fact, the UK government recently updated their physical activity recommendations to include participating in some form of muscle strengthening activity, a minimum of twice per week[1].

Resistance training is fantastic for individuals of all ages and genders. Resistance training is the primary mechanism to increase muscle mass[16,17]. A systematic review of 18 randomised controlled trials showed that resistance training is even beneficial in endurance runners to improve their running performance[18]. Resistance training can also improve physical and cognitive ability, self-esteem, help to prevent type 2 diabetes, improve insulin sensitivity, improve cardiovascular health by reducing resting blood pressure, lower 'bad' LDL-cholesterol, elevate 'good' HDL-cholesterol, increase bone mineral density, potentially help with lower back pain, and reduce anxiety[14,16,19,20]. Resistance training also improves health related quality of life in older people[21]. Resistance training not only promotes improvements in body composition (increased muscle mass, decreased fat mass), but also improves health.

Strength	Usually measured as a 1 rep maximum (1RM), lifting as heavy a load as possible for 1 rep. The athletic discipline is powerlifting for a 1RM in the squat, bench press and deadlift.
Hypertrophy	Usually measured with computed tomography (CT), x-ray, ultrasound or muscle biopsies. The athletic discipline is bodybuilding, to maximise muscle mass whilst simultaneously reducing body fat percentage.
Power	The athletic discipline is weightlifting, with the aim of maximum strength and power in the clean and jerk, and snatch.
Muscular endurance	The number of reps that can be performed regardless of your 1 rep maximum (RM) (absolute). The number of reps that can be performed with a load less than your 1RM (relative).
Strongman/woman competitions	Can utilise all the parameters above.
Maintenance e.g. in older populations	The maintenance of muscle mass and other resistance training performance parameters over time.

Definitions and outcomes of different forms of resistance training.

Focussing on a particular resistance training goal (such as power, strength or hypertrophy) will provide the range of general health benefits associated with resistance training. The choice of training style should be based on any specific goals, and personal preference.

Resistance training during periods of weight loss should feature a structure *similar* to resistance training for muscle gain[22]. The principles that are best to build muscle in a calorie surplus are the *same* principles that are best to preserve and maintain muscle in a calorie deficit. Further nuances with training during weight loss compared to training during weight gain will be discussed.

How muscles work[23]

The body can use proteins, carbohydrates and fats for energy during exercise. The body can also use a range of energy *pathways* to suit different tasks. All of these different energy systems have the same fate, to replenish a molecule called *adenosine triphosphate (ATP)**. ATP provides the energy needed for *all* cellular reactions in the body, including muscular contractions. When we say that you are using carbohydrates or fats to fuel muscles during exercise, what this actually means is that carbohydrates and fats are being broken down and the energy stored within them is being used to replenish ATP. It is this ATP molecule that releases its energy to fuel whatever activity is needed[24].

* The energy in ATP is released when one of the three phosphates breaks away, leaving adenosine diphosphate (ADP) and a separate phosphate molecule. The food we eat provides us with the energy to put ADP and the separate phosphate molecule back together to reform ATP. ATP can then be reused in cells for energy.

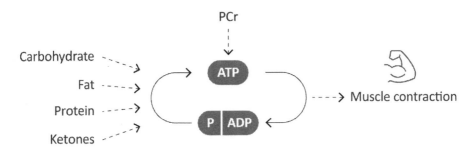

ATP provides the energy for muscles to contract. The energy within the food we eat (protein, carbohydrates and fat) can be used to replenish ATP stores to provide further energy for muscles to contract. Other energy sources such as ketones or phosphocreatine can also replenish ATP. Many factors influence which fuel source is used to replenish ATP at a given time. ATP: Adenosine triphosphate, ADP: Adenosine diphosphate, P: inorganic Phosphate, PCr: Phosphocreatine.

Imagine a catapult. When released, the catapult fires whatever object it holds into the air and into the distance. The catapult performs useful work. However, the catapult now needs to be reset. This is achieved by people putting energy back into the catapult by pulling it back into position. It is now ready to fire another object. The people do *not* directly fire the object, but they *provide* the energy to do so. The catapult is like the ATP in muscles, performing the useful work to make muscles contract. The people resetting it are like the carbohydrates, protein and fat that are used to replenish ATP.

The type of energy used and how it replenishes ATP in the muscle cell depends on how long and how intense the muscle activity is. Below are the energy systems that muscles use, in order of increasing *duration* and descending *intensity* of exercise. During the same period of exercise, these different pathways may be upregulated or downregulated and are not mutually exclusive, depending on the exercise intensity and the energy sources available.

ATP

ATP is the *fundamental energy source* of cells. This is what we use to fuel muscle contractions[24,25]. However, at any given time there is actually a very small amount of it available. So little in fact, that it could provide you with only a few seconds of energy before it would run out. Fortunately, we can use our fuel sources to regenerate ATP.

Phosphocreatine

Muscle cells have a very small supply of ATP ready to go at any time. Exercise beyond a few seconds requires other energy processes. The *ATP-Phosphocreatine (Pcr)* system is used in very short-term high intensity exercise, under 10 seconds. ATP can be reformed by phosphocreatine (creatine and a phosphate) donating its phosphate to ADP, which reforms ATP. This source might provide a few extra seconds of energy production in a 10 second all out, high intensity maximum exertion[25].

Phosphocreatine is a bit like having additional helpers to reset the catapult. When the catapult is fired and needs to be reloaded quickly, these helpers can reset the catapult much faster than the people (carbohydrate, protein or fat) who usually reset it. However, these additional helpers cannot do this for very long.

As the small ATP supplies in muscle are used, phosphocreatine is used to regenerate ATP such that ATP levels are maintained, and phosphocreatine levels drop during intense exercise. This lasts a short period of time before phosphocreatine levels run out. When we stop using our muscles, phosphocreatine levels are replenished by using energy generated from the energy pathways below. The supplement *creatine monohydrate* results in beneficial performance outcomes by increasing phosphocreatine stores (see chapter 25).

Glycolysis: breaking down glycogen stores (carbohydrate) in the muscle

One way that muscles use glycogen and glucose for energy is by *anaerobic glycolysis*[24]. This means using carbohydrate stores without oxygen. This is the fuel source used in short-term high intensity exercise, up to around 60 seconds in duration. Anaerobic glycolysis leads to the production of *lactate* and *protons* (Hydrogen ions) and is quite an inefficient way of making useful energy compared to when using oxygen[26].

Oxidative phosphorylation: using carbohydrate, fat or protein for energy with oxygen

This is just a fancy way to say using carbohydrate, fat or protein stores with oxygen to regenerate the ATP molecule. This is how our cells and muscles create the energy we need to move and stay alive the majority of the time. Even if you are sat on the couch doing absolutely nothing you'll still be burning calories this way. The largest source of energy expenditure is just living and breathing (chapter 5).

This is the primary energy pathway for endurance exercise, such as running, cycling and swimming that lasts longer than a minute, and can last for hours.

We predominantly use fat (fatty acids) and carbohydrate (glucose) to fuel muscle cells to generate the ATP needed for muscles to contract, and the energy needed for other cellular processes such as muscle repair. Muscle cells can use a combination of these energy sources to generate ATP during exercise. Breaking down and using fat molecules is called *fatty acid oxidation*. An important point to note is that fatty acid oxidation requires more oxygen than *glucose* to generate the same amount of useful energy. Fats are a less oxygen efficient method of generating usable energy compared to carbohydrate[27,28].

Exercise intensity: from aerobic to anaerobic

A range of energy sources can be used to fuel aerobic exercise; usually carbohydrates and fats, but less commonly amino acids (protein) and ketone bodies. Due to its relatively large availability, fat is the predominant fuel source when at rest or with low to moderate exercise intensities[24,29]. The higher the intensity, the greater the rate of ATP turnover and therefore the higher the rate of energy use. An increasing proportion of energy is provided via carbohydrates as the intensity of the exercise increases[30]. This does *not* mean that we need to exercise at a lower intensity to lose more fat mass. The overriding factor for fat loss regardless of exercise, is calories in versus calories out (i.e. energy balance). The effect of different exercise intensities on fat loss is discussed in chapter 24.

The *relative* contribution of the energy systems (ATP, phosphocreatine, anaerobic glycolysis or oxidative phosphorylation) will shift, depending on the intensity and duration of the exercise. As exercise intensity increases further such as during resistance training, muscles begin to use carbohydrates (glucose) without oxygen, through anaerobic glycolysis. Fat *cannot* be used to fuel exercise without oxygen. This is related to the fuel source primarily used by different types of muscle fibres[24,25]. High intensity exercise will primarily use ATP, phosphocreatine and anaerobic glycolysis. Moderate intensity exercise will use mainly aerobic energy sources and some glycolytic pathways, and lower intensity exercise will mainly use aerobic energy pathways.

Exercise research limitations[4]

Besides general study limitations that have been discussed in chapter 4 such as recruitment biases, blinding, measurement biases or systematic biases, there are also limitations and considerations specific to research assessing training. There will *always* be limitations to any study. The appropriate questions therefore are, *how many* limitations are there and *how great* are they? This determines how much strength we can place in its findings.

1. **The experience of participants.** Hypertrophy research has primarily been conducted in untrained beginners or moderately trained people. These individuals are at the beginning of their training career and may experience a greater training response to those who have been training for longer[4]. Studies in untrained people are also less relevant to trained people.
2. **Defining training status.** Following from point 1, how was training status defined? Usually studies say participants are either '*untrained*' or '*resistance trained*' and do not make any further differentiation. Was this based on relative strength? Muscle mass? Years training? Consider two people, one with 6 months of experience and the other with 5 years of experience. Both could be considered resistance trained. But, the individual with 6 months of experience could have a much greater relative ability to improve than the person with 5 years of experience, and be more similar to an untrained individual. Being '*resistance trained*' has been defined as having 6 months of resistance training experience[31].
3. **Had participants detrained?** If someone stops training for a while they will lose muscle. But, they may be able to regain muscle mass at a faster rate than a trained or untrained person due to other changes in their muscles from previous training. Similarly, if a participant had a

recent period of training very hard, they may be in a position where muscle growth is less likely[32].

4. **Sex.** Most training research is in males. However, more and more studies are being conducted in females. Nevertheless, the current evidence does not indicate any sex-based differences in training needs nor outcomes[33].

5. **Direct measures of muscle growth.** How was muscle size measured? Did the study use whole-body measurements, muscle specific measurements and muscle biopsies (taking a sample of a muscle and analysing its structure)? Ideally a study will include all three levels of measure, which should be complimentary[4].

6. **Measuring muscle growth.** What device was used to measure muscle growth? Different devices have different advantages and disadvantages, and variable accuracy. Common devices are *dual energy X-ray absorptiometry* (DEXA), *bio impedance assessment* (BIA) *ultrasound* and *magnetic resonance imaging* (MRI). Similarly, was muscle thickness, cross-sectional area or volume measured? *Skinfold callipers* are also common tools to measure changes in body fat percentage, but require training in their use.

7. **Proxy measures.** The use of intermediate and indirect markers of muscle growth instead of direct markers. Studies do not always measure long-term changes in body composition, instead measuring for example, blood samples or acute changes in muscle biomarkers (e.g. levels of muscle protein synthesis (MPS)). Do these markers actually correlate with long-term muscle growth?

8. **Motivation and adherence.** Did the participants perform the training sessions correctly? This is heavily affected by whether the study was conducted under supervision or not.

9. **Execution.** Did the participants perform the exercises correctly? Again, this can be heavily influenced by whether participants were given demonstrations by researchers, whether exercise was supervised, and the training status of individuals (usually trained people will be better at performing a given exercise).

10. **Training plan.** When assessing a specific training variable (such as training frequency) were other training variables optimal for muscle growth? Were other training variables also controlled for?

11. **Length of studies.** The majority of studies are of short duration and rarely last more than 8-12 weeks. Longer studies are needed to see differences in trained individuals, because of a slower rate of growth than in untrained individuals.

12. **Other factors.** How were participants' diets, sleep and stress levels? All will influence hypertrophy. Rarely do exercise studies control the diets of participants, which can heavily influence training outcomes.

A powerful technique being used more and more in exercise research is a *unilateral exercise study design*[34]. This means that a participant undergoes both the experimental intervention and the control intervention. One of their limbs undergoes the treatment plan and the other limb undergoes the control plan. This helps to minimise differences between the experimental group and the control group, such as genetic, environmental and behavioural differences. This can increase the *statistical power* of the study, helping to find small, yet meaningful differences in muscle growth between different interventions.

Your genetics will have the largest impact on how much muscle you can grow.

Unfortunately, some people will be able to grow more muscle on the same training programme than other people because of the large influence genetics has on hypertrophy. Some people can increase muscle mass by up to 60% on a training programme, and some none at all. High and low *responders* to resistance training exist[35-37]. Genetics has been suggested to explain around 50% of muscular training adaptations, but other factors such as diet, training and lifestyle will have further influence[36-38]. There is an incredibly large amount of variability between people in the ability to grow muscle from a given training programme. A recent study using the unilateral exercise study design highlighted that individual *intrinsic* factors have a far greater influence on muscle growth than *extrinsic* factors (manipulating any part of a resistance training programme)[39]. 20 resistance trained participants had one leg undergo a standard resistance training plan. The other leg underwent resistance training whilst varying several training variables (*load, volume, type of contraction* and *rest period*)*. Muscle growth between the legs of each participant was very *similar*. But, the muscle growth between the legs of different participants was very *different*. There was 40-fold greater variability between participants (38% difference in the increase in muscle cross-sectional area between legs of different participants performing the same resistance training plan) than within participants (0.9% difference in the increase in muscle cross-sectional area between the legs of the same participant). Some people will just grow more muscle than others. Unfortunately, this is the cruel hand of genetics[40]. One person may be able to grow more muscle on a sub-optimal programme than someone else who is on a well optimised, individualised plan. However, a more optimal programme will *always* result in improved muscle growth compared to a sub-optimal programme for a given individual. Therefore, the question is to determine what a more optimal programme may look like[40]. Furthermore, the muscle mass an individual has from a previous training programme can predict how much muscle they may build on a new training programme[37]. If you built muscle from previous training, then you are more likely to build muscle with subsequent training (albeit likely less), than someone who did not build much muscle from previous training[37].

The varied programme just assessed manipulating the variables, and not necessarily in a way that is better for muscle growth than a conventional programme. Indeed, the study can also be interpreted as showing that varying too many variables at once does not result in greater hypertrophic benefit.

Training for muscle growth

There is no 'perfect' programme, workout, exercise, rep range etc. We have a rough idea as to what may be optimal for the 'average' person, but this is by far a definitive answer. Much of what will make up your ideal plan comes down to how it suits your lifestyle and your goals. Apart from a few key recommendations, the majority of resistance training variables are largely unimportant and much of it comes down to personal training preference. Most potential variables just need to be kept consistent.

The following pages present a step-by-step summary of key evidence-based recommendations to promote muscle growth[33].

Mechanisms of muscle growth (chapters 17 and 18)[33,41,42]

The main mechanism by which muscle fibres grow is by mechanical tension (the amount of force that a muscle fibre exerts and experiences).
Increasing the amount of mechanical tension over time leads to long-term increases in muscle size.
To increase the amount of mechanical tension over time, there needs to be progressive overload. Lift more weight for the same number of reps, lift more weight or increase training volume (to an extent). Focus on progressively improving on a select choice of exercises for a given muscle group.
Whether metabolic stress (experienced as the muscle pump) or muscle damage (experienced as muscle soreness) directly contribute to muscle growth is still not conclusive, but increasingly appearing less likely with new research. If they do, their role is minor relative to mechanical tension. Current training recommendations focussing on mechanical tension will generate meaningful amounts of metabolic stress. Whether you decide to incorporate training to primarily promote metabolic stress or muscle damage is up to you.

Resistance training for muscle growth (chapters 18 and 19)[33,40-42]

Absolute strength is correlated to muscle fibre size, bigger muscles can produce a greater force. A key principle of muscle growth is getting stronger across high, moderate and low rep ranges. Being strong does not necessarily mean being 'big'. But, being bigger will require some element of being relatively or absolutely stronger.

During intense periods of training or as a beginner, improvements in strength can precede increases in muscle mass.

Muscle growth occurs when training at a high intensity of effort across a wide range of intensities of load.

Training to muscular task failure or just shy of muscular task failure using loads (weights) from an intensity of 30% of your 1 repetition maximum (RM) up to 100% of your 1 repetition maximum will stimulate muscle growth.

The number of weekly sets performed to muscular task failure (or near failure) per muscle group (volume) best correlates with muscle growth, up to a point.

The maximum effective volume to stimulate growth for a muscle in a given training session appears to be lower than the maximum volume for a muscle in a given week.

There appears to be an optimum amount of volume (sets) to perform per muscle group per session and per week. Below this amount, muscles do not receive sufficient stimulus to grow to their maximum potential. Above this, the stimulus is too great for the muscle to effectively recover from and can lead to overtraining. This optimum amount is specific to the individual and muscle group, and can be highly variable. It also does not need to be the same for every workout nor the same for every muscle.

Muscle growth can occur with very low volumes (less than 4 sets per muscle group per week). 10-20 sets per muscle group per week for beginner/intermediate level trainers appears to be an ideal range. Brief periods of high volume above this (20-30 sets) may be useful to break through plateaus for intermediate and advanced trainers.

Resistance training can be utilised to maintain and increase muscle mass. The requirements to maintain muscle mass are significantly less than what is required to increase muscle mass. Unfortunately, improvements do not continue indefinitely in a linear or exponential fashion – plateaus occur. If you have been resistance training for some time, you may have had a period of rapid growth and strength gains when you started training. This is short-lived, and after several months of training the rate of muscle growth decreases. As a beginner, even though you might not need to train optimally to grow muscle, you still need to train *correctly*. Similarly, optimising your training can lead to even greater results. As you become more experienced, with 6-12 months of training experience, it becomes ever more important to ensure that your training is optimised to continue promoting muscle growth.

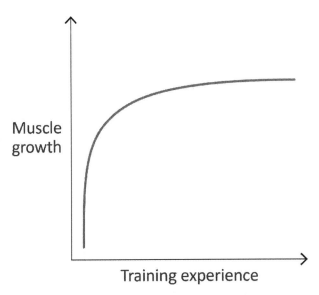

Muscle growth

Training experience

Muscle growth does not continue at the same rate indefinitely. There are diminishing returns in terms of muscle growth with training experience.

As an untrained beginner, begin at the lower ends of these set volumes (i.e. 4 to 5 sets, working up to 10 sets per body part per week), possibly even lower if this volume is too high as a starting point4. Add extra sets once you struggle to increase the number of reps you can perform with a given load in a set, or you struggle to increase the load you can use for a given number of reps in a set. This may occur several weeks or months after you begin training. Work on achieving good *productive* sets, before adding more sets. Aim for the upper ends of these recommendations as an intermediate and experienced weight trainer. However, place this into context of how you feel and your goals. As an intermediate or advanced trainer, if you find more than 10 sets per body part is too fatiguing, then perform fewer sets. The optimal range is *wide*. One weekly set is sub-optimal. 30 or more sets per body part per week is excessive.

Calorie intake will influence your training

When in a calorie deficit for fat loss the ability to recover from workouts is reduced, therefore your training volume may be lower. When in a calorie surplus, you have an increased capacity to recover and grow, and therefore your volume may be higher. This is discussed in chapter 19.

Sex-based differences

Despite less research in females, there is *no* evidence to suggest that females should resistance train any differently to males[33]. Females should use the range of loads, volumes, rep durations and rest periods discussed above. The benefits of protein supplementation also appear to be similar in females[33].

Frequency and rep range for muscle growth (chapters 19, 20 and 22)[33,40,43]

Frequency only appears to be important in facilitating sufficient weekly volume.
Ideally, resistance train at least 3x per week to achieve sufficient weekly volume for all body parts.
Roughly, train each body part 1-3x per week for beginners and intermediate level trainers. Advanced trainers may train specific body parts more frequently than this during high volume periods.
A wide range of reps are effective at building muscle, but the 6-15 rep range is a slightly more ideal rep trade-off for hypertrophy between lower and higher reps. Keep the majority (75%) of training volume around the 6-15 rep maximum (RM) range and the minority (25%) in the 1-6RM or above 15RM range.
Start the workout with heavier weights (higher intensities of load) and lower reps (1-5, then 6-8 reps). As the session progresses, use lighter weights (lower intensity of load) and higher reps (8-15, then 15+ reps)

When training a body part once per week, work up to performing around 8-10 sets per session (e.g. 2-3 exercises per body part, and 2-4 sets for each exercise). When training a body part more than once per week, initially split the volume performed when training the body part once per week, before increasing the volume of each session, using a variety of rep ranges for each session to manage fatigue.

Rest as long as is necessary to perform a subsequent set with sufficient intensity of effort. Shorter rest periods reduce muscle growth for the same number of sets. Rest at least 60 seconds between sets regardless of the number of reps per set performed. Consider additional rest of up to 2-3 minutes, and perhaps up to 5 minutes for low (1-5RM) rep sets. Besides sufficient rest for a subsequent set, variation in rest periods has little influence on muscle growth.

A wide range of rep speeds (i.e. rep durations) build muscle. Choose a consistent rep speed that allows for control of the weight for a given exercise, based on personal preference.

Weekly volume does not have to be equal between body parts nor always increasing. Weekly volumes of body parts of interest that are lagging can be greater than those body parts that are already well developed. Prioritising weekly volume for lagging body parts becomes more important as an intermediate or advanced trainer.

Exercise sequence (chapter 21)[40]

Prioritise exercises for body parts of interest by performing them first in a workout.

Compound and isolation exercises can both effectively promote muscle growth.

Compound exercises can be time-efficient methods to generate volume for multiple muscle groups.

Isolation exercises can be effective methods to generate directed volume to a muscle of interest.

Perform higher intensities of load (lower reps) exercise before lower intensities of load (higher reps) exercise.

How hard to train (chapters 17, 19 and 23)[33,40,43]

Make sure you train hard enough; if you think you could perform many more reps in a given set, then either the weight is too light for that rep range, or you need to perform more reps and get closer to failure. Aim to perform sets to within 5 reps of muscular task failure.

Muscle soreness is not a good indicator of an effective muscle building workout. Soreness is the result of excessive muscle damage, performing a novel exercise, or eccentric (lowering the weight) contractions.

It is not necessary to give everything you have in every session. It can actually be counter-productive. Use training to muscular task failure sparingly to prevent excessive fatigue. Ideally, train to failure with isolation exercises near the end of a workout.

Training beyond failure using advanced training techniques (e.g. drop sets, supersets or forced reps) does not result in greater muscle growth than performing conventional sets. Some techniques can result in similar muscle growth in a shorter amount of time, at the expense of greater perceptions of effort and fatigue.

Aim to be close to failure, but not reaching failure in every set. Within 1 to 5 reps of failure is a good general range to terminate a set.

Periodisation (chapter 18)[40]

Non-periodisation and periodisation (systematically altering training variables over time) appear to be equivocal for muscle growth. Periodisation is more important for strength, and unnecessary as a beginner for muscle growth. As an intermediate or experienced trainer (weight training for more than 6-12 months), some element of periodisation may be considered as a tool to progressively overload.

Aerobic exercise during a period of training for muscle growth (chapter 24)

Aerobic exercise affects strength more than muscle growth. Performing aerobic exercise will not impair muscle growth, so long as the volume performed is not excessive (e.g. several hours every day). Some aerobic exercise can benefit resistance training performance.
To minimise any potentially minor interference effect on muscle growth, consider performing aerobic exercise separately to resistance training, or afterwards. Try and avoid excessively high volume aerobic exercise immediately before.
To minimise any potentially minor interference effect, consider avoiding aerobic exercise that uses the same body part that has just been resistance trained, i.e. after upper body training, consider a lower body form of aerobic exercise (e.g. cycling or running).
There is no superior form of aerobic exercise for weight loss. The primary influence of exercise on weight change is the number of calories burned during the exercise session. Choose the form of aerobic exercise that you enjoy the most and will continue to perform in the long-term.
Fasted exercise is not superior to fed exercise for fat burning or weight loss.
Different intensities of aerobic exercise are not superior for fat burning or weight loss.

If you still feel stuck and are not sure how to plan your training or workouts, then hire *personal trainer*. Find someone willing to sit down and get to know the ins and outs of your lifestyle including work, family, commitments, diet and other factors, so that they can create a plan which suits you. Hiring a trainer can help you to achieve behaviour change, adhere to a plan and motivate you to improve performance[44-47]. This can promote successful changes in body composition.

Muscle

A very in-depth discussion of muscle structure and function is beyond the scope of this book, but if you are interested have a read of *'Skeletal Muscle: A Brief Review of Structure and Function'* by Frontera and Ochela[48].

Muscles stabilise the body and have a functional role in allowing us to move. They attach to bones via tendons. By shortening in length (*concentric* contraction) or increasing in length (*eccentric* contraction) they can cause the skeleton and therefore the body to move. The quadriceps (the muscle used to perform a leg extension) may concentrically contract walking uphill, and eccentrically contract when walking downhill. Muscles can also maintain the same length whilst contracting (*isometric* contraction), such as leg muscles when we are standing, or arm muscles when we are holding something in our hand.

A muscle is made up of many individual *muscle fibres*[49]. Individual muscle fibres are made up of many *myofibrils* which contain the proteins that interact, resulting in a change in the muscle length[50]. Different fibres within a muscle have different properties and are recruited for different tasks. The three main tasks that muscles need to perform are[25]:

- Stabilising joints (e.g. standing upright).
- Long-term, repetitive movements (e.g. walking, chewing, aerobic exercise).
- Short-term, high force movements (e.g. opening a jar, moving furniture, resistance training).

When a muscle contracts, not all of the muscle fibres are necessarily active. Usually, only a fraction of the muscle fibres are active. Our *central nervous system* determines which muscle fibres get activated in a muscle for a given task. The brain activates a *nerve,* which travels to the muscle and connects to a muscle fibre via a *junction.* All the muscle fibres connected to the activated nerve by a junction are then signalled to contract. This coupling is called a *motor unit*[49]. A motor unit is a group of muscle fibres that are controlled and activated by a given nerve. A nerve can activate multiple muscle fibres, but a given muscle fibre is activated by one nerve. The muscle fibres in a given motor unit are similar in structure and function[25,50]. Small motor units controlling a few muscle fibres each are recruited first. With increasing force requirement, there is progressive activation of motor units with tens, then hundreds, and even thousands of fibres under the control of one neuron. Motor units are recruited for a given task based on their size[25]. This is called *Henneman's size principle*[25,51,52]. When low forces are required, the brain stimulates the nerves controlling *low-threshold motor units* (LTMU). Their threshold for activation is low. These are the motor units that are recruited first, regardless of the muscular task (e.g. picking up a pencil and carrying a heavy bag of shopping both recruit low-threshold motor units in the muscles of the fingers). Low-threshold motor units are also active at higher forces. The muscle fibres in low-threshold motor units usually produce low forces for long durations and typically contain what are called *type I fibres*. Low-threshold motor units in the legs are activated when you are walking.

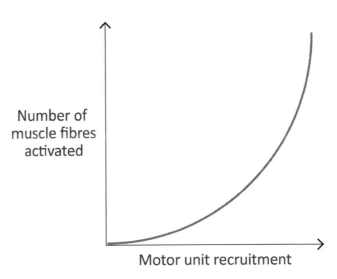

Number of muscle fibres activated

Motor unit recruitment

Henneman's size principle. When low forces are required, few motor units are recruited which control only a small number of muscle fibres. As larger forces are required, more motor units are recruited, which control a large number of muscle fibres.

However, sometimes we need to produce much more force. Imagine we now start to climb a set of stairs. This requires greater forces in the legs. In order to achieve this, the body needs to increase the number of muscle fibres that are active in the leg muscle to produce enough force to climb the stairs. As well as the low-threshold motor units, *high-threshold motor units* (HTMU) are now recruited. High-threshold motor units control many more muscle fibres than low-threshold motor units. One nerve may activate a couple of muscle fibres in a low-threshold motor unit, but a high-threshold motor unit may have one nerve activating thousands of muscle fibres[25]. The muscle fibres in high-threshold motor units usually produce high forces for short durations and typically contain what are called *type II fibres*. High-threshold motor unit recruitment can therefore provide much greater force, but at the expense of only being achievable for a short duration. High-threshold motor units can also be recruited when previously activated low-threshold motor units start to fatigue. *Peripheral fatigue* (fatigue in the muscle) of low-threshold motor units results in recruitment of high-threshold motor units during sustained submaximal contractions[53]. However, *central fatigue* (fatigue of the central nervous system) also occurs. *Central fatigue* has the opposite effect to *peripheral fatigue*, by limiting the recruitment of high-threshold motor units. The central nervous system sends signals via nerves to activate motor units[54]. If the central nervous system is fatigued, fewer signals are sent to motor units, so fewer fibres are activated. Peripheral fatigue results in high-threshold motor unit activation, central nervous system fatigue impairs high-threshold motor unit activation.

Type I fibres are known as *slow twitch fibres*. Type II fibres are known as *fast twitch fibres*. There are three main types of fast twitch muscle fibres[25]. Some muscle fibres have a high contractile ability and can produce lots of force, but only for a short duration. These are called *type IIB fibres*. Some fibres are an intermediate of both the type I and type IIB fibres and are called *type IIA* and *IIX*[25]. Type IIA and IIX fibres produce an intermediate level of force for an intermediate duration of time. Type I fibres are the main form of slow twitch fibre that produce force for extended periods of time. Type IIB fibres are the most responsive fibres to resistance training stimuli, but other muscle fibres are also responsive. Muscle growth can occur in *all* fibre types, but predominantly occurs in fast twitch type II fibres[55,56]. The proportion of type I and type II fibres in the muscles of different people can vary highly, and a significant component of this variation is from genetics. However, fibre type can be altered through training[25].

High-threshold motor units control many muscle fibres and many high force generating type IIB fibres. Type II fibres are most responsive to training and have the greatest potential to grow. They are recruited under heavy weight loads when only a few reps can be completed or near muscular failure after performing reps with lighter loads, when previously recruited low-threshold motor units begin to fatigue.

The body is clever. It only produces as much force as it needs, depending on the task[25]. This means that the body uses as little energy as it has to. When it needs to generate more force or to maintain a force that it is currently producing (to move a heavy object, or from moving a lighter object and the previously active muscle fibres are becoming fatigued), extra muscle fibres within the muscle are recruited by the central nervous system, activating high-threshold motor units. This will become important later as we discuss how and why muscles grow.

Current research suggests that an increase in the size of the muscle fibre (*hypertrophy*) is the main mechanism for muscle growth, rather than an increase in the number of muscle fibres within a muscle (*hyperplasia*)[57,58]. Muscle fibres grow by an increase in the number of contractile proteins within the fibre. This increase can occur in *parallel* or in *series*. The addition of contractile proteins in parallel within muscle fibres increases their diameter, and therefore leads to a greater cross-sectional area[57]. This is the type of hypertrophy we commonly associate with resistance training. However, certain methods and elements of resistance training also lead to the addition of contractile proteins in series (in particular, eccentric contractions involving lowering a weight under control)[59]. This can be a practical and functional form of hypertrophy[41].

There is some evidence to support an increase in muscle size by an increase in the fluid and non-contractile components of the muscle fibre. This is called *sarcoplasmic hypertrophy*. It is likely to be specific to the type of training, such as in weightlifters who use moderate and light loads as opposed to powerlifters focussing primarily on heavy loads and low rep ranges. Whether sarcoplasmic hypertrophy has any functional benefit is yet to be determined[57].

References

1   GOV.UK. *Physical activity guidelines: UK Chief Medical Officers' report.* Available from: https://www.gov.uk/government/publications/physical-activity-guidelines-uk-chief-medical-officers-report (accessed 8 Feb 2020).
2   Loenneke JP, Dankel SJ, Bell ZW, Buckner SL, Mattocks KT, Jessee MB et al. Is muscle growth a mechanism for increasing strength? *Med Hypotheses* 2019; 125: 51–56.
3   Erskine RM, Fletcher G, Folland JP. The contribution of muscle hypertrophy to strength changes following resistance training. *Eur J Appl Physiol* 2014; 114: 1239–1249.
4   Wernbom M, Augustsson J, Thomeé R. The influence of frequency, intensity, volume and mode of strength training on whole muscle cross-sectional area in humans. *Sports Med Auckl NZ* 2007; 37: 225–264.
5   Dankel S, Buckner S, Jessee M, Mouser J, Mattocks K, Abe T et al. Correlations Do Not Show Cause and Effect: Not Even for Changes in Muscle Size and Strength. *Sports Med* 2017; 48. Available from: doi:10.1007/s40279-017-0774-3.
6   Buckner SL, Dankel SJ, Mattocks KT, Jessee MB, Mouser JG, Counts BR et al. The problem Of muscle hypertrophy: Revisited. *Muscle Nerve* 2016; 54: 1012–1014.
7   Dankel SJ, Counts BR, Barnett BE, Buckner SL, Abe T, Loenneke JP. Muscle adaptations following 21 consecutive days of strength test familiarization compared with traditional training. *Muscle Nerve* 2017; 56: 307–314.
8   Nuckols G. *Size vs. Strength: How Important is Muscle Growth For Strength Gains?* Available from: https://www.strongerbyscience.com/size-vs-strength/ (accessed 8 Feb 2020).
9   Lovera M, Keogh J. Anthropometric profile of powerlifters: differences as a function of bodyweight class and competitive success. *J Sports Med Phys Fitness* 2015; 55: 478–487.

10   Brechue WF, Abe T. The role of FFM accumulation and skeletal muscle architecture in powerlifting performance. *Eur J Appl Physiol* 2002; 86: 327–336.

11   Nuckols G. *The Complete Strength Training Guide.* Available from: https://www.strongerbyscience.com/complete-strength-training-guide/ (accessed 8 Feb 2020).

12   Garber CE, Blissmer B, Deschenes MR, Franklin BA, Lamonte MJ, Lee I-M et al. American College of Sports Medicine position stand. Quantity and quality of exercise for developing and maintaining cardiorespiratory, musculoskeletal, and neuromotor fitness in apparently healthy adults: guidance for prescribing exercise. *Med Sci Sports Exerc* 2011; 43: 1334–1359.

13   Stickland MK, Butcher SJ, Marciniuk DD, Bhutani M. Assessing Exercise Limitation Using Cardiopulmonary Exercise Testing. *Pulm Med* 2012; 2012. Available from: doi:10.1155/2012/824091.

14   Phillips SM, Winett RA. Uncomplicated Resistance Training and Health-Related Outcomes: Evidence for a Public Health Mandate. *Curr Sports Med Rep* 2010; 9: 208–213.

15   Winett RA, Carpinelli RN. Potential Health-Related Benefits of Resistance Training. *Prev Med* 2001; 33: 503–513.

16   Westcott WL. Resistance training is medicine: effects of strength training on health. *Curr Sports Med Rep* 2012; 11: 209–216.

17   Grgic J, Mcilvenna L, Fyfe J, Sabol F, Bishop D, Schoenfeld B et al. Does Aerobic Training Promote the Same Skeletal Muscle Hypertrophy as Resistance Training? A Systematic Review and Meta-Analysis. *Sports Med* 2018. Available from: doi:10.1007/s40279-018-1008-z.

18   Alcaraz-Ibañez M, Rodríguez-Pérez M. Effects of resistance training on performance in previously trained endurance runners: A systematic review. *J Sports Sci* 2018; 36: 613–629.

19   Shaw B, Shaw I, Brown G. Resistance exercise is medicine: Strength training in health promotion and rehabilitation. *Int J Ther Rehabil* 2015; 22: 385–389.

20   Gordon BR, McDowell CP, Lyons M, Herring MP. The Effects of Resistance Exercise Training on Anxiety: A Meta-Analysis and Meta-Regression Analysis of Randomized Controlled Trials. *Sports Med Auckl NZ* 2017; 47: 2521–2532.

21   Hart PD, Buck DJ. The effect of resistance training on health-related quality of life in older adults: Systematic review and meta-analysis. *Health Promot Perspect* 2019; 9: 1–12.

22   Lambert CP, Frank LL, Evans WJ. Macronutrient considerations for the sport of bodybuilding. *Sports Med Auckl NZ* 2004; 34: 317–327.

23   American Dietetic Association, Dieticians of Canada, American College of Sports Medicine, Rodriguez NR, Di Marco NM, Langley S. American College of Sports Medicine position stand. Nutrition and Athletic Performance. *Med Sci Sports Exerc* 2009; 41: 709–731.

24 Scott C. Misconceptions about Aerobic and Anaerobic Energy Expenditure. *J Int Soc Sports Nutr* 2005; 2: 32–37.

25 Schiaffino S, Reggiani C. Fiber types in mammalian skeletal muscles. *Physiol Rev* 2011; 91: 1447–1531.

26 Hall M, Rajasekaran S, Thomsen T, Peterson A. Lactate: Friend or Foe. *PM&R* 2016; 8: S8–S15.

27 Lodish H, Berk A, Zipursky SL, Matsudaira P, Baltimore D, Darnell J. *Oxidation of Glucose and Fatty Acids to CO2*. Mol Cell Biol 4th Ed 2000. Available from: https://www.ncbi.nlm.nih.gov/books/NBK21624/ (accessed 23 Feb 2020).

28 Alberts B, Johnson A, Lewis J, Raff M, Roberts K, Walter P. *How Cells Obtain Energy from Food*. Mol Biol Cell 4th Ed 2002. Available from: https://www.ncbi.nlm.nih.gov/books/NBK26882/ (accessed 23 Feb 2020).

29 van Loon LJ, Greenhaff PL, Constantin-Teodosiu D, Saris WH, Wagenmakers AJ. The effects of increasing exercise intensity on muscle fuel utilisation in humans. *J Physiol* 2001; 536: 295–304.

30 Petrick HL, Holloway GP. The regulation of mitochondrial substrate utilization during acute exercise. *Curr Opin Physiol* 2019; 10: 75–80.

31 Nunes JP, Grgic J, Cunha PM, Ribeiro AS, Schoenfeld BJ, Salles BF de et al. What influence does resistance exercise order have on muscular strength gains and muscle hypertrophy? A systematic review and meta-analysis. *Eur J Sport Sci* 2020; 0: 1–22.

32 Kraemer WJ, Ratamess NA. Fundamentals of resistance training: progression and exercise prescription. *Med Sci Sports Exerc* 2004; 36: 674–688.

33 Morton RW, Colenso-Semple L, Phillips SM. Training for strength and hypertrophy: an evidence-based approach. *Curr Opin Physiol* 2019; 10: 90–95.

34 MacInnis MJ, McGlory C, Gibala MJ, Phillips SM. Investigating human skeletal muscle physiology with unilateral exercise models: when one limb is more powerful than two. *Appl Physiol Nutr Metab Physiol Appl Nutr Metab* 2017; 42: 563–570.

35 Erskine RM, Jones DA, Williams AG, Stewart CE, Degens H. Inter-individual variability in the adaptation of human muscle specific tension to progressive resistance training. *Eur J Appl Physiol* 2010; 110: 1117–1125.

36 Timmons JA. Variability in training-induced skeletal muscle adaptation. *J Appl Physiol* 2011; 110: 846–853.

37 Roberts MD, Haun CT, Mobley CB, Mumford PW, Romero MA, Roberson PA et al. Physiological Differences Between Low Versus High Skeletal Muscle Hypertrophic Responders to Resistance Exercise Training: Current Perspectives and Future Research Directions. *Front Physiol* 2018; 9: 834.

38 Mann TN, Lamberts RP, Lambert MI. High responders and low responders: factors associated with individual variation in response to standardized training. *Sports Med Auckl NZ* 2014; 44: 1113–1124.

39 Damas F, Angleri V, Phillips SM, Witard OC, Ugrinowitsch C, Santanielo N et al. Myofibrillar protein synthesis and muscle hypertrophy individualized

responses to systematically changing resistance training variables in trained young men. *J Appl Physiol Bethesda Md* 2019; 127: 806–815.

40   Fisher J, Steele J, Smith D. Evidence-Based Resistance Training Recommendations for Muscular Hypertrophy. *Med Sport* 2013; 17: 217–235.

41   Morton RW, Colenso-Semple L, Phillips SM. Training for strength and hypertrophy: an evidence-based approach. *Curr Opin Physiol* 2019; 11: 149–150.

42   Juneau C-E, Tafur L. Over time, load mediates muscular hypertrophy in resistance training. *Curr Opin Physiol* 2019; 11: 147–148.

43   Carpinelli R, Otto R, Wientt R. A critical analysis of the ACSM position stand on resistance training: Insufficient evidence to support recommended training protocols. *J Exerc Physiol Online* 2004; 7.

44   Rustaden AM, Haakstad LAH, Paulsen G, Bø K. Effects of BodyPump and resistance training with and without a personal trainer on muscle strength and body composition in overweight and obese women-A randomised controlled trial. *Obes Res Clin Pract* 2017; 11: 728–739.

45   Mazzetti SA, Kraemer WJ, Volek JS, Duncan ND, Ratamess NA, Gómez AL et al. The influence of direct supervision of resistance training on strength performance. *Med Sci Sports Exerc* 2000; 32: 1175–1184.

46   Wing RR, Jeffery RW, Pronk N, Hellerstedt WL. Effects of a personal trainer and financial incentives on exercise adherence in overweight women in a behavioral weight loss program. *Obes Res* 1996; 4: 457–462.

47   McClaran SR. The Effectiveness of Personal Training on Changing Attitudes Towards Physical Activity. *J Sports Sci Med* 2003; 2: 10–14.

48   Frontera WR, Ochala J. Skeletal muscle: a brief review of structure and function. *Calcif Tissue Int* 2015; 96: 183–195.

49   Kuo IY, Ehrlich BE. Signaling in Muscle Contraction. *Cold Spring Harb Perspect Biol* 2015; 7. Available from: doi:10.1101/cshperspect.a006023.

50   Scott W, Stevens J, Binder–Macleod SA. Human Skeletal Muscle Fiber Type Classifications. *Phys Ther* 2001; 81: 1810–1816.

51   Henneman E. The size-principle: a deterministic output emerges from a set of probabilistic connections. *J Exp Biol* 1985; 115: 105–112.

52   Henneman E, Clamann HP, Gillies JD, Skinner RD. Rank order of motoneurons within a pool: law of combination. *J Neurophysiol* 1974; 37: 1338–1349.

53   Adam A, De Luca CJ. Recruitment order of motor units in human vastus lateralis muscle is maintained during fatiguing contractions. *J Neurophysiol* 2003; 90: 2919–2927.

54   Wan J-J, Qin Z, Wang P-Y, Sun Y, Liu X. Muscle fatigue: general understanding and treatment. *Exp Mol Med* 2017; 49: e384.

55   van Wessel T, de Haan A, van der Laarse WJ, Jaspers RT. The muscle fiber type–fiber size paradox: hypertrophy or oxidative metabolism? *Eur J Appl Physiol* 2010; 110: 665–694.

56   Verdijk LB, Gleeson BG, Jonkers RAM, Meijer K, Savelberg HHCM, Dendale P et al. Skeletal Muscle Hypertrophy Following Resistance Training Is

Accompanied by a Fiber Type–Specific Increase in Satellite Cell Content in Elderly Men. *J Gerontol A Biol Sci Med Sci* 2009; 64A: 332–339.

57 Schoenfeld BJ. The Mechanisms of Muscle Hypertrophy and Their Application to Resistance Training. *J Strength Cond Res* 2010; 24: 2857–2872.

58 Taylor NA, Wilkinson JG. Exercise-induced skeletal muscle growth. Hypertrophy or hyperplasia? *Sports Med Auckl NZ* 1986; 3: 190–200.

59 Douglas J, Pearson S, Ross A, McGuigan M. Chronic Adaptations to Eccentric Training: A Systematic Review. *Sports Med Auckl NZ* 2017; 47: 917–941.

17. Mechanisms of muscle growth

The original model of mechanical tension, metabolic stress and muscle damage as contributors to muscle growth has been challenged. Previous and recent evidence, emerging findings and the prevailing view amongst academics support mechanical stress as the primary mechanism of muscle growth, with metabolic stress and muscle damage as a driver (metabolic stress) and consequence (muscle damage) of generating mechanical tension. The older model refers to mechanical tension as lifting heavy loads. The newer model of mechanical tension refers to placing sufficient tension on a muscle fibre within the muscle, which can be achieved with light, moderate and heavy loads.

There are currently three proposed mechanisms for hypertrophy;

1. *mechanical tension,*
2. *metabolic stress* and
3. *muscle damage.*

There are two main theories regarding how muscles grow by these mechanisms. Both have mechanical tension as the main driving factor, but the definition of mechanical tension and the role of metabolic stress and muscle damage differs between the two theories[1]. The consensus is that mechanical tension is the primary driver for muscle growth[2,3]. However, the exact stimuli and their relative roles in hypertrophy are still *not* fully understood.

There are 2 main theories of muscle growth (however other and more complex models exist):

1. Theory 1 is the *'old'* original model.
2. Theory 2 is the *'new'* model and the general consensus.

Other models have been proposed that are slight variations of these models.

Theory 1: the old model

Theory 1 states that metabolic stress and muscle damage both have a direct mechanism in muscle growth, albeit a much smaller role than mechanical tension. In this theory, mechanical tension is purely a result of lifting absolutely heavy weights (i.e. mechanical tension only occurs at high intensities of load above 70% of your 1 repetition maximum* (RM)). Hypertrophy results from lifting lighter weights from metabolic stress. Muscle damage also directly promotes muscle growth.

For example, if you can squat 100kg for 1 repetition, 70% of your 1RM would be squatting 70kg.

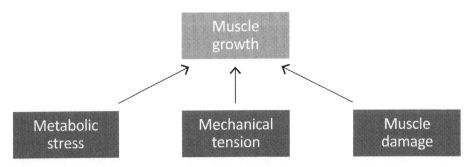

The old model. Metabolic stress, mechanical tension and muscle damage all directly promote muscle growth.

Theory 2: the new model

Theory 2 states that mechanical tension is the *only* mechanism of muscle growth as it is the only mechanism that can explain the results in the literature so far. Mechanical tension here is the result of lifting weights anywhere from 30% to 100% of your 1RM to *failure* (failure being where you are unable to lift a weight for another rep). Metabolic stress indirectly causes muscle growth by resulting in increased mechanical tension from fatigue[3]. Muscle damage does not contribute to muscle growth and is simply a by-product of training.

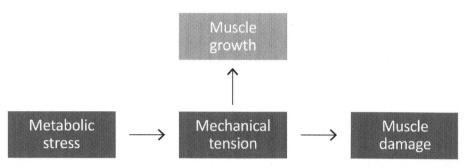

The new model. Only mechanical tension directly promotes muscle growth. Metabolic stress promotes muscle growth by promoting greater mechanical tension. Muscle damage is simply a consequence of training and does not contribute to growth.

Muscle damage and metabolic stress are closely linked to mechanical tension. This makes it very difficult to experimentally isolate these variables to see how they each influence hypertrophy, and hence the uncertainty around what causes muscle growth. However, some studies have shown that hypertrophy can occur independently of metabolic stress and muscle damage[3]. Evidence supporting muscle damage or metabolic stress as mechanisms of muscle growth is mainly indirect. There is also a poor understanding of the molecular mechanisms behind how this might occur[1]. Studies have *not* shown hypertrophy to occur independently of mechanical tension. An excellent publicly available lecture by Menno Henselmans discusses the *'old'* 3 part model and how recent research suggests this model does not adequately explain current research, proposing the *'new'* model[4]. It is important to remember that both models are still *theories,* and *not* conclusive. Other researchers have suggested elements of the old model are still partially correct. For example, there still may be a (albeit small) role of metabolic stress in directly influencing muscle growth, but with the new definition of mechanical tension[1,3]. There is little evidence to support a direct role or even a need for muscle damage in promoting muscle growth[3].

Therefore, the focus of training for muscle growth should be to primarily generate mechanical tension, and possibly metabolic stress, to a lesser extent.

Mechanical tension

According to *Newtons' third law*, mechanical tension is the force exerted and therefore experienced by muscle fibres, which is composed of *active* force generation (by the active contractile proteins in the muscle fibre, producing a force), and *passive* force generation (by the non-contractile proteins in the muscle preventing the muscle fibre from being overstretched, producing a force). Both forms of force are important for muscle growth. Mechanical tension results in activation of *'sensors'* in the muscle fibre. This leads to molecular and cellular responses to increase the size of muscle fibres as an *adaptive response* to a *stimulus*. The exact cellular mechanism is still not fully understood[1,3].

The mechanical tension that appears to be relevant for muscle growth is not the tension on the whole muscle, but the tension placed on individual muscle fibres within the muscle[3]*. This may explain why we can build muscle with heavy, moderate and light weights when training to failure. With heavy weights, high-threshold motor units are recruited from the first rep. With lighter weights, the initial low-threshold motor units fatigue after so many reps, and high-threshold motor units are then recruited near to failure.

* Adjacent muscle fibres are connected together. It has been suggested that lateral force transmission between fibres means a muscle fibre does not actually need to produce the force itself to 'experience' mechanical tension, and can experience tension from neighbouring fibres. This is very much theoretical[3].

The force a muscle experiences is equal and opposite to the force it produces. When contracting, the force a muscle fibre can produce is dependent on the *force-velocity relationship*.

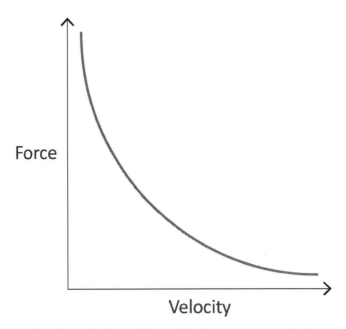

The force-velocity relationship. High forces can only be generated at slow velocities. Fast velocities can only generate low forces. Power (energy used per second) = force × velocity.

Greater forces are produced at *slower* velocities[2]. When attempting to lift a very heavy weight (such as a 1 rep maximum), the weight moves very slowly. Slower velocities allow higher forces to be produced. When lifting light weights to failure, the rep speed gradually slows down as low-threshold motor units fatigue (through metabolic stress) and high-threshold motor units are recruited[3]. Eventually, a muscle can only produce sufficient force at a slow velocity as fatigue accumulates, and fibres experience greater mechanical tension[3].

When looking at the dynamics and electrical activity of muscles in resistance trained males performing the back squat[5], it is clear that:

1. As the amount of weight being lifted increases, the velocity of the concentric (standing up in the squat) portion slows down. As you lift a heavier weight, the maximum speed at which you can lift it slows down.
2. As the amount of weight being lifted increases, the time taken to complete the concentric contraction (standing up in the squat) increases.
3. Lifting light loads at maximum velocity leads to high levels of muscle activation in the quadriceps, hamstrings and glutes, similar to heavy loads.

As we can see in point 1, the velocity at which we can lift heavy weights is slower than the speed at which we can lift lighter weights, because we can only generate sufficient force at slower velocities. High levels of mechanical tension can be generated when the contraction speed needs to be slow to generate sufficient force, in accordance with the *force-velocity relationship*.

When we increase the weight of the load lifted, we need to produce a greater force in order to lift it. We can increase force production by recruiting high-threshold motor units. High-threshold motor units can be recruited with loads lighter than the load for a 1RM. As we can see from point 2, with heavier loads, further increases in force are achieved with slower velocities. This means the exercise duration increases.

In point 3, we can get similar levels of muscle activation with heavier and lighter loads, but not always. Importantly, activation does *not* necessarily result in a stimulus to grow. When lifting light loads, initially there is high muscle activation but with fast velocities, meaning each muscle fibre likely experiences low levels of mechanical tension. We can achieve muscle growth with lighter weights by lifting to failure and thus performing more reps. With lighter weights, there will be a point where fatigue sets in and eventually the weight can only be lifted at a slow speed. This will be a similar speed to that of lifting heavy weights[6]. Another study assessing muscle activity in the triceps and chest with the bench press and triceps pushdown demonstrated that muscle activity increases from the first rep to the last rep for a 10 rep maximum effort[7].

Metabolic stress

Metabolic stress is the result of anaerobic metabolism[3]. Using energy without oxygen leads to the production of *lactate* and other *metabolites* (by-products of metabolism) such as *hydrogen ions, calcium* and *adenosine*. Metabolites interfere with muscular contractions*. Muscular contractions can compress *veins*, preventing the outflow of blood from the muscle back to the heart. The increase in metabolites in the muscle can draw fluid out of the blood and into the muscle tissue, causing cell swelling. This is commonly experienced as the 'muscle pump'[1]. Despite a greater rate of metabolic stress accumulation with high intensity loads, metabolic stress is higher from lifting lighter loads because set durations are much longer, and heavy loads can only be lifted when metabolic stress and fatigue are low[3].

* *The role of lactate in causing fatigue is not as it is commonly believed. Evidence suggests it is not the cause of muscular fatigue[8,9].*

In the newer second theory, it is thought that metabolic stress can lead to hypertrophy with moderate and light loads. This is by fatigue of muscle fibres, leading to high-threshold motor unit recruitment, and activated muscle fibres experiencing greater mechanical tension as the rep velocity slows down. In the original first theory, metabolic stress leads to signalling itself to drive muscle growth as a primary factor, independent of mechanical tension. It may well be that both theories occur to a certain extent.

Muscle damage: exercise-induced muscle damage (EIMD)

Exercise-induced muscle damage is where the muscle tissue itself gets damaged, resulting in very small tears. Muscle damage can occur in different parts of the muscle, such as in the functional contracting units, in the passive units, in connective tissue and in other regions. This leads to injury to the contractile proteins and the muscle cell. The theory is that this damage and injury promotes repair *and* growth of the muscle[1].

Indeed, muscle damage stimulates muscle protein synthesis, but this increase in muscle protein synthesis appears to be directed towards muscle repair, *not* muscle growth. Little evidence supports the role of muscle damage in promoting muscle growth.

In untrained individuals, acute post-resistance training increases in muscle protein synthesis do not seem to correlate with muscle growth when muscle damage is high[10]. The resistance training-induced acute increase in muscle protein synthesis does not correlate with long-term muscle hypertrophy, most likely because this acute increase also incorporates the increase in muscle protein synthesis from muscle damage. Muscle damage elevates muscle protein synthesis which contributes to muscle repair and recovery, but not necessarily growth (as in the brick wall analogy from chapter 9; replacing any damaged bricks but not adding additional new bricks to the wall)[11]. Once an individual has been on a training programme for a few weeks, the extent of muscle damage appears to decline with each session. The resistance training-induced increase in muscle protein synthesis is lower than after sessions at the beginning of the programme, suggesting that elevations in muscle protein synthesis become 'refined' and then begin to correlate with hypertrophy[11]. Over the course of a 10 week training programme, muscle protein synthesis only starts to correlate with long-term muscle growth once the muscle damage that occurs in the initial sessions has attenuated[11]. Therefore, it is the day-to-day elevations in muscle protein synthesis (once muscle damage is lower) that correlates with muscle hypertrophy. Muscle damage does not appear to drive muscle growth.

Eccentric contractions (where the muscle lengthens) cause *more* muscle damage than concentric contractions (where the muscle shortens)[2,12,13]. Novel exercises, large ranges of motion, *advanced training techniques* (e.g. drop sets or forced reps, see chapter 23) and high volume workouts also produce large amounts of muscle damage[3].

Exercise-induced muscle damage may be experienced as significant ache and muscle soreness in the days following the exercise (commonly known as *delayed onset of muscle soreness* (DOMS)). However, DOMS does *not* correlate well with other measures of muscle damage, such as reductions in strength and range of motion. It can tell us when muscle damage has occurred, but it does not give a complete overview of the total damage that has occurred[14]. Furthermore, the evidence does *not* show a direct cause and effect relationship between muscle damage and muscle growth[3,14].

Muscle soreness: delayed onset of muscle soreness (DOMS)

Don't use muscle soreness as an indicator of a good workout.

The primary driver of muscle growth is mechanical tension[3]. Inducing mechanical tension can also induce muscle damage. However, muscle damage is not the aim of the workout. More mechanical tension can generate more muscle damage, but more mechanical tension does not mean more muscle growth. Therefore, tracking DOMS does not track what we are trying to actually achieve[3].

DOMS is a measure of muscle damage, and not a conclusive measure of muscle damage. DOMS can be present for a range of reasons and not necessarily following a workout that stimulates muscle growth. Muscle damage and DOMS can also occur from long distance endurance exercise, and can diminish when repeating the same exercises frequently (novel exercises produce lots of muscle damage). Similarly, different muscles display different levels of DOMs compared to others after a workout. Yet, they can all grow to a similar extent. DOMS also varies greatly between people[15]. Some people get lots of DOMs, and some people get very little. There is also no evidence that not experiencing DOMs impairs muscle growth. Excessive DOMs can be detrimental, reducing range of motion and the motivation to train from discomfort, which may impact on training adherence[14]. Greater DOMS the day after a workout does not mean greater muscle growth compared to no DOMS the day after a workout. *More muscle soreness does not mean more muscle growth.*

Summary

The primary mechanism for muscle growth is mechanical tension. The roles of metabolic stress and muscle damage on muscle growth appear to be less important, but still inconclusive.

Heavy, moderate and light loads can all result in muscle growth.

Heavy loads generate mechanical tension. Light and moderate loads result in metabolic stress and fatigue, leading to subsequent mechanical tension from further motor unit recruitment. Muscle damage is simply a by-product of resistance training.

Muscle ache and soreness after a workout are not useful predictors to determine how good the workout was for stimulating muscle growth.

References

1   Schoenfeld BJ. The Mechanisms of Muscle Hypertrophy and Their Application to Resistance Training. *J Strength Cond Res* 2010; 24: 2857–2872.

2   Wernbom M, Augustsson J, Thomeé R. The influence of frequency, intensity, volume and mode of strength training on whole muscle cross-sectional area in humans. *Sports Med Auckl NZ* 2007; 37: 225–264.

3   Wackerhage H, Schoenfeld B, Hamilton D, Lehti M, Hulmi J. Stimuli and sensors that initiate skeletal muscle hypertrophy following resistance exercise. *J Appl Physiol* 2018; 126. Available from: doi:10.1152/japplphysiol.00685.2018.

4   Henselmans M. *What makes muscle grow?* Available from: https://mennohenselmans.com/mechanisms-muscle-growth-muscle-damage-metabolic-stress-mechanical-tension/ (accessed 9 Feb 2020).

5   Tillaar R van den, Andersen V, Saeterbakken AH. Comparison of muscle activation and kinematics during free-weight back squats with different loads. *PLOS ONE* 2019; 14: e0217044.

6   Taylor JL, Gandevia SC. A comparison of central aspects of fatigue in submaximal and maximal voluntary contractions. *J Appl Physiol* 2008; 104: 542–550.

7   Soares EG, Brown LE, Gomes WA, Corrêa DA, Serpa ÉP, da Silva JJ et al. Comparison Between Pre-Exhaustion and Traditional Exercise Order on Muscle Activation and Performance in Trained Men. *J Sports Sci Med* 2016; 15: 111–117.

8   Cairns S. Lactic Acid and Exercise Performance. *Sports Med Auckl NZ* 2006; 36: 279–91.

9   Hall M, Rajasekaran S, Thomsen T, Peterson A. Lactate: Friend or Foe. *PM&R* 2016; 8: S8–S15.

10   Mitchell CJ, Churchward-Venne TA, Parise G, Bellamy L, Baker SK, Smith K et al. Acute Post-Exercise Myofibrillar Protein Synthesis Is Not Correlated with Resistance Training-Induced Muscle Hypertrophy in Young Men. *PLoS ONE* 2014; 9. Available from: doi:10.1371/journal.pone.0089431.

11   Damas F, Phillips SM, Libardi CA, Vechin FC, Lixandrão ME, Jannig PR et al. Resistance training-induced changes in integrated myofibrillar protein synthesis are related to hypertrophy only after attenuation of muscle damage. *J Physiol* 2016; 594: 5209–5222.

12   Johnston BC, Seivenpiper JL, Vernooij RWM, de Souza RJ, Jenkins DJA, Zeraatkar D et al. The Philosophy of Evidence-Based Principles and Practice in Nutrition. *Mayo Clin Proc Innov Qual Outcomes* 2019; 3: 189–199.

13   Proske U, Morgan DL. Muscle damage from eccentric exercise: mechanism, mechanical signs, adaptation and clinical applications. *J Physiol* 2001; 537: 333–345.

14   Schoenfeld BJ, Contreras B. Is Postexercise Muscle Soreness a Valid Indicator of Muscular Adaptations? *Strength Cond J* 2013; 35: 16–21.

15   Baumert P, Lake MJ, Stewart CE, Drust B, Erskine RM. Genetic variation and exercise-induced muscle damage: implications for athletic performance, injury and ageing. *Eur J Appl Physiol* 2016; 116: 1595–1625.

18. Principles of training

The primary driver of muscle growth is progressive resistance training. When aiming for muscle growth, ensure consistency and adherence to the training plan as a priority, and then work on consistency and adherence to a diet with a caloric surplus and sufficient protein intake.

As with diet, some elements of training have a greater influence on body composition than other elements. Many variables have little influence, if any[1].

The resistance training hierarchy pyramid:

1. **Consistency and adherence to a training programme.**
2. **Volume, intensity and frequency.**
3. **Exercise selection.**
4. **Rest periods and rep duration.**

Some important definitions to know are:

Volume	*Sets*		*The number of sets performed.*
	Sets reps	*x*	*Set workload. The number of reps performed.*
	Sets reps load	*x x*	*Volume workload. The amount of work performed.*
Intensity	*Of load*		*How heavy the load (weight) lifted is, relative to the load that can be lifted for 1 repetition.*
	Of effort		*How much effort is being given to perform a given muscular task.*
Frequency	*Per body part per week*		*How often a specific body part is trained per week.*

Adherence

Just as with your diet, the most important part of a training programme is *consistency* and *adherence;* meaningful amounts of muscle growth occurs over a long period of time, not after one or two big sessions. Don't create a 6 days per week training plan if you can only commit to 3 days. Train at the time you are most likely to commit to going. Don't plan to train early in the morning if you can never get up or you lack motivation at that time. Similarly, don't train after work or in the evenings if you feel too tired, and are highly likely to skip the session. Don't plan to train on Friday nights if you almost always have a social event planned on Fridays. A sub-optimal plan that you can adhere to is always better than a theoretically more optimal plan that you are not consistent with.

Resistance training programming

When planning any good training programme, there are four basic *principles* that should be considered before jumping into the training hierarchy pyramid. Some of these have been briefly mentioned already[2,3].

- Individuality.
- Specificity.
- Progressive overload.
- Variety (Periodisation).

Training that is *individualised* to the person, *specific* to muscle growth and involves *progressive overload* with some *variety*, results in better outcomes.

It is important to note that these principles are still *theories*; the evidence so far shows that when these factors are considered, there are better outcomes than when they are not considered.

Individuality

In order to achieve your desired outcomes, your training must be specific and *individualised* to match those outcomes, based on your preferences. There are certain principles to achieve outcomes relating to strength, power, hypertrophy and muscular endurance. But, there are many ways to implement these certain principles. For example, a principle of muscle growth is lifting more weight over time. But, this could be implemented with barbells, dumbbells, machines, resistance bands, chains and so on[4]. The choice of which should be down to the individual, as no evidence suggests one form is superior to any other for muscle growth[4]. Outcomes are not mutually exclusive. A hypertrophy plan can increase strength, power and muscular endurance. However, a training programme optimised for hypertrophy will not increase strength to the extent that a programme designed for increasing strength could. The way in which to implement these principles should be in a way that suits the *individual; you.* To determine this, you need to ask yourself some questions:

- **What is your primary goal? What are you trying to achieve? (This will affect your overall training programme design)** *Build muscle? Lose fat?*
- **How much time are you willing or able to commit?** *(This will affect your training frequency and training session length)* 3 *days per week, 5 days per week? 30 minute sessions, 90 minute sessions?*
- **What facilities do you have access to? (This will affect your training frequency and exercise selection)** *Home gym? Large extensive commercial gym? Open 24/7? Closed on weekends?*
- **What are your current strengths and weaknesses? (This will affect your training programme and what you prioritise)** *Big legs? Small arms?*
- **Are there any injuries that may limit exercise choice?** *Knee injury preventing squatting? Shoulder injury making bench pressing difficult?*
- **What is your current training experience?** *Have you never trained before or have you been training for years? Have you previously trained, but now haven't trained in a while?*

Specificity

Adaptations (e.g. muscle power, muscle growth, strength and endurance) are *specific* to the resistance training stimulus and will vary with the muscle activated, the range of motion, the energy systems required, and with training intensity and volume[2]. As such, there are principles that apply for different adaptations.

For example, although strength training and hypertrophy training both involve lifting weights with high levels of effort, there are distinct differences in what is trying to be achieved. The aim of strength training (such as powerlifting) is to elicit an adaptive response to be able to lift as much weight as possible for a single rep in a specific exercise (absolute strength for squat, bench and deadlift). The primary outcome is *performance* related. Strength training will involve a narrow repetition range (absolute strength), primarily in low rep ranges for 1-5 rep maximum efforts. On the other hand, the aim of hypertrophy training is to elicit an adaptive response to increase muscle mass. The primary outcome is *body composition* related. Hypertrophy training will involve a wide repetition range (relative strength) and not primarily in low rep ranges for 1-5 rep maximum efforts[5].

Strength training is specific to the exercise. Want a big squat? Then you need to squat. Want a big bench press? Then you need to bench press[5]. One study compared a group of people training only with *isolation* exercises (movement at one joint e.g. biceps curl), with a group of people training only with *compound* exercises (movement at more than one joint e.g. squat). Both groups gained similar amounts of muscle, but the group performing the compound bench press and squat exercises significantly increased their squat and bench 1 rep maximum (RM). This was also significantly greater than the strength increases seen in the isolation group[6]. A plan to improve jumping or sprint performance will have specific exercises and elements that differ from a plan to increase muscle size. For a beginner, the level of specificity can be quite low, such that strength and hypertrophy plans may actually be pretty similar. With training experience, plans need to be more and more specific to the adaptation required.

Muscle growth is specific to the muscle, but *not* to the exercise. Bicep curls build big biceps, not big triceps. But big biceps can be built with dumbbell or barbell bicep curls, for example. Want big quadriceps? Then you could squat, but you could also perform leg extensions, because the quadriceps are the primary muscles used in both exercises. However, building bigger quadriceps via leg extensions and leg presses will not necessarily mean a bigger squat. Want a big chest? Then you could barbell bench press, dumbbell bench press, or perform dips for example, because the chest is the primary mover in all three exercises. But, performing dips and any resulting chest growth doesn't necessarily mean a stronger barbell bench press[5].

Many training variables actually have little influence on muscle growth outcomes[1].

Progressive overload

Progressive overload is the increase in training stress over time to make long-term improvements[1,4,7−9].

Training to, or near to failure results in muscle growth[1]. As sufficient mechanical tension is placed upon a muscle, it then undergoes an adaptive response and increases in size. After the adaptation, lower levels of motor unit recruitment are required to generate the same force in a subsequent session. The same stress (lifting the same weight for the same number of reps) in a subsequent workout produces a smaller adaptive response compared to the previous session. Performing 4 sets of 8 reps of barbell squats with 50kg one week and performing the same number of reps and sets with 50kg the next week will result in a smaller stress and less adaptation. Fewer muscle fibres are required to lift the same weight for the same number of reps and sets, and therefore to further recruit and stimulate high-threshold motor units, a greater tension is required by increasing the *workload*[2]. As discussed later, just increasing workload in itself does not result in more muscle growth, it must be achieved in a certain manner. '*Fewer*' and '*smaller*' are relative terms. On a short timescale (e.g. session to session), the same stress as above may result in a similar stimulus and be a similar effort to perform. Over a long timescale with progression (e.g. months to months), the same stress as above may result in a relatively smaller stimulus, and likely be less effort to perform. In other words, the same rep range and load after the adaptation is now significantly further from failure than when it was first performed. Over time, maintaining sets that are taken to, or near to failure, will require an increase in the load used for a given rep range, for example[4]. The concept follows the *general adaptation syndrome* model of adaptation by Hans Selye[10]:

- **Stressor** (the training session).
- **Adaptation** (the recovery response to the stimuli from the training session).
- **Plateau** (the body now perceives the same stressor as less stressful and there is less of a stimulus to generate a recovery response).

When training to, or near to failure, the muscle adapts and grows[1]. To progressively increase training stress (and therefore continue to grow muscle), the training load needs to increase by[7,9]:

1. Lifting a *heavier* weight for the *same* number of reps.
2. Lifting the *same* weight for a *greater* number of reps.
3. Lifting heavier absolute weight (increasing absolute strength).
4. Increasing training volume (to an extent).

To keep muscles growing over time they need to be placed under greater and greater stress. You need to progressively overload the muscle for long-term muscle growth[4,7]. For progression, you need to get stronger over time across a wide range of rep ranges (increase *relative* strength). In other words, lifting more weight for a given number of reps, such as your 1 repetition maximum (RM), 5RM, 10RM, 20RM lifts and so on for your chosen exercise (lifting more weight in different rep ranges over time)[4,9]. Progression can also be achieved by using the same weight and performing more reps with that weight, or by performing more sets (volume).

For example, if you can squat 50kg x 8 reps for 4 sets in week 1, you can progressively overload by:

1. Adding weight (load):

Week 1: 50kg x 8 reps for 4 sets
Week 2: 52.5kg x 8 reps for 4 sets
Week 3: 55kg x 8 reps for 4 sets

2. Adding reps:

Week 1: 50kg x 8 reps for 4 sets
Week 2: 50kg x 9 reps for 4 sets
Week 3: 50kg x 10 reps for 4 sets

3. Adding sets (volume):

Week 1: 50kg x 8 reps for 4 sets
Week 2: 50kg x 8 reps for 5 sets
Week 3: 50kg x 8 reps for 6 sets

The examples above are in ascending order of the relative increase in stress with each week. Here, adding 2.5kg each week for the same number of reps and sets adds around 5% more workload. Adding 1 extra rep each week increases the workload by around 10%. Adding 1 extra set each week increases the workload by around 15-20%. These are simplifications. As a beginner or intermediate you may indeed be able to make increases as above week on week. More likely, and with training experience, you may only increase the weight on one set, increase the reps on one set, or increase the number of sets every few weeks. Sets, weight (load) or reps are excellent methods to progressively overload. Try to use them all at some point throughout your training (but don't try to increase reps, sets and weight all at the same time, be realistic).

However, which of these variables should be the *focus* of progression is largely unknown[11]. Experts suggest that the most effective method to promote muscle growth is to increase volume through the number of sets performed on a muscle per week, however the evidence is limited[11]. There are many ways of structuring overload to progress in a plan. Two leading experts, Eric Helms and Mike Israetel, have different approaches to progression. *No* studies have compared different progression strategies (i.e. progression through load only, versus progression through set volume) on long-term hypertrophy. It will not be possible to progress in all variables all of the time. Some of which involve smaller increments in stress than others. Adding an extra set adds quite a lot of extra volume. Adding one extra rep to one set is still overloading, but a much smaller increase in workload. How you decide to progress will depend on many factors including training experience, exercise choice and your personal training preference. The two extremes of progressive overload in your training can be:

- **Slow and conservative**. Add a rep at a time or increase the weight by a very small increment. The number of sets per week stays fairly constant but the workload in each set gradually increases.
- **Fast and hard**. This method is based on the fact that volume (chapter 19) appears to be the most important variable for muscle growth. Progression may occur over a period of time (a *mesocycle*) by increasing volume within each session or within each week (a *microcycle*), before reducing volume back down. Set volume is increased for a short period of time before reducing set volume again to allow for adequate recovery, but now using heavier loads for the same number of reps in each set. Over time, you may progress by going from 8 sets, to 10, to 12, to 14 sets per week for a muscle. This can be achieved by adding an extra set to an exercise, or by adding extra exercises. The benefit of using additional exercises to manage fatigue is discussed in chapter 21. After progressively increasing for several weeks you might then reduce volume back to 8 sets to allow full recovery. But, now you are using a heavier weight than when you were originally performing 8 sets. The process is then repeated, adding more sets with the new higher loads. This would create a linear increase in volume, but with a sawtooth profile.

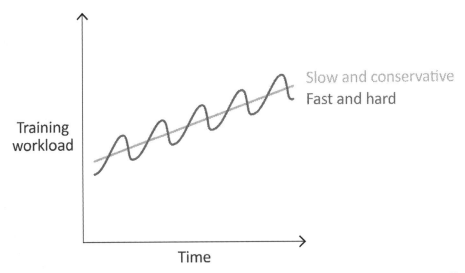

Methods of progression. Fast and hard: set volume increases and decreases over time, but the loads used after each increase and decrease gradually increase for the same rep range. Slow and conservative: set volume is relatively constant, but the loads used gradually increase for the same rep range. Both result in progressive overload over time.

However, which of these methods should be the focus of any progression is largely unknown[11].

There are a range of overload approaches between both extremes. You could maintain the lower weekly set volume after a *'fast and hard'* approach and then switch to the *'slow and conservative'* approach. You could also focus on increasing reps and load, and then set volume, which may be useful as a beginner. There are countless methods. *Periodisation* (discussed next) can be a tool to structure overload. How you overload should take into account your *lifestyle*. The considerable variation in training stress with a hard and fast approach may be difficult to plan around life stresses. The slow and conservative approach results in a similar level of stress from week to week. Also, training stress does not need to continuously increase every session. The stress from training needs to be manageable alongside the stress in the rest of your life, such as a busy period with work or dealing with other stresses. Stress in life can impair recovery and adaptations from resistance training[12,13]. With more general stress, opt for smaller increments in training stress. With less general stress, greater training stresses can be accommodated. Opt for smaller or larger increments based on personal preference.

Similarly, time constraints should be considered. Performing more sets may mean longer workout durations or greater training frequencies, which you may not be able to commit to. In which case, adding weight and reps to your current sets may be more feasible for your training plan.

You can alter the number of sets, reps and weight based on how you feel from session to session and week to week. However, you can also systematically alter the number of sets, reps and weight by planning changes in these training variables.

Variety (periodisation)

Periodisation is the acute and systematic alteration of certain training variables in order to break through plateaus and continue to make long-term improvements. Periodisation is usually used to manipulate volume, frequency and intensity which influence muscle growth. Most training variables should not be varied and should remain consistent because their variation has little to no influence on muscle growth, such as rest periods or rep durations[1,4,14].

Periodisation is not necessary as a beginner. Autoregulating training variables is a sufficient method of periodisation for most people to ensure progression. The limited literature of periodisation on hypertrophy is equivocal on whether periodisation is needed or beneficial[15]. Expert opinion is that the lack of evidence showing a benefit is more a limitation of the current low-quality research, rather than because it is not of benefit to experienced trainers[16]. It may be useful for long-term muscle growth in intermediate or advanced trainers.

A common misconception is that lots of variety is key to maximising muscle growth to 'shock' the muscle. While this may be true to an extent for certain variables, it should not be the case that every workout uses different exercises and rep ranges. This limits the ability to track progression. Also, some variables have little to no influence on muscle growth. Progressive overload with sets taken to, or near to failure is the important determinant for muscle growth. If you keep changing your exercises, rest periods and number of sets, it will be impossible to track this progression. Rapid improvements in new or novel exercises are mainly from neuromuscular improvements in becoming proficient in performing them, and not actually building muscle.

In order to utilise different resistance training variables productively, we need to think of a way to change them, whilst still keeping track. *Periodisation* is the acute and systematic alteration of certain training variables in order to break through plateaus and continue to make long-term improvements[2]. As sufficient mechanical tension (stress) is placed upon a muscle, it undergoes an adaptive response and increases in size. At some point, the stress placed upon the muscle will be insufficient to generate an adaptive response, resulting in a plateau. Periodisation is simply altering training variables to prevent or break through plateaus to continue progressing[2]. The most common variables studied for periodisation are *volume* (sets and reps) and *intensity* (of load).

The majority of periodisation studies however, are focussed on strength training, rather than hypertrophy[15]. With strength training, the aim is to perform a 1 rep maximum on a single pre-planned day at a competition. Even when there is no aim to compete, the aim of any strength training is performance based. Periodisation results in greater improvements in strength training and peak performance on a particular day, compared to a non-periodised approach[17]. Different methods of periodisation can result in similar improvements in muscular strength[18,19]. But, hypertrophy goals are less specific than strength goals. With muscle growth, we do not need to peak on a particular day, just progressively improve over time. The primary outcome is also not performance related. This means there is much more variability with how we can implement periodisation, or whether periodisation is even beneficial for muscle growth. The evidence is still inconclusive as to whether periodisation provides greater hypertrophy compared to no periodisation[15,16]. However, consensus opinion is that it appears to be from a limitation of the current research rather than because it is not of benefit in trained individuals[16]. Most studies are mainly designed to assess changes in strength, with muscle growth as a secondary outcome. Therefore, many studies are not designed to maximise muscle growth in the first instance, and can be statistically *'underpowered'* (chapter 4) to assess muscle growth. And, like many hypertrophy studies, periodisation studies are[16]:

- short in duration,
- mainly in untrained people, and
- few studies directly measure muscle growth.

Studies assessing periodisation are mainly in untrained people, with very few studies in trained people[15]. Untrained people have the greatest potential to increase muscle mass, even on a sub-optimal plan. There are also different forms of periodisation which makes comparison more difficult. Studies are short in duration, with the average study lasting 15 weeks[16]. When considering the slow rate of muscle growth in trained individuals, 15 weeks would likely be too short to be able to demonstrate superior muscle growth between a well-designed *periodised* training plan and a well-designed *non-periodised* training plan through statistical testing[15]. Studies also rarely consider participants' diets, which we know can heavily influence body composition outcomes. Periodisation could provide benefit in intermediate and advanced trainers in the long-term based on existing knowledge from other sporting pursuits (such as strength training and athletics), but more direct research assessing any benefit is needed[2].

Should you periodise for muscle growth?

Autoregulation and non-periodisation are sufficient for muscle growth for most people, especially beginners. Manipulating certain training variables is necessary for progression and muscle growth. Periodisation just means that this manipulation is performed in a systematic, planned manner. There are no negative effects of periodisation beyond the time required to plan training, with no additional cost to implement. There may be a potentially greater benefit for muscle growth, but this has yet to be proven. To progress, training variables will be manipulated anyway regardless of whether it is done randomly (non-periodisation) or systematically (periodisation). If you have reached a plateau from training with non-periodisation, a periodised approach may be useful. Periodisation could be used to 'cover all bases' to maximise any potential benefit it provides. Periodisation can also help to provide a structure to a training programme and guide individual workouts, which may also aid adherence.

As a beginner, periodisation does *not* appear to be necessary[16]. A key focus when starting a training programme is to ensure *repetition,* to promote learning of movement patterns and exercises. Periodisation involves variation. A non-periodised approach may allow sufficient exercise practice without the distraction of manipulating variables and overcomplicating training[16]. However, the ability to grow and improve diminishes with time. If you have been training for some time and are beginning to plateau in your lifts and muscle growth, then structuring your intensity, volume and rep schemes can provide a framework to monitor and achieve progress. The relative ability to grow muscle for someone who has been training for 2 years will be much less than for someone who has just started training. In order to keep making improvements and prevent overtraining as an intermediate or experienced lifter, it would be useful to implement periodisation into your training programme. But, you don't necessarily *need* to, to promote muscle growth.

Progression models

There are multiple periodisation models. Each model manipulates variables in a different, but systematic way with the long-term goal of progressively overloading. In strength training, they are all superior to non-periodised training. For hypertrophy, a systematic review has found the current research to be equivocal[16]. Therefore if considering using periodisation, the best strategy is to try each of them and see which you find best for progression, and which is most enjoyable to adhere to. Even if future research demonstrates superiority of a periodised approach for muscle growth, if this is too stressful or difficult for you to adhere to and removes the enjoyment of training, then a non-periodised approach would still be considered more suitable.

Non-periodisation

Non-periodisation is where training volume is kept high. Here, progression is achieved by adding a rep, set or weight on a particular day based on how you *feel* (*autoregulation*), and more than what you did before. This purely intuitive approach is sufficient for beginners, intermediate and even advanced trainers, with the rate of progression meaning it is feasible to see increases with each session. This is the *autoregulatory* approach[20]. This can be applied by using the strategy to progressively overload from page 334, by increasing or decreasing reps, sets or weight when it *feels* appropriate. Autoregulation can also be used with periodised approaches to training[21]. Chapter 19 will discuss how to use non-periodisation and autoregulation to progress. This includes measuring the intensity of effort, determining *when* it is appropriate to make changes and how to integrate autoregulation into periodised training.

Linear periodisation

Linear periodisation involves increasing the weight (intensity of load increases) whilst decreasing the number of reps (volume decreases) over several weeks. Then you return to the original weight, but now you are able to perform more repetitions. So over time, volume increases and progressive overload has occurred. Linear periodisation can be useful to build strength[16].

Reverse linear periodisation

Reverse linear periodisation involves decreasing the weight (intensity of load decreases) whilst increasing the number of reps (volume increases) over several weeks[16]. Reverse linear periodisation works well with lighter weights and higher rep ranges. It can be difficult to add weight to exercises targeting smaller muscle groups (e.g. biceps), and increasing the number of reps can be easier to achieve. The aim is to use the same weight for a period of time, and to focus on increasing the number of reps per set each session. For example, start at 3 sets of 12 reps. Then in subsequent sessions, do 3 sets of 13 reps, then 14 reps, then 15 reps. Once at 15 reps (or whatever rep you work towards), rather than performing more reps, instead increase the weight and start back on 3 sets of 12 reps. But, now you are performing 3 sets of 12 with a heavier weight, and therefore have progressively overloaded. Now, over time try to progress back up to 3 sets of 15 with the new heavier weight, and repeat. Reverse linear periodisation can be useful for improving *muscular endurance*.

Daily undulating periodisation (DUP)

Daily undulating periodisation is a *non-linear* periodisation approach. Volume and intensity rotate in a non-linear fashion on each training day[16]. High intensity days are low volume and focus on strength (a low number of sets, high intensities of load and low reps). Low intensity days are high volume and focus on hypertrophy (a high number of sets, low to moderate intensities of load and higher reps). Undulating periodisation can also be weekly (weekly undulating periodisation) or biweekly (undulating periodisation)[16].

Block periodisation

Block periodisation splits training into periods focussed on different goals. There can be a period dedicated to strength training, then a period dedicated to hypertrophy training, and then a period dedicated to power training. The similarities between blocks allow for any adaptations from previous blocks to be maintained. Usually periods last for durations of several weeks to months (a *mesocycle*). The specific blocks will depend on the individual. Such a model may be more suited to an individual with multiple goals besides muscle growth, such as sportspersons or athletes. Completing the training for all goals can take up to a year, or several years (a *macrocycle*).

A recent meta-analysis compared linear periodisation with daily undulating periodisation approaches. The analysis from a limited number of studies showed *similar* muscle hypertrophy between the two approaches[22].

Some of these forms of periodisation people do without even realising it. As a beginner, many people will lift the same weight and do more reps over time. People will also find they can lift more weight and perform a similar number of reps. Some people may have days where they try and lift weights near to their 3-5 rep maximum. Other days they may lift weights near to their 10-12 rep maximum.

To build muscle, you need to progressively overload, but you don't need to periodise your training. However, it may be useful for some people.

References

1   Morton RW, Colenso-Semple L, Phillips SM. Training for strength and hypertrophy: an evidence-based approach. *Curr Opin Physiol* 2019; 10: 90–95.
2   Kraemer WJ, Ratamess NA. Fundamentals of resistance training: progression and exercise prescription. *Med Sci Sports Exerc* 2004; 36: 674–688.
3   Fisher J, Steele J, Smith D. Evidence-Based Resistance Training Recommendations for Muscular Hypertrophy. *Med Sport* 2013; 17: 217–235.
4   Carpinelli R, Otto R, Wientt R. A critical analysis of the ACSM position stand on resistance training: Insufficient evidence to support recommended training protocols. *J Exerc Physiol Online* 2004; 7.
5   Fyfe JJ, Loenneke JP. Interpreting Adaptation to Concurrent Compared with Single-Mode Exercise Training: Some Methodological Considerations. *Sports Med Auckl NZ* 2018; 48: 289–297.
6   Paoli A, Gentil P, Moro T, Marcolin G, Bianco A. Resistance Training with Single vs. Multi-joint Exercises at Equal Total Load Volume: Effects on Body Composition, Cardiorespiratory Fitness, and Muscle Strength. *Front Physiol* 2017; 8. Available from: doi:10.3389/fphys.2017.01105.
7   Juneau C-E, Tafur L. Over time, load mediates muscular hypertrophy in resistance training. *Curr Opin Physiol* 2019; 11: 147–148.
8   Zając A, Chalimoniuk M, Maszczyk A, Gołaś A, Lngfort J. Central and Peripheral Fatigue During Resistance Exercise – A Critical Review. *J Hum Kinet* 2015; 49: 159–169.
9   Morton RW, Colenso-Semple L, Phillips SM. Training for strength and hypertrophy: an evidence-based approach. *Curr Opin Physiol* 2019; 11: 149–150.

10   Selye H. Stress and the General Adaptation Syndrome. *Br Med J* 1950; 1: 1383–1392.

11   Israetel M, Feather J, Faleiro TV, Juneau C-E. Mesocycle Progression in Hypertrophy: Volume Versus Intensity. *Strength Cond J* 2020; Publish Ahead of Print. Available from: doi:10.1519/SSC.0000000000000518.

12   Bartholomew JB, Stults-Kolehmainen MA, Elrod CC, Todd JS. Strength gains after resistance training: the effect of stressful, negative life events. *J Strength Cond Res* 2008; 22: 1215–1221.

13   Contreras B. *How important is psychological stress for your gains?* Available from: https://bretcontreras.com/how-important-is-psychological-stress-for-your-gains/ (accessed 9 Feb 2020).

14   Fisher J, Steele J, Bruce-Low S, Smith D. Evidence-Based Resistance Training Recommendations. *Med Sport* 2011; 15: 147–162.

15   Evans JW. Periodized Resistance Training for Enhancing Skeletal Muscle Hypertrophy and Strength: A Mini-Review. *Front Physiol* 2019; 10. Available from: doi:10.3389/fphys.2019.00013.

16   Grgic J, Lazinica B, Mikulic P, Schoenfeld BJ. Should resistance training programs aimed at muscular hypertrophy be periodized? A systematic review of periodized versus non-periodized approaches. *Sci Sports* 2018; 33: e97–e104.

17   Williams TD, Tolusso DV, Fedewa MV, Esco MR. Comparison of Periodized and Non-Periodized Resistance Training on Maximal Strength: A Meta-Analysis. *Sports Med Auckl NZ* 2017; 47: 2083–2100.

18   Bartolomei S, Hoffman JR, Merni F, Stout JR. A comparison of traditional and block periodized strength training programs in trained athletes. *J Strength Cond Res* 2014; 28: 990–997.

19   Harries SK, Lubans DR, Callister R. Systematic review and meta-analysis of linear and undulating periodized resistance training programs on muscular strength. *J Strength Cond Res* 2015; 29: 1113–1125.

20   Ormsbee MJ, Carzoli JP, Klemp A, Allman BR, Zourdos MC, Kim J-S et al. Efficacy of the Repetitions in Reserve-Based Rating of Perceived Exertion for the Bench Press in Experienced and Novice Benchers. *J Strength Cond Res* 2019; 33: 337–345.

21   Zourdos MC, Klemp A, Dolan C, Quiles JM, Schau KA, Jo E et al. Novel Resistance Training-Specific Rating of Perceived Exertion Scale Measuring Repetitions in Reserve. *J Strength Cond Res* 2016; 30: 267–275.

22   Grgic J, Mikulic P, Podnar H, Pedisic Z. Effects of linear and daily undulating periodized resistance training programs on measures of muscle hypertrophy: a systematic review and meta-analysis. *PeerJ* 2017; 5: e3695.

19. Training for muscle growth

With the principles discussed above in mind, it is now time to consider the training programme itself for muscle growth. There is a basic hierarchy of primary factors that should be focussed on, and then other factors which are largely irrelevant.

The training hierarchy pyramid:

1. Consistency and adherence to a training programme.
2. Volume, intensity and frequency.
3. Exercise selection.
4. Rest periods and rep duration.

Training variables: volume, intensity and frequency[1]

Volume, intensity and frequency are tightly related and are the most important training variables for muscle growth. All three cannot be maximised at the same time. Higher intensities take longer to recover from, which can limit volume and frequency. Increasing frequency can increase weekly volume, but at the cost of intensity. Increasing volume per session can limit weekly training frequency and session intensity. The balance of these three variables will vary within a training plan[2]. Due to the fact that all three are linked, it becomes very difficult to separate the individual effects of increasing volume, intensity or frequency, without the effect of altering the other variables.

Volume

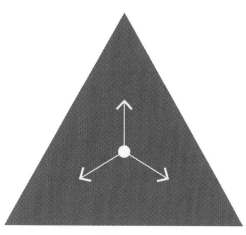

Frequency

Intensity

The volume, intensity, frequency triangle. Maximising all three variables at the same time is not possible. Assessing the effect of changing one variable is confounded by the fact that this will change the other variables as well.

Intensity

There are two measures of intensity: intensity of effort and intensity of load.

Intensity of effort: how 'hard' you train. How close to failure you get regardless of the intensity of load. Where failure is performing the maximum number of reps that you can perform for a give weight. This can be quantified using tools such as the 'Rating of Perceived Exertion' (RPE) or 'Reps in Reserve' (RIR) as measures of effort level and proximity to failure.

Sets should be performed at an RPE >5, and an RIR <5. In other words, at or near failure.

Intensity of load: how close to your 1 repetition maximum (RM) you are, expressed as a percentage of your 1RM. This relates to how many reps you can perform with a given intensity before reaching failure. Very roughly, a 1RM = 100% of your 1RM (high intensity), an 8-12RM = 70-80% of your 1RM (moderate intensity) and a 30-50RM = 30% of your 1RM (low intensity)[3].

Low intensities of load build muscle as well as moderate and high intensities of load. Hypertrophy can occur at any intensity of load from 30% to 100% of your 1RM when sets are taken to, or near to failure (i.e. when the intensity of effort is high)[1,4].

For muscle growth from a practical viewpoint, keep the majority of training volume within moderate intensities of 60-85%, (correlating to the 6-15RM rep range), and the minority of training volumes within high and low intensities of 85-100% and 30-60% (correlating to 1-6 and 15+RM).

The concept of intensity in resistance training can be misunderstood at times. Intensity in aerobic exercise such as high intensity interval training or low intensity steady state cardio refers to your heart rate relative to your maximum heart rate. Instead, intensity of load in resistance training refers to the amount of weight you are lifting relative to your 1 rep maximum (the weight you can lift for only 1 repetition in a given exercise)[1]. For example, lifting 80% of your 1 rep maximum would be a higher intensity than lifting 60% of your 1 rep maximum, even if your heart rate was much higher at 60% than at 80% intensity.

A high intensity of load is above 60% of your 1 rep maximum, but is more often considered to be above 80% of your 1 rep maximum. A low load would be as low as 30% of your 1 rep maximum, and a moderate load in between this[5].

Muscle growth occurs across a wide range of intensities of load.

The literature on training intensity is growing fast. Numerous controlled trials comparing different intensities of load and muscle growth now exist[6,7]. The primary mechanism for muscle growth is mechanical tension. The evidence suggests that this can be achieved with high, moderate and low loads of intensity. Lifting weights above 30% of your 1 rep maximum when taken to failure leads to similar muscle growth as lifting at higher intensities[1,6,8,9]. Training to failure using 20% of your 1RM in comparison to 40, 60 or 80% results in half the amount of hypertrophy, but there is no difference between using 40, 60 or 80%[10]. Therefore, workouts can and should include a wide range of intensities of load, but there is a lower limit.

Moderate intensities of load are a time-efficient optimal trade-off and should make up the majority of your training volume[11,12].

There are advantages and disadvantages to lifting with high and low intensity loads compared to moderate intensities. For most people, all three intensities should be used to maximise growth. High intensity loads and low rep ranges should be included in workouts, especially for individuals who wish to increase absolute strength alongside a muscle building plan. But, high intensity sets may limit the number of working sets in a session[13]. Working with high intensity of load, low rep ranges may require longer rest periods and a longer training session to generate sufficient volume. Low rep ranges such as below 6 reps (very high intensities of load) are also mentally tiring and can be highly demanding on joints. There are only so many sets you can productively perform in a session at such high intensities of load. Higher intensity sets (>80% 1RM) should be completed near the start of a workout.

Conversely, low intensity loads require a large number of reps to be completed. This generates high levels of central nervous system fatigue which can impair high-threshold motor unit activation, requiring longer recovery time after the workout[11,14–16]. A large amount of work is needed to reach the point of failure. The majority of the reps performed in low intensity load sets are non-stimulating, fatiguing volume[11]. A hypertrophic stimulus is not achieved until near the end of the set. It can often be difficult to maintain *focus* during a set with very high reps. Low intensity load sets should be nearer the end of a workout.

This is not to say that lower and higher rep ranges should not be used, but they should be used to a lesser extent than moderate rep ranges. For example, a strength-based low rep protocol could be used at the start of a workout (such as 3 sets of 3 reps, or 5 sets of 5 reps), and a final high rep set (e.g. 30-40 reps) for the last exercise of a workout with the majority of set volume performed within the 6-15 rep range.

The 8-12 rep range or more broadly, the 6-15 rep range is a *practical, optimal trade-off* within the wide range of effective reps and intensities of load. With moderate intensities, sufficient volume can be performed without needing very long rest periods, and non-stimulating volume and unnecessary fatigue are minimised with each set. Of course, personal preference should be considered. Some people prefer training with higher intensities of load and fewer reps. Some people prefer training with lower intensities of load and more reps. Find the rep ranges that you find most effective to achieve a sufficient intensity of effort for each set.

Fibre-type specific hypertrophy

There is no conclusive evidence that different intensities of load result in fibre-type specific hypertrophy. Recommendations are to train across the full range of rep ranges (and corresponding intensities of load) such that any theoretical benefit is already achieved[17].

It has been speculated that muscles with high proportions of type I fibres would benefit from training in higher rep ranges because of functional differences between muscle fibre types[3]. Type I and type II fibres have structural and functional differences. The more reliant a muscle fibre is on using oxygen during exercise, the thinner it is. The more reliant a muscle fibre is on not using oxygen during exercise, the larger it is or can be. Type I fibres are thinner than type II fibres[18]. Type I oxidative fibres contain greater fat stores, and smaller glycogen stores. Type II anaerobic fibres contain smaller fat stores and greater glycogen stores[18]. Phosphocreatine (PCr) content is greater in type II fibres than type I fibres.

Whether higher intensities (of load) result in greater type II fibre hypertrophy compared to type I and vice versa for low loads is unproven, but also inconclusive[3,5,17]. Some studies show differences in type I and type II hypertrophy with different loads, whereas some studies show no differences at all. Differences may just be due to the study design and the high variability of individual responses to resistance training. An argument for shorter rest periods and higher reps is that this form of training targets the type I, oxidative muscle fibres (the lower force producing fibres that can function for a longer duration), whereas lower reps target type II fibres (the higher force producing fibres that can function for a shorter duration). This is an interesting concept. However, it does not seem to hold true from a theoretical or research viewpoint. Recent studies have found no differences in muscle fibre activation or growth of type I and type II fibres with high or low loads lifted to failure[7]. In other words, the load lifted did not influence muscle fibre activation and growth when sets were taken to failure. If different rep ranges caused different muscle fibres to grow, then we would expect hypertrophy in a muscle to occur in different parts of a muscle. However, resistance training with low reps and high reps to failure produce similar levels of hypertrophy, in similar regions of the muscle[19].

From a theoretical viewpoint, type I fibres primarily rely on oxygen to facilitate muscular contractions. If they become too large by increasing in length or diameter, this would impair their functional ability because they need a good blood supply. Type I fibres have a greater ratio of blood vessels to muscle fibres, than type II fibres[18]. Again, the muscle fibres found in high-threshold motor units are typically type II fibres, which are the most responsive fibres to resistance training. Whereas, fibres in low-threshold motor units are mainly type I muscle fibres and show relatively limited muscle growth, however they still have the capacity to meaningfully grow[20]. Type I fibres are commonly recruited during daily activities where low levels of force are required. Because few fibres are active, these type I fibres can experience quite a lot of mechanical tension. In healthy active individuals, some muscle growth in type I fibres has likely already occurred from daily activity. Type II fibres are rarely active during daily activity. They primarily use energy without oxygen. Therefore, having a good blood supply to a type II muscle fibre is less important for its function. This means there is less of a functional constraint on the growth of type II fibres. Because type II fibres are rarely recruited during daily activity, they probably receive minimal stimulus to grow.

In terms of rep ranges, if higher reps caused greater muscle growth in type I fibres, then we would expect highly aerobic muscular contractions such as running or cycling to produce lots of hypertrophy. Aerobic exercise does not produce lots of hypertrophy. In fact, hypertrophy does not appear to significantly occur below 30% of 1RM, even when taken to muscular failure. This could be from aerobic exercise generating high levels central nervous system fatigue[11]. This means that when muscular task failure occurs with very light resistances, insufficient motor units are recruited because the central nervous system is excessively fatigued[21].

There is insufficient evidence to suggest different rep ranges induce differential hypertrophy of muscle fibre types[5,7]. *No* recommendations can be made at this stage regarding specific loads or loading ranges to promote fibre-type specific hypertrophy[3,17,22,23]. Even if this were to be true, it would not be of use to the majority of people. To apply this would require knowledge of someone's muscle fibre type composition. To identify someone's fibre composition would require an invasive muscle biopsy (extracting a sample of the muscle and examining the sample under a microscope), which would have to be performed on *every* muscle in the body[22,23]. Current recommendations are already to train across the full range of muscle building intensities of load, such that any theoretical effect is likely already achieved.

Intensity of load is exercise and gender specific. It is also influenced by training status.

The choice of exercise will affect how many reps you can perform at a given intensity of load. This means that for one exercise you may be able to perform 10 reps at 80% of your 1RM, but for another exercise, only 6 or 7 reps[24]. This is a reason why some coaches suggest basing your training plan on your known 5RM, 6RM, 7RMs and so on for an exercise, instead of using a rep calculator based on your 1RM. Coaches such as Mark Rippetoe have also observed that rep maximum ability differs between males and females, meaning a programme based only on rep maximums is not unisex[25]. Women can generally perform a different number of reps than men for a given intensity of load[26,27]. Endurance and strength trained athletes can also perform a different number of reps at a given RM percentage[27,28]. Rep number at a given intensity is also affected by rep speed. If you perform reps more slowly, you will perform fewer reps than if you lifted the same weight quickly. Rep tempo for a specific exercise may be a training variable that you keep fairly consistent to allow accurate tracking of progression. This is discussed in chapter 22.

Failure: as intense as effort can get

It is the number of sets performed to, or near to muscular task failure per week, per muscle (and thus sets performed with a high intensity of effort), that correlates with muscle growth, up to a point. Therefore, how do we know if we are at or near failure[4,8]?

When we say failure, we mean *muscular task failure*. This is where an exercise cannot be completed by using the same technique with specific muscles, due to fatigue. Fatigue is a reduction in the ability to perform a muscular task, resulting in an increase in the *perception of effort* required[21,29]. Fatigue results in the target muscle(s) being unable to generate sufficient force to, for example, lift a weight. Fatigue from resistance training can occur from both central nervous system fatigue and peripheral fatigue as a result of a range of mechanisms, including metabolic stress and maximal contractions[30-33]. Fatigue also occurs during low intensity aerobic (endurance) exercise[21]. Central fatigue limits the ability to recruit motor units, impairing activation of muscle fibres[21]. Peripheral fatigue limits the ability of recruited and active muscle fibres to contract[29]. The type of fatigue that results in task failure can influence muscle growth. Peripheral and central nervous system fatigue are influenced by the intensity and duration of exercise[33]. Fatigue can accrue at a faster rate at maximal efforts, but can accumulate to a greater extent with sub-maximal efforts due to the longer duration of sub-maximal efforts[29]. Both central and peripheral fatigue accumulates simultaneously during submaximal contractions. It appears that greater peripheral fatigue occurs with shorter, higher intensity exercise, and greater central fatigue occurs with longer, lower intensity exercise[33]. However, the influence of peripheral and central fatigue on muscle performance is still not fully understood[31]. In summary, fatigue is generated when exercise is performed. Fatigue dissipates at rest.

Muscular task failure can be due to:

1. The muscle not being able to generate enough force with all motor units recruited (e.g. a weight heavier than your 1RM or fatigue from multiple reps with a weight lighter than your 1RM).
2. The muscle not being able to generate enough force due to the presence of central fatigue, preventing recruitment of high-threshold motor units[21].
3. The muscle not being able to generate enough force due to the presence of peripheral fatigue, with subsequent recruitment of high-threshold motor units which subsequently also experience peripheral fatigue, leading to point 1[29].

Points 2 and 3 result in slow rep speeds before task failure occurs. However, in point 2, excessive central nervous system fatigue will result in premature muscular task failure because many high-threshold motor units are not recruited[29]. This may limit the mechanical tension experienced by muscle fibres if too many high-threshold motor units are left unrecruited. Central nervous system fatigue accumulates throughout a workout and decays during rest periods between sets[29]. Fatigue can be greater from long duration sub-maximal contractions (i.e. low load, high rep sets)[11]. See chapter 19 for structuring a workout to minimise central nervous system fatigue, and chapter 22 for rest periods to minimise central nervous system fatigue and maximise set performance.

Do effective/stimulating reps exist?

We know that training to, or near to failure is necessary for muscle growth and therefore these final reps in a set have importance. But, whether these reps become important at 5 reps from failure, closer than 5 reps from failure or further than 5 reps from failure is unknown. Whether training 1 or 2 reps from failure, or 3 or 4 reps from failure is better for muscle growth, is also unknown.

If you wish to understand the theoretical argument for effective reps from experimental evidence in more depth, read *'Hypertrophy'* by Chris Beardsley[34].

Effective reps are a theoretical construct to try and explain how resistance training stimulates muscle growth. This model takes theory 2 (chapter 17) one step further. Effective reps are defined as the last 5 or so reps in a set to failure and are the reps in a set that result in muscle growth. This is where the exercise velocity slows down, and muscle fibres experience the highest levels of mechanical tension.

Training to failure or near to failure builds muscle. Ending a set far from failure does not result in much muscle growth at all. It would seem therefore that these final reps in a set to failure are important for muscles to grow. The number of sets performed to failure per week for a given muscle correlates with muscle growth. This concept has been developed further by some researchers. It has been theorised from the current understanding of muscle growth that a strong measure of volume and muscle growth would therefore be the number of stimulating reps within those sets experienced by a muscle across the week. The theory is to only *'count'* the final reps of a set to failure where the rep speed begins to slow down. These are supposedly the reps where the high-threshold motor units are recruited and the exercise velocity is slow. This is when muscle fibres are under a lot of tension and these are the reps that *'stimulate'* muscle growth. The reps that *'count'*, therefore, will be the last 5 or so reps of a set before failure.

So, for example, 4 sets of 5 reps using your 5 rep maximum would generate around 20 stimulating reps. Similarly, 4 sets of 12 reps using your 12 rep maximum would generate 20 stimulating reps. But, 4 sets of 15 reps using your 20 rep maximum would in theory generate 1 or 2, if any stimulating reps. If you remember the force-velocity graph from chapter 17, the greatest forces are generated when a muscle is contracting slowly. Studies show that heavy, moderate and light weights can all cause muscle growth when sets are performed to or near to failure, where exercise velocity slows. The concept of effective reps implies that training closer to failure results in more effective reps, and therefore muscle growth. However, this is not necessarily supported by research findings.

The concept is also used to explain why lifting at intentionally very slow velocities does not result in muscle growth unless taken to failure, because this does not increase mechanical tension. Sub-maximal velocities result in greater motor unit recruitment despite unfatigued low-threshold motor units, so each fibre likely experiences relatively less tension.

Effective reps are *not* a universally accepted model, and others have argued that the effective rep concept is more complex and nuanced than this. As discussed later, training to failure results in more muscle damage, which can be counter-productive. Similarly, muscle activation at light and moderate loads can be similar to muscle activation at heavy loads, suggesting very heavy loads or performing sets to within 5 reps of failure is not necessary for full motor unit recruitment. The model also does not consider how for some compound exercises such as the bench press, there is a large amount of passive tension at the bottom of the movement which will generate high levels of mechanical tension, even when stopping a set far from failure. The effective reps model also implies that mechanical tension experienced by each muscle fibre needs to be very high, when exercise velocity has significantly slowed down. It may well be that sufficiently high tension to promote muscle growth is achieved further from failure than this significant slowing[35]. For an overview of the argument against effective reps, Greg Nuckols has written an excellent publicly available article[36].

At this stage, there is limited evidence to suggest that training can be tracked using the number of effective reps performed.

Failure

The number of sets performed to, or near to failure per week per muscle correlates with muscle growth, up to a point[4,37]. However, reaching failure in a set is highly fatiguing and generates a lot of muscle damage[3]. This can limit volume and frequency, and increase recovery time[14]. This is evident in a study where participants performed on average 11.7, 6.8 and 6.1 reps over 3 sets of back squats, when all sets were taken to failure[38]. The same participants performed on average 11.7, 8.4 and 6.6 reps over 3 sets performed to failure on the bench press[38]. Sets to failure reduces the number of possible reps in subsequent sets. In another study in females, significantly more reps were performed in the first set of squats when training to failure compared to not training to failure (11.58 reps vs 7.58 reps on average)[39]. But, by the fourth set of squats, significantly fewer reps were performed when training to failure compared to not training to failure (3.58 reps vs 5.41 reps on average)[39]. Both groups performed a similar number of reps in total across all 4 sets, all using a 10RM load. Nonetheless, a systematic review of 14 studies demonstrates that training to failure, and training just short of failure leads to similar levels of hypertrophy when volume (number of sets per week) is equal[37,40]. One study of 28 males training to failure or just short of failure found similar increases in muscle growth in all groups. One group performed sets to failure. A second group performed sets near to failure with a fast concentric and controlled eccentric contraction, and a third group performed sets near to failure with a fast concentric and fast eccentric contraction. No difference in muscle growth was seen between the groups, despite one of the non-failure groups performing significantly fewer reps per set[41]. A similar study in females found equivalent muscle growth when performing sets to failure or sets near to failure[40].

Therefore, do we actually need to reach failure? Considering the minimal hypertrophic benefit of training to failure, but the large additional cost of fatigue and detriment in performance, it would make sense to focus on training near to, but not to the point of failure for most sets. This is the consensus recommendation from a range of peer-reviewed articles and experts[3,4,37,42].

However, ending sets too far from failure results in less hypertrophy.

An excellent study demonstrated the importance of the proximity to failure and exerting sufficient intensity of effort to promote hypertrophy[43]. 26 males performed 10 reps of their 10RM. One group performed 10 uninterrupted reps with 1 minute rest between sets. The other group performed 5 reps with 30 seconds of rest before performing the next 5 reps (10 interrupted reps), with 1 minute rest between sets. With equal training volumes, both groups significantly increased muscle mass. But, hypertrophy was far greater in the group performing 10 interrupted reps than the group performing 10 reps with a 30 second rest after 5 reps. Find a weight for an exercise that you can perform 10 reps before reaching failure. Now, complete a set but perform 5 reps before taking a 30 second break, and then complete 5 more reps. Notice how much easier (lower intensity of effort) this 5 + 5 reps set was compared to the straight 10 rep set despite the same workload. Intensity of effort and proximity to failure are important for stimulating growth.

Training to failure causes much more muscle damage and fatigue than not reaching failure. Reaching failure requires more time to recover before the next training session. Training to failure also leads to a subsequent drop in productive set volume in the rest of the workout, from the significant fatigue induced[12]. This means that the muscle being trained can experience less meaningful training volume during the workout, which can reduce the muscle building potential of the session. On the other hand, stopping a set too far from failure results in significantly less muscle growth. Clearly, there is a sweet spot for intensity of effort.

In order to maximise training frequency, maximise stimulation of muscle protein synthesis and minimise muscle damage, it would be advisable to train just shy of failure. Stop 1-5 reps before muscular failure for any set with any intensity of load[3,4]. One argument against the concept of effective reps is that we would expect to see sets performed closer to failure (within 1-2 reps) to produce more muscle growth than sets slightly further from failure (within 3-5 reps). However, this is inconclusive. No differences in muscle growth have been demonstrated between sets performed relatively close to, and very close to failure. Whether effective reps truly exist or not, the bottom line is that you need to train hard enough (within 5 reps of failure), and to ensure progression on your choice of exercises over time.

Implementing failure training

Training to failure is stressful, both mentally and physically[3]. However, training to failure ensures that intensity of effort is sufficiently high. How often you use it depends on your current training goals and general stress levels. Use training to muscular task failure sparingly, in general on the last set of an exercise, a couple of times a week maximum[12]. Consider using failure more near the end of a period of high training volume, where you plan to have a lower volume or recovery period. Or, when weekly volume is low such that there is adequate time and capacity for recovery. Because of the high stress resulting from failure training, some expert coaches suggest to use failure training less, when your general life stresses are high (e.g. work or family stress)[44,45]. Some exercises suit failure training better than others. Generally, failure training is better suited to higher rep, *isolation* exercises (single-joint movements such as bicep curls or shoulder lateral raises) instead of low rep, *compound* exercises (multi-joint movements such as squats or deadlifts)[12]. This is also suggested because when lifting heavy loads, high levels of motor unit recruitment are needed from the first rep to move the weight and failure may not be necessary. Higher rep ranges may only result in full motor-unit recruitment when training to complete failure[45]. When training to failure, it is advisable to have a spotter present to assist you. If you do not have a spotter, then choose exercises where you can achieve failure safely, such as machines, cables or dumbbells where it is much easier to drop the weights and prevent injury when failure has been reached.

It is not advantageous to train to failure on every set. We need to have a tool to work out when we are close enough to failure to achieve sufficient high-threshold motor unit recruitment, but not so close that we accumulate excessive fatigue and muscle damage that will be counterproductive.

Measuring intensity of effort

Most sets need to be performed to within 1-5 reps of failure. How can you gauge that you are exerting enough effort?

There are different methods of gauging how much effort you are putting into your training, or to work out what weight and rep range you need to use for a given level of effort. Two methods are the *percentage of 1 repetition maximum* (RM) and the *repetition maximum range* schemes. You calculate your 1RM for that exercise and choose a weight corresponding to a given percentage of that 1RM or choose the heaviest load possible to complete a number of reps within a given range. Using relative RMs can be a useful tool to gauge the approximate intensity of load and therefore the approximate number of reps per set. Planning workouts based on percentages of your 1RM is a common tool. But, using RMs to choose a specific load and a specific number of reps can be inaccurate. Gauging intensity from RMs can be inaccurate based off a 1RM or 5RM effort, because the number of reps that can be performed at different RMs for an exercise differs between exercises[14,24]. RM also differs between males and females. Females can generally perform more reps at a higher intensity of load. Therefore, using the RM scale for workouts can lead to weights that are too heavy or too light for different people. Use of a single 1RM or 5RM test can also be inaccurate because of relative over- or under-performance in that test set (perhaps longer rest than normal in the days before, or performance of the test in a fatigued state)[14]. Gauging intensity from a RM determines your future performance based on your previous performance. However, the body adapts from previous performances. Therefore, the rep maximum scheme may not accurately reflect what you can now achieve[46]. This may be especially true in untrained people, where progression can occur quickly. Everyone has good and bad training days, where the same weight can feel weightless one day or like a ton of bricks the next. Using RM does not factor in this daily and weekly variation in performance[12]. Untrained and novice individuals are also unlikely to be able to perform a true 1RM effort[47]. In other words, RM schemes do not tell you the intensity of *effort* you need to train with, only the relative intensity of *load*, which can be quite inaccurate.

Rating of perceived exertion (RPE)

First developed by Gunnar Borg, the *rating of perceived exertion (RPE)* is a measure of how much *effort* you are putting into a task, on a scale of 0-10[12,48,49]. As the name suggests, effort is subjectively judged by the effort the individual *feels* they have given. It has been shown that the perception of effort can be dissociated from any perceptions of force, pain or discomfort during exercise[48]. RPE can be judged from the perspective of a whole session, or for each individual set after they have been performed. RPE can also be predetermined, such that an individual performs a number of reps until they perceive a certain RPE[12]. The amount of effort in resistance training will relate to the number of reps performed in a set, relative to the maximum number of reps that could be performed for a given load[14]. The effort required will increase the closer you get to failure, such that performing 1 rep of your 10RM will have an RPE around 1, but performing 9 reps of your 10RM will have an RPE of 9.

RPE Scale	Feeling
10	Very difficult, no more reps possible before failure
9	Difficult, one more rep possible before failure
8	Pretty difficult, two more reps possible before failure
7	
6	
5	Some effort
<5	Little effort
0	At rest

The RPE Scale[48,49].

Training to failure results in a higher RPE, higher session RPE, and higher perceptions of discomfort, compared to not training to failure[39].

Assessment of RPE by an individual during a set appears to be accurate, with increasing accuracy the closer a set is taken to failure. However, studies appear to show that using RPE to gauge intensity underestimates how many reps people can actually perform in a given set. Muscular failure should be achieved at an RPE of 10, however the mean RPE at failure in studies is typically below 10[12,50].

Reps in reserve (RIR)

Following from this, a different but related method called *reps in reserve (RIR)* was developed[47]. RIR is a measure of how many more reps you could have done in that set before reaching failure. The concept is relatively new, and as such the research base is small, but growing. It is suggested that RIR may be more precise in gauging intensity when training near to failure[12]. Therefore, when you perform 1 rep with your 10RM, your RIR is 9 (9 more reps could have been performed).

When you perform 9 reps of your 10RM, your RIR is 1, because you could only perform 1 more rep[47].

RIR	RPE	Example
0	10	1 rep of your 1RM
1	9	1 rep of your 2RM
2	8	2 reps of your 4RM
3	7	1 rep of your 4RM
4	6	6 reps of your 10RM
5	5	4 reps of your 9RM
>5	<5	10 reps of your 20RM
10		

The RIR Scale.

The table below outlines how the intensity you use will affect where the RPE or RIR tool begins (lifting a weight equating to your 1-5RM will mean an RPE of 5 or above, or an RIR of 5 or less), and how the proximity to failure increases RPE, and decreases RIR[47].

Rep maximum	Reps performed	RPE	RIR
1RM	1	9.5-10	0
3RM	2	9	1
5RM	2	7	3
10RM	10	9.5-10	0
20RM	15	5	5

The relationship between RPE and RIR. From Zourdos et al., 2016[47].

The rating of perceived exertion and reps in reserve systems can be very useful in determining how close to failure you are and therefore determining your intensity of effort. As expected, there is an inverse relationship between concentric (muscle shortening) rep velocity and measures of intensity of effort, as velocity decreases with proximity to failure. As RPE increases or RIR decreases, concentric velocity decreases[47,51]. Importantly, experienced trainers and especially those with strength training backgrounds have much slower velocities for their final few reps before failure than untrained lifters[12]. This is because of their experience in movement execution and the ability to recruit all muscle fibres, such that they are able to perform a set much closer to their theoretical performance limit.

Implementing methods to measure intensity of effort

It will take time to learn how to use measures of intensity of effort. Much like it takes time to learn how to properly execute an exercise, it comes down to practice. Learn what being within 4, 3, 2 reps or 1 rep from failure *feels* like for different intensities of load for different exercises. Using a consistent rep tempo (chapter 22) for a given exercise will help to gauge proximity to failure. Unsurprisingly, experienced trainers are better at gauging RPE and RIR than untrained people[12,45,47]. This means trained individuals can more accurately record RIR. As mentioned above, rep velocity at low RIRs is slower for trained people. Practice with your own selected exercises and learn how fast you can perform the exercise before you fail. Therefore, if you have experience, use RIR (or RPE) to gauge training intensity, track progression and guide changes to your reps, sets or weight (as outlined in chapter 18 regarding periodisation models). As a beginner, practice recording RIR (or RPE) for your sets, but do not necessarily use them until you can accurately predict how close to failure you actually are. As a beginner, training closer to failure may help to ensure a sufficient intensity of effort. Helms et al. suggest that a good way to practice this is to perform a set a few reps short of failure and record what you think the RIR or RPE was[12]. Then, perform a second set (with adequate rest) with the same load to failure, and see how close your estimate from the first set was[12]. Rep velocity could similarly be used to measure how close to failure you are, but has the same limitations as using RIR[45].

Autoregulation

Measures of intensity of effort can be used to autoregulate training for both non-periodised and periodised training. RIR can be implemented alongside a rep maximum scheme. This ensures that the intensity of load and intensity of effort are matched to the intended rep range. This prevents performing a set that was too easy, or a set that was too hard. Such a method has mainly been used by strength training coaches. But, it can be effectively used for muscle growth. For example, if your bench press 1RM is 100kg, you might opt to perform sets at 70% of your 1RM (70kg) for sets of 8-12 (see chapter 21 for planning a training workout). You can then use an RIR of 2 (or an RPE of 8), to judge if the load is appropriate for the rep range. If you achieve 8 reps with an RIR of 0-1, then perhaps the weight needs to be lowered. Similarly, if you achieve 12 reps with an RIR of 3-4, then the weight needs to be increased. This is the autoregulation method of adjusting training variables as outlined in chapter 18 as the non-periodised approach[51]. Deciding when to increase the weight, reps or number of sets (to progressively overload) can be determined based on RPE or RIR:

1. Add weight when RIR increases (or RPE decreases):

Week 1: 50kg x 8 reps for 4 sets (RIR = 2, RPE = 8)
Week 2: 50kg x 8 reps for 4 sets (RIR = 4, RPE = 6)
Week 3: 52.5kg x 8 reps for 4 sets (RIR = 2, RPE = 8)

2. Add reps to maintain the same RIR (or same RPE):

Week 1: 50kg x 8 reps for 4 sets (RIR = 2, RPE = 8)
Week 2: 50kg x 8 reps for 4 sets (RIR = 4, RPE = 6)
Week 3: 50kg x 10 reps for 4 sets (RIR = 2, RPE = 8)

3. Add sets (volume): if post-workout RPE decreases, or could be increased:

Week 1: 50kg x 8 reps for 4 sets (Post-workout RPE = 8)
Week 2: 50kg x 8 reps for 4 sets (Post-workout RPE = 6)
Week 3: 50kg x 8 reps for 5 sets (Post-workout RPE = 8)

The use of an RIR of 2 (RPE of 8) here is an example. For heavy loads and compound exercises, an RIR of 2-4 is probably sufficient for muscle growth. As mentioned earlier in the failure chapter, failure is best saved for low load, isolation exercises. For low loads and isolation exercise, an RIR of 0-2 is probably needed[45]. This method can also be used to autoregulate fatigue. Just as much, you could aim for higher RIRs when you have those days where the weight feels like a 'ton of bricks', or when life is a bit more stressful. This would result in lower fatigue from the training session. On the other hand, you could aim for an RIR of 1 or a high post-workout RPE on the days when you are well rested and have plenty of opportunity to sufficiently recover from the additional fatigue. This would result in higher fatigue from the training session. The concept of autoregulation and using measures of effort can just as well be applied to periodised approaches to training. For example, in linear periodisation (increase intensity, decrease volume) you may perform 3 sets of 8 reps with 70kg on the bench press. You record the sets as an RIR of 2. In week 2, you increase the intensity and decrease the volume according to linear periodisation. You decide to perform 3 sets of 6 reps with 80kg on the bench press. However, this week you record the sets as an RIR of 1. Therefore, for week 3 you decide to make a smaller increase in intensity to 85kg and a bigger decrease in volume of 5 reps for 3 sets. This returns your RIR back to 2.

Autoregulation can also be used across sets within a session. If on week 2 you found that the first set of 6 reps with 80kg was much easier than expected (such as an RIR of 3 or 4), then you can increase the weight for the second set to say 82.5kg, which returns RIR back to 2 for a set of 6 reps. If the first set of 6 reps was too hard (such as an RIR of 1), then you can decrease the second set to 77.5kg, which returns the RIR back to 2 for a set of 6 reps.

Measures of intensity of effort are valuable tools that you can use during your training to manage fatigue and track progression.

Volume

Volume is proposed to be the primary driver of muscle growth[22]. On average, 10-20 sets per muscle group per week for beginners and intermediate level trainers appears to be optimal for muscle growth, and for the majority of experienced trainers. There is wide individual variability on what is optimal. Starting at 4-6 sets per muscle group per week as a beginner is a good starting point to prevent excessive fatigue and muscle damage, and provides a good base to add further volume.

With experience, varying volume (periodisation) across weeks and months between high and low volume can allow for muscle-specific increases in mass, whilst maintaining the size of other muscles[22]. Brief periods of very high volume in experienced individuals can be used to 'functionally overreach' before a low volume recovery period to promote hypertrophy[3].

Multiple sets per body part per week is superior to single sets per body part per week for muscle growth. No study has shown a superior benefit of single sets on muscle growth in untrained or trained individuals. However, the number of multiple sets that will be performed will vary based on specific goals, personal preference and throughout a programme to allow for progressive overload. The current view is that there is a weekly upper limit to the amount of volume that can be performed per week per body part, which is likely higher than the upper limit of volume per training session per body part. However, this is still inconclusive.

Volume refers to the amount of work performed by a muscle, usually per session or per week. However, volume has been quantified in different ways in research[1]. Not all definitions correlate with muscle growth, which also tells us what is not important to drive muscle growth. There are several different ways that studies have measured volume, and there is no consensus for which is the best measure[1,52]:

- *Number of sets to failure: most commonly used and correlates with muscle growth.*
- *Number of reps: (sets x reps) does not correlate with muscle growth.*
- *Volume workload: (sets x reps x weight used) does not correlate with muscle growth. High and low intensities of load result in similar hypertrophy but require different amounts of volume load.*

The number of sets to failure is currently the only measure of volume that correlates with muscle growth[22,37]. Studies show that a greater volume of sets to, or near to failure for a muscle per week (up to a point) leads to greater muscle growth[1]. Performing multiple sets per week rather than a single set per week results in more muscle growth[22,53]. A novel study made untrained individuals perform a low volume (1 set) of an exercise for one leg in each session, and a moderate volume (3 sets) for the other leg in each session, 5 times per week. The moderate volume (15 sets per week) resulted in greater muscle growth than the low volume (5 sets per week)[54]. Not all participants benefited from performing a moderate volume, but there was also no detrimental effect. In untrained individuals, fairly low volumes in each training session can result in meaningful muscle growth. A recent review did not find workout volumes equal to or greater than 3 sets per muscle to be more effective for muscle growth than workout volumes fewer than 3 sets for untrained individuals[55]. However as the authors note there is a lack of data, and the exact number you may perform will be down to preference.

Time under tension and workload

The total time under tension for a set does not correlate with muscle growth[8,56].

Variations in rep duration and timing have little influence on hypertrophy. The main focus should be on a high intensity of effort, taking sets to, or near to failure[4,8].

Time under tension refers to the total rep duration of a set (rep duration × number of reps). Despite the large focus on time under tension in muscle building circles, there is very little evidence to suggest that time under tension correlates with muscle growth[4,7,19,57]. This is also evident by the fact that low, moderate and high intensity loads all result in muscle growth with sets taken to, or near to failure. However, low loads require a higher number of reps and more time under tension than high loads with a lower number of reps and therefore less time under tension[7]. Also, varying rep duration has little effect on muscle growth, yet longer rep durations increase time under tension[8,58]. Similarly, progression by adding load to an exercise whilst performing the same number of reps to failure, for the same number of sets would promote hypertrophy[8]. But, this would have no effect on time under tension if rep duration is consistent.

Short rest periods and longer rep durations both reduce the workload (sets × reps × load) performed. However, only short rest periods appear to influence muscle growth even when the intensity of effort is high. Central fatigue may still be high in the subsequent set with shorter rest periods, such that even with high intensities of effort, high-threshold motor units are not recruited. With long rep durations, even though fewer reps are performed, sufficient high-threshold motor units are still recruited at or near failure as central nervous system fatigue is still fairly low, presuming sufficiently long rest periods are used. Workload also does not correlate with muscle growth. An elegant study demonstrated that training with no load at all, but contracting the arm as hard as possible (*a maximal voluntary contraction*) through a full range of motion produced as much muscle growth as using a moderate load[59]. With no load, workload cannot be calculated. On the other hand, performing more reps for the same load will increase time under tension, adding sets will increase session time under tension, and so will increasing training frequency. Changes in time under tension and workload are largely irrelevant and are the consequence of changes in factors that do promote muscle growth, and changes in factors that do not[8].

Currently, the best correlate of training volume with muscle growth is the number of sets taken to, or near to failure per week.

Why might certain measures of volume correlate poorly with hypertrophy?

It may be that workload (sets × reps × load) *only* has relevance within a given set, relative to an individual's potential maximum workload for a given intensity of load, with a given rep duration, lifted to, or near to failure. For example, if someone could bench press 100kg for 10 reps to failure, their maximum *set workload* for this load is 1000kg (1 set × 10 reps × 100kg). If they lifted to, or near to failure, their workload would be around 700-1000kg (i.e. performing 7-10 reps), which would promote hypertrophy. If their set ended far from failure, their set workload may be 300-500kg (i.e. performing 3-5 reps), which from current knowledge would promote little, if any hypertrophy. But, if the individual performed 2 sets that ended further from failure, their total workload for two sets would be comparable to that of one set taken to, or near to failure (2 × 300-500kg = 600-1000kg). The workloads are similar, yet hypertrophy will be greater in the single set performed with a high intensity of effort near to, or to failure. Many research studies try to equate overall volume like this between groups, but clearly this similar overall volume can result in different rates of hypertrophy[43].

Furthermore, with a long rep duration, fewer reps are performed before failure occurs. The maximum workload in a given set is lower with a slower rep speed (1 set × fewer reps × same load). However, a range of rep speeds can result in similar hypertrophy (chapter 22). When a set is taken to or near to failure with a longer rep duration, the set workload is still at or near the theoretical maximum set workload for *that* given rep duration, and hypertrophy still occurs. Meaning, different rep durations will result in different set workloads to failure, with similar hypertrophy. This may provide support as to why there is no superior rep duration and why total workload does not relate to muscle growth.

Very short rest periods result in less hypertrophy. With shorter rest periods, set workload is reduced because fewer reps can be performed before failure. However, this set workload is lower than the theoretical maximum set workload for that load with a given rep duration, as more reps could be performed in that set if the rest period was longer. This may explain why shorter rest periods result in less muscle growth for the same number of sets, because the muscle has not sufficiently recovered (i.e. too much fatigue is still present) to produce a subsequent productive set.

Workload therefore *only* appears relevant to muscle growth when *matched* on a set, load and rep duration basis, when the muscle has sufficiently recovered from a previous workout or set. In fact, workload may just be a proxy for performing sets to, or near to failure (i.e. performing sets with a high intensity of effort). When considered like this, all that needs to be considered is how many reps from failure a set is performed to for a given load, with other variables (such as rep duration) kept consistent. This is basically what the RIR scale achieves. With all else considered, how hard was that set?[16]. This is what research demonstrates. The best correlate with muscle growth is the number of sets taken to, or near to failure per week[8]. In other words, workload is only relevant within a set, relative to the maximum achievable set workload for a given load. Beyond this context, load is largely irrelevant for muscle growth because different loads result in similar hypertrophy. Hence, overall volume workloads do not reflect that high, moderate and low loads all effectively build muscle. *But*, to ensure progressive overload over time, the load used (whether high, moderate or low) for a given rep range needs to increase over time (chapter 17)[8,15]. The use of the RIR and RPE schemes essentially *adjusts* for the use of different loads, such that regardless of the load, a high RPE or low RIR achieved in a given set will promote muscle growth. Meaning, consideration of volume workload is largely *irrelevant* when training for muscle growth[8].

How many sets per session or per week do I need to perform to maximise muscle growth?

A systematic review and meta-analysis of 15 experimental studies comparing the effects of different weekly volumes on muscle growth shows that this dose-response effect appears to hold true up to around 10-20 sets per body part week, where the current consensus is that there is a plateau or decline[60].

Most studies so far have been in untrained people. One of the few studies assessing volume in resistance trained individuals was recently conducted by Brad Schoenfeld[61]. 32 resistance trained males performed either 1, 3 or 5 sets of an exercise per session, for 3 sessions per week (i.e. 1, 9 or 15 sets per body part per week). All training volumes showed a trend for increased muscle size, but there was a significant dose-response trend for greater hypertrophy with greater training volumes[61].

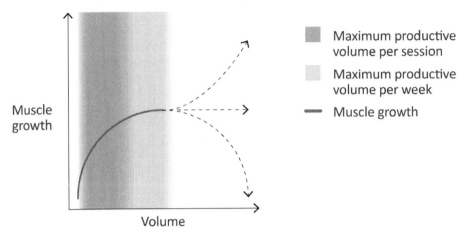

Studies show that a greater volume of sets to, or near to failure for a muscle per week (up to a point) leads to greater muscle growth. It is unclear whether higher volumes are beneficial, equivocal or detrimental (dashed line). There appears to be an upper limit to training volume per body part per session, but contention exists over whether there is a maximum weekly volume. The current general consensus is that the optimum weekly volume per body part is 10-20 sets per week, with no further benefit above 20 sets per week.

Most studies on volume compare two groups of people on a low volume or a high volume training plan. Previous studies assessing a dose-response relationship (more than two study groups) between volume and hypertrophy find a similar trend for greater growth with more volume[62,63]. The effects of different training volumes on hypertrophy have also been studied in females[64]. 40 females underwent a 24 week resistance training programme with 5, 10, 15 or 20 sets per muscle group per session. All groups increased muscle size. However, there was greater growth with 5 or 10 sets than with 15 or 20 sets. Greater growth was achieved with 15 sets than 20 sets, suggesting an inverted-U relationship. However in this study, participants performed all of the weekly volume (5, 10, 15 or 20 sets) for a body part in a *single* session, whereas previous studies split higher weekly volumes across *multiple* sessions. The same researchers suggested an inverted-U relationship in a similarly designed study conducted in males[65]. Another study comparing training frequencies of once or twice a week in trained individuals found a limit to the benefit of additional weekly volume on muscle growth[66]. There was a non-significant trend for greater growth with twice the volume across two sessions per week (9 versus 18 weekly sets), but not with triple the volume across two sessions per week (27 weekly sets). Another study where resistance trained participants performed 12, 18 or 24 sets per week across two sessions (6, 9 or 12 sets per session) for 8 weeks, found a trend for greatest muscle growth with 6 and 9 sets per session, with lowest growth with 12 sets per session[67].

Indeed, there may be an optimum limit to the amount of volume per *session*, which may be lower than the optimum amount per *week*. Menno Henselmans has summed the literature well in a publicly available article[68]. Studies showing that higher weekly volumes result in less muscle growth than lower weekly volumes use a low training frequency. Studies showing that higher weekly volumes result in greater muscle growth than lower weekly volumes use a higher training frequency (i.e. the weekly volume has been split across multiple training sessions). Due to a lack of evidence at higher volumes (>20 sets per week) and conflicting evidence in the few studies conducted at higher volumes (showing greater hypertrophy, equivalent and lower hypertrophy), it is hard to draw any meaningful conclusions about high volumes at this stage[1,22]. A greater training frequency may be necessary to achieve higher volumes that will promote greater muscle growth[13,22]. James Krieger, a prominent researcher studying training volumes for muscle growth has recently released a publicly available article supporting the importance of greater frequencies to generate additional weekly volume[69]. Other experts have also published similar views[13]. The importance of considering frequency in relation to training volume will be discussed next.

Even if much higher volumes can result in greater muscle growth, it is difficult and unnecessary to sustain very high volumes per week for every body part. Periodisation (chapter 17) can be used to plan high volume periods for specific body parts to generate a large training stimulus, followed by a period of lower volume to allow for sufficient recovery (*functional overreaching*)[3]. Other body parts can then be trained at higher volumes. As such, body part specific volume may fluctuate over time between high and low volume, but overall training volume may remain largely consistent. Using measures of intensity of effort can ensure that volume does not become too excessive and to plan when to have lower volume periods.

Some limitations of current studies are that they are short in duration. It probably takes longer than 6-8 weeks for a meaningful difference in hypertrophy to be seen between different weekly volumes. The studies are also fairly small. Having fewer participants increases the risk that there is a true difference in muscle growth with different weekly volumes, but the difference cannot be detected. This gives the appearance of no difference between different volumes (see chapter 4 regarding statistical versus real-life significance). Studies also differ in how they define volume. As mentioned, not all measures of volume are useful for hypertrophy.

Minimum, maximum and optimum levels of volume

The theoretical concept that for a given individual, there are certain amounts of volume (sets per muscle group per week) that are required to maintain muscle mass (minimum), amounts of volume above which are detrimental to muscle building goals (maximum) and a range in between which can meet the needs of the individual, depending on their current training plan (optimum).

The concept was developed by Dr Mike Israetel. For a full discussion of this concept, read 'Scientific Principles of Strength Training' and 'How Much Should I Train?'[70-72].

The amount of training volume (sets per muscle group per week) we need to perform does not need to remain constant, nor should we be continually be striving for increases in volume all the time. Progressive overload can be achieved through variables other than volume (chapter 18). No studies have compared progression with reps, load or sets, and subsequent muscle growth. The amount of volume that should be performed will depend first and foremost on the individual, training status, energy intake and specific training goals. The following discussion is largely theoretical, but is based upon the evidence from research and expert opinion.

Depending on our goal and our relative energy intake (energy surplus, deficit or maintenance), we can in *theory* consider the amount of volume we need based on how the relative energy intake affects our recovery and performance, and how much volume we need to achieve our goal. There currently appears to be a dose-response effect of increasing volume and greater muscle growth, up to a point.

Minimum maintenance volume

The minimum volume required to maintain muscle mass. For a given individual, the minimum volume is likely to be larger in a calorie deficit than in a calorie surplus, regardless of training ability.

As an untrained beginner, the *minimum maintenance volume* is zero. Untrained people do not lose muscle mass (at calorie maintenance). For people who train for a period of time and then detrain (stop lifting weights) they lose their gains in muscle mass over time (at calorie maintenance). This means with training experience, there will be an amount of training volume that is too low to maintain our current muscle mass (i.e. there is a minimum weekly volume that must be performed to maintain muscle). This will be slightly greater in trained people than untrained people or beginners, but regardless of experience, minimum volumes are comparatively similar. In complete beginners, there isn't a minimum threshold. Relative calorie intake also affects the minimum volume. When in a calorie surplus, your body has plenty of energy, storing any of the excess energy (i.e. there is less of a need to break down muscle). It is ready to build new structures, whether that be fat storage or muscle accretion. Your body is in an *anabolic* state and muscle protein synthesis is elevated, such that net protein balance is more positive. In contrast, when in a calorie deficit, your body does *not* have plenty of energy. To meet your daily calorie needs, it needs to utilise stored energy sources, such as fat mass, or fat-free mass (e.g. muscle). Your body is in a *catabolic* state. It wants to break down structures to use the energy stored in them and reduce energy expenditure. Muscle protein synthesis is reduced, such that net protein balance is more negative. Resistance training promotes muscle protein synthesis to promote a more positive net protein balance. Therefore, for a given individual the minimum training volume to maintain muscle mass in a calorie deficit is likely to be larger than at maintenance or in a surplus, regardless of training ability. Say, if 1 to 2 sets per week per body part maintains muscle mass at energy maintenance or in a surplus, then it may require 3 to 4 sets per week to maintain muscle mass in a deficit.

Minimum maintenance volume may be roughly identified by finding the minimum volume required to maintain relative strength in an exercise you are experienced in performing. In other words, if you can usually perform 10 reps on barbell squats with a given load, then if you can achieve this with only 3 sets per week, it may suggest 3 sets per week is near your minimum maintenance volume. Of course, this will also be influenced by recovery.

The *minimum effective volume* is the minimum volume required to not just maintain, but also to build muscle. It will be greater than the minimum maintenance volume, but below the maximum volume.

Maximum effective and recoverable volumes

Maximum volume can include the maximum volume that is optimal for muscle growth, and the maximum volume that it is possible to recover from. Maximum training volume is likely to be higher in a calorie surplus than in a calorie deficit. In a deficit, the body is not primed to build new tissues, and the muscle building potential is attenuated. With fewer resources, the body is less able to recover from the muscle damage incurred from the workout.

We have already mentioned that there appears to be a limit to the amount of weekly volume that leads to increases in muscle growth. We can consider this to be the *maximum effective volume* that can be performed. Volumes above this will not provide a significantly greater muscle growth stimulus, but instead promote greater fatigue, muscle damage, longer recovery times, and likely hinder long-term performance[13]. Similar to minimum volume, maximum volume is likely to be higher for expert level trainers, and lower for beginners and intermediates (with training experience, more effort is required for less reward). It will of course be higher than the minimum volume and will vary greatly between individuals. How does relative calorie intake affect this? In a calorie surplus, the body has a greater potential to grow and respond to any training stimulus. When in a calorie deficit, the body is not primed to build new tissues. With fewer resources, it is less able to recover from the muscle damage incurred from the workout. Therefore, the maximum volume is likely to be higher in a surplus than when in a calorie deficit.

Above the maximum effective volume is the *maximum recoverable volume*[13]. Any greater volume above the maximum recoverable volume is too much to adequately recover from. Very high volumes will lead to *non-functional overreaching*, and if sustained for too long, *overtraining*. This extra volume above the maximum effective volume has been termed *'junk'* volume by some researchers.

If you have training sessions that result in lots of muscle soreness for days on end after a workout, you have high ratings of perceived exertion (RPE), your performance is decreasing and you feel very fatigued after each session, it is likely you are over the maximum recoverable volume.

Overreaching and overtraining

Overreaching and overtraining have primarily been studied in endurance athletes, and partially in strength athletes. Little research has been conducted in training for muscle growth.

Overreaching can be physiologically beneficial (functional overreaching) when planned with a recovery period after a high volume phase.

Overtraining can result from excessively high volumes for long periods of time and is detrimental to performance and health.

The evidence on overreaching and overtraining is very limited, being primarily in endurance exercise, and largely anecdotal in resistance exercise[73,74]. There is only so much training that can be performed with adequate recovery. If training is excessive, it can start to result in a reduction in performance. A single training session will result in a reduction in performance that after several days, results in improved performance following recovery and adaptation. Overreaching is a short-term decline in performance after a period of intense training, at a volume approaching the maximum recoverable volume. Overtraining is a long-term decline in performance after a longer period of intense training. It is currently proposed that overtraining is an extended period of higher training volume, which is subsequent to overreaching[73]. However, very little evidence exists to demonstrate this. There is also little consensus on the signs or measures that can be used to accurately identify overreaching or overtraining, besides declines in performance[74]. Increases in volume may also involve increasing intensity and frequency. Volume and recovery are pushed to the limit so that in the short-term, performance may decrease slightly (e.g. you *feel* close to failure with your usual 10RM load after 5 or 6 reps), but this is followed by a brief period of lower volume or a 'taper' for several days or a couple of weeks[13]. *Functional overreaching* with a subsequent taper (reduced training volume) can result in the body '*supercompensating*', with an increase in performance after a few days or weeks of reduced volume[2,73,75]. The increase in performance can enable progressive overload. If high volumes are used for too long, this can result in *non-functional overreaching*, where performance does not subsequently improve. This has been seen in athletes and in power programmes, but in terms of hypertrophy, it is still speculative as to whether overreaching and overtraining actually occur. A systematic review of overtraining in resistance exercise suggested overtraining most likely occurs with frequent, monotonous, high intensity exercise[74]. One study has shown that overreaching could be a potential mechanism to achieve progressive overload, but more studies are needed[73,76]. As a beginner, you do *not* need to consider overreaching, and should probably be cautious of it as you may end up overtraining if your plan is too rigorous with a high volume. As an intermediate or advanced trainer, it may be something to consider with high volume periods focussing on different body parts, before reducing volume back down to minimum volumes to allow supercompensation and performance improvement. This also gives the muscle and the body time to adequately recover at lower volumes before a subsequent period of planned higher volume training for growth, where the muscle is more responsive to the additional stimuli[13]. On the other hand, you may decide to keep workout volume fairly constant, and opt to increase the load or number of reps performed in each session. These two methods of progression were previously discussed in chapter 18 as '*fast and hard*' and '*slow and conservative*'.

Identifying the volumes that are at or near your maximum ability to recover will require practice and experience. Gauge based on how you feel from:

- slowly increasing weekly volume (sets per muscle per week),
- to the point where recovery begins to slow down, and
- performance begins to stall or decline (which can be measured using the RIR or RPE scales).

Following an acute period of high volume (e.g. 2 to 3 months), a period of much lower volume above the minimum effective volume can then be used to allow for adequate recovery and increases in performance.

Overtraining should be avoided. It is actually described as a medical condition, with tell-tale signs such as restless sleep, very poor workouts and illness. It can take years to recover from[73]. It is much more prevalent in endurance-based disciplines and those competing at an elite level. For most people it should not be a problem, and it is unlikely you will reach this level of excessive volume.

Optimum training volume lies between the minimum and maximum volumes

We can now see that the *'optimum'* amount of volume will be within and inclusive of, the minimum and maximum volumes. Your optimum volume will change over time. What will be the optimum volume will depend on:

- Whether you are aiming to increase or maintain muscle mass.
- Whether you are in a calorie surplus, at calorie maintenance or in a calorie deficit.
- Your training experience.
- Body part specific goals.
- Other factors such as your genetics, stress levels, sleep and ability to tolerate a given amount of volume.

The *'window'* of optimum volume in a calorie deficit is much smaller (a higher minimum volume, and lower maximum volume) than the *'window'* of optimum volume in a calorie surplus (a lower minimum volume, and a higher maximum volume).

Training volume when in a calorie surplus

When in a surplus, we are in a position to build muscle. Therefore, it makes sense to increase training volume to *maximise* the muscle building stimulus. However, we also do not want to perform too much extra *'junk'* volume, because this will only serve to increase muscle damage and recovery time, with no benefit to muscle growth. Therefore, it makes sense to train at, or work towards, a volume at the upper end of the optimum volume range, near to the maximum volume. This can be monitored using the measures of intensity of effort (RIR and RPE), to assess training performance and progression as you add sets and move closer to the maximum effective volume.

Training volume when in a calorie deficit

During a caloric deficit the primary goal is weight loss. Ideally weight loss is from fat mass, and minimal losses from muscle mass. During a deficit, our ability and capacity to perform and recover from training are reduced. It is possible to build muscle during a deficit (usually seen in complete beginners or obese individuals). However, this is much more difficult than in a surplus (and not usually seen in trained individuals). When the goal is fat loss, it is much more realistic to aim to *maintain* or at the very least try to preserve as much muscle mass as possible. The amount of volume needed to maintain muscle mass is much lower than the volume required to promote increases in muscle mass. One study found only one ninth of the initial training volume was needed to preserve the muscle mass that had accrued in the initial training period in individuals aged between 20 and 35[22,77]. However, this was *not* during a calorie deficit. Calorie restriction results in a reduction in muscle protein synthesis, which can result in a more negative net protein balance. Training volume will be important in a calorie deficit to offset reductions in muscle protein synthesis from calorie restriction. Reducing volume to this extent during a caloric deficit where muscle protein synthesis is reduced will likely be insufficient to maintain muscle and also probably unnecessary. Complete detraining results in significant losses in muscle mass, even without a change in calorie intake[77].

In a calorie deficit it is unlikely we will build meaningful amounts of muscle, if at all. The additional stimulus above the minimum required volume to maintain muscle is unlikely to result in any meaningful increases in muscle mass. Therefore, it makes sense to perform as much volume as we need to maintain our current muscle mass, and not to perform too much extra volume to ensure adequate recovery. We also do not want to underestimate how much volume we need to perform to prevent unnecessary muscle loss. Therefore, it makes sense when in a calorie deficit to keep volume above the minimum volume, but lower than the maximum effective volume. This can be gauged by assessing how well you are recovering and feeling after a workout in a caloric deficit, and by estimating the significance of any muscle loss by using relative strength measures in your exercises and visual perceptions. If you are able to maintain your typical rep range for a given load for a given exercise, it suggests that your performance, recovery and muscle are likely being maintained.

If you have been in a calorie surplus for some time, your volume may be near the maximum volume in a surplus. Therefore, if transitioning from a calorie surplus to a calorie deficit, it is likely you may need to decrease your current volume to at least below the maximum volume for a deficit (which will be lower than the maximum volume for a surplus). This may only require a reduction of 1 or 2 sets per week per body part. If performance and recovery are sub-optimal, consider dropping a further set from weekly volume until performance and recovery do not further decline.

Determining your minimum, optimum and maximum volume

Unfortunately, there is *no* magic formula to calculate your required volumes. This is mainly a theoretical construct. The main take home messages are:

- In a *calorie surplus*, you are in more of a position to benefit from greatly increasing training volume and in less of a position to suffer from greatly reducing training volume.
- In a *calorie deficit*, you are in less of a position to benefit from greatly increasing training volume and in more of a position to suffer from greatly reducing training volume.
- With training experience, you will need to do slightly more weekly sets to maintain muscle mass (but not much more than an untrained person) and perform more weekly sets to build further muscle mass.

Specific numbers for minimum or maximum volumes are not possible, because volume will be highly individual to you. Trial and error is key. You should consider:

- **Training experience**. Start with lower volumes as a beginner (anywhere from 4-10 sets per body part per week). When you can no longer increase the load for a given number of reps or increase the number of reps for a given load with each successive session, gradually increase set volume (up to 10 to 20 sets per body part per week). You may then begin to vary weekly volume with higher and lower volume periods to focus on specific body parts[1,13]. As you increase volume, take note of recovery, fatigue and performance to determine when you could perform more volume, or should consider reducing volume.
- **Calorie intake.** When in a calorie deficit, aim for a volume below your maximum effective volume, low enough to ensure adequate recovery but sufficient to maintain muscle mass. When in a calorie surplus, aim for higher volumes.
- **Personal preference.** How does a given volume make you *feel*? You may find that more than 10 sets per body part in one session leaves you feeling overly fatigued and tired. You may find that 20 sets on a body part is easily attainable (although probably unlikely). If you perform a workout and find you have severe muscle ache and significant delayed onset of muscle soreness (DOMS) for several days after the workout, it could be because you used a novel exercise that targeted muscles in a manner they are significantly unaccustomed to. However, if you perform a workout with your usual exercises and find that you have severe muscle ache and significant DOMS for several days after the workout, there is probably a good chance that you performed too much volume. Excessive DOMs means that you have accumulated more muscle damage than the body can adequately recover from. Adjust your volume accordingly.

- **Exercise selection** (chapter 21). Exercise selection can have a large effect on the amount of volume performed and fatigue accrued. One set of squats *'counts'* the same as one set of leg extensions for quadriceps training volume. Yet, squats require far more mental and physical effort, and recruit secondary muscles that may not undergo a sufficient muscle building stimulus, but may still become fatigued[1]. Multiple sets of compound exercises are more demanding than multiple sets of isolation exercises. Achieving higher volumes per workout or per week is probably best achieved by adding additional isolation exercises, rather than additional compound exercises.

It can be useful to consider the typical regime that professionals use. One study conducted a survey in professionals whose aim is to maximise muscle mass (i.e. bodybuilders)[78]. During periods aimed at increasing muscle size, individuals primarily used 4-5 exercises per muscle and 3-6 sets per exercise, corresponding to 12-30 sets per muscle. It is not clear if this volume per muscle was split across weekly sessions.

Deloads

Deloads are where you take a complete break from training to allow for full recovery. It has more use and research in strength training.

Deloads can be *proactively* planned (i.e. in 6 weeks' time, have a break), such as for a holiday, or after a period of high volume. Deloads can also be *reactively* planned (i.e. feeling tired for several days and needing to take a break for the next few days), such as when life stresses are greater, or when training feels counterproductive.

Taking breaks during training will not impair muscle growth, at least in previously untrained people. Two studies show that in untrained people who subsequently take part in a resistance training programme, there is no loss in muscle size with a period of 3 weeks off over 15 weeks, or several periods of 3 weeks off over 6 months, when resuming training after the 3 week break[79,80].

Reducing volume after a planned high volume period to allow for supercompensation (subsequent improvement in performance after training) is better achieved by reducing weekly volume (i.e. fewer weekly sets by having a lower volume training session), than by completely avoiding training altogether (i.e. a deload)[13]. Avoiding long breaks without training is not recommended as this can result in muscle loss and performance decrements. But, having a few days or up to a couple weeks rest is unlikely to have any impact on muscle growth. Whether it is necessary is down to the individual. If a deload is used, keep calorie intake at calorie maintenance and avoid a calorie deficit, as this will increase the risk of muscle loss.

Even if muscle is lost, a detrained muscle has the ability to increase in size at a greater rate than if the muscle was continuously trained. This does not result in greater muscle size with detraining and retraining, but results in comparable muscle size to continuous training[80].

If you find that you need a break from training then have one, but don't feel as though you have to.

Frequency

Volume equated, frequency seems to be unimportant at lower volumes per week. At higher volumes per week, higher frequencies may be required, and subsequently result in greater muscle growth. In other words, higher frequencies allow sufficient or additional volume to be achieved which can result in greater hypertrophy, rather than the effect of a higher frequency of training in itself[81].

Training frequency refers to how often a specific body part is trained per week, not how frequently someone trains[1].

The discussion on what is an optimal frequency is still up for debate and again, dependent on the individual and their goals. Depending on how research has been analysed, it appears there could be an upper limit to the amount of volume performed per session, which is lower than the upper limit of volume per week. This therefore has implications on training frequency. When higher frequencies are used, this can *facilitate* higher weekly volumes, which may allow for greater muscle growth. However, studies are limited at this stage.

Brad Schoenfeld and James Krieger have conducted a systematic review and meta-analysis of 10 experimental studies looking at resistance training frequency and hypertrophy in healthy people. The analysis suggested a training frequency of 2 times per body part per week is best for muscle growth[82]. They argue that whether higher frequencies are more beneficial is unclear. However, their analysis only compared frequencies of 1, 2 or 3 sessions per week per body part, because no study that assessed training a body part more than 3 times per week met the inclusion criteria for the analysis. They concluded that when volume is equated across the week, there is no benefit to training 3 times per week. But, if the weekly volume performed in these studies was near to the maximum *session* volume, but far below the maximum *weekly* volume, then splitting this volume across a greater number of training sessions per week (increasing training frequency) would not be expected to be superior for hypertrophy[82].

Menno Henselmans has questioned the validity of the findings by Schoenfeld and Krieger due to the methods used in the analysis. The inclusion and exclusion criteria of studies may not have been well chosen[83]. In short, due to the grouping of different studies and the methods of reporting used to display the effects of training at different frequencies, some important implications may have been missed. In fact, there may be evidence to support the use of higher training frequencies in individuals with training experience. A recent publicly available, unpublished meta-analysis by Greg Nuckols has conducted the same analysis (to determine the effect of training frequency on muscle hypertrophy)[84]. This was performed with slightly different considerations and approaches to the Schoenfeld review. This analysis found that there was a roughly *linear* increase in the amount of muscle hypertrophy with each additional training session performed on that body part per week. Meaning, increasing training frequency facilitated higher weekly volumes, resulting in greater muscle growth. There was no plateau at or beyond 3 sessions per week. Few studies assess training frequencies over 3 times per week. It would be beneficial for more studies to include frequencies as high as this to confirm findings. In summary, there may be a case to suggest higher frequencies are associated with greater muscle growth[84]. To clarify, this is *not* a peer-reviewed study (see chapter 4 regarding research), but it has been conducted in a similar manner by an author who has previously published peer-reviewed literature. James Krieger, the author of the peer-reviewed meta-analysis has since published a publicly available article supporting the importance of frequency to generate additional weekly volume[69]. The consensus is that greater volumes should be achieved with a frequency of more than once per week. Even so, the question of how to optimise frequency for hypertrophy is still inconclusive.

Are you performing too much volume per body part, per session?

Have you ever been training and found that you are lacking the energy or motivation to perform your last exercise or sets in the session? Quite possibly you performed your final exercise half-heartedly or skipped the exercise altogether. If this exercise was performed first, or on a completely separate day, the set workload and level of effort you would achieve would be far greater. You are *least* fatigued (both central and peripheral fatigue) for the first one or two exercises for a body part in a session. Fatigue accumulates with *every* set, and therefore fatigue is present when performing *any* subsequent exercises and sets later in the workout. Also, motivation to train will decrease with the duration of a workout. Therefore, the load, reps or number of sets you can perform are limited with each successive set. If these latter sets were moved to a separate day of training, it is more than likely you would be able to perform more reps for a given load, use a heavier load for a given number of reps, or perform more sets. These sets would be more conducive to progressive overload. As discussed later in chapter 21, body parts of interest should be prioritised and performed first in a workout. If weekly volume is relatively low (e.g. one or two exercises and 4-6 sets), then spreading this volume across multiple days would make little difference to the set workload performed and stress placed on the muscle, because you are still relatively unfatigued by set 5 or 6. If weekly volume is relatively high (e.g. 4 or more exercises and 12 or more sets), then spreading this volume across multiple days may be beneficial, as a greater set workload and therefore greater meaningful stress can be placed on a muscle than if it were all performed in one single session. This is because say, by the 12th or 13th set for a muscle in a session, you have accumulated a large amount of fatigue, resulting in a reduced set workload compared to if you had performed that 12th or 13th set in the first 1-6 sets of the workout, for example. In other words, you are too tired to train productively. An easy way to gauge if your last exercise and latter sets are 'junk' volume and of little benefit is to perform them at the beginning of a subsequent workout, and compare the number of reps completed to failure for the same load. If you can perform 5 or more additional reps when performing that exercise or set first instead of last in the workout, then those sets at the end of the workout would probably be best performed in a separate workout on another day.

A recent study in young resistance trained males compared training a body part with high weekly volume once per week, or splitting the high training volume for the given body part across 5 sessions per week. The study found meaningfully greater hypertrophy with the 5 days per week split[85]. The 5 days per week group performed significantly more volume across the 8 week training programme. The exercises and number of sets performed were the *same*, with participants instructed to train to muscular task failure. But, by splitting muscle-specific volume across the week, this allowed a greater set workload to be performed (i.e. more reps per set for a given load to failure). Even though sets were equated, if the latter sets in the workouts of the 1 day per week group were performed fatigued, then sets would reach premature failure primarily through central nervous system fatigue, not peripheral fatigue. This would result in an insufficient number of high-threshold motor units being recruited despite the high level of perceived exertion by reaching failure. This could explain why the 5 days per week group gained greater muscle and performed a greater set workload (reps per set) across the 8 weeks. Of note, both groups experienced similar ratings of perceived exertion after each workout. The 5 days per week group performed greater total workload, but with similar perceptions of exertion. Indeed, when studies try to equate workload with different frequencies, this is pretty much *impossible* without the higher frequency group exerting lower intensities of effort. As Henselmans notes, a new meta-analysis needs to equate weekly sets, but not weekly reps or workload[83]. Even if you feel as though you are working very hard, trying to perform as many sets as possible on a specific body part in one session will be counter-productive.

Another theory as to why a greater frequency results in greater muscle growth is that only a relatively low number of sets are needed to stimulate muscle protein synthesis in a muscle in a given session. Splitting training volume for a given body part across several sessions may elevate muscle protein synthesis more efficiently across the week[85].

As discussed during the volume section, there may be an optimum limit to the amount of volume per session, which is likely lower than the optimum amount per week. Menno Henselmans has summed the literature in a publicly available article[68]. Studies using higher weekly volumes with a *worse* outcome in muscle growth use a *low* frequency. Studies using similar or higher weekly volumes with a *better* outcome in muscle growth use a *high* frequency (i.e. the weekly volume has been split across multiple training sessions).

Therefore, any increase in muscle growth when moving from a low training frequency to a moderate training frequency is probably because this increases weekly training volume when individual training session volumes have been maximised. The role of further increases in frequency to increase total weekly volume above 10-20 sets per body part per week, or the role of training frequency itself to drive hypertrophy is still under debate by experts[82–84].

This suggests that when training a given body part with lower weekly volumes (10 sets or less), a lower frequency of training a given body part is sufficient. A higher training frequency for a given body part would not be of superior benefit. For example, training a muscle with 3-4 sets per session over multiple sessions resulting in 10-12 weekly sets would produce similar muscle growth as a single weekly session of 10-12 sets. However, when using higher weekly volumes for a given body part or when reaching the maximum volume for a given body part per session, it may be beneficial to split this volume across more than one session per week (i.e. training a given muscle with 8-10 sets per session, twice per week (16-20 weekly sets), would result in greater muscle growth than a single weekly session of 16-20 sets). When training a given body part with a volume well below the maximum session volume, higher frequencies per week may be required to achieve the same amount of weekly volume as training a given body part once per week at or near the maximum session volume. The weekly *training split* you choose to follow will be based on your personal preference and is discussed next in chapter 20.

There appears to be an upper limit to training volume per body part per session, but contention exists over whether there is a maximum weekly volume. General consensus is that optimum weekly volume per body part is 10-20 sets per week, with no further benefit above 20 sets per week. Further research will reveal if this is the case. There is evidence to suggest that higher volumes may be beneficial. It is highly likely to be dependent on how the volume is generated (i.e. by considering frequency and other variables). At the lower end of weekly volume

(5-10 sets), one session per week is sufficient. At the higher end (10-20 sets), 2 or more sessions per week will be more beneficial to achieve the higher volume. This volume should be split evenly such that each session volume is maximised. If you perform 12 sets for a body part in a session and decide to split this volume across two sessions, split the volume evenly and perform a similar number of sets in each session. Perform 5-7 sets in each session, not 10 in one session and 2 in the other[81]. Then subsequently increase the load, reps and volume to progressively overload.

How to maximise training frequency

If higher frequencies allow for greater muscle growth from greater weekly volumes and therefore greater muscle growth, how can we train a body part as often as possible?

Maximum training frequency requires finding an optimum balance between generating sufficient volume (training stimulus) for a given muscle per workout, without accumulating excessive levels of muscle damage and fatigue. A resistance training workout can elevate muscle protein synthesis in a muscle for 24-72 hours after the workout. There will be diminishing returns in terms of additional sets in the same workout on a given body part to produce stimulating volume versus accumulating fatigue.

Greater fatigue will require greater recovery time.

To maximise training frequency for a particular muscle, avoid excessive volumes per session, slow rep tempos, short rest periods, advanced training techniques, excessive eccentric (muscle lengthening) contractions and reaching failure. These all generate large amounts of muscle damage[1]. Therefore, to maximise training frequency, use a relatively low to moderate volume per body part per session, longer rest periods, fast contractions speeds (tempos) and standard sets close to, but not reaching failure. Frequency will also be influenced by exercise selection and the muscle group trained. Exercise selection is important in maximising the stimulus to grow, and minimising fatigue.

The frequency at which it is possible to train and whether it is or necessary to train a certain muscle again depends on two factors:

1. Whether muscle protein synthesis is still elevated in a muscle.
2. How fatigued the muscle is. When can the next productive workout be performed where progressive overload can be achieved?

Is muscle protein synthesis still elevated in the muscle following the last workout?

The goal of a resistance training session is to stimulate and elevate muscle protein synthesis, which drives muscle growth. Muscle protein synthesis can be elevated for up to 2-3 days after a training session. Resistance training the same muscle during this period would *not* benefit muscle growth as there would be no additional meaningful increase in muscle protein synthesis. Therefore, if protein synthesis is still elevated in a muscle from the last resistance training session, a further resistance training session will not be of benefit to hypertrophy. Therefore, the first consideration for maximising training frequency is to consider the duration of elevated muscle protein synthesis after a training session in the muscle of interest. There is no need to train the muscle again until it returns to, or near to baseline. This is influenced by training status. Post-workout muscle protein synthesis is elevated for longer in untrained than trained individuals[86]. Studies show that in untrained individuals, muscle protein synthesis can still be elevated up to 72 hours after the training session. In trained individuals, the elevation in muscle protein is usually less than 24 hours[86]. With little to no training experience, training twice a week may elevate muscle protein synthesis in a muscle for the whole duration of the week, possibly three times with more experience. With training experience, it is feasible and possibly beneficial to train at higher frequencies. Of course, without invasive tests, this is impossible to measure. Therefore, a more useful method may be to judge how frequently we can train a muscle whilst increasing performance from the previous session. This will be based on fatigue and how long recovery takes.

How fatigued is the muscle?

The second factor for maximising training frequency is to consider how long after the training session does it take for the muscle to fully recover, or at least recover to a state where training is again productive. The main factor determining the second point is the amount of muscle damage that has occurred during the session. Mechanical tension drives muscle growth, but generating sufficient mechanical tension can also result in muscle damage. Other factors also increase muscle damage, including:

- High workout volumes and high rep workouts.
- Training to failure, which can add 1 to 2 days onto recovery time[45].
- Eccentric contractions (lowering the weight)[87].
- Short rest periods.
- Performing novel exercises.
- Advanced training techniques (chapter 23).

If you performed a high volume workout with lots of sets to failure, lots of eccentric reps, short rest periods and some novel exercises, you'll probably find that the trained muscle is aching and sore for several days after the session. Muscle damage can be counter-productive as it can result in DOMS (delayed onset of muscle soreness from exercise-induced muscle damage) and impair performance in the days after a workout (chapter 17 discussed why DOMS is not a useful marker of a good workout for hypertrophy). This can reduce the frequency at which that body part can be trained. It appears that muscle protein synthesis directed towards growth does *not* increase linearly with volume for a given muscle in a workout, but muscle damage will continue to increase. Muscle damage promotes muscle protein synthesis, but this is directed towards repair, not growth (see graph below). There is a point of diminishing returns, where increasing training volume for a given muscle in a workout will result in relatively more muscle damage than stimulation of muscle growth. This can be counter-productive for maximising the frequency of training[1].

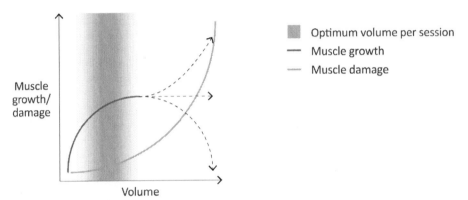

There appears to be an upper limit to training volume per body part per session. A greater number of sets per session results in greater muscle growth, up to a point. A greater number of sets per session results in greater muscle damage.

This theoretical concept has been formalised by Dr. Mike Israetel as the *fitness:fatigue* model, or the *stimulus:fatigue* ratio. For a full discussion of this concept, read the *'Scientific Principles of Strength Training'*[70]. We want to maximise fitness and minimise fatigue with each session and across the week. A greater stimulus and less fatigue means that we can generate the same results with less work and effort, or be able to generate greater results through a greater ability to increase work capacity.

Evidence shows that recovery from muscle damage and muscle growth adaptations involve similar mechanisms (both promoting elevated muscle protein synthesis from disturbing the integrity of the muscle), but greater muscle damage does *not* appear to increase muscle growth (chapter 17)[3]. Eccentric contractions (muscle lengthening), slow rep tempos and short rest periods produce large amounts of muscle damage. Slow rep tempos and short rest periods are of no superior benefit to muscle growth. Therefore, to minimise muscle damage and to maximise the ability to train a particular muscle as frequently as possible:

- Use longer rest periods.
- Use minimal exercise variation.
- Focus on concentric contractions (muscle shortening), avoiding prolonged eccentric contraction (muscle lengthening) durations.

If you train a muscle once per week, the need to minimise muscle damage is probably unnecessary as 6 days rest will be plenty of time to recover from even the most damaging of workouts[45]. If training a body part once per week, you can probably get away with more sets to failure, higher volumes, and advanced training techniques. Any accrued muscle damage will have dissipated by the time you train again next week. Even so, such techniques have *not* been shown to result in greater muscle growth. Just because you may be able to recover from greater muscle damage, does not mean such strategies will benefit muscle growth. If you are splitting your training across 2 or more sessions during the week, minimising excessive muscle damage in each session and maximising stimulating volume will become more important.

The ability to recover from a workout will depend on the individual and the body part being trained. Unsurprisingly, there is large variation between people in how long it takes to recover from the same workout[88]. Decrements in muscle performance following a workout are also body part specific. A study into the ability of the main muscle groups to recover from an exercise session using eccentric contractions (muscle lengthening) in 15 untrained men found that strength was reduced the most in the pectoralis major (chest), elbow flexors (e.g. biceps) and elbow extensors (e.g. triceps). There were large decrements in strength even 2 to 3 days after the workout[88]. Delayed onset of muscle soreness (DOMS) was greatest in the elbow flexors (e.g. biceps), extensors (e.g. triceps) and erector spinae. Muscle damage will attenuate over time when performing the same workout again, with faster rates of recovery after subsequent workouts compared to after the first novel workout (the *repeated bout effect*)[88]. Some muscle groups may require longer than others to recover after a muscle damaging workout. This will largely come down to how you *feel* in the days after your workout and the ability to gauge whether your workout will impair the ability to train that muscle again a few days later. Judging recovery time will come with experience and as you settle into a routine, such that successive sessions become similar in the stimulus and stress they produce. Adequate recovery time can be easily gauged by asking yourself, '*how many days after my last chest workout (or any other body part) do I find I am able to achieve similar or greater performance (i.e. progressive overload of sets, reps or load) in the next chest workout?'.* Bear in mind, this will also be dependent on other factors including your overall training frequency, recovery from other body parts and general life stress.

How to work out the weekly training frequency and volume you need

The frequency and volume you need will depend on how you aim to progress. Your training frequency and volume are not static and can change over time.

Progression with extra sets per week may be benefitted by training a body part with higher frequencies.

Progression by increasing the load and/or reps within the same number of sets at low to moderate volumes will suffice with low training frequencies.

Progression by increasing the load and/or reps within the same number of sets at moderate to high volumes will require higher training frequencies. This is also the highest workload and volume. This may be best suited to intermediate and advanced trainers.

You can use your training experience to guide your training programme. This ensures you are training at a frequency and volume suitable for your experience. Training frequency and total volume will be dependent on what you are personally able to perform, your ability to generally recover and for the specific muscle to recover.

Assessing how *'trained'* someone is, is highly subjective. Training status is often judged either by the duration of training experience, or by the rate of progression. Someone may have been resistance training for several years, but with poor technique. Use the guidelines below as a rough measure. If in doubt, keep things *simpler* (e.g. lower volume and lower frequency) which will aid the ability to *adhere* to any plan.

Beginner or untrained

Someone who has never resistance trained before, or a previously trained individual who has stopped resistance training for a considerable length of time (e.g. 6-12 months of detraining).

Progression in reps and load is possible from session to session.

Following the expert opinion of James Krieger in his publicly available article, achieving 4-6 high quality working sets per body part per week at a high intensity of effort as a beginner may be a lot of volume for some. If so, start as low as 2 to 3 sets per body part per week[69]. Focus on increasing the load and reps within the low volume of sets as a complete beginner. As James Krieger has pointed out, untrained individuals do not respond particularly well to increases in volume[69]. Fewer meaningful, productive sets are more useful for muscle growth (and produce a better *stimulus:fatigue* ratio) than many poor quality, unproductive sets. A lower training volume is also lower commitment, less stressful and easier to adhere to, helping to create the habit of training. Depending on your training split, volume may only be performed once per week per body part. If you prefer, or if you struggle to achieve more than 4-6 productive sets per body part per session, you might choose to say, train the whole body three times per week (with much lower volume per workout per body part). At low volumes, choose the frequency that you can *adhere* to. When the rate of progression with load and/or reps slows down, consider adding sets to increase volume. By which time you will probably be considered an intermediately trained individual after several months of training.

Intermediate

Someone with at least 3 to 6 months of resistance training experience.

Progression in reps, sets and load is possible on a week to week, or month to month basis.

Being *'resistance trained'* has been defined as having at least 6 months of resistance training experience, but definitions vary[89]. As an intermediate, the volume at which you should train should increase from when you were a beginner, and can fluctuate. It will be beneficial to train with a frequency greater than once per week per body part, because this allows for greater weekly volume when training session volume has been maximised. Achieving the upper ends of the optimum training volume of 10-20 sets per muscle per week would probably require multiple sessions across the week.

When transitioning from one session of say, 6-8 sets, to two sessions per week for a body part, split the volume equally between sessions. Start at 3-4 sets for each session (i.e. maintaining your original training volume), and slowly add volume to each session over time whilst monitoring perceptions of exertion after the workouts to ensure adequate recovery.

Again, these are *averages*. You may struggle with more than 2 or 3 sets per body part per session or you may perform 10 sets within one session and adequately recover. Most people will fall within the range of 6-8 sets[69].

Experienced

Someone with at least 24 months of resistance training experience.

Progression in reps, sets and load is possible on a month to month, or on a several monthly basis.

As an experienced trainer, the volume and therefore frequency of training may need to be greater. Phases of increased frequencies to facilitate planned periods of higher weekly volumes above 20 working sets may be useful to develop a lagging body part, or to focus on a body part of particular interest. This can be a useful tool for progression before returning to lower volumes to allow for adequate recovery and adaptation. This would require reduced volume for other body parts to prevent overall volume from becoming excessive. Low training volumes can adequately maintain muscle mass in a calorie surplus. Therefore, during periods of high volume for a given body part, other body parts can be trained at a reduced volume near the *minimum maintenance* or *minimum effective volumes*. This allows extra time to be devoted to training the body part of interest and to help manage overall fatigue. This concept of prioritising certain body parts over others can achieved using periodisation and autoregulation (chapter 18).

A summary of the basic outline for volume and frequency depending on training status:

- **Beginner or untrained:** minimal to no training experience. Start at 4-6 sets per body part per week and increase the reps and load within sets.
- **Intermediate:** at least 3-6 months experience. Progress up to 10-20 sets per body part per week.
- **Experienced**: at least 24+ months experience. 10-20 sets per body part per week with planned high volume periods (>20 sets per week) for given body parts for around 2 to 3 months[69].

Tracking sessions

Clearly, keeping a record and tracking how you perform in each set, each session and each week will become important to monitor whether progressive overload is occurring. What to monitor and how to track has been covered in previous chapters. As an overview, tracking of multiple measures can be achieved in numerous ways:

Tools:

- Pen and paper
- Phone app
- Spreadsheet

Variables:

- Number of sets per session
- Number of sets per week
- Number of reps
- Load used
- Rating of perceived exertion (RPE) / reps in reserve (RIR) at the end of each set and at the end of the session

It can be very useful to make additional notes to aid your training. For example:

- Did that particular set feel lighter than usual? Was the set too heavy or too easy?
- Did you perform more or less reps than expected?
- Were the reps well controlled?
- Did you use momentum in the final few reps?
- Was there a half rep?
- Did you fail a rep?
- Did you use rest pause or other advanced techniques (chapter 23)?
- Did you feel good?

You don't need to consciously track all these variables all of the time, but being aware of them can help you to focus on following the basic training principles. Some key variables to consider tracking would be the number of sets performed per week for a muscle, and the reps and loads used within those sets. This can help to see if progressive overload is taking place, and whether you may need to make changes.

References

1   Wernbom M, Augustsson J, Thomeé R. The influence of frequency, intensity, volume and mode of strength training on whole muscle cross-sectional area in humans. *Sports Med Auckl NZ* 2007; 37: 225–264.

2   Kraemer WJ, Ratamess NA. Fundamentals of resistance training: progression and exercise prescription. *Med Sci Sports Exerc* 2004; 36: 674–688.

3   Schoenfeld BJ. The Mechanisms of Muscle Hypertrophy and Their Application to Resistance Training. *J Strength Cond Res* 2010; 24: 2857–2872.

4   Carpinelli R, Otto R, Wientt R. A critical analysis of the ACSM position stand on resistance training: Insufficient evidence to support recommended training protocols. *J Exerc Physiol Online* 2004; 7.

5   Grgic J, Schoenfeld BJ. Higher effort, rather than higher load, for resistance exercise-induced activation of muscle fibres. *J Physiol* 2019; 597: 4691–4692.

6   Schoenfeld BJ, Peterson MD, Ogborn D, Contreras B, Sonmez GT. Effects of Low- vs. High-Load Resistance Training on Muscle Strength and Hypertrophy in Well-Trained Men. *J Strength Cond Res* 2015; 29: 2954–2963.

7   Morton RW, Sonne MW, Farias Zuniga A, Mohammad IYZ, Jones A, McGlory C et al. Muscle fibre activation is unaffected by load and repetition duration when resistance exercise is performed to task failure. *J Physiol* 2019; 597: 4601–4613.

8   Morton RW, Colenso-Semple L, Phillips SM. Training for strength and hypertrophy: an evidence-based approach. *Curr Opin Physiol* 2019; 10: 90–95.

9   Varela-Sanz A, Tuimil JL, Abreu L, Boullosa DA. Does Concurrent Training Intensity Distribution Matter? *J Strength Cond Res* 2017; 31: 181–195.

10   Lasevicius T, Ugrinowitsch C, Schoenfeld BJ, Roschel H, Tavares LD, De Souza EO et al. Effects of different intensities of resistance training with equated volume load on muscle strength and hypertrophy. *Eur J Sport Sci* 2018; 18: 772–780.

11   Haun CT, Mumford PW, Roberson PA, Romero MA, Mobley CB, Kephart WC et al. Molecular, neuromuscular, and recovery responses to light versus heavy resistance exercise in young men. *Physiol Rep* 2017; 5: e13457.

12   Helms ER, Cronin J, Storey A, Zourdos MC. Application of the Repetitions in Reserve-Based Rating of Perceived Exertion Scale for Resistance Training. *Strength Cond J* 2016; 38: 42–49.

13   Israetel M, Feather J, Faleiro TV, Juneau C-E. Mesocycle Progression in Hypertrophy: Volume Versus Intensity. *Strength Cond J* 2020; Publish Ahead of Print. Available from: doi:10.1519/SSC.0000000000000518.

14   Pareja-Blanco F, Villalba-Fernández A, Cornejo-Daza PJ, Sánchez-Valdepeñas J, González-Badillo JJ. Time Course of Recovery Following Resistance Exercise with Different Loading Magnitudes and Velocity Loss in the Set. *Sports Basel Switz* 2019; 7. Available from: doi:10.3390/sports7030059.

15   Juneau C-E, Tafur L. Over time, load mediates muscular hypertrophy in resistance training. *Curr Opin Physiol* 2019; 11: 147–148.

16   Rodríguez-Rosell D, Yáñez-García JM, Torres-Torrelo J, Mora-Custodio R, Marques MC, González-Badillo JJ. Effort Index as a Novel Variable for Monitoring the Level of Effort During Resistance Exercises. *J Strength Cond Res* 2018; 32: 2139–2153.

17   Grgic J, Schoenfeld BJ. Are the Hypertrophic Adaptations to High and Low-Load Resistance Training Muscle Fiber Type Specific? *Front. Physiol.* 2018 Available from: doi:10.3389/fphys.2018.00402.

18   Schiaffino S, Reggiani C. Fiber types in mammalian skeletal muscles. *Physiol Rev* 2011; 91: 1447–1531.

19   Fisher J, Steele J, Bruce-Low S, Smith D. Evidence-Based Resistance Training Recommendations. *Med Sport* 2011; 15: 147–162.

20   Ogborn D, Schoenfeld BJ. The Role of Fiber Types in Muscle Hypertrophy: Implications for Loading Strategies. *Strength Cond J* 2014; 36: 20–25.

21   Sadri K, Khani M, Sadri I. Role of Central Fatigue in Resistance and Endurance Exercises: An Emphasis on Mechanisms and Potential Sites. *Sportlogia* 2014; 10: 65–80.

22   Schoenfeld B, Grgic J. Evidence-Based Guidelines for Resistance Training Volume to Maximize Muscle Hypertrophy. *J Strength Cond Res* 2017 Available from: doi:10.1519/SSC.0000000000000363.

23   Nuckols G. *Training Based On Muscle Fiber Type: Are You Missing Out?* 2016. Available from: https://www.strongerbyscience.com/muscle-fiber-type/ (accessed 9 Feb 2020).

24   Shimano T, Kraemer WJ, Spiering BA, Volek JS, Hatfield DL, Silvestre R et al. Relationship between the number of repetitions and selected percentages of one repetition maximum in free weight exercises in trained and untrained men. *J Strength Cond Res* 2006; 20: 819–823.

25   Rippetoe M. *Training Female Lifters: Neuromuscular Efficiency.* Available from: https://startingstrength.com/article/training_female_lifters_neuromuscular_efficiency (accessed 10 Feb 2020).

26   Flanagan SD, Mills MD, Sterczala AJ, Mala J, Comstock BA, Szivak TK et al. The relationship between muscle action and repetition maximum on the squat and bench press in men and women. *J Strength Cond Res* 2014; 28: 2437–2442.

27   Hoeger WWK, Hopkins DR, Barette SL, Hale DF. Relationship between Repetitions and Selected percentages of One Repetition Maximum: A Comparison between Untrained and Trained Males and Females. *J Strength Cond Res* 1990; 4: 47–54.

28   Richens B, Cleather DJ. The relationship between the number of repetitions performed at given intensities is different in endurance and strength trained athletes. *Biol Sport* 2014; 31: 157–161.

29   Taylor JL, Gandevia SC. A comparison of central aspects of fatigue in submaximal and maximal voluntary contractions. *J Appl Physiol Bethesda Md* 2008; 104: 542–550.

30   Thomas K, Brownstein CG, Dent J, Parker P, Goodall S, Howatson G. Neuromuscular Fatigue and Recovery after Heavy Resistance, Jump, and Sprint Training. *Med Sci Sports Exerc* 2018; 50: 2526–2535.

31   Zając A, Chalimoniuk M, Maszczyk A, Gołaś A, Lngfort J. Central and Peripheral Fatigue During Resistance Exercise – A Critical Review. *J Hum Kinet* 2015; 49: 159–169.

32   Sundberg CW, Fitts RH. Bioenergetic basis of skeletal muscle fatigue. *Curr Opin Physiol* 2019; 10: 118–127.

33   Weavil JC, Amann M. Neuromuscular fatigue during whole body exercise. *Curr Opin Physiol* 2019; 10: 128–136.

34   Beardsley C. *Hypertrophy: Muscle fiber growth caused by mechanical tension*. Strength and Conditioning Research Limited, 2019. Available from: https://www.strengthandconditioningresearch.com (accessed 5 Feb 2020)

35   Tillaar R van den, Andersen V, Saeterbakken AH. Comparison of muscle activation and kinematics during free-weight back squats with different loads. *PLOS ONE* 2019; 14: e0217044.

36   Nuckols G. *The Evidence is Lacking for 'Effective Reps'*. 2019. Available from: https://www.strongerbyscience.com/effective-reps/ (accessed 10 Feb 2020).

37   Baz-Valle E, Fontes-Villalba M, Santos-Concejero J. Total Number of Sets as a Training Volume Quantification Method for Muscle Hypertrophy: A Systematic Review. *J Strength Cond Res* 2018. Available from: doi:10.1519/JSC.0000000000002776.

38   Duncan MJ, Weldon A, Price MJ. The Effect of Sodium Bicarbonate Ingestion on Back Squat and Bench Press Exercise to Failure. *J Strength Cond Res* 2014; 28: 1358–1366.

39   Santos WDND, Vieira CA, Bottaro M, Nunes VA, Ramirez-Campillo R, Steele J et al. Resistance Training Performed to Failure or Not to Failure Results in Similar Total Volume, but With Different Fatigue and Discomfort Levels. *J Strength Cond Res* 2019. Available from: doi:10.1519/JSC.0000000000002915.

40   Martorelli S, Cadore EL, Izquierdo M, Celes R, Martorelli A, Cleto VA et al. Strength Training with Repetitions to Failure does not Provide Additional Strength and Muscle Hypertrophy Gains in Young Women. *Eur J Transl Myol* 2017; 27. Available from: doi:10.4081/ejtm.2017.6339.

41   Sampson JA, Groeller H. Is repetition failure critical for the development of muscle hypertrophy and strength? *Scand J Med Sci Sports* 2016; 26: 375–383.

42   Nóbrega SR, Libardi CA. Is Resistance Training to Muscular Failure Necessary? *Front Physiol* 2016; 7. Available from: doi:10.3389/fphys.2016.00010.

43   Goto K, Ishii N, Kizuka T, Takamatsu K. The impact of metabolic stress on hormonal responses and muscular adaptations. *Med Sci Sports Exerc* 2005; 37: 955–963.

44   Contreras B. *How important is psychological stress for your gains?* 2015. Available from: https://bretcontreras.com/how-important-is-psychological-stress-for-your-gains/ (accessed 9 Feb 2020).

45   Schoenfeld BJ, Grgic J. Does Training to Failure Maximize Muscle Hypertrophy? *Strength Cond J* 2019; 41: 108–113.

46   Timmons JA. Variability in training-induced skeletal muscle adaptation. *J Appl Physiol* 2011; 110: 846–853.

47   Zourdos MC, Klemp A, Dolan C, Quiles JM, Schau KA, Jo E et al. Novel Resistance Training-Specific Rating of Perceived Exertion Scale Measuring Repetitions in Reserve. *J Strength Cond Res* 2016; 30: 267–275.

48   Pageaux B. Perception of effort in Exercise Science: Definition, measurement and perspectives. *Eur J Sport Sci* 2016; 16: 885–894.

49   Borg G. *Borg's Perceived Exertion And Pain Scales*. Human Kinetics 1998.

50   Hackett DA, Johnson NA, Halaki M, Chow C-M. A novel scale to assess resistance-exercise effort. *J Sports Sci* 2012; 30: 1405–1413.

51   Ormsbee MJ, Carzoli JP, Klemp A, Allman BR, Zourdos MC, Kim J-S et al. Efficacy of the Repetitions in Reserve-Based Rating of Perceived Exertion for the Bench Press in Experienced and Novice Benchers. *J Strength Cond Res* 2019; 33: 337–345.

52   Schoenfeld B, Grgic J, Ogborn D, Krieger J. Strength and hypertrophy adaptations between low- versus high-load resistance training: A systematic review and meta-analysis. *J Strength Cond Res* 2017. Available from: doi:10.1519/JSC.0000000000002200.

53   Krieger JW. Single vs. multiple sets of resistance exercise for muscle hypertrophy: a meta-analysis. *J Strength Cond Res* 2010; 24: 1150–1159.

54   Hammarström D, Øfsteng S, Koll L, Hanestadhaugen M, Hollan I, Apró W et al. Benefits of higher resistance-training volume are related to ribosome biogenesis. *J Physiol* 2020; 598: 543–565.

55   La Scala Teixeira CV, Motoyama Y, de Azevedo PHSM, Evangelista AL, Steele J, Bocalini DS. Effect of resistance training set volume on upper body muscle hypertrophy: are more sets really better than less? *Clin Physiol Funct Imaging* 2018; 38: 727–732.

56   Morton RW, Colenso-Semple L, Phillips SM. Training for strength and hypertrophy: an evidence-based approach. *Curr Opin Physiol* 2019; 11: 149–150.

57   Carlson L, Jonker B, Westcott WL, Steele J, Fisher JP. Neither repetition duration nor number of muscle actions affect strength increases, body composition, muscle size, or fasted blood glucose in trained males and females. *Appl Physiol Nutr Metab Physiol Appl Nutr Metab* 2019; 44: 200–207.

58   Wilk M, Golas A, Stastny P, Nawrocka M, Krzysztofik M, Zajac A. Does Tempo of Resistance Exercise Impact Training Volume? *J Hum Kinet* 2018; 62: 241–250.

59   Counts BR, Buckner SL, Dankel SJ, Jessee MB, Mattocks KT, Mouser JG et al. The acute and chronic effects of "NO LOAD" resistance training. *Physiol Behav* 2016; 164: 345–352.

60   Schoenfeld BJ, Ogborn D, Krieger JW. Dose-response relationship between weekly resistance training volume and increases in muscle mass: A systematic review and meta-analysis. *J Sports Sci* 2017; 35: 1073–1082.

61   Schoenfeld BJ, Contreras B, Krieger J, Grgic J, Delcastillo K, Belliard R et al. Resistance Training Volume Enhances Muscle Hypertrophy but Not Strength in Trained Men. *Med Sci Sports Exerc* 2019; 51: 94–103.

62   Ostrowski K, Wilson G, Weatherby R, Murphy P, Lyttle A. The Effect of Weight Training Volume on Hormonal Output and Muscular Size and Function. *J Strength Cond Res* 1997; 11. Available from: doi:10.1519/1533-4287(1997)011<0148:TEOWTV>2.3.CO;2.

63   Radaelli R, Fleck SJ, Leite T, Leite RD, Pinto RS, Fernandes L et al. Dose-response of 1, 3, and 5 sets of resistance exercise on strength, local muscular endurance, and hypertrophy. *J Strength Cond Res* 2015; 29: 1349–1358.

64   Barbalho M, Coswig VS, Steele J, Fisher JP, Paoli A, Gentil P. Evidence for an Upper Threshold for Resistance Training Volume in Trained Women. *Med Sci Sports Exerc* 2019; 51: 515–522.

65   Barbalho M, Coswig VS, Steele J, Fisher JP, Giessing J, Gentil P. Evidence of a Ceiling Effect for Training Volume in Muscle Hypertrophy and Strength in Trained Men—Less is More? *Int J Sports Physiol Perform* 2020; 15: 268–277.

66   Heaselgrave SR, Blacker J, Smeuninx B, McKendry J, Breen L. Dose-Response Relationship of Weekly Resistance-Training Volume and Frequency on Muscular Adaptations in Trained Men. *Int J Sports Physiol Perform* 2019; 14: 360–368.

67   Aube D, Wadhi T, Rauch J, Anand A, Barakat C, Pearson J et al. Progressive Resistance Training Volume: Effects on Muscle Thickness, Mass, and Strength Adaptations in Resistance-Trained Individuals. *J Strength Cond Res* 2020; Publish Ahead of Print. Available from: doi:10.1519/JSC.0000000000003524.

68   Henselmans M. *Is there a maximum productive training volume per session?* 2019. Available from: https://mennohenselmans.com/maximum-productive-training-volume-per-session/ (accessed 10 Feb 2020).

69   Krieger J. *Set Volume for Muscle Size: The Ultimate Evidence Based Bible.* Available from: https://weightology.net/the-members-area/evidence-based-guides/set-volume-for-muscle-size-the-ultimate-evidence-based-bible/ (accessed 10 Feb 2020).

70   Renaissance Periodization. *Scientific Principles of Strength Training.* Available from: https://renaissanceperiodization.com/scientific-principles-of-strength-training (accessed 10 Feb 2020).

71   Renaissance Periodization. *Training Volume Landmarks for Muscle Growth.* Available from: https://renaissanceperiodization.com/expert-advice/training-volume-landmarks-muscle-growth (accessed 10 Feb 2020).

72   Renaissance Periodization. *How Much Should I Train?* Available from: https://renaissanceperiodization.com/shop/how-much-should-i-train/ (accessed 11 Feb 2020).

73   Halson SL, Jeukendrup AE. Does overtraining exist? An analysis of overreaching and overtraining research. *Sports Med Auckl NZ* 2004; 34: 967–981.

74   Grandou C, Wallace L, Impellizzeri FM, Allen NG, Coutts AJ. Overtraining in Resistance Exercise: An Exploratory Systematic Review and Methodological Appraisal of the Literature. *Sports Med Auckl NZ* 2019. Available from: doi:10.1007/s40279-019-01242-2.

75   Aubry A, Hausswirth C, Louis J, Coutts AJ, Buchheit M, Le Meur Y. The Development of Functional Overreaching Is Associated with a Faster Heart Rate Recovery in Endurance Athletes. *PLoS ONE* 2015; 10. Available from: doi:10.1371/journal.pone.0139754.

76   Bjørnsen T, Wernbom M, Løvstad A, Paulsen G, D'Souza RF, Cameron-Smith D et al. Delayed myonuclear addition, myofiber hypertrophy, and increases in strength with high-frequency low-load blood flow restricted training to volitional failure. *J Appl Physiol Bethesda Md* 2019; 126: 578–592.

77   Bickel CS, Cross JM, Bamman MM. Exercise dosing to retain resistance training adaptations in young and older adults. *Med Sci Sports Exerc* 2011; 43: 1177–1187.

78   Hackett DA, Johnson NA, Chow C-M. Training practices and ergogenic aids used by male bodybuilders. *J Strength Cond Res* 2013; 27: 1609–1617.

79   Ogasawara R, Yasuda T, Sakamaki M, Ozaki H, Abe T. Effects of periodic and continued resistance training on muscle CSA and strength in previously untrained men. *Clin Physiol Funct Imaging* 2011; 31: 399–404.

80   Ogasawara R, Yasuda T, Ishii N, Abe T. Comparison of muscle hypertrophy following 6-month of continuous and periodic strength training. *Eur J Appl Physiol* 2013; 113: 975–985.

81   Grgic J, Schoenfeld BJ, Latella C. Resistance training frequency and skeletal muscle hypertrophy: A review of available evidence. *J Sci Med Sport* 2019; 22: 361–370.

82   Schoenfeld BJ, Ogborn D, Krieger JW. Effects of Resistance Training Frequency on Measures of Muscle Hypertrophy: A Systematic Review and Meta-Analysis. *Sports Med Auckl NZ* 2016; 46: 1689–1697.

83   Henselmans M. *How many times per week should a muscle be trained to maximize muscle hypertrophy? New meta-analysis review.* 2019. Available from: https://mennohenselmans.com/training-frequency-2018-meta-analysis-review/ (accessed 10 Feb 2020).

84   Nuckols G. *Training Frequency for Muscle Growth: What the Data Say.* 2018. Available from: https://www.strongerbyscience.com/frequency-muscle/ (accessed 10 Feb 2020).

85   Zaroni RS, Brigatto FA, Schoenfeld BJ, Braz TV, Benvenutti JC, Germano MD et al. High Resistance-Training Frequency Enhances Muscle Thickness in Resistance-Trained Men. *J Strength Cond Res* 2019; 33: S140.

86   Damas F, Phillips S, Vechin FC, Ugrinowitsch C. A review of resistance training-induced changes in skeletal muscle protein synthesis and their contribution to hypertrophy. *Sports Med Auckl NZ* 2015; 45: 801–807.

87   Nikolaidis MG. The Effects of Resistance Exercise on Muscle Damage, Position Sense, and Blood Redox Status in Young and Elderly Individuals. *Geriatrics* 2017; 2. Available from: doi:10.3390/geriatrics2030020.

88   Chen TC, Yang T-J, Huang M-J, Wang H-S, Tseng K-W, Chen H-L et al. Damage and the repeated bout effect of arm, leg, and trunk muscles induced by eccentric resistance exercises. *Scand J Med Sci Sports* 2019; 29: 725–735.

89   Nunes JP, Grgic J, Cunha PM, Ribeiro AS, Schoenfeld BJ, Salles BF de et al. What influence does resistance exercise order have on muscular strength gains and muscle hypertrophy? A systematic review and meta-analysis. *Eur J Sport Sci* 2020; 0: 1–22.

20. Training splits

How to work out the training split that suits your lifestyle and matches your estimated volume and frequency

In the same way that there is no perfect diet, there is also no perfect workout split. There are just splits that better suit different people and different muscle building goals.

When starting, choose a simpler, less frequent, lower volume split to begin with. This makes it much easier to adhere to and helps to create the habit of regularly training. This also provides a wide scope to progress and generate long term overload.

If you already have a plan, look at the various possibilities and see whether a different split may better suit you. Your current split may be adequate, but your current volume and exercise selection may need shifting.

We now know how to train for muscle growth, how much volume we need to perform to promote muscle growth and how to split this volume across the week. It is time to now identify your training plan. The weekly training split you use will depend on your training experience, your goals, personal preference and lifestyle. As such, it does *not* need to be fixed indefinitely and *can* change. However, consistently changing volume, frequency and therefore training plans will limit muscle building success. Your plan of choice depends on how much time you have to go to the gym, and how many times per week and how long per session you can commit to training. There is no point planning a 2x per week *push, pull, legs split* (6 sessions per week), if your work and life commitments mean you can only adequately train three times per week. Similarly, if you have been training for some time and you are struggling to see improvements when training 3x per week with a *whole-body split* or by training each body part once per week, it may be time to try a new split.

There are *advantages* and *disadvantages* to each split. Some allow greater volume and frequency per week, but lower volumes per muscle per session. Some are better for focussing on a specific muscle group, but at the detriment of training frequency. When the same volume (sets per muscle per week) is achieved, different training splits result in the *same* changes in body composition[1-4]. Therefore, a split is just a schedule of *when* during the week you perform your weekly volume per muscle. Imagine revising for an exam. You might decide to create a *revision timetable* to plan which topics you will revise at certain times. A revision timetable is like a training split; it simply provides a structure for you to adhere to.

There are four main weekly training setups[5]:

- **Whole-body (WB).**
- **Upper, lower (UL).**
- **Push, pull, legs (PPL).**
- **Individual body parts per training session: the 'bro' split.**

These are interchangeable. It is possible have whole-body sessions or individual body part sessions in the same plan, such as when adding extra weekly volume for a certain body part.

Read through each training split and decide which is most likely to fit into your lifestyle, your training goals, and most importantly the one you can enjoy *adhering* to. You might find training the whole body each session very tiring, but training each body part by itself fun. You might find training each body part by itself too fatiguing, and the whole-body sessions more enjoyable. For each split, there are a range of set ups suitable for beginners, intermediates and advanced trainers.

Things to consider:

- How many times per week you can commit to training?
- How long can your training sessions be due to other commitments and training ability?
- When is your gym open?
- How do you enjoy training? Do you prefer training lots of muscles in one session, or focussing on a specific muscle?
- How long does it typically take for you to recover after a workout?
- How much volume do you need or think you can perform?
- What is your training experience?
- Do you have any specific body parts you wish to develop, or are you looking to train all body parts consistently?

The splits are in roughly ascending order of training session specificity; the splits descend in order of fewer and fewer body parts trained in each training session.

Whole-body split (WB):

- All main body parts are trained in every session, or at least exercise choice is not focussed (e.g. not a push, pull or legs focussed session).
- A great split to use if you can only train a few times a week, or you are new to resistance training. As a beginner, you may find that one exercise per body part for 2 to 3 sets per session is a sufficient stimulus, and any more training is counterproductive, producing excessive delayed onset of muscle soreness (DOMS). Therefore, spreading the volume for a body part across three sessions can allow for greater weekly volume by allowing adequate recovery time.
- Each body part (e.g. legs, back, chest, shoulders) is trained with one exercise (possibly two), which ideally should be a compound exercise to time-efficiently train a range of muscles (a multi-joint exercise such as a squat or row). Initially, triceps and biceps may not be directly trained as they are stimulated by upper body compound exercises, but they may be added towards the end of a workout for enjoyment and variation, which can improve adherence.
- Whole-body splits can be varied in several ways, but are limited in frequency because for most people there generally needs to be a rest day in between training sessions to allow for adequate recovery. Training on consecutive days can be utilised by carefully considering exercise choice (chapter 21). This may be difficult to easily implement without significant training experience, and may just end up resembling a push, pull, legs split.
- Your performance will be greatest in the first one or two exercises before fatigue builds up. Each session can begin with a different body part first, such as a leg, chest, back or shoulder exercise. This ensures body parts progress in tandem and prevents over- or under-development.

	Split 1	Split 2	Split 3	Split 4	Split 5
Monday	WB	WB	WB	WB	WB
Tuesday					WB
Wednesday	WB	WB	WB	WB	
Thursday					WB
Friday	WB	WB	WB	WB	WB
Saturday					
Sunday		WB	Lagging body part	WB	WB

Split 1: beginner. Equal volume, 3 times per week. Despite a training frequency of 3 times per week, the volume per body part, per session is low (e.g. only one exercise per body part), so weekly volume is not high.

Split 2: beginner/intermediate. Equal volume 4 times per week (rest day after the WB session on Sunday). This can be a split to progress to from split 1, to increase weekly set volume.

Split 3: beginner/intermediate. Equal volume 3 times per week, but a lagging body part has an extra day to itself to increase its weekly training volume. For example, this day could be used as a dedicated arm day if it is not directly trained during the whole-body sessions.

Split 4: intermediate. Every session begins with the most underdeveloped body part. For example, every session starts with a leg exercise first to maximise training on this muscle group. Or, every session has two exercises for the lagging body part, compared to one for other body parts.

Split 5: intermediate/advanced. Whole body training on consecutive days. This will require good knowledge of balancing sufficient volume with minimising muscle damage, and also careful exercise selection. For example, Monday may involve exercises for the chest, biceps and calves. Tuesday may involve the back, triceps and hamstrings. Thursday may involve shoulders, quads and glutes. Friday may use exercises for abs, hamstrings and chest. Sunday can be used to train the back, triceps and quadriceps, with a rest day after Sunday. The key is to choose exercises that minimise interference and fatigue of the muscles that will be trained in the successive day.

Upper, lower body split (UL)

- The UL split is an intermediate between PPL and WB splits. Therefore, each session is more body part specific than WB, but less specific than PPL.
- It involves one session of upper body training such as the chest, shoulders, back, arms and abs. The other lower body session trains leg muscles such as calves, quads, glutes and hamstrings.
- Training upper or lower sessions multiple times per week means that each session can focus on specific upper or lower body parts. As such, this can start to resemble a PPL or a 'bro' style split.

	Split 1	Split 2	Split 3	Split 4	Split 5	Split 6
Monday	Upper	Lower	Upper	Lower	Upper	Lower
Tuesday	Lower		Lower	Upper	Lower	Upper
Wednesday		Upper	Upper	Lower	Upper specific	Lower specific
Thursday	Upper					
Friday	Lower	Lower	Lower	Upper	Lower	Upper
Saturday			Upper	Lower	Upper specific	Lower specific
Sunday		Upper				

Split 1: beginner. Equal frequency, twice per week. If really pushed for time, UL once per week may be used in complete beginners. But, it will quickly limit weekly volume and progression. However, committing and training twice per week is far better than committing to 3 or 4 days per week and being inconsistent (i.e. performing 0 days per week).

Split 2: beginner. Equal frequency, twice per week. But, with a rest day between sessions if it takes longer to recover between sessions. This would suit longer, higher volume sessions, requiring greater recovery time.

Split 3: intermediate. Upper body focus with 3 upper body sessions and 2 lower body sessions. Upper body volume can be increased from splits 1 or 2 by simply adding in the extra session. This would suit hard and fast progression by adding set volume (chapter 18). Or, the extra upper body session could be used to spread upper volume across the week, keeping weekly volume the same. This would suit slow and conservative progression by increasing volume through greater reps and loads per set.

Split 4: intermediate. Same as split 3, but with a lower body focus.

Split 5: intermediate/advanced. The overall programme is an upper/lower focus. But, some days are specific to an upper body part, such as shoulders or back. This allows focussed training for any lagging body parts.

Split 6: intermediate/advanced. Same as split 5, but with a lower body focus.

Push, pull, legs split (PPL)

- A commonly used split because it allows you to train all body parts in just three sessions, training similar muscles and movements in the same session.
- Push: training session focussing on pressing or pushing exercises, which involves the chest, shoulders and triceps.
- Pull: training session focussing on pulling or rowing exercises, which involves the back and biceps.
- Legs: training session focussing on leg exercises, which involves the glutes, quads, hamstrings and calves (more generally, also the hip flexors, knee extensors, adductors and abductors).

	Split 1	Split 2	Split 3	Split 4	Split 5	Split 6
Monday	Push	Push	Legs	Legs	Push	Push
Tuesday		Pull	Push	Push	Pull	Pull
Wednesday	Pull	Legs	Pull			Legs
Thursday				Legs	Pull	
Friday	Legs	Legs	Legs	Pull	Push	Legs
Saturday		Pull	Push		Legs	Push
Sunday		Push	Pull	Legs		Pull

Split 1: beginner. Equal focus and volume once per week.

Split 2: beginner/intermediate. Equal focus and volume twice per week (note the reverse order of push, pull and legs following each rest day). A beginner may use lower volumes per session.

Split 3: beginner/intermediate. Leg day focus but equal volume (leg day after the rest day when you are most recovered). Push or pull days can also be the focus. A beginner may use lower volumes per session.

Split 4: intermediate. Leg day focus with a greater frequency and volume than push or pull sessions. For when legs are an underdeveloped body part (there is a rest day after the Sunday leg day, so weekly frequency varies between 5 and 6 sessions per week).

Split 5: intermediate. Upper body focus, with a greater upper body frequency and volume for when the upper body is underdeveloped.

Split 6: advanced. The same splits used in splits 2, 3, 4 and 5, but with greater workout volumes.

Body part specific split: the 'bro' split

- Each session is dedicated to usually one or possibly two body parts. The second body part can often be additional accessory work (e.g. abdominals, biceps or triceps after the main body part).

- Each session may specifically focus on the chest, back, shoulders, legs, arms or abs. Sessions can be as specific as the hamstrings and calves, or quadriceps and glutes. Training volume per body part is high in a given session, but low to moderate across the week because the body part is trained only once. Weekly volume is achieved by completing the same number of sets in the one dedicated session that is achieved in multiple push, pull, legs or whole-body sessions across the week.

- One factor determining whether this is a suitable split for you is your weekly volume per body part. At low to moderate weekly volumes, training a body part once per week is sufficient. As you increase volume, it may be more practical to split the volume across multiple sessions.

- The bro split allows you to focus on each body part across the week without too much thought for optimising recovery. The muscles or exercises that are trained or performed at the start of a workout make more improvements than those later in the workout. The bro split allows for each body part to receive equal focus during the week without having to vary exercise order, as would be needed for PPL or WB splits. This can make planning the programme easier.

- The bro split also allows for a lot of flexibility in terms of training frequency and body part focus. Consecutive days will train completely different body parts. Therefore, any muscle-specific fatigue (provided it is not too excessive) should not impair the session for a different muscle on the following day. Sessions can be added to increase weekly volume for a body part, or removed to have a lower weekly volume for a recovery period (i.e. a taper).

- The bro split may also suit the personal preference of those who enjoy the sensation of the 'muscle pump'. Although not the primary mechanism of muscle growth, metabolic stress may still be important (chapter 17). Also, adherence is key to long-term progress and the sensation of the muscle pump can be satisfying. If a PPL or WB split doesn't *feel* as enjoyable, then by all means work with a bro split.

- Generally, bro split programmes require a high weekly training frequency in order to hit every muscle group once, but a low weekly frequency for each muscle. For example, a typical chest, shoulders, back, legs and arms split would require a minimum of 5 training days, but each muscle is trained once. If you choose this plan, make sure you have the time to commit to it.

- Caution should be taken when training the chest and shoulders (the front shoulder is highly recruited in both), or shoulders and back (the rear shoulder is heavily active in both) on consecutive days. The shoulder joint may have insufficient rest between sessions. Consider training them on the same day. This would then be more comparable to a PPL split.

	Split 1	Split 2	Split 3	Split 4	Split 5	Split 6
Monday	SH	Legs	Chest	Back	Chest	Chest
Tuesday	Legs	SH, abs	Legs	Chest	Back	Legs, abs
Wednesday			SH	Legs	Legs	Chest
Thursday	Back	Back, biceps			SH	
Friday	Chest	Chest, triceps	Chest, triceps	Back	Back	Chest
Saturday	Arms, abs	Legs	Back, biceps	SH	Chest	Back, SH
Sunday						

SH: Shoulders.

Split 1: beginner/intermediate. Equal volume for each body part, once per week. This works well as a beginner if you can train most days and train for only a short amount of time each day (i.e. 30 minute sessions). But, it does require a high frequency across the week compared to other splits where you could train 3 times per week. As a beginner, a relatively low volume is sufficient to stimulate growth, and the training novelty may mean it takes the best part of a week for a body part to recover. Higher training volumes may lead to excessive muscle damage and impair the ability to train. As an intermediate, sets can be added to each body part session. This works well to increase from beginner levels of low weekly volume to moderate weekly volume. As such, sessions will increase in length towards 60-90 minutes to complete more sets.

Split 2: intermediate/advanced. This split is a leg focussed split with twice the weekly training volume for legs as any other body part. This is achieved by moving arms onto the upper body sessions and adding in an extra leg day. This principle can be repeated for any other lagging body part, as in split 3 or 4. This can be a useful method to increase training volume when progressing from beginner to intermediate experience, when a specific body part appears to be underdeveloped.

Split 3: intermediate/advanced. Similar to split 3, but chest focussed. Notice how rest days are before the body part of interest. If a body part is lagging, move it to the start of the week or to the day after a rest day where you are better recovered and less fatigued.

Split 4: intermediate/advanced. Same as split 3 and 4 but with a back focus.

Split 5: advanced. This is a 6 times per week training frequency which may not be necessary for most individuals, especially beginners. It will also require high levels of adherence. It is most suitable for those with extensive training experience where the extra session is needed to promote growth to increase weekly volume. Care needs to be taken to plan workouts to prevent overtraining and injury. The *rotator cuff* muscles that act to stabilise the shoulder joint can be heavily fatigued with successive chest, back and shoulder workouts. The Wednesday shoulder day could focus more on front and middle shoulders (e.g. shoulder press and upright row). This would keep the rear shoulders relatively unfatigued to train back the next day. This then allows 48 hours rest before the front shoulders are trained during the chest session on Saturday. This would require good knowledge of exercise selection (chapter 21), how to maximise training frequency, and how to perform sessions that minimise excessive muscle damage (chapter 19).

Split 6: advanced. This is a high volume split for a specific body part (in this case for chest). Depending on the training volume used for the body part of interest, this may exceed 20 sets per week. This split can be used in the short term to maximise weekly volume to functionally overreach, before reducing the volume for the specific body part for several weeks, facilitating adequate recovery and adaptation (chapter 19 discussed overreaching).

Summary

Hopefully from the splits discussed above you can see at least one split that suits your training style and personal preference. Splits are a plan of how you will manage to perform the weekly volume you need to build muscle; they are just constructs and do not need to be followed rigidly. There is also significant overlap between different splits, they can be combined across the week and can vary over time. In reality, there are limitless ways to plan your training and the above just covers the main methods to do so. The key point is to ensure adherence to a given split for a sufficient amount of time to allow for progression. If you do decide to change your split, make sure it is because it meets the needs of your training, and not because one week you cannot be bothered to train. However, be adaptive. If you know you have a busy week ahead with work or social events such that your usual training of 5 days per week now has to be 3 or 4, then look to shift your split to ensure you still achieve the same volume in fewer sessions.

You may begin with a body part specific split, but find you struggle with the training session volume on upper body exercises. As such, you may move to a PPL split. With more experience, you want to further increase volume by increasing frequency, so you switch to an UL split. You also want to build big arms, so you add in a body part specific arm day into your UL split.

Below is a basic outline for volume and frequency depending on training status, and how these can be incorporated into different splits:

- **Beginner or untrained:** minimal to no training experience. Start at 4-6 sets per body part per week and increase the reps and load within sets.
  - Body part frequency of 1x per week e.g. PPL split, body part specific split.
  - Body part frequency of 2-3x per week e.g. WB split (higher frequency with less volume per session).

- **Intermediate:** at least 3-6 months of training experience. Progress up to 10-20 sets per body part per week.
  - Body part frequency of 1x per week e.g. PPL split, body part specific split.
  - Body part frequency of 2x per week e.g. PPL split, multi-body part split, UL split.
  - Body part frequency of 3-4x per week e.g. WB split, UL split.

- **Experienced**: at least 24+ months of training experience. 10-20 sets per body part per week with planned high-volume periods (>20 sets per week) for given body parts for around 2 to 3 months.
  - Body part frequency 1-4x per week e.g. PPL split, multi-body part split, UL split (4x for a lagging body part, 1x for developed body parts) with brief phases of high volumes.

References

1   Heke TO. *The effect of Two-equal Volume Training Protocols upon strength, body composition and salivary hormones in strength trained males.* 2011. Available from: https://openrepository.aut.ac.nz/handle/10292/1173 (accessed 11 Feb 2020).

2   Gentil P, Fisher J, Steele J, Campos MH, Silva MH, Paoli A et al. Effects of equal-volume resistance training with different training frequencies in muscle size and strength in trained men. *PeerJ* 2018; 6: e5020.

3   Buford TW, Rossi SJ, Smith DB, Warren AJ. A comparison of periodization models during nine weeks with equated volume and intensity for strength. *J Strength Cond Res* 2007; 21: 1245–1250.

4   Candow DG, Burke DG. Effect of short-term equal-volume resistance training with different workout frequency on muscle mass and strength in untrained men and women. *J Strength Cond Res* 2007; 21: 204–207.

5   Kraemer WJ, Ratamess NA. Fundamentals of resistance training: progression and exercise prescription. *Med Sci Sports Exerc* 2004; 36: 674–688.

21. Exercise selection: variation

Initial exercise choice should focus on a range of exercises that cover all the main movement patterns. For muscle growth, no exercise must be performed. The exact exercises you choose will depend on personal preference, equipment availability, muscle building goals and fatigue management. Both compound and isolation exercises can effectively promote muscle growth. Compound exercises may provide a time-effective method to simultaneously train multiple muscle groups, especially in beginners. Isolation exercises can provide an effective method to generate volume for a specific muscle. Any form of resistance (e.g. free weights, machines or cable machines) can effectively promote muscle growth. Focus on improving and progressively overloading on a select few exercises for each movement pattern and body part. Add or use other exercises to increase weekly volume, to prevent training from becoming monotonous and stale and to provide a novel training stimulus from time to time.

Now that we know how to train for muscle growth, how much volume you need to perform, and identified the weekly split that suits you and your lifestyle, it is now time to choose the exercises to use in your plan. Despite there being many 100s of exercises, they all involve motion through specific *movement patterns*. The body actually has only a small number of basic movement patterns, which includes:

- Squat pattern (simultaneous hip extension and knee flexion).
- Hip hinge pattern (e.g. deadlift).
- Lunge.
- Horizontal press (e.g. bench press).
- Horizontal pull (e.g. row).
- Vertical press (e.g. shoulder press).
- Vertical pull (e.g. pull up).

Any basic or advanced programme should cover the main movement patterns with exercises that suit the individual, and then with additional exercises for specific muscles. This can be achieved by focussing on the main muscle used in each movement pattern or focussing on the movement pattern itself.

Compound and isolation exercises

Compound exercises are forms of basic movement patterns. *Isolation exercises* can train specific components of movement patterns.

Compound exercises are also called *multi-joint exercises*. The movement requires motion at more than one joint in the body. This includes exercises such as the squat, deadlift, bench press, pull up, row and shoulder press.

Isolation exercises are also called *single-joint exercises*. The movement requires motion at only one joint in the body. This includes exercises such as bicep curls, leg extensions, leg curls, and triceps extensions.

A review of 23 studies assessing isolation and compound exercises show that both forms of exercise can result in *similar* increases in muscle growth for a given muscle[1]. A recent systematic review and meta-analysis identified that the order of isolation or compound exercises for a given muscle in a workout did *not* influence muscle growth[2]. Compound exercises can allow for a time-efficient method to achieve weekly set volume for multiple muscle groups. Isolation exercises allow for an efficient method to achieve weekly set volume for a specific muscle, without fatiguing other muscles that may be active during compound exercises. Leading experts and coaches have a similar view on using compound movements to train the basic movement patterns as a fundamental part of a training programme[3-5]. Health benefits relating to resistance exercise have been proposed through the use of compound exercises[6].

The main factor determining muscle growth is the mechanical tension exerted and therefore experienced by the fibres of a muscle. Metabolic stress may play a minor role. Muscle growth can occur across a wide range of loads. However, isolation exercises *tend* to be better suited to higher rep ranges and lighter intensity loads, and compound exercises *tend* to be better suited to lower rep ranges and higher intensity loads. Compound exercises generally *tend* to have a greater scope to progressively overload with in the long term. As previously discussed, higher intensities of load and lower rep sets should be performed near the beginning of the workout, and lower intensities of load and higher rep sets should be performed near the end of the workout. This tends towards performing compound exercises before isolation exercises. But, this doesn't *always* have to be the case, especially with training experience, where a training session may focus on a specific muscle through isolation exercises.

Compound exercises

When performing a compound exercise, multiple muscles are involved. Many of the muscles can undergo a muscle building stimulus, especially in beginners. However, there is a difference between a muscle being *active*, and a muscle being *stimulated* to grow during an exercise. The examples below are for the horizontal press movement pattern (e.g. bench press exercise). Muscles can be classed as[7]:

- **Agonists/primary movers** (chest): the muscle that carries out the movement.
- **Synergists/secondary movers** (triceps and anterior deltoids): the muscle that contracts along with the primary mover to aid in the movement.
- **Stabilisers** (abdominals, legs and the rotator cuff): muscles that are isometrically active to provide support (muscles do not change length but are producing tension).
- **Antagonists** (biceps, upper back): a muscle that acts to move in the opposite direction to the primary mover. They can be eccentrically contracting (biceps) or isometrically active (upper back) to act as stabilisers during the movement.

For beginners, the additional muscles that are recruited as secondary movers and stabilisers in compound exercises may undergo sufficient tension to promote muscle growth[7,8]. Using compound exercises therefore provides a time- and fatigue-efficient manner to generate weekly volume for multiple body parts. Over time, this stimulus may be insufficient and more directed training with isolation exercises may be necessary[8,9]. For example as a beginner, pull ups may be a time-efficient method to train both the back and elbow flexors (e.g. the biceps). With experience, the individual may improve their ability to recruit the back muscles and the stimulus to the elbow flexors may become insufficient, such that a set of biceps curls is much more effective at promoting biceps muscle growth than a set of pull ups.

Stabilising muscles (such as the core during squats or rows) or secondary movers (such as the triceps during the bench press, or biceps during pull ups) will be active during certain exercises, especially compound exercises. Just because a muscle is active, contracting, or 'burns', does *not* mean that the muscle is undergoing a stimulus that will lead to muscle growth. Muscle 'burn' and fatigue also occurs in aerobic exercise, which does not build muscle. This is more likely with increasing training experience, such that muscles will require direct stimulation. Despite not promoting growth, this indirect activation can still result in subsequent fatigue and muscle soreness in the days after, especially with novel exercises. This has important implications for planning what is being trained on certain days. For example, the core is active during a squat to help ensure correct posture. Therefore, if you plan an abdominal workout the day before leg day, you may be compromising your ability to perform your sets of squats. This is where exercise choice is *strategic*. You could train abs and then the day after train legs, but use leg exercises with less core requirement, such as a leg press or leg extension. Smart exercise selection can *optimise* weekly volume. This is how it may be possible to perform whole-body workouts on consecutive days.

With training experience, only one of the active muscle groups will be the *limiting factor* dictating the weight, reps and number of sets that can be performed for a given compound exercise. This does not necessarily have to be the primary mover. If the primary mover or secondary mover fatigues, this can be seen as muscular task failure. If a synergist fails, this can result in technical failure. This is where a stabilising muscle is fatigued (such as the erectors in the back or forearms during a bent over row), but the primary mover is not completely fatigued (the lats and upper back in a bent over row). This means that you are unable to maintain the correct posture and perform any further reps, even though you have the capacity to do so. Depending on how close to failure the primary mover reaches when the synergist fails will influence how effective that set is for promoting muscle growth in the primary mover. If the primary mover is far from muscular failure, then this exercise would again be inefficient as the target muscle is not being effectively trained. Exercises strengthening the stabilisers (e.g. back hyperextensions to strengthen the erectors or forearm exercises to improve grip strength) or exercise choices which eliminate the use of stabilisers (e.g. chest-supported rows to reduce the recruitment of the erectors, or using wrist wraps to reduce forearm recruitment) can allow for progression of the primary movers recruited in a given compound exercise.

Compound exercises may not be particularly useful to activate certain muscles, despite their apparent utility. *Surface electromyography* (EMG) (studying the electrical activity of the muscle) provides information about the electrical activity of the motor units in a muscle[10]*. When a muscle is activated it produces an electrical signal, which can be detected. In these studies, electrodes are placed on the skin above muscles of interest, and the electrical activity is measured during the exercise. As leading researchers have stated, when the muscle is unfatigued, the size of the EMG signal relates to the force produced by the muscle. This can give information on how hard a muscle is working relative to other muscles that are active in the same exercise, for a given load[11-13]. Higher electrical activity when the muscle is not fatigued indicates higher muscle activity. Low electrical activity indicates that a muscle is not generating much force and not working very hard[14]. Measuring the electrical activity on the skin surface of the leg during the squat shows that the quadriceps have the highest electrical activity of any leg muscle in any squat variation, followed by the gluteal muscles[15]. However, the hamstrings have relatively low electrical activity in the squat (which is due to the biomechanics of the squat and how the hamstring attaches to the skeleton)[10,15-17]. Long term studies show that individuals performing the squat produce significantly greater quadriceps growth, than hamstrings growth[7]. To maximise hamstring muscle development, other compound exercises that lead to high electrical activity in the hamstrings (e.g. deadlifts) should be included, which typically utilise a hip hinge movement pattern[15,18].

* Levels of electrical activity do not imply greater motor unit recruitment or muscle growth, but provide an insight into how much work the muscle is performing during the movement[7,19,20].

Isolation exercises

Isolation exercises have their place in a workout. Some have argued for and against their use in a resistance training programme that utilises compound exercises[1,9,21]. With training experience, exercises to target specific muscles (i.e. single-joint isolation exercises) can be used to efficiently generate sufficient weekly volume. Many sets of compound exercises can be mentally and physically fatiguing. Motivation to do so can also be lacking. The additional rest that may be required to perform a subsequent productive set with a compound exercise may prolong a workout session. Performing 4 sets of squats followed by 4 sets of leg extensions may provide better overall fatigue management compared to 8 sets of squats, whilst still maintaining quadricep training volume. This would reduce the training demands of other muscles active in the squat (e.g. gluteal muscles and core) Similarly, isolation exercises are efficient methods to add muscle-specific volume to a session and therefore across the week. Isolation exercises tend to better suit low to moderate intensities of load with moderate to high rep ranges. Thus, isolation exercises are a fatigue efficient method of adding volume to a specific body part, producing similar muscle growth as performing the same set volume with compound exercises[7].

Isolation exercises can provide a safe means with which to reach failure. Compound exercises can be technically difficult. Performing incorrect movement patterns may mean the target muscle is not sufficiently recruited and other muscles may dominate, meaning the muscle of interest is not stimulated to grow. If uncorrected, this may result in injury or the incorrect perception of progression, when actually, performance has changed because technique has changed. Muscular failure and poor technique can result in *technical failure* (being unable to perform a rep due to poor technique or technique breakdown). Technical failure and muscular task failure can be risky and unsafe in compound exercises[22]. Even with perfect technique, muscular task failure in compound exercises such as the squat can also be dangerous, especially when heavy loads are used. As discussed in chapter 19, failure is unlikely to be necessary for muscle growth. If training to muscular task failure, isolation exercises such as leg extensions are much safer methods to do so than compound exercises.

Isolation exercises are useful tools to track progression. Due to the often fixed position of isolation exercises, it is much easier to maintain proper correct technique when approaching failure. With their lower technical requirement, isolation exercises can be practical tools to add volume near to the end of the workout when fatigue is greater, and motivation and focus may start to decline. Progression in isolation exercises is largely due to increased mass in the isolated muscle and less dependent on improved movement coordination and neural recruitment.

Does 1 set of a compound exercise *count* the same as 1 set of an isolation exercise?

Isolation and compound exercises are currently considered *equal* on a set by set basis for promoting muscle growth for a given body part[7]. Compound exercises initially may provide a good stimulus for multiple muscles, but with time may become less effective for some secondary muscle groups. Isolation exercises may then be needed to provide direct stimulation.

As a beginner, pull ups provide effective stimulation to both the back and biceps. However with experience, whether a set of pull ups *'counts'* as one set for the biceps in the same way as one set of bicep curls *'counts'* has not been formalised in the research, largely due to limitations in the current evidence[7]. The effect is likely to be exercise specific (i.e. to what extent are different muscles recruited in the exercise), and variable between people and their experience. Isolation and compound exercises are currently considered equivalent due to insufficient evidence to recommend otherwise, however there is a strong theoretical case to be made that in trained individuals, a 1:1 relationship is unlikely to remain. This is also suggestive from assessing muscle activity in surface electromyography (EMG) studies[7]. As demonstrated with the squat and deadlift (both considered as *'leg'* exercises) and hamstring activation, different compound leg exercises do not stimulate leg muscles to the same extent. This can be partially adjusted for by considering the muscles that an exercise primarily trains. In other words, the squat counts towards quadricep and glute volume, and the deadlift contributes towards hamstring and glute volume. Of course, this means a more detailed approach to determining weekly set volume which may make it harder to track and adhere to.

From a pure muscle building perspective, a given muscle of interest should be trained first in a workout, *regardless* of its size or whether it is trained with isolation or compound exercises[23]. A systematic review and meta-analysis shows that the order of isolation or compound exercises for that given muscle does not appear to influence muscle growth[2]. But, *exercises* performed first in a workout show the greatest improvements in performance (i.e. strength)[2,23]. This follows the principle of specificity (chapter 18). Improvements in strength are specific to the *exercise*, but increases in muscle mass are specific to the *muscle*, not the exercise. Exercises where there is also an aim to increase strength should be performed first in a workout. For example, if you wanted to build big quadriceps, you could perform leg extensions and then squats. But to get stronger at squatting, you should perform squats first. The limited evidence suggests that exercise order does not have a meaningful influence on energy expenditure from a resistance training session[23]. However, when using compound exercises for a given body part, it makes *practical* sense to perform them first or earlier in the workout to ensure *technical proficiency*, such as in the quadriceps example above. Compound exercises may also have more functional carry over to some sporting disciplines, which should be considered if there are goals besides muscle growth[23]. Exercise technique can deteriorate with fatigue which can influence injury risk and reduce the efficacy of an exercise to promote growth[23]. Performing isolation exercises before a compound exercise does not increase muscle activation (chapter 23), and instead can increase the recruitment of secondary muscles due to fatigue of the primary muscle[23].

Train body parts of interest first in a workout. *Local* and *non-local* muscular fatigue occurs in a workout, such that performance in each subsequent set, whether targeting the same muscle or not, is reduced[2]. For example, greater upper body strength improvements occur when training the upper body before the lower body. But, greater lower body strength improvements occur when training the lower body before the upper body[24].

As a general starting point, train all major muscle groups with compound exercises targeting the main movement patterns to ensure complete muscle development, and use isolation exercises when needed to achieve sufficient weekly volume.

There are countless exercises available. Most exercises are just *variations* of the *same* movement pattern. For example, a simultaneous hip extension and knee flexion movement (a squat) can be performed with goblet squats, barbell squats (front and back) or smith machine squats, to name a few. Variations of a horizontal push can be performed with a dumbbell press, smith machine press, barbell bench press or machine press, for example. One reason for performing different exercises however, is to prevent training staleness and to target specific muscles. 10 sets of the same exercise can get boring. Switching to other exercises can also help to manage fatigue whilst adding volume. Variations of a similar exercise can change the exercise biomechanics, which *theoretically* may promote muscle growth in different muscles, or regions of a muscle. For muscle growth, reaching the maximum training session volume with 2-5 sets of a compound exercise and a further 2-5 sets of an isolation exercise for a given muscle may be much more efficient and optimal than performing all sets with a compound exercise. The compound exercise may be used to train in the low to moderate rep ranges, and the isolation exercise used to train in the moderate to high rep ranges.

Choose 1 to 3 compound exercises that primarily target a movement pattern or body part. Become *technically* proficient at performing them (using the correct muscles and movement pattern) *before* aiming to progressively overload with them across the week and over time.

For each body part or movement pattern:

1. One (possibly two) main compound exercise(s) to achieve long-term progression. To train a muscle or movement pattern across low to moderate rep ranges.

2. A small selection of secondary compound exercises that may be included in workouts depending on the amount of volume needed per body part in a given session, or in the week. To increase overall training volume for general muscle growth. To train a muscle or movement pattern across low, moderate and high rep ranges.

3. A small selection of isolation exercises for each body part. To be used to increase volume, manage fatigue and focus on specific lagging areas. To train a muscle or movement pattern across moderate to high rep ranges.

As an example, if you want to focus on your shoulders, then your main compound exercise could be a vertical press movement pattern such as a barbell, dumbbell or machine shoulder press. Secondary compound exercises may include some form of upright row or cable face pulls. Isolation exercises could include lateral raises or rear deltoid (shoulder) flye exercises.

Exercise choice is an important factor influencing the amount of muscle growth that may occur with your training programme. How often you vary these exercises can be considered alongside. Which exercises should you focus on? And how often should you change exercises?

Some of the exercises you choose may change over time but should be consistent for a sufficient amount of time to allow tracking of progression.

No single exercise will make or break you. There will always be another exercise or variation of that exercise that will be just as effective for muscle growth.

When choosing which exercises to include in your programme, consider:

- **Which exercises do you enjoy performing and feel good to you?** This should be a combination of finding exercises that you like to perform, and also exercises that allow you to *feel* the target muscle working. For example, if you prefer barbell back squats to front squats as you can feel your quadriceps working much more and it feels more enjoyable to perform, then stick with back squats. If dumbbell chest flyes feel awkward and hurt your shoulder, then choose another chest exercise, such as cable or machine flyes.

- **Is that exercise good for long-term progression?** To build muscle over time, the load you use to perform a given number of reps and sets will have to increase, or the number of reps you perform for a given load will have to increase. However, some exercises are better suited to increased loads, and some less so. There is only so much load you can add to isolation exercises, compared to compound exercises[25]. Practically, compound exercises may better suit sets performed in the lower rep ranges, and isolation exercises may better suit sets performed in the higher rep ranges. The instability of some movements will always limit the load you can lift (have you ever tried to perform a cable chest flye and struggle to get into position, feeling off balance whilst performing it?). Whereas, a dumbbell, barbell or smith machine press can be heavily loaded with stability from the bench. This will also influence the method of progression you use with an exercise (e.g. increasing the number of reps for a given load tends to work better for lighter loads, or increase the load used for a given number of reps tends to work better for heavier loads) and the rep range you primarily train the muscle with that exercise (e.g. low to moderate rep ranges for the barbell bench press, but moderate to high rep ranges for the cable chest flye).

- **What equipment does your gym have?** Are there sufficient weights to load up barbells and sufficiently heavy dumbbells to allow you to progress? For example, if your gym only has dumbbells up to 30kg and you can already dumbbell bench press 30kg for 10 reps, it may be wise to choose another horizontal press or chest exercise at your gym.

- **Which body parts do you want to build most?** For example, if you want to build your hamstrings but you only train legs with squats, then it may be worthwhile to consider other exercises. Squats are primarily a quadricep and glute dominant exercise. A hip hinge movement pattern (e.g. a deadlift) would target the hamstrings, and an exercise for this movement pattern should be prioritised in a workout.

- **How long do you have for a gym session?** Some exercises take longer than others to get to a first *'working set'*. It may take you over half an hour to get fully warm and ready to perform a working set of squats. However, it may only take 5 minutes to get ready to perform a first working set of leg extensions. If you are short on time, pick exercises you can warm up for and get productive sets completed *quickly*, rather than reducing productive volume.

- **How busy is your gym when you train?** If you often find all the equipment in the gym is being used when you train, then consider choosing exercises where you can easily switch in between another gym user (such as a machine) or choose exercises where there is plenty of equipment available, so you do not have to wait (such as dumbbells or barbells).
- **Do you dislike the weights section and prefer to train in the studio room?** Gyms can be intimidating places. If you find them daunting, then if you can find a nice quiet area to train in it will mean that you are more likely to adhere to training and commit to a plan. Choose exercises that can be successfully performed and progressively overloaded with the equipment available in such areas. For example, choosing box lunges or goblet squats instead of barbell back squats in a studio room. With no squat rack, barbell back squats in a studio room will require you to pick the bar up off the floor and overhead press it onto your back, which will always be less than what you could squat.
- **Do you use multiple gyms and travel a lot?** If you use multiple gyms, it may be beneficial to choose barbell or dumbbell exercises, which allows consistency and progression across gyms with different equipment. Barbells and dumbbells are pretty similar at any gym, but machines and cables can vary greatly between gyms. Training with different machines and different cables makes tracking of progression very difficult.

Exercise variation

Exercise variation is not superior to consistent exercise selection for muscle growth, but it may increase the motivation to train.

It has often been mentioned that muscles get accustomed to an exercise, and in order to progress, there is a need to continually rotate around different exercises to provide a new stimulus and produce '*muscle confusion*'. In other words, using the same exercises results in less muscle growth than varying them. However, there is *no* evidence to suggest this is the case. Furthermore, a recent study compared the effect of using randomly varied exercises compared to a fixed exercise selection. 21 resistance trained males were randomised to perform 8 weeks of either: a varied training programme, or a programme with consistent exercise selection. Both programmes consisted of performing 3 sets for 6 exercises, 4 times per week. One group performed the same 6 upper body and 6 lower body exercises. The other group performed exercises randomly chosen from a database of 80 exercises, which were matched to the consistent group in each session for upper and lower exercises, and movement pattern (e.g. pulling and pushing exercises). Resistance training variables (weekly set volume, intensity of effort and load and rest intervals) were controlled for between groups[26]. Both groups significantly increased muscle mass, but no difference was seen between groups. Varied, random exercise selection is *not* superior for muscle growth. However, exercise selection can be important to provide *enjoyment* to training. For many, using the same exercises can become monotonous and reduce the motivation to train. Indeed, the authors noted that the participants who performed the varied exercise programme increased their *intrinsic motivation* to train. Other studies have demonstrated that a moderate level of *autoregulating* exercise variation may have some benefit for muscle growth[27,28]. In other words, if the motivation to train is lacking, then using a new exercise may aid motivation to train. If adherence to a training plan is an issue, exercise variation may be an important tool to achieve consistency, which is far more important than any specific training-related variable[26]. The authors of the study suggest that compound exercises that have a high level of neuromotor learning and technical skill (e.g. squats or bench press) should be regularly trained to practice technique, and less complex exercises such as isolation exercises can be more frequently switched in and out[26].

Consistent exercise choice is necessary to allow for accurate tracking of progressive overload. However, exercise variation can improve training motivation, but with no benefit to muscle growth. Only using one exercise is probably sub-optimal, and always varying exercises is probably sub-optimal. As such, how consistent or varied your exercise choices are should be down to personal preference, primarily to ensure adherence to training, and then secondly to ensure productive training sessions.

Below provides a simple guide to balancing consistent exercise choice with varied exercise choice, when training one body part in a session:

- **Keep one or two exercises per body part the same for every workout.** Start the workout with a compound exercise that focuses on a movement pattern with the body part of interest as the primary muscle. For example, a squat pattern: use squats to target quadriceps and glutes. Horizontal press: use the bench press to target chest. Vertical pull: use pull ups to target the back. Aim to progress in each workout. As a beginner this could be one more rep or slightly more weight, before adding an extra set.
- **Once you have completed your main one or two exercises, consider one or two exercises that you perform frequently, but not necessarily every workout.** Use additional compound exercises to increase overall weekly volume for multiple muscles, or isolation exercises to target an underdeveloped muscle. For these exercises, you should have a good idea of the weight you can use and the reps for that weight, so progression can be tracked. For example, if your

quads are lagging, choose leg extensions. If your chest is lagging, choose another chest exercise.

- **For the last exercise, you could choose a novel exercise.** This does not need to be performed every session. The aim of this exercise would be to target the muscle group of choice from a different angle to usual. Remember that muscles have a 3D shape, yet an exercise movement is often in one plane. For example, you could perform a seated leg curl rather than a lying leg curl to target different aspects of the hamstring, or perform a close grip bench press to theoretically change muscle fibre recruitment. The focus here is on hitting the muscle in a different way, and also to just have a bit of fun. This can also be a good exercise to use if you *choose* to train to maximise metabolic stress (i.e. the muscle pump) (chapter 23).

With experience, you may decide to start workouts with, or focus on progressing with isolation exercises.

A body part specific workout therefore may involve as little as 3 sets with 1 exercise, or as much as 20+ sets across 5 exercises. However, note that the current evidence does not appear to support using volumes greater than around 8-10 sets per body part per session for muscle growth[29,30]. However, this is an average, and hence the wide variability in possible training session volumes outlined above. The primary focus should be the number of sets performed. The number of exercises, choice of exercises and number of sets per exercise are just tools to achieve the required volume. Higher body part specific session volumes should be used sparingly and be based on personal preference.

As a guide when training more than one body part in a session:

- **Keep the same overall structure as above for each body part in the session. But, use the lower end of the exercise and set recommendations (reduce the number of exercises and/or sets) per body part as a starting point.** If training two body parts, the number of exercises per session could be halved. If training three, a third of the volume can be used. Let's say, if training one body part in a session, you use 2-3 exercises, and anywhere between 6-12 sets depending on experience. If training two body parts, you may aim for between 1-2 exercises and 3-6 sets per body part per session, and therefore a total weekly volume of 6-12 sets per body part. For three body parts, you may use 1-2 exercises, and 2-4 sets per body part per session, and therefore a total weekly volume of 6-12 sets. Note how session volume per body part quickly becomes very low with increasing frequency, for the *same* overall weekly volume. But, the higher frequencies mean that set volume can then be slowly increased in each session to generate *higher* weekly volumes. If training a body part multiple times per week, consider having sessions with varying rep ranges and intensities, such as starting one session within the 4-6 rep range, and another day within the 8-12 rep range.

Exercise variation to target specific parts of a muscle

The level of evidence for exercise selection to promote muscle region specific growth is of low quality. Evidence is primarily from small scale indirect studies of muscle growth, expert opinion and theoretical considerations. It is likely that different exercises can target different regions of a muscle, but whether this results in meaningful differences in muscle growth has not been formally studied. However, it may be likely[31,32].

Despite the loads typically used for isolation exercises generally being lighter than those in compound exercises, they both result in similar muscle growth when performing the same number of sets to failure[7]. Low, moderate and high intensity loads can all produce similar muscle growth with sets taken to, or near to failure. Isolation exercises allow not just *specific* muscles to be targeted, but different *regions* of a muscle to be targeted[33]. Large muscle groups are made up of *muscle heads*. Muscle heads are part of the same muscle, but attach to different parts of the skeleton. A muscle and its muscle heads can be stronger or weaker at different points in the range of motion of an exercise. Also, muscle fibres do not span the whole length of the muscle, meaning that fibres in proximal and distal regions of a muscle can be targeted. The variation in the function of a given muscle at different lengths and positions has been theoretically proposed to be a reason for using a range of exercises for the muscle. Regions of a muscle can be targeted by changing hand, foot and limb positions, and with different variations of an exercise. This is also possible with compound exercise variations[33].

For example, proximal and distal hamstring muscle activation differs with different hamstring exercises, demonstrating region-specific activity[14]. On the other hand, the incline bench press is proposed to better recruit upper chest muscle fibres compared to the flat bench press. The theory is that there is better alignment and recruitment of the upper chest, which would result in greater upper chest growth. However, studies comparing upper chest muscle fibre activation in an incline bench press compared to a flat bench press are conflicting, with some suggesting greater and some suggesting similar activation[34]. However, *no* study has formally compared exercises for a given muscle that generate region-specific differences in muscle activation, and subsequent region-specific hypertrophy. Surface electromyography (EMG) of the pectoralis major (a muscle of the chest) is similar for the barbell bench press, dumbbell bench press and dumbbell flye[35]. Given that a range of exercises for a given muscle result in similar muscle growth, if region specific hypertrophy did occur, it would be much less meaningful than simply performing a given weekly set volume for that body part with any suitable exercise. A muscle does not need to be maximally stimulated for muscle growth to occur. Surface EMG measurements (which assess muscle activation) ignore any passive mechanical tension a muscle may experience when in a stretched position, such as the passive tension that the chest may experience at the bottom of a bench press rep. To build a bigger chest, progressively overload on a selection of chest exercises. It may be a good idea to include a variety of exercises training different angles for training enjoyment and for any theoretical benefit, but whether this has any meaningful benefit on hypertrophy is *not* definitive nor proven.

If regions of a muscle can be specifically targeted to grow more than other regions, then muscle cross-sectional area would not correlate with muscle volume after a training period. However, studies show that the cross-sectional area from the middle of a muscle can predict muscle volume[31]. Regional hypertrophy may well be possible. But, it would mainly be of benefit to experienced individuals. Given the slow rate of growth, it is unlikely that any controlled study could identify a significant difference between programmes using exercises targeting different parts of a muscle, especially considering interindividual variation. As such, exercise selection to target specific parts of a muscle should only be considered once established as an intermediate or advanced trainer. Overall exercise selection and weekly volume for the muscle should be the primary focus.

Dumbbells, barbells and machines: which is best?

All three are excellent forms of resistance in their own right, each with advantages and disadvantages. None of the three are superior for everyone. Different forms will suit different people at different times, both within a workout and across a training programme.

To progress, we will need tools that allow for a resistance to be produced that we can act against. Is there a superior form of resistance that should be used? Common forms of resistance include dumbbells, barbells, fixed machines and our own body weight. Most body weight exercises quickly become too 'light' with training experience (e.g. being able to perform far more than 30 press ups or body weight squats before fatigue occurs), meaning additional resistance is necessary to maintain a sufficient intensity of load. The number of studies comparing different forms of resistance is very small. Few studies compare dumbbells to smith machines to barbells. Most compare their short-term effects on muscle activation or muscle damage after a single session, rather than their long-term effects on muscle growth. Many studies assess strength, not muscle growth[36,37].

A study comparing muscle activation of the barbell bench press compared to a smith machine press found similar chest EMG activation, but increased activation of stabilisers (middle deltoid) on the barbell bench press[38]. Barbell bench, dumbbell bench and dumbbell flye exercises all produce similar chest activation[35]. Smith machines, dumbbells and barbells also all produce similar amounts of muscle damage following a single workout[39]. Free weights or machines result in similar muscle growth with the same resistance training programme[31].

The studies discussed so far that assess volume, intensity and frequency utilise *different* training modalities and result in *similar* muscle growth. There are no recommendations to use one exercise modality over another[14,29,40].

The tables below outline some elements you may wish to consider.

Free weights (e.g. barbells, dumbbells)	Fixed machines
Can increase muscle size	Can increase muscle size
Can be multi-joint or single-joint	Can be multi-joint or single-joint
Can increase strength	Can increase strength
Requires activation of stabilising muscles. Higher risk of incorrect technique and injury	Fixed position. Requires less stabilisation. Lower risk of incorrect technique and injury
Can be used in periodisation and for progressive overload	Can be used in periodisation and for progressive overload
Easier to track progress between gyms. The effect of slightly different barbells and dumbbells is minimal	Harder to track progress between gyms. Different machines will mean different movement patterns, different load increments etc

Pros and cons of free weights and fixed machines[22,29,42].

Compound / multi-joint (e.g. squat) exercise	Isolation / single-joint (e.g. leg extension) exercise
Can increase muscle size	Can increase muscle size
Can be free weights or fixed machines	Can be free weights or fixed machines
Can increase strength	Can increase strength[42]
Recruits multiple muscle groups, but may only be an effective muscle building stimulus for one muscle	Targets a specific muscle
Can be used in periodisation and for progressive overload	Can be used in periodisation and for progressive overload
More complex neuromotor activation and movement pattern; higher risk of injury due to greater technical difficulty and skill involved. A greater learning curve	Simpler neuromotor activation; one muscle group to focus on. Lower risk of injury due to less technique and skill required
Generally involve higher absolute loads and lower rep ranges. Best used at the start of workouts when fatigue is minimum to prevent injury	Generally involve lower absolute loads and higher rep ranges. Best used at the end of workouts to target lagging body parts and increase weekly volume whilst minimising fatigue

Pros and cons of compound and isolation exercises[22,29,42].

There is no reason (or at least a lack of evidence suggesting otherwise) to support any unanimous preferential use of barbells, dumbbells or machine exercises over the other for muscle growth. By following the general evidence-based recommendations for resistance training for muscle growth outlined in chapter 16 (i.e. sufficient tension being placed on the muscle with sets taken close enough to failure (intensity of effort) and progressive overload is achieved), muscle growth will occur with *any* training modality. There is no major theoretical reason why any form of resistance should be superior or inferior to another. The decision should rest on personal preference[41]. If you are worried about exercise safety, then perhaps opt for the fixed machines such as the smith machine. If barbells cause pain, then use dumbbells. If you enjoy powerlifting and weightlifting style exercises, then maybe choose barbell exercises.

Accommodating resistance (i.e. chains and resistance bands)

There is very limited research on the use of accommodating resistance to promote hypertrophy. Most evidence is from small scale studies and expert opinion following from theoretical considerations. No evidence suggests accommodating resistance is superior to typical fixed resistance. Following the same principles of progression and overload, accommodating resistance can promote muscle growth. However, tracking progression, the availability of equipment, setting up equipment and the relative ease of other forms of resistance means it is probably more practical to use other forms of resistance (i.e. fixed resistances such as dumbbells, barbells and machines), especially as a beginner or intermediate.

Accommodating resistance is where the amount of load changes as the lift is performed. This can be achieved by using *resistance bands*. When they are stretched, tension increases. Or, *chains* can be used that are in contact with the floor during the exercise, such that with increasing height in a lift, more of the chains are off the floor and therefore a greater load is placed on muscles.

The supposed benefit of accommodating resistance is that it allows a better match between the *strength profile* of a muscle (muscles are not always capable of producing the same amount of force throughout its range of motion) and the load placed on the muscle throughout the range of motion for an exercise. For example, squats are *'hardest'* when at the bottom of the movement, but relatively *'easier'* near the top. Adding bands means that a greater load can be applied at the top part of the squat where the lift is *'easier'*. This means the lift is *'hard'* throughout the entire range of motion and not just at the bottom. Therefore, tension better matches force production through the range of motion[31]. But, does this better match result in greater muscle growth?

Many studies compare conventional resistance training to accommodating resistance, but assess changes in strength and not hypertrophy[14,37]. A systematic review and meta-analysis of 8 studies comparing conventional resistance training to elastic resistance training found neither were superior and just as good as each other for strength improvements[43]. The analysis did not assess muscle growth.

It is suggested that mechanical tension and total time under tension are increased when using accommodating resistance, which would increase muscle growth or provide a novel stimulus. There are *no* high quality randomised or controlled studies comparing accommodating resistance to typical fixed resistances (e.g. dumbbells, barbells or machines) and muscle growth outcomes. The limited evidence from a systematic review finds accommodating resistance to be as effective, but not superior to fixed resistance for hypertrophy[31]. Whether you choose to use accommodating resistance or not should be down to preference. Consider the time requirement to set up the equipment and how the exercise *'feels'*. Furthermore, accommodating resistance may make it more difficult to track progression. It is best reserved for intermediate or advanced trainers alongside typical resistance modalities, rather than instead of.

Summary

Muscle growth is specific to the muscle. Strength is specific to the exercise.

Exercise choice should largely be driven by personal preference, based on the specific goals of the individual.

Prioritise what you want to improve on most; train the muscle or body part of interest first in a workout.

Exercises do not need to be varied for muscle growth, but exercise variation can benefit the motivation to train and therefore improve adherence.

Multi-joint (compound) and single-joint (isolation) exercises both effectively build muscle.

Multi-joint (compound) exercises do not have to be performed before single-joint (isolation) exercises, but they are technically more difficult. Therefore, it may be more practical to perform them first when using both types of exercise.

Resistance is just the tool to generate an adaptive stimulus in a muscle. Any form of resistance is effective for muscle growth when following the basic principles. The form of resistance should largely be driven by personal preference.

References

1   Gentil P, Fisher J, Steele J. A Review of the Acute Effects and Long-Term Adaptations of Single- and Multi-Joint Exercises during Resistance Training. *Sports Med Auckl NZ* 2017; 47: 843–855.

2   Nunes JP, Grgic J, Cunha PM, Ribeiro AS, Schoenfeld BJ, Salles BF de et al. What influence does resistance exercise order have on muscular strength

gains and muscle hypertrophy? A systematic review and meta-analysis. *Eur J Sport Sci* 2020; 0: 1–22.

3   Helms E, Morgan A, Valdez A. *A 6-Step Guide to Building Training Programs.* 2019. Available from: https://rippedbody.com/how-to-build-training-programs/ (accessed 11 Feb 2020).

4   Naoto, Kengo. *A Guide to Exercise Selection When You Don't Have Access to a Coach.* 2016. Available from: https://rippedbody.com/exercise-selection/ (accessed 11 Feb 2020).

5   Helms E, Morgan A, Valdez A. The *Muscle and Strength Pyramid: Training.* Available from: https://muscleandstrengthpyramids.com/ (accessed 11 Feb 2020).

6   Phillips SM, Winett RA. Uncomplicated Resistance Training and Health-Related Outcomes: Evidence for a Public Health Mandate. *Curr Sports Med Rep* 2010; 9: 208–213.

7   Schoenfeld BJ, Grgic J, Haun C, Itagaki T, Helms ER. Calculating Set-Volume for the Limb Muscles with the Performance of Multi-Joint Exercises: Implications for Resistance Training Prescription. *Sports* 2019; 7. Available from: doi:10.3390/sports7070177.

8   Ogasawara R, Yasuda T, Ishii N, Abe T. Comparison of muscle hypertrophy following 6-month of continuous and periodic strength training. *Eur J Appl Physiol* 2013; 113: 975–985.

9   Ribeiro A, Schoenfeld B, Sardinha L. Comment on: "A Review of the Acute Effects and Long-Term Adaptations of Single- and Multi-Joint Exercises During Resistance Training". *Sports Med* 2016; 47: 1–3.

10   Chowdhury RH, Reaz MBI, Ali MABM, Bakar AAA, Chellappan K, Chang TG. Surface Electromyography Signal Processing and Classification Techniques. *Sensors* 2013; 13: 12431–12466.

11   Contreras B. *Can motor unit recruitment be inferred from EMG amplitude?* 2015. Available from: https://bretcontreras.com/can-motor-unit-recruitment-be-inferred-from-emg-amplitude/ (accessed 11 Feb 2020).

12   Contreras B. *What's All the Fuss About EMG?* 2014. Available from: https://bretcontreras.com/whats-fuss-emg/ (accessed 11 Feb 2020).

13   Beardsley C. *Electromyography (EMG).* 2015. Available from: https://www.strengthandconditioningresearch.com/biomechanics/electromyography-emg/ (accessed 11 Feb 2020).

14   Hegyi A, Csala D, Péter A, Finni T, Cronin NJ. High-density electromyography activity in various hamstring exercises. *Scand J Med Sci Sports* 2019; 29: 34–43.

15   Ebben WP. Hamstring activation during lower body resistance training exercises. *Int J Sports Physiol Perform* 2009; 4: 84–96.

16   Nishiwaki GA, Urabe Y, Tanaka K. EMG Analysis of Lower Extremity Muscles in Three Different Squat Exercises. *J Jpn Phys Ther Assoc* 2006; 9: 21–26.

17   Isear JA, Erickson JC, Worrell TW. EMG analysis of lower extremity muscle recruitment patterns during an unloaded squat. *Med Sci Sports Exerc* 1997; 29: 532–539.

18   Lee S, Schultz J, Timgren J, Staelgraeve K, Miller M, Liu Y. An electromyographic and kinetic comparison of conventional and Romanian deadlifts. *J Exerc Sci Fit* 2018; 16: 87–93.

19   Vigotsky AD, Ogborn D, Phillips SM. Motor unit recruitment cannot be inferred from surface EMG amplitude and basic reporting standards must be adhered to. *Eur J Appl Physiol* 2016; 116: 657–658.

20   Vigotsky AD, Beardsley C, Contreras B, Steele J, Ogborn D, Phillips SM. Greater electromyographic responses do not imply greater motor unit recruitment and 'hypertrophic potential' cannot be inferred. *J Strength Cond Res* 2017; 31: e1–e4.

21   Gentil P, Steele J, Fisher J. Authors' Reply to Ribeiro et al.: 'A Review of the Acute Effects and Long-Term Adaptations of Single- and Multi-Joint Exercises During Resistance Training'. *Sports Med Auckl NZ* 2017; 47: 795–798.

22   Kraemer WJ, Ratamess NA. Fundamentals of resistance training: progression and exercise prescription. *Med Sci Sports Exerc* 2004; 36: 674–688.

23   Simão R, de Salles BF, Figueiredo T, Dias I, Willardson JM. Exercise order in resistance training. *Sports Med Auckl NZ* 2012; 42: 251–265.

24   Saraiva A, Pinto G, Costa e Silva G, Bentes C, Miranda H, Novaes J. Influence of exercise order on strength in Judo athletes. *Gazzetta Medica Ital Arch Sci Mediche* 2014; 173: 251–7.

25   Ogborn D, Schoenfeld BJ. The Role of Fiber Types in Muscle Hypertrophy: Implications for Loading Strategies. *Strength Cond J* 2014; 36: 20–25.

26   Baz-Valle E, Schoenfeld BJ, Torres-Unda J, Santos-Concejero J, Balsalobre-Fernández C. The effects of exercise variation in muscle thickness, maximal strength and motivation in resistance trained men. *PLOS ONE* 2019; 14: e0226989.

27   Fonseca RM, Roschel H, Tricoli V, de Souza EO, Wilson JM, Laurentino GC et al. Changes in exercises are more effective than in loading schemes to improve muscle strength. *J Strength Cond Res* 2014; 28: 3085–3092.

28   Rauch JT, Ugrinowitsch C, Barakat CI, Alvarez MR, Brummert DL, Aube DW et al. Auto-regulated exercise selection training regimen produces small increases in lean body mass and maximal strength adaptations in strength-trained individuals. *J Strength Cond Res* 2017. Available from: doi:10.1519/JSC.0000000000002272.

29   Morton RW, Colenso-Semple L, Phillips SM. Training for strength and hypertrophy: an evidence-based approach. *Curr Opin Physiol* 2019; 10: 90–95.

30   Krieger J. *Set Volume for Muscle Size: The Ultimate Evidence Based Bible*. Weightology. Available from: https://weightology.net/the-members-area/evidence-based-guides/set-volume-for-muscle-size-the-ultimate-evidence-based-bible/ (accessed 10 Feb 2020).

31   Wernbom M, Augustsson J, Thomeé R. The influence of frequency, intensity, volume and mode of strength training on whole muscle cross-sectional area in humans. *Sports Med Auckl NZ* 2007; 37: 225–264.

32   Schoenfeld B, Grgic J. Evidence-Based Guidelines for Resistance Training Volume to Maximize Muscle Hypertrophy. *Strength Cond J* 2018; 40: 107–112.

33   Fisher J, Steele J, Bruce-Low S, Smith D. Evidence-Based Resistance Training Recommendations. *Med Sport* 2011; 15: 147–162.

34   Saeterbakken AH, Mo D-A, Scott S, Andersen V. The Effects of Bench Press Variations in Competitive Athletes on Muscle Activity and Performance. *J Hum Kinet* 2017; 57: 61–71.

35   Welsch EA, Bird M, Mayhew JL. Electromyographic activity of the pectoralis major and anterior deltoid muscles during three upper-body lifts. *J Strength Cond Res* 2005; 19: 449–452.

36   Farias D de A, Willardson JM, Paz GA, Bezerra E de S, Miranda H. Maximal Strength Performance and Muscle Activation for the Bench Press and Triceps Extension Exercises Adopting Dumbbell, Barbell, and Machine Modalities Over Multiple Sets. *J Strength Cond Res* 2017; 31: 1879–1887.

37   Ghigiarelli JJ, Nagle EF, Gross FL, Robertson RJ, Irrgang JJ, Myslinski T. The effects of a 7-week heavy elastic band and weight chain program on upper-body strength and upper-body power in a sample of division 1-AA football players. *J Strength Cond Res* 2009; 23: 756–764.

38   Schick EE, Coburn JW, Brown LE, Judelson DA, Khamoui AV, Tran TT et al. A comparison of muscle activation between a Smith machine and free weight bench press. *J Strength Cond Res* 2010; 24: 779–784.

39   Ferreira DV, Ferreira-Júnior JB, Soares SRS, Cadore EL, Izquierdo M, Brown LE et al. Chest Press Exercises With Different Stability Requirements Result in Similar Muscle Damage Recovery in Resistance-Trained Men. *J Strength Cond Res* 2017; 31: 71–79.

40   Carpinelli R, Otto R, Wientt R. A critical analysis of the ACSM position stand on resistance training: Insufficient evidence to support recommended training protocols. *J Exerc Physiol Online* 2004; 7.

41   Fisher J, Steele J, Smith D. Evidence-Based Resistance Training Recommendations for Muscular Hypertrophy. *Med Sport* 2013; 17: 217–235.

42   Paoli A, Gentil P, Moro T, Marcolin G, Bianco A. Resistance Training with Single vs. Multi-joint Exercises at Equal Total Load Volume: Effects on Body Composition, Cardiorespiratory Fitness, and Muscle Strength. *Front Physiol* 2017; 8. Available from: doi:10.3389/fphys.2017.01105.

43   Lopes JSS, Machado AF, Micheletti JK, Almeida AC de, Cavina AP, Pastre CM. Effects of training with elastic resistance versus conventional resistance on muscular strength: A systematic review and meta-analysis: *SAGE Open Med* 2019. Available from: doi:10.1177/2050312119831116.

22. Timing: the time of the rest, the time of the rep and the time of the session

Muscle growth can occur using any intensity of load from 30% of your 1 repetition maximum (RM) up to 100% of your 1RM when training to, or near to failure. This corresponds to building muscle from 1 rep per set, up to 30-50 reps per set.

Your personal preference as to when you feel 'ready' to perform a subsequent productive set should be the primary factor for determining your rest period[1].

Rest periods shorter than 60 seconds result in less muscle growth than rest periods longer than 60 seconds, when set volume is equated. There is no benefit to resting less than 60 seconds between sets, and likely not less than 2 minutes. Rest at least 2 minutes between sets, possibly up to 3-5 minutes for sets with a high intensity of load (i.e. 1-6RM rep range). Rest periods do not need to be consistent from set to set.

There is an *inverse relationship* between the intensity of load (the weight you lift as a % of your 1 repetition maximum (RM)), and the number of reps that can be performed to failure. You can perform 1 rep at 100% of your 1RM (a low number of reps at a high intensity of load) and around 30-50 reps at 30-50% of your 1RM (a high number of reps at a low intensity of load). When sets are performed to or near to failure, long-term muscle growth is similar for a range of intensities of load. As such, sets within a workout are important. But, we need a break between sets to allow acute recovery from fatigue, such that another productive set may be performed[2]. But, how long should a rest period be to allow for a subsequent productive set? It is commonly thought that rep ranges and rest periods go hand in hand, such that higher reps require shorter rest, and lower reps require longer rest. A long-held belief is that rest periods need to be short when performing high rep sets so that metabolic stress can build up in the muscle. This is to promote the 'muscle pump'. Early evidence suggested that short rest periods also result in acute hormonal changes around a workout that would help with muscle growth.

However, it appears that neither are major nor meaningful factors for long-term hypertrophy[1]. Older, outdated recommendations suggested that different rep ranges and rest periods can be summarised into three broad categories for different muscular adaptations[3]:

- Use 1-6 reps for strength and rest for 3-5 minutes.
- Use 8-12 reps for hypertrophy and rest for 1-3 minutes.
- Use 15+ reps for muscular endurance and rest for 30-60 seconds.

These are also the recommendations that are commonly reported in the media and in general fitness circles. There is also discontinuity between the different ranges. Many anecdotal recommendations seem to ignore the 7th, 13th and 14th reps. The research on rep ranges, rest periods and hypertrophy does *not* suggest the model above is true. Firstly, the concept of the 8-12 rep range as being the *'hypertrophy rep range'* for muscle growth is outdated. Hypertrophy can occur using heavy, moderate and light weights; therefore hypertrophy can also occur with low and high rep ranges[4-8].

Therefore, the rep ranges can be rewritten as:

- Use 1-6 reps for hypertrophy.
- Use 6-15 reps for hypertrophy.
- Use 15+ reps for hypertrophy.

Considering hypertrophy can occur across a wide range of reps, does the rest period still need to change for a given rep range?

Rest Period

Longer rest periods allow for greater muscle growth when set volume is equated. Shorter rest periods (30 seconds to 2 minutes) still result in muscle growth. But, more sets are required to achieve the same amount of volume and the same amount of growth as sets performed with longer rest periods.

It was previously thought that to stimulate hypertrophy, shorter rest periods from anywhere between 30 seconds and 2 minutes were needed to allow metabolic stress to accumulate[1] and to promote favourable acute changes in certain hormones. However, studies comparing short rest periods (30 seconds to 2 minutes) to long rest periods (2 to 5 minutes) have shown that longer rest periods allow for greater volume to be performed, and *greater* muscle growth[1,9,10]. *No* study to date has demonstrated superior muscle growth with shorter rest periods compared to longer rest periods[1]. A systematic review of 6 studies demonstrated that rest periods longer than 60 seconds were more beneficial for muscle growth[11]. A limitation of this systematic review however, is that they only assessed the cut-off at 60 seconds and did not assess a dose-response relationship (i.e. was there more muscle growth with 2 minute rests, or 3 minute rests and so on). This is partly due to a lack of studies.

Shorter rest periods compromise the ability of muscles to perform; short rest periods result in fewer reps being performed per set.

When you reduce the rest period between sets, the number of reps you can perform per set is reduced[3]. Every set in a workout results in peripheral and central nervous system fatigue[2,12]. Peripheral and central nervous system fatigue dissipate during the rest period between sets, but some level of fatigue will remain until there is complete rest (i.e. rest in the days after the workout)[12]. After multiple sets, there is an amount of fatigue that prevents any further productive sets in that session. Shorter rest periods will mean a greater presence of central nervous system fatigue for any given set after the first set. A greater presence of central nervous system fatigue will mean the high-threshold motor units controlling the muscle fibres that are most responsive to resistance training are not recruited. Hence, fewer reps are performed before muscular task failure. As such, each set after a shorter rest period results in fewer reps, less workload per set and less hypertrophy[10]. When sets are equated, using longer rest periods results in greater muscle growth[10]. The reduction in set workload from short rest periods was demonstrated in a study where males and females performed 3 sets of the bench press with different rest periods. Rest periods shorter than 3 minutes (either 1 minute or 2 minutes) resulted in fewer reps being performed for a predicted 10RM. *All* individuals performed 10 reps on the first set. By the third set, men resting for 1 minute between sets could only perform 4 reps on average. With 2 minutes rest, 5.9 reps were performed in the third set. With 3 minutes rest, 7.7 reps in the third set. Comparing the set workload, resting for 3 minutes resulted in an extra 3.7 reps in the third set compared to resting for 1 minute (7.7 reps compared to 4 reps)[13]. In women, resting for 3 minutes resulted in an extra 1.9 reps in the third set compared to resting for 1 minute (9.6 reps compared to 7.7 reps). There is *no* optimum rest period. But, it appears that it requires at least a couple of minutes of rest for fatigue to dissipate to a level where a sufficient number of reps can be performed in a subsequent set.

We can now rewrite the rep ranges along with their corresponding rest periods categories for muscle growth as the following[3,9,10]:

- 1-6 reps for hypertrophy, rest at least 60 seconds, up to 3-5 minutes.
- 6-15 reps for hypertrophy, rest at least 60 seconds, up to 2-3 minutes.
- 15+ reps for hypertrophy, rest at least 60 seconds, up to 2-3 minutes.

The length of your rest periods should come down to personal preference, by *autoregulating* when to begin the next set when you *feel* ready[1]. Rest long enough such that you have recovered sufficiently to perform a productive set, but not so long that you lose focus, get cold and your training session takes 4 hours. As an example, say you *feel* 90% ready (if 100% ready is prior to your first set) for the next set after 2 minutes, 95% ready after 5 minutes and 99% ready after 10 minutes. Unless you are aiming for 1 rep maximum attempts, 2 minutes rest will probably be optimal between insufficient rest and a workout taking too long.

Rest periods do not need to be kept constant

Resting for exactly the same amount of time between every set is probably unnecessary, because the amount of rest you need to *feel* 90% ready will vary, being dependent on[1]:

- The intensity of effort of your last set (higher effort will require longer rest).
- The intensity of the load used and therefore the rep range performed (higher loads will require longer rest).
- The exercise performed. A longer rest period may be required for more complex and technically difficult exercises such as compound or free weight (barbells and dumbbells) exercises, than less technical isolation or machine exercises.
- Your general levels of fatigue (higher levels of general fatigue will require longer rest).
- Age.
- Gender.

For example, a set of squats at 90% of your 1RM taken one rep short of failure (i.e. 1 rep in reserve (RIR)) (see chapter 19 regarding intensity of effort) will require much longer rest before the next set than a set of bicep curls at 60% of your 1RM taken 3 or 4 reps short of failure (RIR = 3-4).

As such, the optimal rest you need may differ between sets. That being said, a regimented 2-3 minute rest period can help to keep a workout efficient especially when time-limited. In contrast, autoregulating rest periods can help to ensure that each set is as productive as possible[1]. This will largely be dependent on how you like to train, and how much time you can commit to training. That being said, for most sets the rest period needed will likely be quite similar.

Shorter rest periods do not result in a time efficient workout for muscle growth.

One argument for using shorter rest periods is that it allows you to complete a workout in less time. Indeed, you may be able to complete a given number of sets in shorter time, but this does *not* translate to the same amount of muscle growth.

Shorter rest periods do not allow as many reps to be completed for a given intensity[3]. Shorter rest periods result in a reduced set workload (fewer reps for that set with a given load and rep duration). This is due to the presence of significant central nervous system fatigue from the previous set, limiting high-threshold motor unit recruitment, resulting in muscular task failure with fewer reps performed. For example, say you aim to perform 4 sets of 10 reps with your 10-11RM for a given exercise. With long rest periods you might achieve 8-10 reps per set. Using a shorter rest period may result in only 6-8 reps per set. Very short rest periods may only allow 4-6 reps per set. This means comparatively fewer reps per set (with the same load and rep duration) when resting for very short periods of time, even though the perceived effort may still be high (a rating of perceived exertion (RPE) >8)[2]. An in-depth discussion of why shorter rest periods and the resulting reduction in workload result in lower muscle growth was discussed in chapter 19 on page 362. *Shorter* rests will mean your workout is quicker, but *less* effective for muscle growth[9]. The data for sets 1, 2 and 3 in the table below are the averages (rounded to the nearest rep) from the bench press study discussed on the previous page[13]. It is clear to see how set workload is significantly reduced with reductions in rest period, such that subsequent sets become less and less productive. Where the cut-off lies between a rest period being sufficient or insufficient for a subsequent productive set is inconclusive. It is currently suggested to be at least 1 minute in length, but it may well be longer.

Rest period	Set 1	Set 2	Set 3	Total reps	Relative workload in set 3 compared to 3 minutes rest (matched for load and rep duration)
1 minute	10	7	4	21	50%
2 minutes	10	8	6	24	75%
3 minutes	10	9	8	27	100%

How rest period can influence rep performance in a given set in males. From Ratamess et al., 2012[13].

If you wanted to achieve a similar amount of volume workload (albeit not a good measure of muscle growth) as a longer rest period when training with a shorter rest period, then you would need to perform more sets (how many extra sets would relate to how many fewer reps you achieved per set compared to a longer rest period). The result is that you would probably end up with a similar workout duration. You would also undergo *greater* effort to achieve that *same* volume. Short rest periods are not a more efficient method to generate volume for hypertrophy, compared to longer rest periods.

If you are short on time and looking to maximise muscle growth from your session, still focus on longer rest periods (at least 1-2 minutes) and achieving a rating of perceived exertion (RPE) above

5, or reps in reserve (RIR) below 5. Reduce workout time by using rep ranges and exercises that allow you to perform your normal set volume in as short a time as possible. Such as, choosing moderate to high rep ranges or choosing exercises that require less warm-up preparation (e.g. isolation or machine exercises). Reduce the number of sets performed in the workout as a last resort to reduce workout time, after first ensuring the training session has been optimised. If you just want to get a pump and a sweat on, then by all means cut your rest periods down. Just don't expect to grow as much. One other solution may be to use the advanced training technique known as a 'drop set'. This is discussed in chapter 23.

It is most important to ensure you rest at least 1-2 minutes rather than 30s to 1 minute[3,7]. Whether resting up to 3-5 minutes is more beneficial for all rep ranges is unclear. Longer rest periods will be beneficial for high intensities of load such as when lifting in the 1-6 rep range. To determine how long you should rest, try rest periods of at least 2-3 minutes for a few weeks and see how well you perform. Then, try a few weeks with longer rest periods of 4 to 5 minutes and see how your training differs. The additional rest may allow you to be more mentally prepared and rested, or they may result in you losing focus between sets. Whether you find 2 minutes of rest to be sufficient is up to you to experiment and discover. If you prefer to experience the muscle pump with shorter rest periods, then consider performing more of your sets with higher rep ranges, or reserve shorter rests for later in a workout.

Besides not letting your body cool down too much or losing focus, there probably isn't a detrimental effect to resting for longer, besides your workout taking longer. It would probably be unwise to rest up to 10 minutes between sets. But from what we know, resting for an extra minute or two may be beneficial, but unlikely to be detrimental. No studies to date have assessed the effect of using rest periods longer than 5 minutes on muscle growth.

Rest periods for metabolic stress

Metabolic stress may promote muscle growth, but to a much lesser extent than mechanical tension. Metabolic stress may adequately promote muscle growth with current recommendations of performing sets to, or near to failure. There is little evidence to recommend training to maximise metabolic stress and the sensation of a muscle pump for muscle growth.

If choosing to train for the muscle pump (via metabolic stress), keep it to the end of your workouts.

Experiment with some short rest periods at the end of your workout and see how you find it, but don't let it become the focus of your workout.

The prior conversation has focussed on training with mechanical tension as the primary focus. Indeed, mechanical tension appears to be the primary mechanism for muscle growth and is the basis for evidence-based recommendations. Despite this, metabolic stress may still play a minor role. Metabolic stress-mediated muscle growth may be adequately achieved within the context of current recommendations of performing sets to, or near to failure. Higher rep, low load sets with longer rest periods performed to, or near to failure will still generate significant amounts of metabolic stress and the sensation of the *'muscle pump'*. Metabolic stress *will* accumulate with the recommendations discussed above and therefore any theoretical benefit of metabolic stress for hypertrophy may already be achieved. Whether it is necessary to train in a manner as to maximise metabolic stress, is unknown. Training specifically to promote metabolic stress for muscle growth is not supported by current research. Maximising metabolic stress may be of no benefit and be detrimental. But, you may wish to add this style of training to your workout to *'cover all bases'* and for personal preference, because it can be an enjoyable training style. Metabolic stress can be increased by using higher reps, lower intensities of load and shorter rest periods. For the higher rep range component of your workout (which should be at or near the end of your session), you would simply reduce the rest period to 30-60 seconds. Metabolic stress may also be important for some individuals for adherence. Inducing and experiencing metabolic stress as the muscle pump can itself be fun, and part of the enjoyment of training. If it allows you to adhere to training, then by all means perform such sets at the end of a workout. However, use the technique sparingly as there is limited evidence to support its benefit in muscle growth, and as it can generate large amounts of fatigue.

Rep speed and rep duration

Rep duration refers to how long it takes to complete a lift. A faster rep speed means a shorter rep duration. Rep duration can be different for different parts of the movement.

As a training variable, rep duration is a minor consideration and should not be manipulated. The optimal rep duration is yet to be determined, and a wide range of rep durations can effectively build muscle. Some exercises may better suit a faster rep speed, and some exercises may better suit a slower rep speed. Choose the rep duration for your chosen exercises that allows for consistency across reps, sets and sessions.

Older recommendations suggest most people should use a fast (1-2s) concentric duration, and a moderately controlled (1 to 4s) eccentric duration[9]. However, the evidence for this is very limited and there is little to no evidence for a superior rep duration[14]. It does appear that very slow rep durations (>10s) are suboptimal if muscle growth is the goal.

There is no evidence that varying the rep speed benefits muscle growth. Varying speed adds complexity to a programme and is a variable that most people do not need to alter. Varying speed should be reserved for experienced resistance trainers and considered an advanced training variable to theoretically 'cover all bases', but is not supported by research. Varying rep speed can detract away from the main goal of lifting to, or near to failure. As stated before, choose the rep duration for your chosen exercises that allows for consistency across reps, sets and sessions.

Rep speed refers to the rate at which different portions of the lift are conducted. The rep duration refers to the number of seconds it takes to perform a lift. A lift can be split into 4 distinct parts:

1. The first* is the lowering portion of the lift, where the muscle lengthens (*eccentric contraction*).
2. The second is where the muscle is not changing length but still producing force at the bottom of the lift (*isometric contraction*). The muscle is at its peak length.
3. The third is the lifting of the weight where the muscle shortens (*concentric contraction*).
4. The fourth is the second *isometric contraction* at the top of the lift. The muscle is at its shortest length.

* Technically the first portion of a lift can be eccentric or concentric, depending on the exercise. The first part of a squat is an eccentric contraction as you squat down, whereas the first part of a shoulder press is a concentric contraction as you press up.

A systematic review and meta-analysis of 8 studies demonstrated that rep durations between 0.5 and 8 seconds result in similar muscle growth. The data suggested that very slow rep speeds (>10s) are probably sub-optimal for muscle growth. But, the data is very limited and of lower quality in terms of how muscle growth was measured[14]. The analysis only considered the whole rep duration and did not consider the 4 parts of the lift in isolation. The importance of rep speeds in different portions of the lift may be important for hypertrophy, but this is still largely unknown. Older recommendations are to use a fast concentric, and a controlled but not slow eccentric contraction[9,15,16]. However, the limited evidence has *not* demonstrated a superior rep duration for hypertrophy[4]. For example, a recent study in males and females demonstrated no difference in muscle growth after 10 weeks when using a 2s-4s or a 10s-10s concentric-eccentric contraction rep durations. However, both groups gained minimal muscle mass compared to the start of the plan, limiting the utility of the study[17]. This may have been due to the fact participants were trained, the training was of low volume and their diets were not controlled for[17].

If differences in rep durations affect muscle growth, it is likely they are limited by the same factors as other variables, such as study duration and slow rates of muscle growth in trained individuals (see chapter 16 regarding exercise research limitations).

Concentric contraction duration

Older recommendations are to lift a weight with a duration of around 1-2 seconds. But, the evidence does not suggest a superior benefit with using faster rep speeds compared to slower rep speeds. A fast rep speed may allow for better consistency by not unconsciously shortening the rep duration to increase the number of reps performed as fatigue kicks in. But ultimately, rep duration should be based on personal preference to maintain consistent form[4].

Maximum concentric rep velocity is inversely related to the intensity of load[3]. Because of the force-velocity relationship for a muscle (chapter 17), to move very heavy (>80% 1RM) weights, the contraction speed must be slow. Therefore, rep tempo can *only* be unintentionally slow at high intensity loads. However, maximal concentric contractions with lighter weights will lead to fast velocities because less force is needed. As you complete reps with lighter loads, fatigue will occur. Rep velocities with lighter loads will eventually slow down when approaching failure to a velocity *comparable* to lifting a heavy weight[2]. It is possible to lift lighter loads at an intentionally fast *or* intentionally slow rep tempo[3].

Completing a rep with a deliberately slow concentric tempo rep speed does *not* lead to increased muscle stimulation. It results in fewer reps being performed in the set. The slower the concentric contraction, the greater the reduction in workload and reps performed[18]. Very slow tempos may require a drop of 40% in the intensity of load to perform the same number of reps, or a reduction in reps performed at a given load compared to a fast tempo[19]. Given the experimental evidence showing a sub-optimal response to very slow rep speeds (>10s), and the observed reduction in the work performed when using slow rep speeds compared to fast rep speeds, it has been experimentally and theoretically deduced that fast concentric rep speeds should be used for muscle growth. But, this has *not* been proven experimentally. In fact, studies demonstrate that a wide range of concentric rep speeds result in similar muscle growth[4,7,14]. Currently, a 1 second concentric contraction speed appears comparable to a 3 or 5 second contraction speed for muscle growth[17]. It is unknown whether slow rep tempos must be taken to failure or not, as studies included in the previously mentioned meta-analysis required all sets to be taken to failure[14]. Are slower rep tempos only effective when sets are taken to muscular failure? Currently, it is clear that lifting across a range of fast and moderate tempos will lead to hypertrophy. The concentric rep speed chosen should be the one of personal preference that allows for consistency[7,14].

Eccentric contraction duration

Older recommendations are to lower a weight with a controlled tempo of around 2-4 seconds. Eccentric contractions produce muscle growth when the weight is lowered in a controlled manner. But, the evidence does not suggest a superior benefit to fast rep speeds compared to slower speeds. Rep duration should be based on personal preference to maintain consistent form.

The evidence for an optimal eccentric contraction rep speed is fairly inconclusive. What is considered a *fast* rep tempo and what is considered *slow* is not standardised[20]. Eccentric contractions can result in hypertrophy that is distinct from concentric contractions[21,22]. From a theoretical viewpoint, when using a very fast eccentric contraction speed, the load is essentially being *dropped*. This may limit eccentric contraction-mediated muscle growth because there is very little tension on the muscle when the weight is dropped. This may also influence the concentric portion of the lift by promoting poor technique and the use of other muscles, as the weight is not under control[23]. On the other hand, very slow eccentric contractions require significant drops in the intensity of load to produce a given number of reps, and fewer reps for the same load, reducing workout volume[20]. Slow eccentric contractions also reduce motor unit activity[14,20] and result in greater muscle damage after the workout. Extending the duration of a set spent where the muscle is lengthening can increase muscle damage[9]. As such, recommendations have suggested that the eccentric portion should be controlled, such that the lengthening of the muscle takes around 2-4 seconds. This is to ensure that the weight is not dropped to maintain tension on the muscle, but also to ensure that the rep speed is not excessively slow, which would reduce set workload and induce excessive muscle damage[3,9]. Despite this theoretical consideration, a wide range of eccentric durations have been shown to be suitable in achieving muscle growth[17]. Further studies are needed to identify the role of eccentric rep speed on muscle growth[20]. Ideally, the weight should not be dropped to maintain proper control throughout the set and to prevent injury. But again, the eccentric rep duration chosen should be the one of personal preference.

Your personal rep tempo

The rep tempo you use should be one that allows for best *control* of the weight and *maintenance* of form. One consideration from a consistency perspective is that it may be more consistent to lift as fast as possible (i.e. lifting with *intent*) and then controlling the weight back down (i.e. not dropping the weight and losing tension). This is a tempo that can be accurately *replicated* across reps, sets and sessions without having to overthink. When a set starts to get hard (i.e. approaching failure), it may become more and more difficult to focus on proper form *and* maintaining a given tempo that deviates from this. The reduction in rep velocity may also aid in gauging how close you are to reaching failure. This is not superior, and only preferable if form cannot be kept consistent with another rep duration. Rep durations may also vary with exercise choice and exercise modality (e.g. machine or free weights). Some exercises may better suit a faster rep tempo, and some may better suit a slower rep tempo. Find the right tempo for *each* of your chosen exercises and stick to it, so that you can accurately track progression[17].

As a beginner or intermediate, rep tempo should be kept consistent for a given exercise to allow accurate tracking of progressive overload. There is little to no evidence that varying rep durations influences muscle growth[4].

As an advanced lifter, varying the rep tempo may provide a theoretical novel stimulus to increase muscle growth, although there is little to no evidence to support this. If used, it should be used sparingly to ensure reliable monitoring of progression[4].

Isometric contraction duration: paused reps

There is very little research assessing paused reps and muscle growth. Given the lack of evidence suggesting variation in rep durations on muscle growth, there is little to no evidence to suggest paused reps are superior for muscle growth compared to reps with pauses.

Paused reps can be useful to ensure consistency and that concentric contractions are the result of the muscle contracting, and not as a result of momentum or elastic recoil.

Paused reps are a basic example of manipulating rep tempo. After completing each rep, there is a momentary pause before the next rep is completed during the second phase (the isometric contraction in the stretched position). This can either be an actual isometric hold (such as holding the bottom position of a squat) or coming to a complete rest between reps to take the load off the muscle (such as letting the load on a machine come back to rest). The idea is that the brief pause means each rep must be completed *solely* by the muscle contracting, without being aided by the force generated from the elastic energy stored in connective tissues (*tendons*) at the bottom of each rep. This can occur with fast rep tempos. The pause means that the target muscle has to generate the necessary force throughout the whole range of motion and therefore *potentially* experiences greater mechanical tension. Consider the calf raise. After the eccentric (heels lowering) phase, using a pause at the bottom before contracting and pushing the heels up should be noticeably harder to execute the rep, because you can no longer *bounce* up by utilising some of the stored elastic energy. Studies utilising a pause between the eccentric and concentric contractions find that it results in more reliable strength tests[24]. Paused reps can be an effective way to ensure that proper form is used, consistency is maintained and that concentric contractions are achieved by using the target muscles. But, if this can already be achieved without a pause, there is unlikely to be a benefit with paused reps when training with a sufficient intensity of effort.

Given that the intensity of effort and proximity to failure are the main set-specific factors to consider for muscle growth, whether this were achieved with or without a pause between portions of a lift is unlikely to influence muscle growth. Including a brief (1 second pause) at the top or bottom of the rep can ensure good form and consistency to measure progression, if this is an issue. However, if using a controlled eccentric contraction, the load should be under control throughout the entire range of the movement. Again, whether this significantly affects muscle growth is unknown and probably unlikely, and its use should primarily come down to personal preference.

The time of day: when to train

Train at the time of day that suits you. The evidence currently suggests there is no meaningful effect on muscle growth with training at different times of the day. Timing has more of an effect on strength. Completing a training session (adherence) and performing sufficient volume is more important than the timing of it[7].

Is there a best time to train? It has been suggested that training in the afternoon or evening is better than training in the morning. If you are training for strength, then it appears so. If the primary goal is muscle growth, timing appears relatively unimportant[25,26]. In the morning, your body is at a lower temperature than in the evening. Some hormones in the body such as *testosterone* and *cortisol* are under a *circadian* rhythm (their levels vary depending on the time of day or night). It has been suggested that these factors may mean greater strength improvements and more muscle growth when training in the evenings, or at least training later on in the day. A recent systematic review and meta-analysis of 11 studies has indeed shown that at the beginning of a training programme, individuals have lower strength in morning sessions than in evening sessions[25-27]. However, individuals who trained in the morning had comparable strength and muscle growth as those who trained in the afternoon by the end of the programme. Strength improvements were the same, regardless of whether individuals trained in the morning or in the evening. Muscle growth was also the same, regardless of whether they trained in the morning or evening. Training in the evening however, maintained the difference in strength between morning and evenings[25]. If you want to be bigger or stronger it doesn't matter what time of day you train. Training frequency and volume were equated between mornings and evenings, so the similar effect was not due to one group training more. Despite a wide age range, most people in the analysis were young untrained men. Therefore, the applicability to other ages and to females may be limited. With the current evidence, train at the time that suits you and your lifestyle. If you do prefer to train in the evenings then do so, but don't feel as though you must avoid morning sessions if this is the only time you can train.

The fact that morning training led to similar strength levels as the evening suggests a possible adaptation of the body to morning sessions. The authors suggest that this may mean that the body is *'primed'* to train in the mornings. This seems plausible, when considering that people become accustomed to new routines. Something that would need to be proven in a future study is if this priming of the body to morning sessions means that the body becomes less primed to train in the evenings. Does training both in the morning *and* the evening across the week influence muscle growth compared to only training in the morning *or* the evening? Given the lack of any influence so far, any difference is likely to be fairly insignificant for most people.

One final point is that the studies in this analysis did not consider the effect of *'chronotype'*. This is more commonly referred to as larks and owls, or morning people and evening people. Do morning people train better in the mornings, and evening people train better in the evenings? Even if this were true, if the timing of training was based on personal preference, individuals would train to suit their lifestyle, such that they probably already train at their ideal time.

So, if you're an early bird and like to wake up at 5am for leg day, then go for it, you'll make as much progress as the person who rocks up to the gym at 9pm. Similarly, if an early morning workout fills you with dread, save your session for the afternoon or evening when you feel ready, and are mentally and physically ready to train with a high intensity of effort.

References

1   Henselmans M, Schoenfeld BJ. The effect of inter-set rest intervals on resistance exercise-induced muscle hypertrophy. *Sports Med Auckl NZ* 2014; 44: 1635–1643.

2   Sadri K, Khani M, Sadri I. Role of Central Fatigue in Resistance and Endurance Exercises: An Emphasis on Mechanisms and Potential Sites. *Sportlogia* 2014; 10: 65–80.

3   American College of Sports Medicine. American College of Sports Medicine position stand. Progression models in resistance training for healthy adults. *Med Sci Sports Exerc* 2009; 41: 687–708.

4   Carpinelli R, Otto R, Wientt R. A critical analysis of the ACSM position stand on resistance training: Insufficient evidence to support recommended training protocols. *J Exerc Physiol Online* 2004; 7.

5   Mitchell CJ, Churchward-Venne TA, West DWD, Burd NA, Breen L, Baker SK et al. Resistance exercise load does not determine training-mediated hypertrophic gains in young men. *J Appl Physiol* 2012; 113: 71–77.

6   Nuckols G. *The 'Hypertrophy Rep Range' – Fact or Fiction?* 2016. Available from: https://www.strongerbyscience.com/hypertrophy-range-fact-fiction/ (accessed 11 Feb 2020).

7   Morton RW, Colenso-Semple L, Phillips SM. Training for strength and hypertrophy: an evidence-based approach. *Curr Opin Physiol* 2019; 10: 90–95.

8   Morton RW, Colenso-Semple L, Phillips SM. Training for strength and hypertrophy: an evidence-based approach. *Curr Opin Physiol* 2019; 11: 149–150.

9   Wernbom M, Augustsson J, Thomeé R. The influence of frequency, intensity, volume and mode of strength training on whole muscle cross-sectional area in humans. *Sports Med Auckl NZ* 2007; 37: 225–264.

10   Schoenfeld BJ, Pope ZK, Benik FM, Hester GM, Sellers J, Nooner JL et al. Longer Interset Rest Periods Enhance Muscle Strength and Hypertrophy in Resistance-Trained Men. *J Strength Cond Res* 2016; 30: 1805–1812.

11   Grgic J, Lazinica B, Mikulic P, Krieger J, Schoenfeld B. The effects of short versus long inter-set rest intervals in resistance training on measures of muscle hypertrophy: A systematic review. *Eur J Sport Sci* 2017; 17: 1–11.

12   Wan J-J, Qin Z, Wang P-Y, Sun Y, Liu X. Muscle fatigue: general understanding and treatment. *Exp Mol Med* 2017; 49: e384.

13   Ratamess N, Chiarello C, Sacco A, Hoffman J, Faigenbaum A, Ross R et al. The Effects of Rest Interval Length on Acute Bench Press Performance: The Influence of Gender and Muscle Strength. *J Strength Cond Res* 2012; 26: 1817–1826.

14   Schoenfeld BJ, Ogborn DI, Krieger JW. Effect of repetition duration during resistance training on muscle hypertrophy: a systematic review and meta-analysis. *Sports Med Auckl NZ* 2015; 45: 577–585.

15   Kraemer WJ, Ratamess NA. Fundamentals of resistance training: progression and exercise prescription. *Med Sci Sports Exerc* 2004; 36: 674–688.

16   Kraemer WJ, Adams K, Cafarelli E, Dudley GA, Dooly C, Feigenbaum MS et al. American College of Sports Medicine position stand. Progression models in resistance training for healthy adults. *Med Sci Sports Exerc* 2002; 34: 364–380.

17   Carlson L, Jonker B, Westcott WL, Steele J, Fisher JP. Neither repetition duration nor number of muscle actions affect strength increases, body composition, muscle size, or fasted blood glucose in trained males and females. *Appl Physiol Nutr Metab Physiol Appl Nutr Metab* 2019; 44: 200–207.

18   Mårtensson G. *The effect of lifting speed on factors related to resistance training: A study on muscle activity, amount of repetitions performed, and time under tension during bench press in young males.* 2015 Available from: http://urn.kb.se/resolve?urn=urn:nbn:se:hh:diva-28522 (accessed 12 Feb 2020).

19   Wilk M, Golas A, Stastny P, Nawrocka M, Krzysztofik M, Zajac A. Does Tempo of Resistance Exercise Impact Training Volume? *J Hum Kinet* 2018; 62: 241–250.

20   Suchomel TJ, Wagle JP, Douglas J, Taber CB, Harden M, Haff GG et al. Implementing Eccentric Resistance Training—Part 1: A Brief Review of Existing Methods. *J Funct Morphol Kinesiol* 2019; 4: 38.

21   Douglas J, Pearson S, Ross A, McGuigan M. Chronic Adaptations to Eccentric Training: A Systematic Review. *Sports Med Auckl NZ* 2017; 47: 917–941.

22   Schoenfeld BJ, Ogborn DI, Vigotsky AD, Franchi MV, Krieger JW. Hypertrophic Effects of Concentric vs. Eccentric Muscle Actions: A Systematic Review and Meta-analysis. *J Strength Cond Res* 2017; 31: 2599–2608.

23   Marzilger R, Bohm S, Mersmann F, Arampatzis A. Effects of Lengthening Velocity During Eccentric Training on Vastus Lateralis Muscle Hypertrophy. *Front Physiol* 2019; 10. Available from: doi:10.3389/fphys.2019.00957.

24   Pallarés JG, Sánchez-Medina L, Pérez CE, De La Cruz-Sánchez E, Mora-Rodriguez R. Imposing a pause between the eccentric and concentric phases increases the reliability of isoinertial strength assessments. *J Sports Sci* 2014; 32: 1165–1175.

25   Grgic J, Lazinica B, Garofolini A, Schoenfeld BJ, Saner NJ, Mikulic P. The effects of time of day-specific resistance training on adaptations in skeletal muscle hypertrophy and muscle strength: A systematic review and meta-analysis. *Chronobiol Int* 2019; 36: 449–460.

26   Sedliak M, Finni T, Cheng S, Lind M, Häkkinen K. Effect of time-of-day-specific strength training on muscular hypertrophy in men. *J Strength Cond Res* 2009; 23: 2451–2457.

27   Guette M, Gondin J, Martin A. Time-of-Day Effect on the Torque and Neuromuscular Properties of Dominant and Non-Dominant Quadriceps Femoris. *Chronobiol Int* 2005; 22: 541–558.

23. Advanced training techniques

Standard conventional sets to, or near to failure builds significant muscle mass and should be the basis of any resistance training plan for hypertrophy. There is no conclusive evidence that advanced training techniques (that extend a set beyond failure) can promote greater muscle growth than conventional sets to, or near to failure[1,2]. Some advanced training techniques may be useful to promote hypertrophy in some individuals.

The rationale for using advanced training techniques is based largely on non-scientific literature, anecdote, theoretical assumptions and expert opinion. Considering the general lack of research in resistance training for hypertrophy, it is unsurprising that there are even fewer studies on advanced training techniques[3].

Some advanced training techniques have been shown to be equivalent to, but not superior to standard sets for muscle growth. Some techniques can be very useful when short on time and there is a need to complete a productive session quickly. But, they are not necessary nor additive to performing conventional sets. Advanced training techniques should be considered as an adjunct to conventional training, rather than a replacement of conventional training. Advanced techniques are highly fatiguing and can cause a lot of muscle damage. There is an increased risk of overtraining and injury with using advanced training techniques compared to conventional training. Some techniques push muscles beyond standard concentric failure. Therefore, if utilised, they should not be performed in every workout. If they are used, save them for the last set of an exercise. They are also more difficult to track progression with compared to straight sets. Some techniques suit compound exercises and others suit isolation exercises. As a beginner, advanced techniques are not necessary, and may only potentially be of benefit in intermediate and advanced trainers.

Consider the fact that there is little evidence to support their benefit, but definite evidence that they result in greater fatigue and muscle damage. In other words, a possible but unconfirmed small benefit, but a definite and potentially large cost.

A conventional set is where a load is lifted (concentric contraction) and lowered (eccentric contraction) to, or near to failure as discussed so far, and as outlined in chapter 22 regarding rep tempo. The rationale behind advanced training techniques is that with training experience, the muscle needs to undergo a greater stimulus which cannot be achieved with conventional sets alone. But is this actually true? A large part of the reasoning for advanced training techniques is to further increase metabolic stress and muscle damage, as mechanisms to increase muscle growth[4]. However, as discussed in chapter 17, metabolic stress and muscle damage appear to be much less relevant to muscle growth than mechanical tension. Given hypertrophy is equivocal between sets taken to failure, and sets taken near to failure, there is unlikely to be any benefit through mechanical tension by taking sets beyond failure.

In terms of recovery, one study in trained individuals with 6 years' experience found on average that a single session involving 10 sets of advanced training techniques (*pre-exhaust* and *super sets*) did not negatively impact performance 48 hours later compared to conventional sets[4]. However, this study only assessed the effect of a single bout of advanced training techniques within a moderate session volume in young trained males, and the conventional sets were also taken to failure, which would *also* be highly fatiguing. Occasional use of advanced training techniques is unlikely to impact performance, but excessive use likely will.

Blood-flow restriction training (BFR)

Blood-flow restriction involves placing a cuff around the arms or legs, to limit blood flow during resistance exercise.

Blood-flow restriction with light loads is as effective as using heavy loads to build muscle. It is not superior. It can be used to reduce stress on joints and tendons and results in increased metabolic stress and muscle activity. Consider using blood-flow restriction when returning from an injury, or to prevent excessive joint strain by avoiding heavy loads. Use a load from 20-50% of your 1 repetition maximum (RM) with higher reps (15 to 30 per set) for 2 to 4 sets, with exercises targeting the arms or legs at the end of a workout[5]. If there is no reason to avoid using heavy loads, there is little benefit to using blood-flow restriction.

Blood-flow restriction is one of the better studied advanced training techniques. Guidelines have even been developed for its proper application[6]. Unlike many of the other advanced training techniques, blood-flow restriction training does *not* aim to push a set *beyond* failure. Blood-flow restriction involves reducing the circulation of blood flow in order to increase fatigue and promote metabolic stress. Multiple suggestions have been made as to how blood-flow restriction can promote muscle growth, including increased muscle activation, stimulating muscle protein synthesis, cellular signalling or muscle swelling[5,7]. The aim of blood-flow restriction is to prevent venous blood flow, but not to prevent arterial blood flow *into* the arm or leg[5]. The venous system takes blood *away* from the arm and back to the heart. It is a much lower pressure system than the arterial system, making this practically possible. This is usually achieved by using tourniquets, pressure cuffs or elastic bands that can tighten on the upper arm or leg[5]. Cuffs are tightened to be sufficiently tight, but not so tight that it feels as though the arm is going numb. Blood-flow restriction training poses *no* greater safety risks than conventional resistance training[5,7].

Blood-flow restriction at lower intensities of load is beneficial in promoting hypertrophy and strength to a similar extent as hypertrophy from training with heavy loads[5,8]. It is already known that light loads to failure increase muscle mass to the same extent as heavy loads to failure when volume is equated[9]. When training to failure using blood-flow restriction with light loads, or the same light load alone (in this study, 40% of 1RM), muscle growth is the same[10]. Using blood-flow restriction reduces the volume of work performed for the same load (i.e. fewer reps are performed in a given set with a given load)[10]. Conventional training can produce similar hypertrophy at loads as low as 30% of 1RM compared to 80 or 90% of 1RM. However with blood-flow restriction, it appears that the minimum load threshold for hypertrophy shifts from 30% of 1RM, *down* to 20% of 1RM[7,9,11]. In fact, blood-flow restriction can even result in muscle growth when used in conjunction with walking or cycling, however to a much lesser extent than with higher resistance loads[5]. Despite the use of much lighter weights, blood-flow restriction training results in similar levels of muscle damage and higher levels of delayed onset of muscle soreness (DOMS) as conventional training with heavy loads[12]. However, this is neither long lasting nor excessive. Therefore when considering recovery and training frequency, it can be considered similarly to conventional sets[5]. It is recommended to not maintain blood-flow restriction continuously between sets to allow reperfusion of muscles with blood. Use blood-flow restriction during the set, then remove the pressure during the rest period.

Blood-flow restriction can easily be implemented by using a cuff that can be tightened around the arm or leg before performing the exercise. It should be considered when you may need to *avoid* using heavy loads, but training is still possible[9]. The same hypertrophic effect can be achieved as traditional training to failure, but with much lighter weights. Blood-flow restriction can therefore be useful during rehabilitation or to reduce stress on joints, muscles and tendons[9]. There is no evidence that blood-flow restriction results in a different form of hypertrophy to conventional training. Therefore, the benefit to using blood-flow restriction is limited if there is no need to avoid using heavier loads, especially considering the requirement of additional equipment, and the effort in setting it up for each set.

Current recommendations for blood-flow restriction are to use a load from 20-50% of your 1RM with higher reps (15 to 30 per set) for 2 to 4 sets, with exercises targeting the arms or legs. Use a concentric and eccentric contraction duration of 1 to 2 seconds. Suggestions are to keep rest periods shorter than those used for conventional sets with 30-60 second rests. Blood-flow restriction can be used 2 to 3 times per week and can promote muscle growth over a few weeks and longer. If using blood-flow restriction as an additional technique to conventional training, perform blood-flow restriction sets at the end of a workout after sets with moderate to heavy loads[5,6].

Rest-pause

Rest-pause is a technique whereby in a set, you take a rest 1 or 2 reps before failure, for around 10-15 seconds. This brief recovery allows you to perform an extra 4 or 5 reps. This can be taken further by only performing 3 or 4 reps after the first rest (i.e. resting 1 or 2 reps before failure again), resting another 10-15 seconds and performing another 2 to 3 reps. Whether this is superior to conventional sets is inconclusive, with a lack of long-term studies assessing rest-pause and muscle growth[13-15].

Again, this is highly demanding and should not be used in every set, but can be a useful tool to generate workout volume in a short amount of time[15]. Rest-pause can be used on both compound and isolation exercises. The rest should be taken at the point of least tension to allow some level of recovery. For the bench press, this would be with arms extended, or in a squat when standing upright. This can easily be achieved with machines by letting the weights return back onto the stack, whilst still holding the load and maintaining a low level of tension.

Eccentric training

Eccentric (lengthening) contractions can result in distinct muscle growth that differs from concentric contractions.

Eccentric contractions result in muscle growth during a typical conventional set where the same weight is lifted and lowered under control.

Additional eccentric training techniques have yet to be shown to result in greater muscle growth in addition to conventional training.

Eccentric contractions result in significant muscle growth that is different to muscle growth from concentric contractions[16]. Eccentric contractions tend to result in more muscle fibre elements in *series* at the distal portion of the muscle. Concentric contractions tend to add muscle fibre elements in *parallel* around the middle of the muscle[16,17]. Eccentric contractions usually occur during conventional resistance training by controlling the weight down. This results in eccentric contraction-mediated hypertrophy[16,18].

As such, sub-maximal (lighter than what you could lift for 1 rep) eccentric contractions typically form part of a standard training programme. However, a muscle can be up 20-50% stronger when lengthening than when shortening[19]. Muscles are stronger in the eccentric portion of a rep. With a very heavy weight, you might not be able to lift it, but you can lower it slowly. Consider your first ever attempt at a pull up. You cannot pull yourself up, but you are able to slowly lower yourself down.

Mechanical tension is considered the primary driver of muscle growth. Therefore, it has been suggested that this ability to add greater load during the eccentric phase may lead to greater muscle growth[18]. Supramaximal loads (heavier than what you could lift for 1 rep) during eccentric training have also been called *"overload eccentric"*, *"heavy negatives"* or *"accentuated eccentric loading"*[3]. This form of training has been studied to assess whether it may offer an additional hypertrophic benefit to conventional training.

Overload eccentric / accentuated eccentric loading

Overload eccentrics involve lowering a weight that is heavier than what can be lifted. This is possible because muscles are stronger when lengthening than when shortening.

Overload eccentrics have been found to be beneficial for improving strength, however it does not appear to be superior to a conventional training programme for building muscle[16,17]. Overload eccentrics can be practically difficult to implement and may produce large amounts of muscle damage that may limit training frequency. There is no consensus on the load, reps or sets that should be used. Most studies use a load around 110-120% of an individuals' concentric 1RM. If overload eccentrics are utilised, it should be considered by intermediate to advanced trainers in addition to conventional resistance training.

Eccentric training can involve eccentric and concentric contractions with greater load during the eccentric contraction, or eccentric-only contractions with no concentric component[16].

Overload eccentrics can be achieved with:

- **Body weight exercises** (eccentric-only contractions such as *'negatives'* on pull-ups by jumping up and lowering the body down slowly under control).
- Using a **spotter** to assist on concentric phases (which can be either eccentric-only contractions or eccentric and assisted concentric contractions).
- Using **machines** (with eccentric and concentric contractions with bilateral concentric motions, and unilateral eccentric motions. For example, lifting the weight with both arms or legs, and lowering it with one arm or leg).
- With specially designed machines such as **fly-wheels**[19].

Eccentric (lowering the weight and the muscle lengthens) contractions can result in significant hypertrophy[19,20]. However, the research on supramaximal eccentric loads (lowering a weight that is heavier than what can be lifted) is very limited. Two meta-analyses, one assessing 15 studies and the other 20 studies, found slightly greater muscle growth with eccentric-*only* training compared to concentric-*only* training[19,21]. The difference was marginal and demonstrated only a small advantage with eccentric training. Another review found no difference in hypertrophy between eccentric and concentric training, but different regional hypertrophy as mentioned previously[18]. Importantly, analyses did *not* differentiate between sub-maximal and supra-maximal eccentric loads (because some studies did not report this) and workload was not equated. Sub-maximal eccentric contractions are already performed in conventional resistance training. The utility of eccentric-only training compared to concentric-only training also has very *limited* real-life utility. Most people already train concentrically and eccentrically through conventional training, because it is a practical method of training. What is more relevant therefore, is whether eccentric training *in addition* to conventional training is beneficial. Unfortunately, no studies have compared conventional training to conventional training with overload eccentrics. This is more informative, as overload eccentrics are more likely to be used alongside conventional training, rather than instead of conventional training[16]. As such, conclusions are far from definitive and much more research is needed before recommendations can be made.

Studies have compared overload eccentrics to conventional training or concentric-only contractions. A systematic review found no superior benefit of overload eccentrics in either comparison[16]. Overload eccentrics do not result in greater muscle growth than conventional training for muscle growth. Most studies find no difference in muscle growth compared to conventional sets[18,22-28].

Greater work can be performed in eccentric contractions because a muscle is up to 50% stronger when lengthening than contracting. When workload is equated, eccentric and concentric training forms appear to result in similar amounts of hypertrophy[18]. Greater tension can be placed on a muscle when lowering a load, which may explain the muscle growth seen[19]. However, other theories have been suggested, such as muscle growth as a result of greater exercise-induced muscle damage from eccentric training[16,19]. However, it is unlikely that exercise-induced muscle damage actually drives muscle growth, as studies have shown that muscle growth can occur independent of muscle damage[29]. The practicality of performing eccentric-only or overload eccentric training is difficult. Eccentric contractions also result in a large amount of muscle damage[19]. Overload eccentric training may limit the frequency at which a body part can be trained.

The focus should remain on conventional training with concentric and eccentric contractions. Whether additional overload eccentrics result in additional hypertrophy is not clear. Studies suggest this is a possibility, but direct evidence is lacking. Considering the practical challenge of overload eccentrics and its effect on training frequency, it should only be considered by those with training experience who are looking to theoretically maximise the training stimulus on a particular muscle.

Overload eccentric training can be most easily performed on machines. This allows placement of more tension on the lengthening part of the exercise by lifting a weight using both limbs (e.g. both arms or both legs) before removing one limb and lowering with the other limb. This essentially doubles the eccentric tension compared to the concentric tension. Machine exercises allow you to safely and effectively remove tension from one limb. For example, whilst using a leg extension machine you can use both legs to lift the weight up. Then, let one leg rest, leaving all the tension on the other leg, before slowly lowering the weight back to the start. This works well on other isolation machine movements (e.g. bicep curl machine, calf raise machine, hamstring curl machine). This form of overload would be best avoided on compound movements because of the increased requirement of stability.

Supra-maximal eccentric loads without concentric contractions can be performed with a spotter to lift the weight on the concentric portion, such as eccentric dumbbell curls. For a bicep curl, a heavy dumbbell can be lowered before a spotter picks the weight back up. Most studies to date use a weight between 105-125% of 1RM[3]. Alternatively for heavier loads, overload eccentric and concentric training can be performed with a spotter to help assist in the concentric portion, such as for the barbell bench press. Either the spotter can assist on the concentric portion or provide additional load on the eccentric portion by pushing down on the bar. However, this form of overload is hard to monitor progression with as it is highly dependent on how hard the spotter presses down. Given the lack of superiority of a rep duration, there is also no evidence for what rep duration overload eccentrics should be performed with.

Specific machines (such as flywheels) have been developed to overload eccentric contractions. Their availability is limited and so will not be discussed any further.

Eccentric contractions within conventional resistance training can result in hypertrophy. Whether additional eccentric focused exercise in addition to this promotes further muscle growth is unknown. The decision as to whether it is used should also take into consideration equipment availability, total weekly volume, and recoverability.

Forced reps and drop sets

Forced reps and drop sets involve taking a standard set beyond conventional muscular task failure. There are few studies that assess these advanced training techniques and muscle growth.

There is no evidence that taking a set beyond failure results in greater muscle growth than sets taken to, or near to failure[3].

Sets performed to, or near to failure correlate with muscle growth. However, the muscle is *not* completely fatigued at this point, because the muscle can still produce force at lower intensities of load[30]. Therefore, pushing a muscle beyond the initial point of failure by reducing the concentric load is suggested to increase tension, metabolic stress and supposedly increase growth.

This can be achieved with:

- **Forced reps:** *indirectly* lowering the load by having someone assist on the concentric contraction.
- **Drop sets:** *directly* lowering the load by taking weight off the barbell, using a lighter dumbbell or reducing the weight on a machine.

Forced reps

There are limited studies assessing the effect of forced reps on muscle growth. They do not appear to be superior to performing conventional sets.

When failure has been achieved from a standard set, the muscle is not actually completely fatigued. It can still produce force, but below the level required to lift the current load. By having someone assist in lifting the weight, this reduces the force required by the muscle and allows more reps to be completed. This results in further fatigue and tension to be placed on the muscle. Pushing a muscle beyond failure will result in increased metabolic stress and muscle damage[3,4].

The subsequent load that is lifted after failure is highly dependent on how much assistance someone is adding to the lift. Tracking progression will be difficult, and it is likely that there will be inconsistency from session to session when using forced reps. Each subsequent rep after failure will have high ratings of perceived exertion (RPE), because the individual will only assist to the minimum required to allow for the trainer to lift the weight[4].

There is a lack of evidence and no suggestion that a set of forced reps promotes greater muscle growth than a set taken to, or near to failure.

Drop sets

Drop sets result in similar muscle growth to conventional sets. They can be performed much more quickly, but at the expense of higher levels of effort and greater muscle damage. Consider using drop sets if you are short on workout time, and if you have several days before you train the body part again to allow for sufficient recovery from any additional muscle damage. Drop sets may also be a useful tool to increase training volume within a typical conventional workout without significantly increasing training time. This may be useful during periods of high volume training in intermediate or advanced trainers.

A drop set is where at the point of failure, you lower the load used in the exercise by 20-30% before continuing the set. 'Drops' can be performed several times. However, one drop set (perform a first set to failure, drop the weight and then perform further reps to a second failure) is the most common format. It is suggested that drop sets result in greater muscle growth by increasing motor unit fatigue. If you drop the weight after hitting failure on the first set, then more reps can be completed before reaching subsequent failure. Drop sets result in similar muscle growth to conventional sets, *but* can be performed in a shorter amount of time[31]. However, they also result in significantly greater muscle damage. Every additional drop to failure will generate more and more muscle damage.

One study found performing a drop set can increase hypertrophy above conventional sets. Set volumes were *not* equated however, with the drop set group essentially performing 5 sets compared to the conventional group performing 4 sets. As such, it may just be that the additional volume performed resulted in greater muscle growth[30,32].

Another study where volume was not equated (the drop set group performed drop sets on all of their sets, which was the same number of sets as the conventional training group, who stopped at the first muscular task failure) in resistance trained individuals, found no difference between conventional and drop set training. However, the method of measuring body composition was not specific to measure muscle mass and diets were not assessed, which can heavily influence muscle growth[30,33].

When volume *has* been equated between conventional training and drop set training, there is generally *no* difference in muscle growth[30,31,34,35]. One study did equate volume and found a non-significant, but potentially meaningfully greater increase in muscle growth with drop sets than conventional sets[35]. However, volume was equated as workload (load x reps). Performing a drop set significantly reduces the number of subsequent reps at the lighter load. If the mechanism by which drop sets increase muscle growth is by achieving greater tension and fatigue of high-threshold motor units, then the number of times that failure was achieved would provide a better measure of volume. As such, the drop set group reached failure 4 times, but only 3 times in the conventional training group. The slightly higher muscle growth may therefore once again be due to a greater volume of *sets* performed to failure[35].

A pilot study (a small study to assess the feasibility to perform a bigger study) found similar improvements in muscle growth, but less workout time was required when using drop sets compared to either high or low load conventional sets in untrained males[31]. The high and low load participants performed three sets to failure. The drop set group performed one set to failure, and then performed four drop sets immediately after. Drop sets build muscle, but no more so than a similar set volume of conventional training[36].

The main benefit of drop sets is that they allow *similar* muscle growth to conventional sets, but in a much *shorter* period of time. Some studies found workouts were less than half the length of sessions with conventional training[31,35]. However, this is at the expense of *higher* intensities of effort (i.e. higher rating of perceived exertion (RPE)), *increased* metabolic stress, and *greater* muscle damage[35]. As such, drop sets are useful tools. But like other advanced training techniques, they are *not* superior to conventional training and should be used sparingly to prevent excessive muscle damage and high perceived levels of effort.

Drop sets do not require an assistant and can be quickly achieved with dumbbells or machines with a pin-stack, minimising time between drops. This also means tracking progression with drop sets is easier, as the loads and reps performed for each drop can be tracked. Another point to add is that drop sets have largely been studied using isolation exercises, such as tricep extensions and bicep curls. Some studies have assessed drop sets with the leg press, chest press and lateral pull down, however[30].

To implement a drop set, select your usual load for say, your 10 repetition maximum. Perform 10 reps to failure, and then lower the weight by 20-30% (drops smaller than this limit the number of subsequent reps, and drops larger than this make it difficult to reach subsequent failure) and immediately perform reps to a second failure with minimal rest between drops. Repeat this process as many times as desired. Use a similar rep duration as you usually perform for conventional reps. Multi-joint and single-joint exercises can be used, but due to the high levels of effort and fatigue, it may be more suitable to choose single-joint isolation exercises to perform drop sets[30].

Pre-exhaust training

Few studies have assessed pre-exhaust training; there appears to be no benefit above conventional training for increasing muscle activation or muscle growth.

Pre-exhaust training involves fatiguing a muscle with a single-joint isolation exercise before performing a multi-joint compound exercise[4]. The theoretical rationale is to supposedly increase activation of the target muscle in the subsequent multi-joint exercise. The idea is that the single-joint exercise will fatigue muscle fibres, and any unfatigued fibres will need to be recruited in order to lift the weight in the multi-joint exercise, and therefore result in increased motor unit recruitment[4,37]. For example, first performing leg extensions to failure to fatigue the quadriceps, and then performing squats, such that the quadriceps will be the first muscle to fatigue in the compound exercise. Or, performing chest flyes to failure to pre-fatigue the chest, before performing the bench press.

Studies have compared multi-joint exercise followed by single-joint exercise training to pre-exhaust training (a single-joint exercise followed by a multi-joint exercise) and have found *similar* levels of muscle activation in both[37-39]. One study found reduced muscle activation via surface electromyography (EMG) in the quadriceps in the leg press *after* pre-exhausting with leg extensions[40]. In other words, pre-exhaustion does *not* increase muscle electrical activity[38,39]. Activity was measured by surface electromyography (EMG). Higher surface EMG does not imply greater motor unit recruitment nor greater muscle building potential, especially in fatigued conditions[41]. Even if greater muscle activation was seen with pre-exhaustion, it does not necessarily mean greater muscle growth. Muscle activation will already be high for the given body part in the compound exercise, if it is the primary mover. Some studies find that pre-fatiguing the chest with chest flyes instead results in increased activation of the triceps, not the chest, in the subsequent bench press, most likely to compensate for the reduced force producing ability of the chest[38,39]. Interestingly, pre-exhaust did not limit the total workload that was performed for both exercises. However, the exercise performed first (flye or press) achieved a greater number of reps, and the exercise that was performed second achieved fewer reps[42]. Pre-exhaust also does not appear to influence perceptions of effort (RPE), most likely because similar levels of fatigue and failure are achieved[37,42]. As with multi- then single-joint training, pre-exhaust training results in a decrease in the number of reps performed in the second exercise.

As such, pre-exhaust training for muscle growth is a technique that should largely be avoided if the *sole* aim of doing so is to increase activation of a target muscle[38,42]. Given that muscle growth correlates with the number of sets performed to, or near to failure, isolation and compound exercises targeting a specific muscle can both be used to promote muscle growth, and the order does not appear to be important[43].

If there is particular interest to grow a specific muscle, train it earlier or first in the workout rather than later, whether that be with compound or isolation exercises[42]. But, don't use an isolation exercise first if the only reason is to try and increase the activation of a muscle in subsequent exercises.

Supersets

No long-term studies comparing supersets to traditional sets on direct measures of muscle growth exist. If training session duration is not constrained, there is little benefit to performing supersets.

Supersets can be performed as two exercises targeting the same muscle back to back (agonist-agonist supersets), two exercises for antagonistic muscles back to back (agonist-antagonist supersets) or two completely unrelated exercises, with minimal rest in between. Supersets in general result in greater fatigue, metabolic stress and muscle damage than conventional sets. Agonist-agonist supersets do not result in greater muscle growth than conventional sets. Agonist-antagonist supersets allow similar or greater training volumes to be performed in a shorter duration but at the expense of greater fatigue, metabolic stress and muscle damage[4,44]. Supersets can increase perceptions of effort and may require a longer recovery time[44,45].

Supersets are where two exercises are performed back to back, typically with no rest in between exercises, with rest in between each superset. Supersets can be categorised based on the exercises that are used.

Agonist-agonist sets

Agonist-agonist sets use exercises that target the *same* muscle. For example, performing a set of barbell bench press followed by a set of chest flyes, with minimal rest in between. Agonist-agonist sets produce greater fatigue and metabolic stress than conventional sets, due to the reduced rest period[3,4]. Agonist-agonist supersets result in larger reductions in performance across a workout compared to other superset formats[45]. From the perspective of increasing mechanical tension, agonist-agonist supersets are not very effective. Whether this accumulation in fatigue results in muscle growth has not been studied. But, considering the minor role at best that metabolic stress may have in muscle growth, it would be best to limit the use agonist-agonist sets. Shorter rest periods are sub-optimal for muscle growth, and strategies that take a muscle beyond failure have not been demonstrated to be superior for muscle growth. As such, it is unlikely that performing a subsequent exercise immediately after a fatiguing exercise on the same muscle will promote any further muscle growth.

Agonist-antagonist sets

Agonist-antagonist sets may have potential. Such sets use exercises that target muscles with opposing actions. For example, a pushing (i.e. chest) exercise followed by a pulling (i.e. back) exercise. It has been shown that performing antagonistic exercises back to back can increase force output[3]. However, *no* studies have directly compared agonist-antagonist sets to conventional sets for muscle growth. Studies have compared agonist-antagonist sets to traditional sets during and after a training session. Performing the seated row before the bench press can increase the number of reps performed on the bench press. Performing the bench press before the seated row can increase the number of reps performed on the seated row[3,46]. It appears that performing an antagonistic set (e.g. a press before a row, or a leg curl before a leg extension) can increase the volume load performed for the subsequent agonist exercise (e.g. the row or leg extension)[46,47]. This could theoretically increase mechanical tension on the muscle and promote greater muscle growth, but this has *not* been formally studied. Increased training volume also does not necessarily result in greater muscle growth, and the existing knowledge also suggests that greater mechanical tension in a set does not imply greater muscle growth. Other studies have found no effect of antagonist sets on subsequent agonist exercises. The same bench/row study found no effect on bench press volume following a preceding antagonist set of rows[46].

Agonist-antagonist sets can result in similar or greater training volume to traditional training in a shorter period of time by performing agonist and antagonist sets immediately back to back (whereas conventional sets perform one exercise for several sets with rest, before performing the next exercise). However, this comes at the cost of greater fatigue when using agonist-antagonist sets[44,48]. Increased fatigue can result in reduced performance the day after using supersets[45]. Supersets have usually been performed with 2 minutes rest between supersets (i.e. bench press then immediately performing a seated row, followed by 2 minutes rest before the next bench press and seated row superset). Performing agonist-antagonist supersets with longer rest (4 minutes instead of 2 minutes) reduces perceptions of effort without any difference in the number of reps performed[49]. This of course would then take a similar duration of time to complete as conventional sets.

If training session duration is not limited, there is not much benefit if any, with using agonist-antagonist sets. Agonist-antagonist sets may be useful when training with multiple body parts per session and when limited for time. For example, if using an upper, lower split with a low training frequency (see chapter 20 regarding training splits), agonist-antagonist sets could be useful with sufficient recovery time until the subsequent session. Given the minimal effect of rest periods on volume but the large effect on perceptions of effort, when you are feeling good, rest periods can be shorter. Potentially when you are feeling more fatigued, longer rest periods can be used[49].

Unrelated exercise supersets

Unrelated exercise supersets are a third and much less common form of supersets. It is the least researched form of all supersets. For example, performing a shoulder press immediately followed by leg extensions[45]. In a similar manner to agonist-antagonist sets, the likely benefit is in performing workout volume in a shorter duration. The effect is most likely dependent on the choice of exercises; a highly demanding first exercise (e.g. deadlifts or squats) will heavily limit performance in the exercise immediately following. Again, unless workout duration is a limiting factor, there is unlikely to be any benefit to this form of training.

Other training techniques to influence performance

Internal vs external focus

Focussing on lifting the weight (external focus) results in greater strength, but focussing on contracting the muscle (internal focus) leads to greater muscle activation. The long-term significance of this on muscle growth is still inconclusive due to a lack of evidence.

What an individual focusses on during a lift can influence muscle growth. Attentional focus can either be *external* or *internal*. An external focus would be to think about *moving* the load or the body relative to the environment, such as pushing the floor away in a squat, or reaching up in a pull up. An internal focus would be to think about *contracting* the muscle of interest. For example, thinking about *squeezing* and contracting the biceps in a bicep curl. A novel study compared the focus of participants and resulting changes in strength and muscle growth[50]. There was an increase in muscle size of the elbow flexors (e.g. the biceps) with an internal rather than an external focus, but no difference in quadriceps size with a different attentional focus. The authors suggest that this may be related to the upper limbs being used for fine motor movements (e.g. holding a pencil), whereas the lower limbs are used for gross movements (e.g. moving the body). This may mean that internal focus during lower limb exercises has little benefit. Participants also generally found it easier to internally focus on the elbow flexors rather than the quadriceps[50]. This may explain why the study from chapter 19 on page 362 that demonstrated training with *'no load'* resulted in as much muscle growth as using a *'load'*, due to the internal focus used by *'no load'* participants to focus on contracting the muscle[51]. A *mind-muscle connection* has long been suggested in training to *feel* the muscle contracting. The long-term consequence of focussing on the muscle contracting rather than the weight itself on muscle growth is inconclusive however, given the paucity of evidence[52].

Post-activation potentiation

Post-activation potentiation is where you perform a single rep at a higher intensity of load than the load of your working set. This can result in more reps being performed in an exercise in a given set for a given load. It has been shown to result in greater performance. But, whether it has any effect or significance for muscle growth is unknown.

Post-activation potentiation is the *"increase in muscle force and rate of force development (RFD) that occurs as a result of previous activation of the muscle"*[53]. It is achieved by performing 1 rep with a heavier weight than the weight used for working sets, which primes the muscle and makes the working weight *'feel'* lighter[53]. Performing exercise induces fatigue, but performing exercise can also *prime* a muscle and improve subsequent performance[54]. This is dependent on the amount of work performed. Typical working sets fatigue a muscle more than they prime it. But brief, high-intensity contractions that are minimally fatiguing (i.e. one rep at a higher load than the load to be used for working sets) may improve muscular performance[53,54]. The force a muscle can produce is influenced by its previous contraction[54]. The theory is that this either increases neural drive to the muscle, or the active proteins in a muscle become more sensitive to stimulation, meaning muscle fibres can produce greater force from the same stimulus. Most evidence is currently within the fields of strength and power performance and sports rehabilitation. However, in one study of 14 trained males, using post-activation potentiation significantly increased the number of reps performed in 3 sets of bench press at an intensity of load of 75% of 1RM[55]. This has been demonstrated in similar studies using back squats[56].

However, there is *no* long-term evidence on whether post-activation potentiation can be of benefit to muscle growth. Any benefit is purely theoretical or indirect at this stage and no recommendations can be made[53,54]. Does the greater number of reps in a given set with a given load mean greater mechanical tension, stimulus and growth? Or is mechanical tension already sufficient for growth without post-activation potentiation? It may well be that there is no benefit of post-activation potentiation on muscle growth, provided progressive overload occurs. Whether it is used should be down to personal preference. If you can perform at or near maximal performance without post-activation potentiation, then there would be little benefit. If your sets *feel* good and you can feel the target muscle working better after post-activation potentiation, then you might like to use it.

Summary: advanced training techniques

Advanced training techniques generate greater fatigue and damage compared to conventional sets, but are of limited benefit, if any. They should be considered within the context of a conventional training programme. They are not necessary for muscle growth. Little evidence suggests that any are superior to conventional sets, and only some have been demonstrated to result in similar muscle growth. They may be used to *'cover all bases'*, as the current evidence is still very limited. As with training to failure, limit their use, aligning with lower and higher training volume periods and around general life stresses[3].

References

1 Carlson L, Jonker B, Westcott WL, Steele J, Fisher JP. Neither repetition duration nor number of muscle actions affect strength increases, body

composition, muscle size, or fasted blood glucose in trained males and females. *Appl Physiol Nutr Metab Physiol Appl Nutr Metab* 2019; 44: 200–207.

2   Carpinelli R, Otto R, Wientt R. A critical analysis of the ACSM position stand on resistance training: Insufficient evidence to support recommended training protocols. *J Exerc Physiol Online* 2004; 7.

3   Schoenfeld B. The Use of Specialized Training Techniques to Maximize Muscle Hypertrophy. *Strength Cond J* 2011; 33: 60–65.

4   Wallace W, Ugrinowitsch C, Stefan M, Rauch J, Barakat C, Shields K et al. Repeated Bouts of Advanced Strength Training Techniques: Effects on Volume Load, Metabolic Responses, and Muscle Activation in Trained Individuals. *Sports Basel Switz* 2019; 7. Available from: doi:10.3390/sports7010014.

5   Pope ZK, Willardson JM, Schoenfeld BJ. Exercise and blood flow restriction. *J Strength Cond Res* 2013; 27: 2914–2926.

6   Patterson SD, Hughes L, Warmington S, Burr J, Scott BR, Owens J et al. Blood Flow Restriction Exercise: Considerations of Methodology, Application, and Safety. *Front Physiol* 2019; 10. Available from: doi:10.3389/fphys.2019.00533.

7   Loenneke JP, Wilson JM, Marín PJ, Zourdos MC, Bemben MG. Low intensity blood flow restriction training: a meta-analysis. *Eur J Appl Physiol* 2012; 112: 1849–1859.

8   Lixandrão ME, Ugrinowitsch C, Berton R, Vechin FC, Conceição MS, Damas F et al. Magnitude of Muscle Strength and Mass Adaptations Between High-Load Resistance Training Versus Low-Load Resistance Training Associated with Blood-Flow Restriction: A Systematic Review and Meta-Analysis. *Sports Med Auckl NZ* 2018; 48: 361–378.

9   Slysz J, Stultz J, Burr JF. The efficacy of blood flow restricted exercise: A systematic review & meta-analysis. *J Sci Med Sport* 2016; 19: 669–675.

10   Farup J, de Paoli F, Bjerg K, Riis S, Ringgard S, Vissing K. Blood flow restricted and traditional resistance training performed to fatigue produce equal muscle hypertrophy. *Scand J Med Sci Sports* 2015; 25: 754–763.

11   Takarada Y, Tsuruta T, Ishii N. Cooperative effects of exercise and occlusive stimuli on muscular function in low-intensity resistance exercise with moderate vascular occlusion. *Jpn J Physiol* 2004; 54: 585–592.

12   Alvarez IF, Damas F, Biazon TMP de, Miquelini M, Doma K, Libardi CA. Muscle damage responses to resistance exercise performed with high-load versus low-load associated with partial blood flow restriction in young women. *Eur J Sport Sci* 2020; 20: 125–134.

13   Marshall PWM, Robbins DA, Wrightson AW, Siegler JC. Acute neuromuscular and fatigue responses to the rest-pause method. *J Sci Med Sport* 2012; 15: 153–158.

14   Korak JA, Paquette MR, Brooks J, Fuller DK, Coons JM. Effect of rest-pause vs. traditional bench press training on muscle strength, electromyography, and lifting volume in randomized trial protocols. *Eur J Appl Physiol* 2017; 117: 1891–1896.

15   Prestes J, A Tibana R, de Araujo Sousa E, da Cunha Nascimento D, de Oliveira Rocha P, F Camarço N et al. Strength and Muscular Adaptations After 6 Weeks of Rest-Pause vs. Traditional Multiple-Sets Resistance Training in Trained Subjects. *J Strength Cond Res* 2019; 33 Suppl 1: S113–S121.

16   Douglas J, Pearson S, Ross A, McGuigan M. Chronic Adaptations to Eccentric Training: A Systematic Review. *Sports Med Auckl NZ* 2017; 47: 917–941.

17   Wagle JP, Taber CB, Cunanan AJ, Bingham GE, Carroll KM, DeWeese BH et al. Accentuated Eccentric Loading for Training and Performance: A Review. *Sports Med Auckl NZ* 2017; 47: 2473–2495.

18   Franchi MV, Reeves ND, Narici MV. Skeletal Muscle Remodeling in Response to Eccentric vs. Concentric Loading: Morphological, Molecular, and Metabolic Adaptations. *Front Physiol* 2017; 8. Available from: doi:10.3389/fphys.2017.00447.

19   Schoenfeld BJ, Ogborn DI, Vigotsky AD, Franchi MV, Krieger JW. Hypertrophic Effects of Concentric vs. Eccentric Muscle Actions: A Systematic Review and Meta-analysis. *J Strength Cond Res* 2017; 31: 2599–2608.

20   Wernbom M, Augustsson J, Thomeé R. The influence of frequency, intensity, volume and mode of strength training on whole muscle cross-sectional area in humans. *Sports Med Auckl NZ* 2007; 37: 225–264.

21   Roig M, O'Brien K, Kirk G, Murray R, McKinnon P, Shadgan B et al. The effects of eccentric versus concentric resistance training on muscle strength and mass in healthy adults: a systematic review with meta-analysis. *Br J Sports Med* 2009; 43: 556–568.

22   Suchomel TJ, Wagle JP, Douglas J, Taber CB, Harden M, Haff GG et al. Implementing Eccentric Resistance Training—Part 1: A Brief Review of Existing Methods. *J Funct Morphol Kinesiol* 2019; 4: 38.

23   Walker S, Blazevich AJ, Haff GG, Tufano JJ, Newton RU, Häkkinen K. Greater Strength Gains after Training with Accentuated Eccentric than Traditional Isoinertial Loads in Already Strength-Trained Men. *Front Physiol* 2016; 7: 149.

24   Higbie EJ, Cureton KJ, Warren GL, Prior BM. Effects of concentric and eccentric training on muscle strength, cross-sectional area, and neural activation. *J Appl Physiol Bethesda Md* 1996; 81: 2173–2181.

25   Vikne H, Refsnes PE, Ekmark M, Medbø JI, Gundersen V, Gundersen K. Muscular performance after concentric and eccentric exercise in trained men. *Med Sci Sports Exerc* 2006; 38: 1770–1781.

26   Friedmann B, Kinscherf R, Vorwald S, Müller H, Kucera K, Borisch S et al. Muscular adaptations to computer-guided strength training with eccentric overload. *Acta Physiol Scand* 2004; 182: 77–88.

27   Brandenburg JP, Docherty D. The effects of accentuated eccentric loading on strength, muscle hypertrophy, and neural adaptations in trained individuals. *J Strength Cond Res* 2002; 16: 25–32.

28   Friedmann-Bette B, Bauer T, Kinscherf R, Vorwald S, Klute K, Bischoff D et al. Effects of strength training with eccentric overload on muscle adaptation in male athletes. *Eur J Appl Physiol* 2010; 108: 821–836.

29   Schoenfeld BJ. Does exercise-induced muscle damage play a role in skeletal muscle hypertrophy? *J Strength Cond Res* 2012; 26: 1441–1453.

30   Schoenfeld BJ, Grgic J. Can Drop Set Training Enhance Muscle Growth? *Strength Cond J* 2018; 40: 95–98.

31   Ozaki H, Kubota A, Natsume T, Loenneke JP, Abe T, Machida S et al. Effects of drop sets with resistance training on increases in muscle CSA, strength, and endurance: a pilot study. *J Sports Sci* 2018; 36: 691–696.

32   Goto K, Nagasawa M, Yanagisawa O, Kizuka T, Ishii N, Takamatsu K. Muscular adaptations to combinations of high- and low-intensity resistance exercises. *J Strength Cond Res* 2004; 18: 730–737.

33   Fisher JP, Carlson L, Steele J. The Effects of Breakdown Set Resistance Training on Muscular Performance and Body Composition in Young Men and Women. *J Strength Cond Res* 2016; 30: 1425–1432.

34   Angleri V, Ugrinowitsch C, Libardi CA. Crescent pyramid and drop-set systems do not promote greater strength gains, muscle hypertrophy, and changes on muscle architecture compared with traditional resistance training in well-trained men. *Eur J Appl Physiol* 2017; 117: 359–369.

35   Fink J, Schoenfeld B, Kikuchi N, Nakazato K. Effects of drop set resistance training on acute stress indicators and long-term muscle hypertrophy and strength. *J Sports Med Phys Fitness* 2017. Available from: doi:10.23736/S0022-4707.17.06838-4.

36   Johannsmeyer S, Candow DG, Brahms CM, Michel D, Zello GA. Effect of creatine supplementation and drop-set resistance training in untrained aging adults. *Exp Gerontol* 2016; 83: 112–119.

37   Soares EG, Brown LE, Gomes WA, Corrêa DA, Serpa ÉP, da Silva JJ et al. Comparison Between Pre-Exhaustion and Traditional Exercise Order on Muscle Activation and Performance in Trained Men. *J Sports Sci Med* 2016; 15: 111–117.

38   Brennecke A, Guimarães TM, Leone R, Cadarci M, Mochizuki L, Simão R et al. Neuromuscular activity during bench press exercise performed with and without the preexhaustion method. *J Strength Cond Res* 2009; 23: 1933–1940.

39   Gentil P, Oliveira E, de Araújo Rocha Júnior V, do Carmo J, Bottaro M. Effects of exercise order on upper-body muscle activation and exercise performance. *J Strength Cond Res* 2007; 21: 1082–1086.

40   Augustsson J, Thomeé R, Hörnstedt P, Lindblom J, Karlsson J, Grimby G. Effect of pre-exhaustion exercise on lower-extremity muscle activation during a leg press exercise. *J Strength Cond Res* 2003; 17: 411–416.

41   Vigotsky AD, Beardsley C, Contreras B, Steele J, Ogborn D, Phillips SM. Greater electromyographic responses do not imply greater motor unit recruitment and 'hypertrophic potential' cannot be inferred. *J Strength Cond Res* 2017; 31: e1–e4.

42   Simão R, de Salles BF, Figueiredo T, Dias I, Willardson JM. Exercise order in resistance training. *Sports Med Auckl NZ* 2012; 42: 251–265.

43   Nunes JP, Grgic J, Cunha PM, Ribeiro AS, Schoenfeld BJ, Salles BF de et al. What influence does resistance exercise order have on muscular strength gains and muscle hypertrophy? A systematic review and meta-analysis. *Eur J Sport Sci* 2020; 0: 1–22.

44   Weakley JJS, Till K, Read DB, Roe GAB, Darrall-Jones J, Phibbs PJ et al. The effects of traditional, superset, and tri-set resistance training structures on perceived intensity and physiological responses. *Eur J Appl Physiol* 2017; 117: 1877–1889.

45   Weakley JJS, Till K, Read DB, Phibbs PJ, Roe G, Darrall-Jones J et al. The Effects of Superset Configuration on Kinetic, Kinematic, and Perceived Exertion in the Barbell Bench Press. *J Strength Cond Res* 2020; 34: 65–72.

46   Maia M, Paz G, Souza J, Miranda H. Strength performance parameters when adopting different exercise sequences during agonist–antagonist paired sets. *Apunts Med Esport* 2015; 50. Available from: doi:10.1016/j.apunts.2015.01.001.

47   Paz G, Willardson J, Simão R, Miranda H. Effects of different antagonist protocols on repetition performance and muscle activation. *Med Sport* 2013; 17: 362–370.

48   Paz GA, Robbins DW, de Oliveira CG, Bottaro M, Miranda H. Volume Load and Neuromuscular Fatigue During an Acute Bout of Agonist-Antagonist Paired-Set vs. Traditional-Set Training. *J Strength Cond Res* 2017; 31: 2777–2784.

49   de Freitas Maia M, Paz GA, Miranda H, Lima V, Bentes CM, da Silva Novaes J et al. Maximal repetition performance, rating of perceived exertion, and muscle fatigue during paired set training performed with different rest intervals. *J Exerc Sci Fit* 2015; 13: 104–110.

50   Schoenfeld BJ, Vigotsky A, Contreras B, Golden S, Alto A, Larson R et al. Differential effects of attentional focus strategies during long-term resistance training. *Eur J Sport Sci* 2018; 18: 705–712.

51   Counts BR, Buckner SL, Dankel SJ, Jessee MB, Mattocks KT, Mouser JG et al. The acute and chronic effects of "NO LOAD" resistance training. *Physiol Behav* 2016; 164: 345–352.

52   Juneau C-E, Tafur L. Over time, load mediates muscular hypertrophy in resistance training. *Curr Opin Physiol* 2019; 11: 147–148.

53   Lorenz D. Postactivation potentiation: an introduction. *Int J Sports Phys Ther* 2011; 6: 234–240.

54   Hodgson M, Docherty D, Robbins D. Post-activation potentiation: underlying physiology and implications for motor performance. *Sports Med Auckl NZ* 2005; 35: 585–595.

55   Alves RR, Viana RB, Silva MH, Guimarães TC, Vieira CA, Santos D de AT et al. Postactivation Potentiation Improves Performance in a Resistance Training Session in Trained Men. *J Strength Cond Res* 2019. Available from: doi:10.1519/JSC.0000000000003367.

56   Conrado de Freitas M, Rossi FE, Colognesi LA, de Oliveira JVNS, Zanchi NE, Lira FS et al. Postactivation Potentiation Improves Acute Resistance Exercise Performance and Muscular Force in Trained Men. *J Strength Cond Res* 2018. Available from: doi:10.1519/JSC.0000000000002897.

24. Aerobic exercise

Should you perform aerobic exercise for good health? Yes.
Do you *need* to perform aerobic exercise to lose weight? No.
Do you *need* to avoid aerobic exercise to build muscle? No.

The majority of exercise research is in obese individuals. However, there are many studies looking at the effects of aerobic exercise in healthy individuals.

Aerobic exercise for weight loss

You should participate in aerobic exercise primarily to stay healthy, not as a tool to promote weight loss.

Dietary changes should be the primary mechanism to promote fat loss. On average, exercise interventions alone result in less weight loss than dietary interventions. If the primary focus is to lose fat mass, aerobic exercise is not fundamental. But, aerobic exercise can be used to help create or maintain a caloric deficit.

There is no 'best' exercise for weight loss. Adherence to an exercise plan is far more important than the type, duration or intensity of aerobic exercise performed.

From a weight loss perspective, exercise is just a tool to increase energy expenditure. High intensity and moderate intensity exercise are as effective as each other. They are not inherently better than simply 'moving more' during the day for calorie burning; exercise intensity should be dictated by personal preference. Instead, ask yourself, 'What's the easiest and most enjoyable way for me to expend additional calories?'. Once your diet is in place, then consider adding or increasing aerobic exercise, or moving more.

Choose the exercise or movement you enjoy the most and can adhere to in the long-term. This could be outside (e.g. walking, cycling, running), in the gym (e.g. treadmill, stationary bike, stair climber, rowing machine), a sport (e.g. football, tennis, hockey) or an exercise class. It could be high intensity (e.g. sprints), it could be moderate intensity (e.g. cycling, a dance class) or it could be low intensity (e.g. walking). It can be a specific training session, or it can just be moving more, and not a dedicated part of your day (e.g. moving more at work, walking or cycling to work or taking the stairs instead of the lift).

Excessive aerobic exercise (either by performing a high volume of aerobic exercise in itself, or by performing a high volume which increases energy expenditure alongside a reduced energy intake, generating a large calorie deficit), may increase losses in muscle mass, which will make fat loss harder in the long run.

What's the most efficient exercise for weight loss?

This depends on what is meant by 'efficient'. The higher the intensity of exercise, the faster the rate at which you use energy, but also the higher the levels of effort and fatigue. Some people want to burn as much energy as possible in the shortest time; the 'get in, get it done, and get out' mentality. However, this is also very tiring and taxing and requires a lot of effort. If you want to burn calories faster, you have to work harder. Other people would rather perform much lower intensity exercise, because high intensity work is too stressful or may impact their ability to perform during a resistance training session. It may also be because they have more free time, and therefore do not need to complete it quickly. Choosing an exercise that is enjoyable to perform is most important.

If the aim is to burn more calories through exercise, either exercise for longer (an absolute increase in calories burnt) or exercise at a higher intensity (a relative increase in calories burnt per unit time).

Exercise modality should primarily be based on personal preference. If the aim is to burn as many calories as possible with the least amount of effort, then treadmill exercise appears to burn calories at the highest rate at any level of effort compared to other exercises (such as rowing, stationary bike or ski erg) and appears to be more significant at higher exercise intensities. This should be a minor consideration.

If the aim is to burn calories whilst minimising fatigue and any impact on resistance training sessions, consider fewer high intensity sessions and more low to moderate intensity sessions (especially if your programme has a high frequency of resistance training).

If the aim is to burn calories as quickly as possible, consider high intensity exercise using whole body movements (such as sprints).

If the aim is to burn calories with the least amount of perceived effort (RPE), consider low to moderate intensity aerobic exercise. This will require a longer exercise duration to burn an equivalent number of calories as a higher intensity.

Non-exercise activity thermogenesis (NEAT) is also important and can significantly increase total daily energy expenditure (TDEE). If the aim is to burn calories, try and move more during the day besides any planned exercise.

Aerobic exercise can be considered from different perspectives:

- The benefits of aerobic exercise for health.
- The benefits of aerobic exercise to improve body composition.
- Aerobic exercise to improve aerobic exercise performance.

As previously discussed in chapter 16, the health benefits of aerobic exercise are numerous, and recommended by many health organisations. This discussion will focus on the role of aerobic exercise to influence body composition.

As a starting point, use health organisation recommendations of 3 x 20 minute runs, or 5 x 30 minute brisk walks per week for the health benefits of aerobic exercise.

Consider recommendations from health organisations as a starting point. These recommendations are for the amount of exercise that should be performed to benefit from exercise-induced health improvements; however there is *no* minimum threshold of exercise that needs to be performed to benefit from exercise. Health organisations and the UK government recommend moderate aerobic exercise for 30 minutes, 5 times per week (150 minutes of moderate intensity exercise per week), or vigorous intensity aerobic exercise for 20 minutes, 3 times per week. Shorter durations suit higher intensity activity (such as sprints). Individuals should avoid being sedentary, and where possible move around with at least some light exercise, such as walking[1]. A combination of moderate and vigorous intensity exercise can be used to meet recommendations. Moderate activity includes brisk walking. Vigorous activity includes jogging, with an elevation in breathing and heart rate. Recommendations also include participating in resistance or strength training at least twice per week[1,2].

With changes in exercise intensity, the duration of recommended exercise per week changes. Aerobic exercise can therefore be categorised based on the intensity[3]:

- **High intensity.** Near maximal efforts where exercise is performed above 80% of maximum heart rate*, interspersed with periods of recovery at a lower intensity. This is commonly referred to as *high intensity interval training* (HIIT). The duration of intervals, rest periods, the number of intervals and the exercises chosen for the training are highly variable, both in real-life and in research[4]. Intervals can last from 5 seconds to 4 minutes. Rest periods can last from 9 seconds to 10 minutes. Training sessions can last from 20 seconds to 50 minutes[4]. The intervals are typically above the *anaerobic threshold* (using energy without oxygen, see chapter 16), such that intervals cannot be maintained and hence the need for rest periods[5]. For example, *sprint interval training* (SIT) is where intervals are *supra-maximal* (above maximum rates of oxygen consumption), which requires using energy without oxygen. Health related benefits can be achieved in the shortest amount of time with HIIT and SIT[1].
- **Moderate intensity.** Exercise that raises heart rate above the resting heart rate and can be maintained for a long duration of time. Intensities are usually around 40-80% of maximum heart rate[4]. It is generally performed at the same intensity for the duration of the exercise period. This is commonly referred to as moderate intensity, steady state cardio.
- **Low intensity.** Exercise resulting in minimal elevations in heart rate, such as walking.

Your maximum heart rate is 220 - age. So, a 25 year old has a maximum heart rate of 195. Therefore 156 beats per minute would equal an 80% intensity.

Exercise for weight loss

Exercise activity thermogenesis will contribute to generating a calorie deficit, or aid ensuring caloric maintenance. The effect of exercise on weight loss is highly variable between individuals. The influence of exercise on weight loss is smaller than the influence of diet on weight loss.

Numerous systematic reviews and meta-analyses comparing high intensity or sprint interval style training versus moderate intensity exercise show HIIT is *not* superior for fat loss in lean or obese people[6–10]. Many of these meta-analyses actually find little influence of exercise on body composition or weight loss. However, these studies generally find minimal weight loss with a low volume or short duration exercise intervention. Differences in the outcomes of many exercise studies are because of variations in the type, intensity and duration of the exercise performed, the tools used to measure metabolic rate, the characteristics of participants and the statistical tools used to compare groups[11]. One major limitation of exercise-only studies is the lack of a dietary intervention or dietary control, which as discussed in the diet chapter will significantly impact outcomes. Increasing energy expenditure through exercise often produces less weight change than is expected. It has been suggested that increasing energy expenditure via exercise activity thermogenesis (EAT) may result in some compensatory decrease in non-exercise activity thermogenesis (NEAT) or increase in energy intake when diet is not controlled[12].

Small increases in energy expenditure may be compensated for, but larger increases may not. Indeed, one study compared low and high volume exercise on weight loss over 12 weeks in overweight individuals, where participants were able to consume energy freely. One group expended 1500kcal per week (300kcal x 5 sessions), and another group expended 3000kcal per week (600kcal x 5 sessions)[13]. Both groups had a similar absolute compensation of energy expenditure from their diet (an increase of 1500kcal per week), such that the 3000kcal group generated a much larger calorie deficit. Over 12 weeks, the 3000kcal/week group lost weight, but the 1500kcal/week group did not. A small volume of exercise may be compensated for with energy intake, but larger volumes likely do not. Successful weight loss has been demonstrated in other randomised controlled exercise intervention trials that use larger volumes of weekly exercise[14-16]. However, other studies have found energy compensation to still increase further with higher exercise volumes (greater compensation with 3600kcal/week of exercise compared to 1800kcal/week)[17]. Performing exercise can help to generate a calorie deficit to promote weight loss, but exercise volume likely needs to be above a minimum volume to be of meaningful benefit[12]. Any resultant compensatory effect from performing exercise will be highly individual; some people might have modest weight loss from exercise, some may not lose any weight at all[12].

Evidence from meta-analyses of randomised controlled trials show that exercise interventions alone usually result in far *less* weight change compared to a diet intervention, or a combined diet and exercise intervention[18-23]. Weight loss is most likely achieved through *dietary* caloric restriction[12]. Of course, this is highly dependent on the calorie deficit generated by such interventions. And, it is important to remember that *more* weight change isn't necessarily *better* weight change. Despite exercise not being crucial for weight loss, exercise does appear to be important for weight maintenance and the prevention of weight gain[12]. Such a concept to aid weight maintenance has been termed 'high energy flux'[24]. In other words, it may be beneficial to keep energy expenditure high to facilitate greater freedom with energy intake, especially in a modern society with many energy dense foods. A systematic review of 67 observational and controlled trials show that greater levels of physical activity is associated with maintenance of weight loss[25-27].

It is important to emphasise that even if exercise does not result in weight loss, exercise still results in a wide range of improvements in health[12,13,28].

Which intensity should I exercise at?

In terms of enjoyment, choose the type and modality that you enjoy the most. If you like it (or at least do not dislike it), you are more likely to adhere to it.

As with dietary changes, the greatest success in weight loss with exercise interventions is in the individuals who adhere to the plan, whether recorded with measures such as minutes exercising, or step counts[18].

The table below provides a very general guide on the benefits and drawbacks of high intensity, moderate intensity, or low intensity exercise for weight loss.

	Low intensity	Moderate intensity	High intensity
Calorie expenditure equated, is there a superior benefit with this intensity for body composition?	No. But for health benefits, ideally heart rate should be elevated, which may not occur with low intensity activity	No	No
How fatiguing is the intensity?	Not very fatiguing	Slightly fatiguing	Very fatiguing, resulting in more muscle damage and increasing recovery time
Time required to burn the same calories	Longer	Moderate	Shorter
Frequency	Very feasible to perform daily	Feasible to perform daily	Harder to perform daily, especially alongside resistance training
Is there a benefit to performance?	Useful for those currently performing no exercise, looking to create a habit of exercising regularly	Useful for individuals with other sports or performance related goals	Useful for individuals with other sports or performance related goals
Can I perform this exercise on any diet?	Less difficult on a very low carbohydrate diet	Moderately difficult on a very low carbohydrate diet	More difficult on a very low carbohydrate diet
Fasted or fed?	Fed. There is no benefit to fasted exercise for weight loss and possibly reduces performance	Fed. There is no benefit to fasted exercise for weight loss and possibly reduces performance	Fed. There is no benefit to fasted exercise for weight loss and possibly reduces performance

Exercise intensity and duration

When calorie expenditure is equated, high intensity exercise can generally be performed in a shorter duration than moderate intensity aerobic exercise. But, this is at the expense of greater fatigue and perceptions of effort (RPE).

High intensity interval training (HIIT) training requires rest periods in between high intensity bursts to allow for recovery. During these rest periods, fewer calories are burnt. But, the energy cost of performing the high intensity intervals is much greater than for steady state exercise. Meta-analyses show that HIIT allows for the same number of calories to be expended in a shorter duration of time compared to moderate intensity exercise[4,10]. One study compared HIIT to moderate intensity exercise and assessed 24 hour energy expenditure. Despite requiring less time to complete the HIIT protocol, 24 hour energy expenditure was the same[29]. A systematic review and meta-analysis of studies comparing HIIT to moderate intensity aerobic exercise for weight loss showed that when HIIT and moderate intensity aerobic exercise were equated for energy expenditure, they resulted in the *same* weight loss[6]. In studies where HIIT duration was much shorter, such that less energy was expended per session than moderate intensity aerobic exercise, *less* weight loss was achieved with HIIT[6]. Exercise intensity should be based on personal preference. When pushed for time, HIIT may be more suitable to burn energy in a limited time. HIIT may be more time effective, but only as effective if sufficient exercise is performed. 20 minutes of sprints may burn a similar number of calories as a 30 to 40 minute run, but a 60 minute run will burn more energy than 5 minutes of sprints. Burning calories at a faster rate with HIIT has drawbacks. HIIT is performed at the expense of training at higher perceptions of effort, greater fatigue and more muscle damage[30]. Hence, HIIT may be a time-efficient form of burning calories, but from the perspective of fatigue management, lower intensities may be more efficient, especially if muscle ache and fatigue reduce motivation and impact on adherence. This is important to consider when factoring in resistance training sessions at high intensities. Performing additional high intensity interval training increases the possibility of fatigue, muscle damage and overtraining. When utilising HIIT, take into account how many resistance training sessions you perform per week, and how HIIT makes you feel during the resistance training sessions[5]. Also consider that HIIT may require a longer warm up and cool down than exercise of a moderate intensity.

Does HIIT build muscle?

Some have speculated that HIIT can be used as a method to build muscle. Indeed, individual studies have found that HIIT training results in fat loss and muscle growth in untrained beginners and overweight or obese people (including the only study to date assessing alcohol intake and body composition with a HIIT training plan from chapter 13)[31-34]. However, a meta-analysis showed HIIT has no impact on muscle mass compared to moderate intensity exercise[7]. The findings of individual studies can be explained by considering the nature and novelty of HIIT in untrained people. Untrained individuals are highly responsive to any training stimulus for muscle growth. HIIT involves short durations of high intensity at maximal levels of effort, followed by periods of rest before repeating for several sets. As such, HIIT is not too dissimilar from resistance training. The higher levels of effort can result in fatigue and activation of high-threshold motor units (HTMUs). For example, one study in resistance training naïve females compared two forms of HIIT. Both groups performed 6 sets of 60 second bouts at maximal intensity, with 3 minute rests between sets, 3 times per week for 12 weeks. One group used intervals of rowing, whilst the other used a multi-modal approach. The multi-modal approach used resistance exercises with barbells, dumbbells and other exercises with low rep ranges during the 60 second bouts. 8 different sessions were used with different exercise movements over the 12 weeks. Such a training session does not look that different to a resistance training session typically utilised for muscle growth[32]. Both groups similarly increased muscle mass. The sub-optimal 'resistance training style' HIIT compared to a conventional HIIT plan with a rowing machine resulted in similar increases in muscle mass. Another study compared high intensity interval training on a cycle ergometer in overweight and obese individuals. One group performed 5 sets of 2 minute intervals, the other group completed 10 sets of 1 minute intervals, both with 1 minute rests[31]. Only the 1 minute sprint group increased quadriceps muscle size above the control group who performed no exercise. It is feasible to perform at a sufficient intensity for muscle growth for 1 minute, generating significant peripheral fatigue. However, it is unlikely that a sufficiently high intensity for muscle growth can be maintained for 2 minutes, generating significant central fatigue. Meaning, the 1 minute group may have more closely resembled traditional resistance training, with short intense efforts relative to the rest period[31]. HIIT therefore can result in muscle growth in complete beginners, because some aspects of HIIT resemble conventional resistance training, but a sub-optimal form of it. HIIT does not build meaningful amounts of muscle in resistance trained individuals.

Excess post-exercise oxygen consumption (EPOC)

The vast majority of calories burnt from exercise are during the exercise activity, not after. The calories burnt after exercise are relatively insignificant and account for only 6-15% of calories burnt from performing the exercise in total (during and after).

Excess post-exercise oxygen consumption (EPOC) is greater with higher intensities of exercise, showing a curvilinear relationship. The greatest EPOC is from heavy resistance training, followed by high intensity, moderate intensity and then low intensity aerobic exercise. EPOC also increases linearly with exercise duration. The duration of EPOC also appears to be shorter in trained compared to untrained individuals[35].

Performing exercise burns calories (called exercise activity thermogenesis, EAT). But, we also burn additional calories above our basal metabolic rate (BMR) even after we have stopped exercising. This is related to recovery-related increases in energy use[35]. This increase in oxygen consumption and energy use can last for several hours after exercise. On average, excess post-exercise oxygen consumption (EPOC) accounts for 6-15% of the total energy expended from performing exercise (which includes energy expenditure during and after exercise). After we perform high intensity exercise, we burn more calories than after steady state lower intensity exercise. In fact, high intensity (of load) resistance training results in the greatest increase in EPOC[35]. EPOC can be elevated after a resistance training session for almost 2 days[36]. Most of the differences seen in EPOC between exercise are generally due to variations in the intensity and duration of different exercise forms, which have not been considered[35]. For example in one study, EPOC accounted for 7.1% of the total calories burnt when running at 70% of VO_2 max (the maximum rate of oxygen consumed, 100% = maximum aerobic exercise capacity) compared to 13.8% from sprint training at 105% of VO_2 max[37]. Regardless, differences in EPOC between exercises are small. One study compared resistance training, intermittent training and steady state training on EPOC for 24 hours after the training session[38]. Each session was performed to burn the same number of calories whilst exercising, such that any differences in EPOC are due to exercise intensity. Despite finding statistically significantly greater EPOC with resistance training or interval training compared to steady state, this was *not* meaningfully significant in the context of total daily energy expenditure (TDEE).

"Despite the significant results of the present study, practitioners should remain focused primarily on the caloric expenditure achieved during the exercise session and should continually inquire as to what modes and intensities of exercise their clients find most enjoyable and use this information to guide their training plans."
Greer et al., 2015[38].

EPOC also decreases with training experience, such that any differences in EPOC between exercises will diminish with repeated training bouts[38].

Considering exercise-activity thermogenesis (EAT) usually accounts for around 10% of total daily energy expenditure, EPOC only contributes around 1-2% to total daily energy expenditure. The difference in total daily energy expenditure due to differences in EPOC between different exercise intensities and durations when work is equated is therefore less than 1%. *Meaningless* for weight loss[7]. EPOC itself does contribute to total daily energy expenditure, but it is just relatively small compared to what is burnt during exercise. The main determinants of how many calories we burn from exercise are the *duration* of time spent exercising, and the *intensity* of the exercise performed[35,39].

"EPEE [excess post-exercise oxygen consumption] is therefore of negligible physiological significance as far as weight loss is concerned."
Laforgia et al., 1997[37].

Exercise efficiency and training status

The body does get more efficient over time with exercise, but never to the extent that you need to factor it into your plan.

It is important when reading research on exercise efficiency (reductions in the rate of energy expenditure with training experience) to consider the influence of any weight change from a training programme. Muscles become more efficient with weight loss.

Muscle economy and efficiency depend on a range of factors, including metabolism, biomechanics, cardiorespiratory function, ambient temperature and neuromuscular changes[40,41].

Muscle economy refers to the rate of energy expenditure during exercise. *Muscle efficiency* refers to the proportion of energy expenditure that is useful energy and not dissipated as heat[40].

With training experience, you can become more economical or more efficient at performing an exercise[42]. Improvements can just be down to improved coordination in performing the movement[41]. But, you can only get so economical and efficient at an exercise, movement requires energy. If you continually become more and more efficient, you would eventually not burn any additional energy from performing exercise, which clearly does not happen. Maximum efficiency of a muscle is around 32% of total energy use[42,43]. Whole body efficiency is typically lower than this, at around 25%[41]. Muscles are actually quite inefficient; over two thirds of the energy used during exercise is lost as heat. Any training related improvements in economy and efficiency are *meaningless* in the context of the volume of exercise performed and in the context of total daily energy expenditure.

Calorie expenditure from aerobic exercise compared to resistance training

One study compared the energy expenditure from 30 minutes of moderate intensity exercise at 70% maximum heart rate to 30 minutes of resistance training[44]. Moderate intensity exercise was performed on a treadmill and a cycle ergometer. The resistance training session involved 3 sets of 10 reps at 75% of participants' 1 rep maximum (RM) (note this intensity is relative to 1RM, *not* relative to maximum heart rate) for the squat, chest press, leg extension, shoulder press, leg curl and seated row. Participants completed all three exercise forms. 30 minutes of cycling, 30 minutes of running on a treadmill and 30 minutes of resistance exercise all burnt the *same* number of calories (roughly 9kcal per minute for each form of exercise). However, resistance training did result in slightly higher perceptions of effort (higher RPE). Even so, the rate of energy expenditure will be highly dependent on the tasks being performed when resistance training, such as exercise choice, load, reps and the rest periods used[45].

Exercise choice

An important consideration for how many calories are burnt from exercise, is exercise choice. Exercises that involve larger amounts of muscle mass (such as whole-body exercises) will burn energy at a faster rate than exercises using specific body parts. However, other factors besides active muscle mass influence energy expenditure during exercise[46]. It appears that the rate of energy expenditure may differ between exercise modalities when perceptions of effort or exercise intensity are matched[47-49]. However, there are also studies showing minimal differences between exercise modalities at the same level of effort[50]. Studies show that when intensity of effort is equated (same rating of perceived exertion), greater rates of energy expenditure are achieved with treadmill exercise compared to a ski ergometer, rowing machine or stair stepper exercise, which all had greater rates of energy expenditure than the stationary bike, which had the lowest rate of energy expenditure[47,49]. One study found similar energy expenditure with a stationary bike, rowing machine, ski ergometer and treadmill walking at 65% of maximum heart rate for 60 minutes. Although not statistically significant, exercising with the treadmill expended 220kcal (+24%) more than the stationary bike, 310kcal (+36%) more than the rowing machine, and 100kcal (+9%) more than the ski ergometer[48]. When not controlling for heart rate or perceptions of effort, one study found that participants tended to exercise at a higher self-selected rate of energy expenditure when exercising on a treadmill compared to the ski ergometer and stationary bike[46]. Ratings of effort were similar between all exercise forms. It appears that as the duration of exercise increases and the intensity decreases, the difference in energy expenditures between modalities decreases[46]. Similarly for resistance training, a couple of sets of bicep curls will clearly expend much less energy than some heavy sets of squats or deadlifts. Even if differences exist between aerobic exercise modalities, the difference is far less important than performing *any* exercise for a given duration to burn a given number of calories. Such that, *personal preference* of exercise choice should be the priority.

The power of non-exercise activity thermogenesis (NEAT)

The main focus of aerobic exercise for influencing body composition is to increase the energy expended during the day, to maintain a caloric deficit for weight loss. Aerobic exercise is a form exercise activity thermogenesis (EAT) which contributes to total daily energy expenditure. However, a very large component of total daily energy expenditure that is often overlooked is non-exercise activity thermogenesis (NEAT). NEAT can constitute pretty much *any* random little movement you might perform during the day such as chewing, foot tapping, arm waving, cleaning or moving around at work. NEAT can have a significant influence on your total daily energy expenditure. If the aim is to expend additional calories, consider the influence of these small daily movements as a potential source to increase total daily energy expenditure. Similarly, when performing fatiguing exercise or an increased volume of exercise, it has been suggested that this increase in energy expenditure is compensated for in part, by a reduction in NEAT and other forms of EAT performed during the day[19,51]. Think about a time you may have performed a long, strenuous run or intense gym session and collapsed on the sofa afterwards with very little movement. Just moving around more during the day (i.e. low intensity exercise) can significantly increase your daily energy expenditure. A classic example is ensuring a daily *'step count'* of so many (e.g. 10,000) steps per day.

Fat burning versus fat loss: fasted exercise and exercise intensity

Greater fat oxidation (using fat) during the exercise session does not mean more fat loss.

Fasted vs fed exercise

At best, fasted exercise is equivalent to fed exercise for fat loss. At worst, fasted exercise is detrimental to fat loss compared to fed exercise.

Fasted exercise does not result in greater fat loss. It can possibly impair performance and result in lower energy expenditure during the exercise session.

The evidence does *not* support fasted exercise in the morning for greater fat loss than fed exercise[52]. A systematic review and meta-analysis of 5 studies has shown no benefit of performing fasted exercise compared to fed exercise for body composition, or weight loss[8]. It should be noted however that fairly few studies exist that compare the effect of fed exercise or fasted exercise on body composition, and like other studies of exercise on weight change, participant diets were largely uncontrolled. This may mean that increases in exercise activity thermogenesis (EAT) were unconsciously mitigated through other changes in energy intake or expenditure.

A high quality randomised trial by Brad Schoenfeld and Alan Aragon showed that fasted exercise is *not* superior and at best, is as effective as fed exercise for weight loss. They compared the effect of fasted or fed exercise on body composition in females[53]. Participants performed 1 hour of steady state exercise 3 times per week, for 4 weeks. One group performed exercise in a fasted state, and the other group in a fed state. Groups consumed the same pre-exercise (fed) or post-exercise (fasted) meal at different times, such that energy intake was *matched*. Participant diets were monitored to ensure that they were in a calorie deficit to promote fat loss. After 4 weeks, both groups lost weight and fat mass, but *no* difference was seen between groups. Other studies have also shown *no* difference between fasted and fed exercise and body composition[34,53].

One study found reduced weight gain in a calorie surplus with fasted exercise compared to fed exercise over 6 weeks. However, the study only measured body weight and there was no significant increase in skinfold measurements (a measure of body fat percentage) for fed exercise, meaning the additional weight gain with fed exercise may have resulted from an increase in muscle mass[54]. Even so, in another study, the same researchers found no difference between fasted exercise and fed exercise for body composition at caloric maintenance[34,55].

The main argument for exercising in a fasted state is that not eating before exercise increases the fat burning (fat oxidation) potential of the exercise. The body uses carbohydrates and fats for energy at different rates throughout the day. Fat oxidation is greatest after an overnight fast, and carbohydrate oxidation is greatest after a meal[22]. Some have speculated that because there is potentially greater fat oxidation when performing fasted exercise, this means that a 20 minute fasted exercise session will burn more fat than say, a 60 minute fed exercise session, leading to greater fat loss[8,52]. In other words, their rationale is that by burning more fat *during* exercise, more fat loss will occur[8]. Unfortunately, performing fasted exercise does *not* increase fat loss[56]. This concept ignores the bigger and more important picture of total daily energy intake, total daily energy expenditure and less importantly, daily fluctuations in fat oxidation. The main factor for weight change is calories in versus calories out, *regardless* of exercise intensity, duration, modality or how much fat is being burned during exercise[57]. When energy expenditure from exercise is *equated, all* forms of aerobic exercise result in the *same* amount of weight loss. As discussed in the comparison between low fat and low carbohydrate diets in chapter 8, whether fat is gained or stored is a balance between fat storage and fat oxidation (using fat for energy)[57]. Storage and oxidation vary across the day and with relative energy balance. Greater fat oxidation occurs when in a calorie deficit, and lower oxidation in a calorie surplus[57]. Only considering changes in fat oxidation during a 20 minute exercise session does not factor in the variations in fat oxidation and storage that occur across the day[52,58,59]. Skipping breakfast does not influence fat or carbohydrate metabolism over the course of the day, nor does it influence the amount of energy expended when calorie intake is equated[60]. The only difference is that fat and carbohydrate are used at different times of the day, depending on when food is consumed. Low to moderate intensity exercise will result in greater fat oxidation during exercise than high intensity exercise, but high intensity exercise results in relatively greater fat oxidation after exercise[61]. Similarly, fasted exercise results in lower fat oxidation in the post-exercise period compared to fed exercise[8,22,60,62]. In other words, having a meal before exercise can result in greater fat oxidation later in the day, after exercise. Fat oxidation also varies with diet composition. High fat, low carbohydrate diets result in greater fat oxidation during exercise, but this is because the body is using the greater proportion of fats that are being consumed[63]. Even so, altering fat content in the diet does not influence fat loss beyond whether energy intake is below energy expenditure[22]. Many exercise studies do not take into account participants' dietary composition. The main focus should be on how many total calories were expended to complete the exercise task, *not* where those calories originated from.

The amount of glycogen (carbohydrate stores) in muscles and in the liver limits endurance exercise. Marathon runners hit the *'wall'* when their muscles are depleted of glycogen. This is why carbohydrate feeding during endurance exercise benefits performance. An overnight fast can deplete muscle and liver glycogen stores, placing a limit on the volume of aerobic exercise that can be performed before the next meal[64]. Consuming carbohydrates before exercise does indeed reduce the amount of fat that is released (lipolysis) from adipose tissue (fat stores) during exercise, but this does not impact on fat use for energy in muscles (fat oxidation)[52,56,65]. As discussed in chapter 5, carbohydrate consumption elevates blood sugar levels. Insulin then acts to return blood sugar levels back to resting (fasted) levels by promoting the use and storage of sugar, and simultaneously preventing fat release (lipolysis). However, recent studies show that differences in fat oxidation between fasted and fed exercise (whether it be pre-exercise protein or carbohydrate) are minimal[56,66]. In moderately and well trained people, exercising fasted or fed may not even have a large influence on fat oxidation during exercise[56,59]. When performing fasted exercise, the body releases more fat (lipolysis) from fat stores (adipose tissue) than it can use (oxidation), such that any effect of consuming carbohydrates on fat release may not significantly impact on how much fat is being used in the muscle, even though lipolysis is lower[52,59]. One randomised *cross-over* study (participants underwent both fasted and fed exercise interventions) found greater fat oxidation from fasted exercise compared to fed exercise[67]. However, another randomised crossover pilot study found greater fat oxidation when consuming 25g of whey or casein protein prior to moderate intensity treadmill exercise, compared to the same exercise in a fasted state[56]. There was *no* difference in total energy expenditure between conditions in *any* of these studies.

At the level of *acute fat oxidation* and *energy use*, the findings from fasted and fed exercise studies are inconclusive and conflicting. But, at the level of *long-term total energy balance* and *body composition*, the findings from *all* fasted and fed exercise studies demonstrate that differences in *acute fat oxidation* and *energy use* are *irrelevant* for weight loss, when equating 24 hour energy expenditure between conditions.

Differences in fat oxidation are likely to be due to the factors discussed such as diet composition, meal timing, meal quantity, energy balance, training status and exercise intensity[56]. Any theoretical benefit of increased fat oxidation with fasted exercise is *not* meaningful in the context of total daily energy balance. Energy balance dictates weight change. Rather than adding extra calories prior to exercise, consume some of the calories you usually have later in the day after exercise, before.

Muscles do not rely alone on adipose tissue as the only source of fat to fuel exercise. Muscles can use the fat stores within them as well (*intramuscular triglycerides* (IMTG)), and fats circulating in the blood. Type I fibres have greater IMTG stores than type II fibres. IMTG stores can increase with endurance training experience[57]. And by experience, this means compared to someone who is completely untrained; as little as a few weeks of exercise can result in an endurance 'trained' status[52]. Endurance training experience also increases the fat oxidation capabilities of muscle[57]. There may be a greater reliance on intramuscular fat stores or circulating fat to fuel exercise, but this is still inconclusive. The supposed increase in fat oxidation during exercise being superior for fat loss from adipose stores (fat cells) does not consider that there will be fat oxidation from other sources of fat[52]. Regardless, these factors are irrelevant beyond the context of total daily energy intake and expenditure for weight change.

Cross-over studies show energy expenditure (from EPOC) is also generally greater several hours after performing exercise in the fed state, than in the fasted state[8,11,61,68]. However, energy expenditure acutely (<2 hours) after exercise has also been shown to be higher with fasted exercise[67]. Although not significant in itself for weight loss, differences in post-exercise fat oxidation in part may explain why any differences in fat oxidation during exercise do not relate to fat loss. A pre-exercise meal increases the thermogenic effect of the subsequent exercise session for several hours afterwards. This means that greater energy is expended after the meal and after the exercise. In fact, consuming a meal without exercise results in similar elevations in energy expenditure (via thermogenesis) as exercising in the fasted state (excluding the energy expended performing the actual exercise)[11]. There appears to be no advantage to performing exercise fasted, with the hope of increasing EPOC or energy expenditure after exercise[11].

*Consider if two identical people consumed 2000kcal per day with the same macronutrients and with the same calorie deficit. They both perform 20 minutes of exercise at the same intensity. One person performed 20 minutes of fasted exercise in the morning before eating breakfast. The other person performed 20 minutes of fed exercise after eating breakfast. **Both people would lose the same amount of fat.** Imagine now, that one individual instead performed HIIT, and the other performed moderate intensity exercise. Both individuals burned the same number of calories from exercise (such that the individual performing HIIT was exercising for less time). **Both individuals would lose the same amount of fat.** The main factor determining the influence of aerobic exercise on promoting fat loss will be down to how many calories are expended (i.e. how much exercise activity thermogenesis contributes to total daily energy expenditure, relative to energy intake).*

There is no evidence that fasted exercise can improve performance compared to fed exercise. Most evidence suggests that both fasted endurance exercise or fasted resistance exercise can impair performance[69–72]. Interestingly, a systematic review and meta-analysis of Ramadan fasting in amateur and elite athletes (food intake restricted to the hours of darkness) demonstrated that this form of intermittent fasting generally did not impair aerobic or strength exercise performance or workload, but did affect power and sprint performance[73]. Limitations of this analysis have been discussed in chapter 11. Even so, there was no benefit from performing exercise in a fasted state. Impaired performance means fewer calories are being burned during exercise, or a reduced muscle building stimulus if performing resistance exercise fasted. Both outcomes may reduce the efficacy of exercise-induced energy expenditure (EAT) or impair the ability to preserve muscle in a calorie deficit. Fed exercise may also increase energy expenditure during exercise from the thermic effect of food (TEF)[66]. When glycogen stores are depleted (such as after an overnight fast), exercise may also be detrimental for muscle growth from an increase in protein catabolism and a reduction in muscle protein synthesis during fasted exercise[8,74,75]. This acute change has *not* been formally related to long-term changes in muscle size, but it will influence day-to-day variations in net protein balance, which is important for muscle growth and maintenance. Frequent (e.g. daily) bouts of fasted exercise *may* significantly impact net protein balance and impact muscle mass. Again, even if fasted exercise does not negatively impact energy expenditure or muscle mass, it would be at best equivocal to fed exercise, and *not* be of benefit. Rather than increasing carbohydrate or protein consumption, consider consuming calories that you usually consume later in the day, first thing in the morning, before exercise.

It may be that you perform exercise fasted in the morning because you do not have time to consume a large meal. If so, even just a small amount of carbohydrate (as little as 30g of carbohydrates, roughly 120kcal) or a protein shake (20-40g of protein) 30 minutes before exercise can improve performance and increase post-exercise energy expenditure[56,64].

Lower intensity exercise: 'the fat burning zone'

Greater fat oxidation during the exercise session does not result in more fat loss. 24 hour fat oxidation is not influenced by the intensity of any exercise performed. The intensity of exercise does not influence weight loss beyond the total number of calories expended from the exercise.

Fat oxidation varies with the intensity of exercise. The higher the intensity, the greater the reliance on carbohydrate to fuel exercise[76]. The longer the duration of exercise, the greater the utilisation of fat to fuel the exercise[5,57]. Even so, there is evidence that intramuscular fats (IMTG) are still used as an energy source during high intensity resistance exercise[77].

There is increased fat burning (fat oxidation) during lower intensity exercise, but this does not mean low to moderate intensity exercise results in greater fat loss than HIIT or resistance training. 24 hour fat oxidation does *not* vary between low, moderate or high intensity exercise, nor with resistance training, or compared to 24 hours without exercise[57]. Any difference in fat oxidation *during* exercise is compensated for *after* exercise, such that daily fat oxidation is equivocal.

The theory for low to moderate intensity aerobic exercise being a tool for greater fat loss is based on the same argument that is made for fasted exercise, and is incorrect for the same reasons that fasted exercise does not result in greater fat loss.

Exercise will *only* result in greater weight loss when *more* calories are expended performing exercise, with all other factors *unchanged* (energy intake and other forms of energy expenditure). This is achieved by exercising for longer, or by exercising for the same length of time, but at a higher intensity.

All things considered, the biggest factor that should influence the type, duration, intensity and modality of any exercise you perform should be down to personal preference.

James Krieger and Bret Contreras have noted that your decision to use aerobic exercise for weight loss should take into account[78]:

- How aerobic exercise affects your appetite and hunger. Despite a meta-analysis showing no apparent effect of exercise on subsequent food intake, this is an average[21]. Some people will increase their intake, some will decrease their intake and others have an unchanged intake[79]. Find how aerobic exercise influences your intake.
- How fatigued you are across the rest of the day, and how exercise affects your non-exercise activity thermogenesis (NEAT) (random movement during the day). If you train so hard that you then limit your activity for the rest of the day compared to your habitual activity, this can negate any energy expenditure from the exercise performed[80].
- How does aerobic exercise affect your resistance training sessions?
- How does aerobic exercise affect your sleep? Exercise for most people usually helps with sleep. However for some, exercise can impair sleep.
- How does aerobic exercise affect your self-discipline, does aerobic exercise make you less controlled with any other exercise you do or your diet? Does the stress of adhering to an exercise plan cause you to become less adherent to your diet or exercise later in the day?

Aerobic exercise and muscle gain: concurrent exercise training and the 'interference effect'

How much aerobic exercise should I perform during a period of muscle growth?

The interference effect is more important in pure strength and power-based disciplines and less so on muscle growth. The strength of evidence for an interference effect of aerobic exercise on muscle growth is weak, and many variables (e.g. training status) have not been fully examined. Unless you are competing in purely strength-based sports or competitions at a high level (such as a powerlifting competition), it is unnecessary to avoid aerobic exercise whilst aiming to build muscle. In fact, evidence suggests that some endurance exercise may benefit muscle growth.

The effect depends on the frequency, duration and intensity of aerobic exercise, and its proximity to the resistance training session. Longer durations and higher frequencies of aerobic exercise are more likely to have an effect. To minimise any possible effect on muscle growth or if there are strength-related goals, avoid performing excessive aerobic exercise immediately before a resistance training session and ideally after or well before, or on a separate day. Simply, avoid a high volume of endurance exercise, which might be considered to be several hours of aerobic exercise more than 3-4 times per week.

To maximise muscle, there is no need to exclude aerobic exercise. Stick to health organisation recommendations to maintain and improve health. This consists of 3 x 20 minute vigorous (e.g. running), or 5 x 30 minute moderate (e.g. brisk walk) exercise sessions per week.

Choose the form of aerobic exercise that suits you, whether that be low, moderate or high intensity exercise.

More importantly, consider at what volume does the aerobic exercise you perform start to impair your resistance training sessions. For some this could be a lot, for some not much at all. The amount, type and frequency of aerobic exercise you perform will be highly individualised.

Performing both strength-based exercise and endurance-based exercise is common for many individuals, especially in sports (such as rugby) and for people trying to stay fit. *Concurrent training* (endurance and resistance exercise) has been shown to be superior to endurance or resistance training alone for health-related benefits and improvements in performance-related adaptations (e.g. aerobic capacity, hypertrophy and strength). The benefits of concurrent training for the general population far outweigh any potential performance or training-related risks[81–83]. Both forms of exercise are recommended by a range of health authorities[1,84].

However, a long-held belief by many who try to build muscle is that '*cardio kills gains*', or more formally, performing aerobic exercise alongside resistance training limits muscle growth. As such, some have suggested that little to no aerobic exercise is necessary to promote muscle growth. This idea is called the '*interference effect*' from concurrent training (aerobic and resistance training in the same plan), such that aerobic exercise '*interferes*' with resistance training adaptations. The concept of interference from concurrent training arose from studies in the 1980's[85]. Adaptations to the training stimulus are *specific* to the exercise. It was found that endurance training alongside resistance training impaired resistance training adaptations (e.g. strength) compared to resistance training alone[81]. This was supported by mechanistic, cellular and theoretical evidence that the specific adaptations of endurance and resistance training require different and conflicting pathways in cells. Numerous studies have been performed since then into concurrent training and subsequent adaptations (including power, strength, hypertrophy and aerobic performance).

Despite theoretical suggestions and acute post-workout mechanistic evidence to suggest an interference effect, the collective body of evidence suggests that the interference effect is minimal to non-existent for muscle growth, and concurrent training can even be beneficial in some circumstances[83,86]. Acute cellular changes do not necessarily correlate with long-term training adaptations (as seen with acute post-workout elevations in muscle protein synthesis and muscle growth in chapter 9)[86]. The interference effect does however, appear to affect strength and power to a greater extent (such as a 1 repetition maximum test)[86].

Two meta-analyses have been performed that assess the interference effect and muscle growth[83,86–88]. Neither found any difference in muscle growth between concurrent training and resistance training alone. One meta-analysis from 2018 compared concurrent cycling or running-based HIIT with resistance training, to resistance training alone[88]. An analysis of 7 studies showed concurrent training did not affect hypertrophy or upper body strength, and an analysis of 12 studies showed a trend for impaired lower body strength. The other meta-analysis from 2012 compared any form of concurrent endurance exercise alongside resistance training[87]. They found that the overall effect of resistance training alone compared to concurrent training was not significantly different for muscle growth or strength. There was also no difference between the three training types (endurance-only, concurrent and resistance-only) and changes in body fat levels.

As always, there are limitations to both meta-analyses. For example, several important variables were not analysed, including:

1. Exercise sequence (order of aerobic or resistance training).
2. Volume, intensity, duration and frequency of aerobic exercise.
3. Recovery period between exercise forms (e.g. minutes, hours or days between endurance and resistance training sessions).

Most studies are on untrained individuals, who are highly responsive to training stimuli. Concurrent training may not be detrimental for untrained individuals as both endurance and resistance training related adaptations can occur simultaneously. Similarly, most studies do not extend beyond 4 to 5 months. Whether concurrent training has a long-term detrimental effect is unknown[81,82]. Also, the time-course for improvements in strength appears to occur faster than the time-course for increases in muscle size. This means studies are better able to identify interference effects on strength than muscle growth. This could be an explanation as to why the interference effect is evident for strength outcomes, but not for muscle growth. Potentially if studies were conducted for longer, similar effects would be seen on muscle growth[83]. However, considering meta-analyses (which increase the overall ability to detect interference effects) still find no influence on muscle growth, suggests that this may be an unimportant methodological consideration. A muscle building plan may incorporate high intensity of load and low rep training alongside moderate and low intensity of loads (see chapter 16 for a summary of evidence-based training recommendations). The effect on strength may be a more important point to consider for some individuals when planning training.

Muscle growth can occur when performing endurance exercise alongside resistance training. The overall effect of concurrent training on muscle growth appears minimal. But, when analysing the data further it is clear that certain variables increase and decrease the risk of interference occurring. Some studies show a reduction, some no effect, and some even an improvement in resistance training adaptations with endurance exercise[81]. The question is, which variables within a concurrent training plan interfere with muscle growth? An important analysis is determining *how* to perform concurrent training to the *benefit* and not to the potential *detriment* of muscle growth[82]. The effect of concurrent training on muscle growth will depend on the timing, volume, intensity and frequency of endurance exercise, resistance exercise variables, the body parts trained, training status and the intrinsic variability in adaptive responses between people. Due to the numerous variables, it is currently not possible to quantify the amount of aerobic exercise that will cause a given effect on muscle growth[81,82,86].

Therefore, some important variables need to be clarified:

- Was aerobic exercise performed before or after resistance training?
- What was the volume (frequency, intensity and duration) and modality of aerobic exercise?
- What was the training experience of participants?
- What are the adaptations of interest from training?

We can consider specific studies to see how these variables may influence the interference effect.

Another point to consider is that there could be *no* interference effect at all. It could just be that poorer outcomes in some studies are simply the result of overtraining with far too much volume (i.e. simply a result of the additional workload from performing both forms of exercise)[87,88].

Exercise sequence

Intra-session exercise order (whether resistance training is performed first, or aerobic exercise first) has been suggested to influence interference. It has been suggested that performing aerobic exercise first generates fatigue, which limits the subsequent resistance training session and therefore impacts on growth. Even so, the 2018 meta-analysis demonstrated that intra-session exercise order had no impact on muscle growth compared to resistance training alone. However, the volume of both resistance and endurance exercise was low. Endurance exercise was only around 30 minutes in duration, with training frequencies of only 2 to 3 days per week. Most studies were also on untrained people[89]. As such, it is not unsurprising that no interference effect was seen. Performing endurance exercise before resistance training can have no effect on muscle growth[81]. But, both meta-analyses show that exercise order does influence 1 repetition maximum strength, especially in trained individuals[89,90]. Therefore, exercise order may impact strength development, but any effect on muscle growth appears to be small, at least in untrained people with a low volume of training.

The fact that intra-session exercise sequence has little influence of muscle growth suggests that acute cellular changes noted in earlier studies have little long-term consequence on muscular adaptation[86].

Despite the equivocal findings, the general consensus is to *prioritise* what is important, especially with training experience. The greatest performance is in the exercises performed first in a workout. Hence, performing exercises that train the body parts of interest first will produce the greatest adaptations in those muscles. If your goal was to build the chest, you would perform chest exercises first and not last after other body parts. Likewise, if muscle growth is the goal, perform resistance training before endurance training. If endurance training was your goal, then you would perform that first.

But it does mean, if you did perform aerobic exercise for some reason soon before you planned to resistance train, then this would likely have a minimal effect on your session for muscle growth.

Aerobic exercise and resistance training on separate days

Most studies compare concurrent training in the same session (as above), although concurrent training can be performed in the morning and afternoon, or on separate days. It appears the larger the time gap, the less of any possible effect. Again, the influence is more prominent on strength-based outcomes[82,86,91,92].

A longer duration between aerobic exercise and resistance exercise allows for greater performance in the resistance training session[93]. When resistance training 4, 8 or 24 hours after aerobic exercise, lower body leg press resistance training performance was impaired 4 and 8 hours after, but not 24 hours after lower body aerobic exercise. There was no effect on upper body bench press performance at any time point after lower body aerobic exercise. Whether this has any importance for muscle growth is unclear.

Interference is body part specific

The 2012 meta-analysis found the overall effect of resistance training compared to concurrent training to not be significantly different for muscle growth and strength[87]. However, looking more closely, the effects of concurrent training are specific to the body part. The effects of concurrent endurance exercise reduced muscle strength in the lower body compared to resistance training alone. No effect of concurrent training was found for upper body muscle growth or strength, compared to resistance training alone. This is probably because the majority of endurance exercise modalities are lower body dominant (e.g. running and cycling). Few endurance exercise modalities utilise the upper body, besides rowing and the hand-bike.

It is likely that the interference effect will be specific to the body parts being concurrently trained; a lower body HIIT and lower body resistance training session will result in greater interference than a lower body HIIT and upper body resistance training session[93]. As demonstrated in the study above for training on separate days, resistance training after lower body aerobic training impaired lower body leg press resistance training performance, but had no effect on upper body bench press performance. Lower body HIIT only influenced lower body strength, not upper body strength[93]. However, further work needs to confirm this and whether it is meaningful for muscle growth.

Performing aerobic exercise (which is usually a lower body modality such as running or cycling) on a separate day to a lower body resistance training session may be beneficial for performance. If resistance training the upper body, separating aerobic exercise may provide less benefit.

Exercise modality

The type of endurance exercise performed may have a significant effect on strength, but again less so on muscle mass. The 2018 meta-analysis found a greater effect of high intensity cycling intervals (HIIT) on strength, whereas the 2012 analysis found a greater effect of moderate intensity running on strength[82]. The long-term implications of this on muscle growth are uncertain, especially when resistance training with higher intensities of load and lower reps (i.e. a more strength-based period of resistance training). The contrasting influence of exercise modality on strength, but no effect on muscle growth means no strong recommendations can be made regarding whether one modality is preferred to another. As such, the modality used should be the one of *personal preference*[82]. Indeed, whether rowing would result in a greater interference effect of the back musculature when the back is concurrently resistance trained, is unknown.

Aerobic intensity

It has been suggested that the similarities between HIIT and resistance training means there is less of an interference effect than with moderate intensity training[86]. However, it has similarly been suggested that HIIT or sprint interval training (SIT) results in a greater interference effect than moderate intensity training, because both HIIT and resistance training recruit high-threshold motor units, resulting in high-threshold motor unit fatigue and metabolic stress. Fatigue would then in theory limit muscle performance compared to resistance training alone[86,88]. However, a meta-analysis showed no effect of concurrent HIIT on muscle growth compared to resistance training alone, and overall, the evidence finds no effect of HIIT on muscle growth.[86,88].

Furthermore, meta-analyses comparing concurrent HIIT and moderate intensity exercise find no effect of exercise intensity on muscle growth, at least with low volumes. Therefore, the intensity of aerobic exercise is likely to have a minimal effect on muscle growth[87,88]. Studies specifically comparing high intensity to moderate intensity aerobic exercise alongside resistance training also find that the intensity of the exercise did not influence any changes in resistance training performance[93–95].

Choose the aerobic intensity that suits you.

Aerobic volume (duration and frequency)

Greater frequencies and durations of aerobic exercise are correlated with lower levels of muscle growth[87]. Studies finding greater muscle growth with concurrent training generally use lower volumes and lower frequencies of aerobic and resistance training[86]. However, there are still many unknowns. Clearly, a 5 hour run before resistance training will impair performance and likely muscle growth. A 5 minute warm-up on the treadmill will clearly have a beneficial (if any) effect on performance and muscle growth, yet both examples would be considered concurrent training. HIIT every day will be highly fatiguing and limit resistance training far more than HIIT training once or twice per week. Where the *transition* from benefit to detriment occurs is unknown and will be highly individual. As such, overall training volume (to avoid overtraining) may be the main overall consideration for concurrent training and planning how much endurance exercise to perform.

The volumes that can be performed will vary greatly between people. Some people may be able to build lots of muscle from resistance training alongside hours of aerobic exercise. Others may find any volume of aerobic training blunts resistance training performance and growth. However, more volume will likely mean more interference. How much is too much depends on the individual.

Training status

The interference effect appears to be greater in trained individuals[81,83,88]. Untrained individuals and beginners are highly responsive to training stimuli. With experience, training needs to become more specific in order to illicit the specific training adaptations that are desired. Given the increase in volume needed for further growth with training experience, endurance training volume may place a limit on this resistance training capacity without overtraining. Again, the limit of effective volume will vary between people.

Summary

Some individuals may suggest that to optimise gains in muscle size, one would not do any endurance exercise at all. However, this would not optimise general health and the limited evidence does not suggest this. It is your choice as to whether you choose to do endurance exercise, and how much you choose to do whilst trying to build muscle. To acquire the health benefits of endurance exercise, consider how active you are during the day in relation to the recommended amounts of moderate exercise, and add in as much as is necessary to achieve these goals. If you are active all day, (such as a builder), then you might not need to add in much aerobic activity. Whereas, if you spend all day at a desk, it may be worthwhile to perform some endurance exercise throughout the week.

Although small, any risk of interference will be greater with certain variables. A greater risk of an interference effect on muscle growth will occur with:

- High volume, long distance exercise.
- Exercise with high energy demands.
- Longer duration (over 20-30 minutes) exercise.
- Greater aerobic exercise-induced muscle damage and fatigue (e.g. downhill running, which involves large amounts of eccentric contractions).

- Excessive endurance exercise performed immediately before resistance training.
- Intermediate or advanced training experience.

A smaller risk of an interference effect or a potentially beneficial effect on muscle growth will occur with:

- Low volume (<20 minutes) aerobic exercise (e.g. a warm up prior to resistance training).
- Exercise performed several hours apart from resistance training, or on a completely separate day[82].
- Aerobic exercise using a different body part to that being resistance trained on the same day.
- Little to no training experience (i.e. in untrained individuals).

Greater consideration of these variables should be considered if you have strength-related goals alongside any muscle building goals.

For muscle growth, you probably don't want to be doing hours of endurance exercise every day, but there's no evidence to support doing none at all. There's no strong evidence that a particular form of aerobic exercise is better or worse than another for muscle building. It does appear that more frequent, longer duration aerobic exercise with greater training experience is more likely to impact muscle growth.

Nutritional considerations when adding endurance exercise to a muscle building resistance training programme.

An important point to add is that muscle growth is optimised in a caloric surplus. Any additional energy expenditure via aerobic exercise needs to be factored into your caloric needs to ensure you achieve a surplus[86]. If you already struggle to consume sufficient energy, this may be a factor to consider, especially if you tend to not compensate for any exercise-related energy expenditure (EAT) with additional energy intake. There is no influence of concurrent training on muscle growth when adequate protein is consumed[96]. Protein intake should already be optimised (at 1.6g/kg of body weight per day) and fat intake above the minimum recommendations (above 0.5g/kg of body weight per day, or at least 15-20% of daily calorie intake). Considering the strong evidence showing the benefit of carbohydrate intake on endurance performance, it is likely that any additional calorie intake to account for endurance exercise may benefit from being predominantly carbohydrate in origin, especially when adopting a diet that is relatively low in carbohydrate intake already[97]. A lack of carbohydrate before, during and after endurance exercise can limit performance and lower markers of muscle protein synthesis[69,97]. The carbohydrate recommendations made in chapter 8 presume that only resistance training is being performed. If performing concurrent aerobic and resistance training sessions, then additional carbohydrate will become more important to prevent glycogen depletion. This will ensure adequate energy for resistance training sessions, especially with longer durations and higher frequencies of aerobic exercise[86]. If a significant volume of aerobic exercise has been performed, it may be beneficial to consume 1-1.5g/kg of body weight of carbohydrate in the hours after the workout (note again the relative unimportance of immediate consumption). This can easily be achieved with a mixed meal in the hours after the concurrent workout[86,98,99].

If utilising a ketogenic diet (see chapter 8), consider that concurrent studies rarely consider participant diets. *No* concurrent studies have utilised a ketogenic diet. High intensity exercise will be limited with a ketogenic diet due to the limited carbohydrate availability. Inadequate carbohydrate intake with exercise-induced glycogen depletion may then further limit resistance training performance and muscle growth. This is largely a theoretical consideration.

To maximise muscle growth whilst performing aerobic exercise, two researchers recommend that aerobic exercise should be[86]:

- Performed with a frequency of up to 3x per week.
- Of a shorter duration, up to 30-40 minutes per session.

However, what works for you will be highly individual. Consider your training and how much progression you are making with your current aerobic exercise and resistance training volume. At what point does the aerobic exercise you perform start to impair your resistance training sessions? For some this could be a lot, for some not much at all. Some people can build muscle with large volumes of endurance training, some can perform very little and still struggle to build muscle. Whether concurrent training is impairing your muscle growth can be judged by considering:

- Are you progressively overloading in your resistance training?
- Are you increasing in body weight? Does this weight appear to be muscle or fat?
- Do you feel fresh and ready, or fatigued and tired for your resistance training sessions?
- Do you feel well rested?
- Are you definitely in a calorie surplus (have you considered the additional energy expenditure from aerobic exercise)? A more conscious approach to energy intake may help to determine if you are or not (discussed in chapter 6).

How frequently you resistance train, how frequently you perform aerobic exercise and how strenuous both activities are will also have an influence. This needs to be considered for overall management of fatigue and recovery. When muscle growth is the goal, *prioritise* resistance sessions over endurance sessions. Bearing in mind the greater interference effect on strength, consider limiting aerobic training near to resistance sessions where you will be performing sets with a greater strength-based focus (i.e. higher intensity loads within the 1-6 rep range).

If you really enjoy aerobic exercise and enjoy exercising for hours then by all means do so, especially if you find that it does not impact on your resistance training. If you find that more than 10 to 20 minutes of aerobic exercise impairs your ability and motivation to resistance train, then seriously consider performing aerobic exercise on a separate day or reducing the volume of aerobic exercise you perform (duration and/or frequency).

References

1   GOV.UK. *Physical activity guidelines: UK Chief Medical Officers' report.*   Available   from: https://www.gov.uk/government/publications/physical-activity-guidelines-uk-chief-medical-officers-report (accessed 12 Feb 2020).
2   Haskell WL, Lee I-M, Pate RR, Powell KE, Blair SN, Franklin BA et al. Physical activity and public health: updated recommendation for adults from the American College of Sports Medicine and the American Heart Association. *Circulation* 2007; 116: 1081–1093.
3   MacInnis MJ, Gibala MJ. Physiological adaptations to interval training and the role of exercise intensity. *J Physiol* 2017; 595: 2915–2930.
4   Maillard F, Pereira B, Boisseau N. Effect of High-Intensity Interval Training on Total, Abdominal and Visceral Fat Mass: A Meta-Analysis. *Sports Med Auckl NZ* 2018; 48: 269–288.
5   Schoenfeld B, Dawes J. High-Intensity Interval Training: Applications for General Fitness Training. *Strength Cond J* 2009; 31: 44–46.
6   Keating SE, Johnson NA, Mielke GI, Coombes JS. A systematic review and meta-analysis of interval training versus moderate-intensity continuous training on body adiposity. *Obes Rev Off J Int Assoc Study Obes* 2017; 18: 943–964.
7   Sultana RN, Sabag A, Keating SE, Johnson NA. The Effect of Low-Volume High-Intensity Interval Training on Body Composition and Cardiorespiratory Fitness: A Systematic Review and Meta-Analysis. *Sports Med Auckl NZ* 2019; 49: 1687–1721.
8   Hackett D, Hagstrom AD. Effect of Overnight Fasted Exercise on Weight Loss and Body Composition: A Systematic Review and Meta-Analysis. *J Funct Morphol Kinesiol* 2017; 2: 43.

9   Taylor J, Keating SE, Holland DJ, Coombes JS, Leveritt MD. The Chronic Effect of Interval Training on Energy Intake: A Systematic Review and Meta-Analysis. *J Obes* 2018; 2018: 6903208.

10   Wewege M, van den Berg R, Ward RE, Keech A. The effects of high-intensity interval training vs. moderate-intensity continuous training on body composition in overweight and obese adults: a systematic review and meta-analysis. *Obes Rev Off J Int Assoc Study Obes* 2017; 18: 635–646.

11   Davis JM, Sadri S, Sargent RG, Ward D. Weight control and calorie expenditure: thermogenic effects of pre-prandial and post-prandial exercise. *Addict Behav* 1989; 14: 347–351.

12   Swift DL, Johannsen NM, Lavie CJ, Earnest CP, Church TS. The Role of Exercise and Physical Activity in Weight Loss and Maintenance. *Prog Cardiovasc Dis* 2014; 56: 441–447.

13   Flack KD, Ufholz K, Johnson L, Fitzgerald JS, Roemmich JN. Energy compensation in response to aerobic exercise training in overweight adults. *Am J Physiol Regul Integr Comp Physiol* 2018; 315: R619–R626.

14   Slentz CA, Duscha BD, Johnson JL, Ketchum K, Aiken LB, Samsa GP et al. Effects of the amount of exercise on body weight, body composition, and measures of central obesity: STRRIDE--a randomized controlled study. *Arch Intern Med* 2004; 164: 31–39.

15   Donnelly JE, Honas JJ, Smith BK, Mayo MS, Gibson CA, Sullivan DK et al. Aerobic exercise alone results in clinically significant weight loss for men and women: midwest exercise trial 2. *Obes Silver Spring Md* 2013; 21: E219-228.

16   Ross R, Janssen I, Dawson J, Kungl A-M, Kuk JL, Wong SL et al. Exercise-induced reduction in obesity and insulin resistance in women: a randomized controlled trial. *Obes Res* 2004; 12: 789–798.

17   Rosenkilde M, Auerbach P, Reichkendler MH, Ploug T, Stallknecht BM, Sjödin A. Body fat loss and compensatory mechanisms in response to different doses of aerobic exercise--a randomized controlled trial in overweight sedentary males. *Am J Physiol Regul Integr Comp Physiol* 2012; 303: R571-579.

18   Foster-Schubert K, Alfano C, Duggan C, Xiao L, Campbell K, Kong A et al. Effect of diet and exercise, alone or combined, on weight and body composition in overweight-to-obese post-menopausal women. *Obes Silver Spring Md* 2012; 20: 1628–1638.

19   Hall KD, Heymsfield SB, Kemnitz JW, Klein S, Schoeller DA, Speakman JR. Energy balance and its components: implications for body weight regulation. *Am J Clin Nutr* 2012; 95: 989–994.

20   Wing RR. Physical activity in the treatment of the adulthood overweight and obesity: current evidence and research issues. *Med Sci Sports Exerc* 1999; 31: S547-552.

21   Schubert MM, Desbrow B, Sabapathy S, Leveritt M. Acute exercise and subsequent energy intake. A meta-analysis. *Appetite* 2013; 63: 92–104.

22   Smith SR. Beyond the Bout - New Perspectives on Exercise and Fat Oxidation. *Exerc Sport Sci Rev* 2009; 37: 58–59.

23   Miller WC, Koceja DM, Hamilton EJ. A meta-analysis of the past 25 years of weight loss research using diet, exercise or diet plus exercise intervention. *Int J Obes Relat Metab Disord J Int Assoc Study Obes* 1997; 21: 941–947.

24   Melby CL, Paris HL, Sayer RD, Bell C, Hill JO. Increasing Energy Flux to Maintain Diet-Induced Weight Loss. *Nutrients* 2019; 11. Available from: doi:10.3390/nu11102533.

25   Varkevisser RDM, Stralen MM van, Kroeze W, Ket JCF, Steenhuis IHM. Determinants of weight loss maintenance: a systematic review. *Obes Rev* 2019; 20: 171–211.

26   Institute of Medicine (US) Subcommittee on Military Weight Management. *Weight-Loss and Maintenance Strategies.* National Academies Press, 2004. Available from: https://www.ncbi.nlm.nih.gov/books/NBK221839/ (accessed 12 Feb 2020).

27   Klem ML, Wing RR, McGuire MT, Seagle HM, Hill JO. A descriptive study of individuals successful at long-term maintenance of substantial weight loss. *Am J Clin Nutr* 1997; 66: 239–246.

28   Church TS, Earnest CP, Skinner JS, Blair SN. Effects of Different Doses of Physical Activity on Cardiorespiratory Fitness Among Sedentary, Overweight or Obese Postmenopausal Women With Elevated Blood Pressure: A Randomized Controlled Trial. *JAMA* 2007; 297: 2081–2091.

29   Skelly LE, Andrews PC, Gillen JB, Martin BJ, Percival ME, Gibala MJ. High-intensity interval exercise induces 24-h energy expenditure similar to traditional endurance exercise despite reduced time commitment. *Appl Physiol Nutr Metab* 2014; 39: 845–848.

30   Alansare A, Alford K, Lee S, Church T, Jung HC. The Effects of High-Intensity Interval Training vs. Moderate-Intensity Continuous Training on Heart Rate Variability in Physically Inactive Adults. *Int J Environ Res Public Health* 2018; 15. Available from: doi:10.3390/ijerph15071508.

31   Blue MNM, Smith-Ryan AE, Trexler ET, Hirsch KR. The effects of high intensity interval training on muscle size and quality in overweight and obese adults. *J Sci Med Sport* 2018; 21: 207–212.

32   Brown EC, Hew-Butler T, Marks CRC, Butcher SJ, Choi MD. The Impact of Different High-Intensity Interval Training Protocols on Body Composition and Physical Fitness in Healthy Young Adult Females. *BioResearch Open Access* 2018; 7: 177–185.

33   Molina-Hidalgo C, De-la-O A, Jurado-Fasoli L, Amaro-Gahete FJ, Castillo MJ. Beer or Ethanol Effects on the Body Composition Response to High-Intensity Interval Training. The BEER-HIIT Study. *Nutrients* 2019; 11. Available from: doi:10.3390/nu11040909.

34   Gillen JB, Percival ME, Ludzki A, Tarnopolsky MA, Gibala MJ. Interval training in the fed or fasted state improves body composition and muscle oxidative capacity in overweight women. *Obesity* 2013; 21: 2249–2255.

35   Børsheim E, Bahr R. Effect of exercise intensity, duration and mode on post-exercise oxygen consumption. *Sports Med Auckl NZ* 2003; 33: 1037–1060.

36   Schuenke MD, Mikat RP, McBride JM. Effect of an acute period of resistance exercise on excess post-exercise oxygen consumption: implications for body mass management. *Eur J Appl Physiol* 2002; 86: 411–417.

37   Laforgia J, Withers RT, Shipp NJ, Gore CJ. Comparison of energy expenditure elevations after submaximal and supramaximal running. *J Appl Physiol Bethesda* 1997; 82: 661–666.

38   Greer BK, Sirithienthad P, Moffatt RJ, Marcello RT, Panton LB. EPOC Comparison Between Isocaloric Bouts of Steady-State Aerobic, Intermittent Aerobic, and Resistance Training. *Res Q Exerc Sport* 2015; 86: 190–195.

39   LaForgia J, Withers RT, Gore CJ. Effects of exercise intensity and duration on the excess post-exercise oxygen consumption. *J Sports Sci* 2006; 24: 1247–1264.

40   Barnes KR, Kilding AE. Running economy: measurement, norms, and determining factors. *Sports Med Open* 2015; 1. Available from: doi:10.1186/s40798-015-0007-y.

41   Böning D, Maassen N, Steinach M. The efficiency of muscular exercise. *Dtsch Z Für Sportmed* 2017; 2017: 203–214.

42   Broskey NT, Boss A, Fares E-J, Greggio C, Gremion G, Schlüter L et al. Exercise efficiency relates with mitochondrial content and function in older adults. *Physiol Rep* 2015; 3. Available from: doi:10.14814/phy2.12418.

43   Whipp BJ, Wasserman K. Efficiency of muscular work. *J Appl Physiol* 1969; 26: 644–648.

44   Falcone PH, Tai C-Y, Carson LR, Joy JM, Mosman MM, McCann TR et al. Caloric Expenditure of Aerobic, Resistance, or Combined High-Intensity Interval Training Using a Hydraulic Resistance System in Healthy Men. *J Strength Cond Res* 2015; 29: 779–785.

45   Tiggemann CL, Pinto RS, Noll M, Schoenell MCW, Kruel LFM. Energy expenditure in strength training: a critical approach. Available from: https://www.researchgate.net/publication/318239530_ENERGY_EXPENDIT URE_IN_STRENGTH_TRAINING_A_CRITICAL_APPROACH (accessed 4 Mar 2020).

46   Kravitz L, Robergs RA, Heyward VH, Wagner DR, Powers K. Exercise mode and gender comparisons of energy expenditure at self-selected intensities. *Med Sci Sports Exerc* 1997; 29: 1028–1035.

47   Zeni AI, Hoffman MD, Clifford PS. Energy expenditure with indoor exercise machines. *JAMA* 1996; 275: 1424–1427.

48   Thomas TR, Feiock CW, Araujo J. Metabolic responses associated with four modes of prolonged exercise. *J Sports Med Phys Fitness* 1989; 29: 77–82.

49   Moyna NM, Robertson RJ, Meckes CL, Peoples JA, Millich NB, Thompson PD. Intermodal comparison of energy expenditure at exercise intensities corresponding to the perceptual preference range. *Med Sci Sports Exerc* 2001; 33: 1404–1410.

50   Brown GA, Cook CM, Krueger RD, Heelan KA. Comparison of Energy Expenditure on a Treadmill vs. an Elliptical Device at a Self-Selected Exercise Intensity. *J Strength Cond Res* 2010; 24: 1643–1649.

51   Stiegler P, Cunliffe A. The Role of Diet and Exercise for the Maintenance of Fat-Free Mass and Resting Metabolic Rate During Weight Loss. *Sports Med* 2006. Available from: doi:10.2165/00007256-200636030-00005.

52   Schoenfeld B. Does Cardio After an Overnight Fast Maximize Fat Loss? *Strength Cond J* 2011; 33: 23–25.

53   Schoenfeld BJ, Aragon AA, Wilborn CD, Krieger JW, Sonmez GT. Body composition changes associated with fasted versus non-fasted aerobic exercise. *J Int Soc Sports Nutr* 2014; 11: 54.

54   Van Proeyen K, Szlufcik K, Nielens H, Pelgrim K, Deldicque L, Hesselink M et al. Training in the fasted state improves glucose tolerance during fat-rich diet. *J Physiol* 2010; 588: 4289–4302.

55   Van Proeyen K, Szlufcik K, Nielens H, Ramaekers M, Hespel P. Beneficial metabolic adaptations due to endurance exercise training in the fasted state. *J Appl Physiol* 2011; 110: 236–245.

56   Gieske B, Stecker R, Smith C, Witherbee K, Harty P, Wildman R et al. Metabolic impact of protein feeding prior to moderate-intensity treadmill exercise in a fasted state: A pilot study. *J Int Soc Sports Nutr* 2018; 15. Available from: doi:10.1186/s12970-018-0263-6.

57   Melanson EL, MacLean PS, Hill JO. Exercise improves fat metabolism in muscle but does not increase 24-h fat oxidation. *Exerc Sport Sci Rev* 2009; 37: 93–101.

58   Febbraio MA, Chiu A, Angus DJ, Arkinstall MJ, Hawley JA. Effects of carbohydrate ingestion before and during exercise on glucose kinetics and performance. *J Appl Physiol Bethesda* 2000; 89: 2220–2226.

59   Horowitz JF, Mora-Rodriguez R, Byerley LO, Coyle EF. Lipolytic suppression following carbohydrate ingestion limits fat oxidation during exercise. *Am J Physiol* 1997; 273: E768-775.

60   Ogata H, Kayaba M, Tanaka Y, Yajima K, Iwayama K, Ando A et al. Effect of skipping breakfast for 6 days on energy metabolism and diurnal rhythm of blood glucose in young healthy Japanese males. *Am J Clin Nutr* 2019; 110: 41–52.

61   Lee YS, Ha MS, Lee YJ. The effects of various intensities and durations of exercise with and without glucose in milk ingestion on postexercise oxygen consumption. *J Sports Med Phys Fitness* 1999; 39: 341–347.

62   Paoli A, Marcolin G, Zonin F, Neri M, Sivieri A, Pacelli QF. Exercising fasting or fed to enhance fat loss? Influence of food intake on respiratory ratio and excess postexercise oxygen consumption after a bout of endurance training. *Int J Sport Nutr Exerc Metab* 2011. Available from: doi:10.1123/ijsnem.21.1.48.

63   Patterson R, Potteiger JA. A comparison of normal versus low dietary carbohydrate intake on substrate oxidation during and after moderate intensity exercise in women. *Eur J Appl Physiol* 2011; 111: 3143–3150.

64   Rosenbloom C. Food and Fluid Guidelines Before, During, and After Exercise. *Nutr Today* 2012; 47: 63–69.

65   Ahlborg G, Felig P. Influence of glucose ingestion on fuel-hormone response during prolonged exercise. *J Appl Physiol* 1976; 41: 683–688.

66   Perez WJ. The Effect of Fasted vs Fed High-Intensity Interval Exercise on Metabolism and Diet. *Old Dominion University* 2016. Available from: https://digitalcommons.odu.edu/cgi/viewcontent.cgi?article=1007&context=h ms_etds (accessed 5 Feb 2020).

67   Bennard P, Doucet E. Acute effects of exercise timing and breakfast meal glycemic index on exercise-induced fat oxidation. *Appl Physiol Nutr Metab Physiol Appl Nutr Metab* 2006; 31: 502–511.

68   Goben KW, Sforzo GA, Frye PA. Exercise intensity and the thermic effect of food. *Int J Sport Nutr* 1992; 2: 87–95.

69   Impey SG, Hammond KM, Shepherd SO, Sharples AP, Stewart C, Limb M et al. Fuel for the work required: a practical approach to amalgamating train-low paradigms for endurance athletes. *Physiol Rep* 2016; 4. Available from: doi:10.14814/phy2.12803.

70   Bin Naharudin MN, Yusof A, Shaw H, Stockton M, Clayton DJ, James LJ. Breakfast Omission Reduces Subsequent Resistance Exercise Performance. *J Strength Cond Res* 2019; 33: 1766–1772.

71   Wright DA, Sherman WM, Dernbach AR. Carbohydrate feedings before, during, or in combination improve cycling endurance performance. *J Appl Physiol Bethesda* 1991; 71: 1082–1088.

72   Schabort EJ, Bosch AN, Weltan SM, Noakes TD. The effect of a preexercise meal on time to fatigue during prolonged cycling exercise. *Med Sci Sports Exerc* 1999; 31: 464–471.

73   Abaïdia A-E, Daab W, Bouzid MA. Effects of Ramadan Fasting on Physical Performance: A Systematic Review with Meta-analysis. *Sports Med Auckl NZ* 2020. Available from: doi:10.1007/s40279-020-01257-0.

74   Howarth KR, Phillips SM, MacDonald MJ, Richards D, Moreau NA, Gibala MJ. Effect of glycogen availability on human skeletal muscle protein turnover during exercise and recovery. *J Appl Physiol Bethesda* 2010; 109: 431–438.

75   Lemon PW, Mullin JP. Effect of initial muscle glycogen levels on protein catabolism during exercise. *J Appl Physiol* 1980; 48: 624–629.

76   Romijn JA, Coyle EF, Sidossis LS, Gastaldelli A, Horowitz JF, Endert E et al. Regulation of endogenous fat and carbohydrate metabolism in relation to exercise intensity and duration. *Am J Physiol* 1993; 265: E380-391.

77   Essén-Gustavsson B, Tesch PA. Glycogen and triglyceride utilization in relation to muscle metabolic characteristics in men performing heavy-resistance exercise. *Eur J Appl Physiol* 1990; 61: 5–10.

78   Contreras B. *Individual Differences: The Most Important Consideration for Your Fitness Results that Science Doesn't Tell You.* 2017. Available from: https://bretcontreras.com/individual-differences-important-consideration-fitness-results-science-doesnt-tell/ (accessed 13 Feb 2020).

79   Finlayson G, Bryant E, Blundell JE, King NA. Acute compensatory eating following exercise is associated with implicit hedonic wanting for food. *Physiol Behav* 2009; 97: 62–67.

80   Di Blasio A, Ripari P, Bucci I, Di Donato F, Izzicupo P, D'Angelo E et al. Walking training in postmenopause: effects on both spontaneous physical activity and training-induced body adaptations. *Menopause N Y N* 2012; 19: 23–32.

81   Methenitis S. A Brief Review on Concurrent Training: From Laboratory to the Field. *Sports Basel Switz* 2018; 6. Available from: doi:10.3390/sports6040127.

82   Berryman N, Mujika I, Bosquet L. Concurrent Training for Sports Performance: The Two Sides of the Medal. *Int J Sports Physiol Perform* 2018; 14: 1–22.

83   Fyfe JJ, Loenneke JP. Interpreting Adaptation to Concurrent Compared with Single-Mode Exercise Training: Some Methodological Considerations. *Sports Med Auckl NZ* 2018; 48: 289–297.

84   Garber CE, Blissmer B, Deschenes MR, Franklin BA, Lamonte MJ, Lee I-M et al. American College of Sports Medicine position stand. Quantity and quality of exercise for developing and maintaining cardiorespiratory, musculoskeletal, and neuromotor fitness in apparently healthy adults: guidance for prescribing exercise. *Med Sci Sports Exerc* 2011; 43: 1334–1359.

85   Hickson RC. Interference of strength development by simultaneously training for strength and endurance. *Eur J Appl Physiol* 1980; 45: 255–263.

86   Murach KA, Bagley JR. Skeletal Muscle Hypertrophy with Concurrent Exercise Training: Contrary Evidence for an Interference Effect. *Sports Med Auckl NZ* 2016; 46: 1029–1039.

87   Wilson JM, Marin PJ, Rhea MR, Wilson SMC, Loenneke JP, Anderson JC. Concurrent training: a meta-analysis examining interference of aerobic and resistance exercises. *J Strength Cond Res* 2012; 26: 2293–2307.

88   Sabag A, Najafi A, Michael S, Esgin T, Halaki M, Hackett D. The compatibility of concurrent high intensity interval training and resistance training for muscular strength and hypertrophy: a systematic review and meta-analysis. *J Sports Sci* 2018; 36: 2472–2483.

89   Eddens L, van Someren K, Howatson G. The Role of Intra-Session Exercise Sequence in the Interference Effect: A Systematic Review with Meta-Analysis. *Sports Med Auckl NZ* 2018; 48: 177–188.

90   Murlasits Z, Kneffel Z, Thalib L. The physiological effects of concurrent strength and endurance training sequence: A systematic review and meta-analysis. *J Sports Sci* 2018; 36: 1212–1219.

91   Schumann M, Yli-Peltola K, Abbiss CR, Häkkinen K. Cardiorespiratory Adaptations during Concurrent Aerobic and Strength Training in Men and Women. *PloS One* 2015; 10: e0139279.

92   Sale DG, Jacobs I, MacDougall JD, Garner S. Comparison of two regimens of concurrent strength and endurance training. *Med Sci Sports Exerc* 1990; 22: 348–356.

93   Sporer BC, Wenger HA. Effects of aerobic exercise on strength performance following various periods of recovery. *J Strength Cond Res* 2003; 17: 638–644.

94   Fyfe JJ, Bartlett JD, Hanson ED, Stepto NK, Bishop DJ. Endurance Training Intensity Does Not Mediate Interference to Maximal Lower-Body Strength Gain during Short-Term Concurrent Training. *Front Physiol* 2016; 7. Available from: doi:10.3389/fphys.2016.00487.

95   Petré H, Löfving P, Psilander N. The Effect of Two Different Concurrent Training Programs on Strength and Power Gains in Highly-Trained Individuals. *J Sports Sci Med* 2018; 17: 167–173.

96   Shamim B, Devlin BL, Timmins RG, Tofari P, Lee Dow C, Coffey VG et al. Adaptations to Concurrent Training in Combination with High Protein Availability: A Comparative Trial in Healthy, Recreationally Active Men. *Sports Med Auckl NZ* 2018; 48: 2869–2883.

97   Kerksick CM, Wilborn CD, Roberts MD, Smith-Ryan A, Kleiner SM, Jäger R et al. ISSN exercise & sports nutrition review update: research & recommendations. *J Int Soc Sports Nutr* 2018; 15. Available from: doi:10.1186/s12970-018-0242-y.

98   Perez-Schindler J, Hamilton DL, Moore DR, Baar K, Philp A. Nutritional strategies to support concurrent training. *Eur J Sport Sci* 2015; 15: 41–52.

99   Mata F, Valenzuela PL, Gimenez J, Tur C, Ferreria D, Domínguez R et al. Carbohydrate Availability and Physical Performance: Physiological Overview and Practical Recommendations. *Nutrients* 2019; 11. Available from: doi:10.3390/nu11051084.

25. Supplements

Supplements are largely unnecessary and should only be considered once your diet and training plan are in place. Few supplements have any high quality evidence that they are of a benefit to muscle growth. No supplements have conclusive evidence that they can promote greater fat loss for a given calorie deficit.

The discussion on supplements has been left to the end of the book for good reason. They are arguably the *least* important factor for muscle gain or fat loss. The role of supplements has been overinflated by the media, giving the impression that many body composition transformations are the result of simply using supplements, when in actual fact it is the hard work and adherence of individuals to a given plan. Despite this, the sports nutrition industry is worth over €3 billion in the European Union alone[1].

The aim of a supplement is to increase performance (e.g. muscle strength, size, endurance or power), aid recovery, or prevent injury[2]. From the perspective of body composition, all three will have utility for long-term success. A supplement can be *acutely ergogenic* (provide benefit for a specific session) or *chronically ergogenic* (providing benefit from multiple sessions).

Several supplements have been extensively studied. Many others have very little science behind them. Up to date reviews on the effectiveness and safety of the most commonly used supplements are included in this chapter.

What is defined as a *'supplement'* is highly variable. Some suggest the term supplement can only be given to those products that have been *proven* to have ergogenic benefit[2]. Supplements can take many forms, including carbohydrate, fat, protein, vitamins, minerals, plant extracts, metabolic intermediates, and others[2]. Supplements can often just be convenient forms of food. Unfortunately for supplement companies, only a small minority of *'supplements'* have been shown to have any benefit in improving body composition. As with diet and exercise, whether a supplement works or not should be proven through rigorous randomised controlled trials, not because a high-profile individual promotes it.

When choosing to use a supplement, the main initial concerns should be whether it is *safe, legal* and *ergogenic*[2].

- Is there a sound mechanistic or theoretical pathway for the supplement to have an effect? As we have seen from a range of examples (e.g. low carbohydrate versus low fat diets for weight loss, or fasted low intensity exercise for fat loss), a theoretical or mechanistic rationale for a supplement based on lab data does not mean it actually has benefit in humans. But, a complete lack of any theoretical reasoning puts into question whether the supplement has any effect at all.
- Are there any randomised controlled trials demonstrating the efficacy of the supplement? (see chapter 4 regarding research quality). Are the studies in sedentary people, obese people, athletes or healthy active individuals? The more similar the individuals being studied are to the population we want to give the supplement to, the more relevant the findings. If you are a trained young healthy female and a study shows greater muscle growth with a supplement in trained young healthy females, then that would be a useful study. If you are a trained young healthy female and a study shows greater muscle growth with a supplement in elderly males with heart disease, then that would be a less useful study.
- Strong evidence would include randomised controlled trials and human studies showing its efficacy, backed up by theoretical evidence and lab studies. This would be considered good evidence for the use of a supplement. *Very few* supplements have this high level of evidence. A proposed theoretical mechanism with limited evidence from lab, cell or animal studies and no human studies, or human studies showing no benefit is poor quality evidence. *Most* supplements have this low level of evidence, backed up with anecdotal claims[3].

Whether you consider taking a new supplement or not should be a *cost-benefit* analysis. Ask yourself some questions:

- Has this supplement been proven to be safe for consumption in healthy individuals?
- What are the benefits of this supplement?
- Have these benefits been proven in high quality studies (as opposed to reported benefits from unreliable media sources)?
- Do these benefits align with my goals?
- Are there any potential negative effects from taking the supplement and do they apply to me?
- Is the supplement expensive?
- Am I purchasing a high quality grade of this supplement? Does the ingredient list state many other products, or just the supplement of

interest and possibly an artificial sweetener (e.g. sucralose or aspartame)?

It is worth taking the time to research, or at least read about a supplement before purchasing and using it, considering the financial cost that many supplements involve.

Whilst most supplements commonly found in health and fitness shops are safe for consumption, very few actually have any concrete evidence that they provide a benefit. Therefore, knowing which supplements will benefit you and knowing which supplements provide no benefit and are burning a hole in your pocket will save you time, effort and money.

This chapter will discuss the most extensively researched supplements available that are considered beneficial for improvements in body composition: supplements that will aid muscle gain and/or fat loss. Supplements that can improve performance will also be covered as they may facilitate greater training adaptations. Supplements where the current evidence base suggests it is of no benefit will also be covered.

Supplements with strong evidence that they can promote muscle growth:

- Protein.
- Creatine monohydrate.
- Beta-hydroxy-beta-methylbutyrate (HMB) (in beginners).

Supplements that have not been shown to promote muscle growth, but have strong evidence that they can improve performance relevant to a muscle building plan:

- Caffeine.
- Beta-alanine.

There are currently no supplements that are safe and promote greater weight loss at a given calorie deficit. Weight loss supplements (i.e. fat burners) do not work.

Despite the fact that many supplements are marketed with the aim of increasing fat burning and supporting weight loss, currently, *no* supplements have strong evidence that they can promote fat loss[4,5]. A systematic review of systematic reviews demonstrated that there is no benefit to using supplements for weight loss, including green tea, calcium, conjugated linoleic acid and glucomannan[6]. 5 systematic reviews and meta-analyses show *no* convincing evidence of a benefit of a range of commonly marketed *'fat loss'* supplements for weight loss[4,7].

If the aim is weight loss, focus on generating a caloric deficit.

Multi-ingredient supplements

Multi-ingredient supplements promote muscle growth, but no more so than just a protein supplement alone. Usually this is because the additional ingredients are not proven to have any benefit, or any additional ingredients that are proven to have a benefit are added at sub-optimal doses.

As the name suggests, multi-ingredient supplements contain several ingredients. Some of the ingredients are well established with ergogenic benefit, and some less so. The *quantity* and *composition* of the ingredients in such supplements varies wildly. All contain some form of protein, and most also contain some form of creatine. A meta-analysis of 35 randomised controlled trials comparing multi-ingredient supplements to a control alongside a resistance training plan found greater muscle growth when compared to placebo, but no benefit when compared to a protein supplement[8]. All of the multi-ingredient supplements studied contained protein. Unsurprisingly compared to a placebo control, multi-ingredient supplements improved body composition because most individuals consumed a sub-optimal amount of protein. Other ingredient content varied based on the supplement studied, ranging from creatine (page 508), carbohydrate, vitamin D, different amino acids (the building blocks of protein), HMB (page 510), polyunsaturated fatty acids, beta-alanine and caffeine. Again, it is important to remember whether the doses used were at efficacious levels or not. The variations in doses used may have limited the ability to determine significant effects from these additional supplements. As the authors noted, there was a general trend for greater muscle growth with the multi-ingredient supplement over protein only. However, this was not significant, again highlighting the minor consideration of supplements in relation to sufficient protein intake and a resistance training programme. Multi-ingredient supplements are often much more expensive than individual supplements. Protein supplementation may be of use, but whether the additional ingredients are beneficial needs to be determined by assessing the efficacy of each of the other ingredients in isolation. Even so, it is probably more cost effective to purchase the individual supplements separately and use them at the doses proven to be efficacious.

Protein

Protein supplements are beneficial when consuming less than 1.6g of protein per kg of body weight per day. They are no more effective than using any other protein source to meet daily protein needs. But, they can be more convenient and cost effective[3,9].

The protein supplement industry is big business. People drink protein shakes everywhere. Supplementing with protein makes theoretical sense; it is well established that higher protein intakes can result in favourable changes in body composition (as discussed in chapter 8 and 9). As such, it has been proposed that supplementing with protein can lead to further improvements in body composition.

Protein supplementation can aid both muscle gain (with progressive resistance training) and fat loss[2,3]. But, whether supplementation is beneficial *depends* on your current total daily protein intake.

The most recent and largest systematic review and meta-analysis on protein supplementation for muscle growth to date was of 49 randomised controlled trials in 2018[10]. Previous studies and analyses have shown conflicting findings. However, previous studies often did not control for potentially influential variables, such as training experience, daily protein intake and participant age. By considering these factors and conducting more detailed analyses, the 2018 meta-analysis found protein supplementation does indeed result in greater increases in fat-free mass when daily protein intakes are low. The benefit to fat-free mass only occurs until daily protein consumption reaches 1.62g/kg of body weight per day (g/kg/day), the recommended daily intake for muscle growth (as previously discussed in chapter 9). Of note, the average pre-supplementation protein intake of participants was 1.4g/kg/day. Therefore, even a small addition of around 35g of protein per day, or 0.2g/kg/day still had significant effects on strength and fat free mass[10]. The last meta-analysis assessing protein supplementation from 2012 demonstrated similar findings[11]. This meta-analysis assessed the effect of protein supplementation compared to placebo on fat mass, lean muscle mass, 1 repetition maximum (absolute) strength and muscle fibre type during a resistance training programme (over 6-24 weeks depending on the specific study). The analysis found that protein supplementation led to greater increases in fat-free mass regardless of age, or whether the individual was trained or untrained. However, the analysis did not find an effect on fat mass. Both type I and type II muscle fibres significantly increased in size with protein supplementation compared to placebo for younger individuals, but not older individuals. Protein supplementation also led to greater increases in 1 rep maximum (RM) than placebo, regardless of age. These effects were the same, irrespective of the type of protein supplement used. The majority of studies compared whey and casein protein to a carbohydrate placebo. Some studies assessed consumption of essential amino acids (EAA), egg protein and milk protein, and one study looked at dietary increases in protein. Other placebos and comparators used were water, low protein diets or exercise only. The individuals in the studies were all consuming over 1.2g/kg/day of protein, which would already be considered a relatively adequate amount. Considering there was no difference between using different protein supplements and given what we already know about higher protein diets for body composition, it is most likely that the benefits seen in these studies were simply due to a higher total daily protein intake, rather than the effect of a specific protein supplement.

In other words, protein supplements are essentially just convenient forms of protein, providing no superior benefit once total daily protein intake has been optimised[12]. The study also further highlights how the role of protein timing, source, dose or post-exercise protein timing all have minimal effects on body composition once total protein intake has been optimised[10].

Over the course of 12 weeks, healthy males can add on average, 1.5kg of lean mass whilst participating in a resistance training programme and supplementing with protein[10,13]. To put supplementation into context, consuming an additional 50g of protein per day via supplements in healthy people already consuming 1.2g/kg/day contributed 300-800g to total gains in lean mass over a period of 12 weeks, compared to not supplementing with protein[10,11]. Individuals trained on average, 3 times per week. Such an effect could also be achieved by simply consuming more protein from whole food sources.

Should you use a protein supplement?

Ask yourself these questions:

- Do you need to increase your protein intake? Do you currently consume the minimum recommended protein intake for muscle growth or fat loss (1.6g/kg/day), or for fat loss as a trained individual (1.8g/kg/day or 2.2g/kg of lean body mass per day)?
- Do you struggle to consume sufficient protein through whole food-based protein sources alone (e.g. meat, fish, dairy, leguminous vegetables)?
- Is your lifestyle too busy to prepare meals, and a quick protein source would be more convenient?
- Is there a long duration around your workout (several hours before and after) where you do not consume any protein?

If you answer yes to any of the above questions (especially regarding daily protein intake), you might want to consider using a protein supplement, or consider increasing protein intake through whole food sources. The more questions that you answered yes, the more likely that supplementation will be of benefit.

Vitamin and mineral supplementation

There is no benefit to consuming above the daily recommended intakes of vitamins or minerals. A varied, balanced diet including for example, grains, nuts, fruit and vegetables provides all the vitamins and minerals needed. Further supplementation does not provide an additional benefit. Additional supplementation can in fact be counter-productive and detrimental to body composition goals. Supplementation is not needed when at caloric maintenance or in a surplus with a varied, balanced diet. Supplementation may become useful when in a caloric deficit due to reduced food consumption or when food groups are excluded (e.g. vegan or vegetarian diets). Where there is potentially a vitamin or mineral deficiency, contacting a medical professional (GP) should be the priority to address the dietary insufficiency.

Consuming vitamins over and above the recommended daily allowance does *not* result in any performance benefits[2]. However, if there is a deficiency in a particular vitamin, then supplementation or dietary changes may improve performance[2,9]. In other words, if you eat a healthy balanced diet, there is *no* need to supplement micronutrients. However, excluding food groups can lead to deficiencies, such as in a vegan diet (discussed in chapter 8). In this scenario there may be a case to supplement or change dietary choices. This is a health-related concern, and therefore contacting a medical professional such as your GP is recommended in the first instance to identify if this is the case, to rectify any deficiency.

Several vitamins have *antioxidant* properties including vitamin C and E, which have received the most attention regarding resistance training. Antioxidant vitamin supplementation is *not* beneficial for muscle growth. Resistance training induces an adaptive response, resulting in some inflammation. This inflammation is a response to exercise and is needed as part of the adaptive response to recover. Consuming high levels of antioxidants reduces inflammation, blunting the repair response. Vitamin E or C supplementation does not mitigate the performance decrements or muscle damage that occur after resistance training[2,14-16].

Studies find either no benefit or impaired muscle growth with vitamin supplementation. A randomised controlled trial in trained men and women found no benefit of vitamin C and E supplementation on muscle growth[14]. One study in young females found that long-term supplementation with vitamin C and E impaired the ability to grow muscle and lose fat, compared to a placebo[17]. Another randomised controlled trial in young females found no difference in muscle growth with a resistance training programme between participants either consuming a vitamin C and E supplement or a group consuming a placebo[18].

There is also no evidence to suggest mineral supplementation improves performance or body composition[2,19-22].

A multivitamin supplement may be considered when in a calorie deficit for an extended period of time, however. When calorie intake is restricted, this may limit the ability to consume sufficient food sources containing vitamins and minerals. A supplement may help to prevent inadvertently becoming deficient[12].

Regardless, if you do believe that you have a deficiency for any reason, then consult your GP in the first instance.

Caffeine

Strong evidence shows that caffeine can enhance performance. It may aid the ability to train with a high intensity of effort. There is no direct evidence for a benefit on muscle growth.

Caffeine is the most commonly consumed stimulant worldwide, found in coffee, tea, soft drinks and chocolate[2,23]. Caffeine actually has no essential function in the body and provides no nutritional value[23]. As a stimulant, caffeine consumption is often used in a wide range of scenarios, including sports and training. Caffeine exerts its effect by acting as an antagonist of *adenosine receptors*. Caffeine increases mental awareness and increases the release of *endorphins*, which may reduce perceptions of pain[3,24]. The International Society of Sports Nutrition (ISSN) have conducted a review on caffeine consumption and exercise, which has been incorporated into this discussion[24].

A 2019 *umbrella review* (a very high quality form of evidence, analysing systematic reviews and meta-analyses[25]) of 21 meta-analyses shows that caffeine consumption is beneficial for a broad range of exercise types including[26]:

- Muscular strength[3,27,28].
- Anaerobic power[27].
- Muscular endurance[3].
- Aerobic exercise.

However, *no* studies to date have assessed whether caffeine consumption can promote muscle protein synthesis or increase muscle mass[29].

Current evidence shows that:

- Caffeine is safe[30]. Caffeine may also reduce the rating of perceived exertion (RPE) (the effort experienced to complete a physical task), which may lead to some of the performance enhancing effects[3,29].
- Caffeine can also lead to acute elevations in blood pressure. Therefore, caution should be taken of excessive caffeine intake in individuals with high blood pressure.
- The majority of ingested caffeine is absorbed and enters the bloodstream within one hour[23]. Peak caffeine levels in the blood are usually around 60 minutes after ingestion[31]. 3-9mg/kg of body weight 60 minutes before exercise provides sufficient ergogenic benefits without leading to excessive side effects such as insomnia, anxiety and irritation[2,3,24]. Caffeine consumption anywhere from immediately before exercise, to 2 hours before exercise appears to provide an ergogenic benefit[32].
- 6mg/kg of body weight is commonly used for ergogenic effects in research studies (equivalent to 4 or 5 cups of coffee)[26].
- Whether becoming habituated (needing more caffeine for the same desired effect) negatively affects the ergogenic benefits of caffeine is unclear, especially with resistance training[26,29].
- Most studies so far have been conducted in young males, so whether similar benefits are found in females is not clear[26].
- Most caffeine research assesses its acute effects on a single training session. The long-term benefit of caffeine intake on performance and body composition is understudied[26].
- Most research studies assess the ergogenic effect of caffeine in the form of caffeine powder, rather than in liquid forms (such as caffeine in coffee or energy drinks)[26].
- The evidence suggests that the consumption of caffeine via coffee is equally as ergogenic (improving physical performance) as caffeine via capsules or powders. Limited studies show a similar ergogenic benefit from coffee consumption compared to caffeine powder, when caffeine content is equated. The biggest limitation with coffee for caffeine consumption is the high variability in caffeine content with different forms of coffee[26]. However, on average it is expected that two cups of coffee would provide around 200mg (0.2g) of caffeine.
- Other forms of caffeine such as gum or energy drinks are understudied.

The effect of caffeine is highly variable between people. This is largely down to differences in the ability to metabolise caffeine. This is influenced by genetic, environmental and lifestyle factors[23].

Like many other outcomes discussed (such as muscle growth or concurrent training effects), the influence of caffeine varies greatly between people. Some people experience little performance benefit, whereas others experience large improvements. But on average, caffeine consumption improves performance over placebo. Caffeine is ergogenic regardless of whether people are *high* or *low responders*[33].

The effect of caffeine is dependent on its concentration in the blood. After ingestion, concentrations peak around 60 minutes later, and then slowly decline as caffeine is broken down by the liver. In humans, caffeine has an average *half-life* of 4 hours[30]. The half-life time is a measure of how fast the body can clear a substance from the blood, such as caffeine. This means that every 4 hours, the concentration of caffeine in your blood halves. So that on average, after 8 hours, the concentration of caffeine in your blood is a quarter (½ at 4 hours, ½ of ½ after 8 hours) of the original level. However, there is considerable variation around this average. Some people have a caffeine half-life as fast as 2 hours and some as slow as 10 hours[23,34,35]. Saying the average half-life of caffeine is 4 hours is a bit like saying the average height of a man and woman is 171cm and 159cm, respectively[36]. This is true, but the variability around this average height is enormous, and even more so with caffeine metabolism. There can be 5 to 11-fold differences in caffeine concentrations in the blood of different people in the hours after consuming the same amount of caffeine[23]. Indeed, it appears there are *'fast'* and *'slow'* caffeine metabolisers, due to variability in the gene (CYP1A2) coding for the enzyme (cytochrome P450) that is primarily responsible for breaking down caffeine (i.e. genetics affect how long caffeine remains in your blood)[23,30,37]. The ability of this enzyme to metabolise caffeine can also be influenced by alcohol, vegetable consumption, coffee intake, gender, body mass index and smoking[23,37]. The majority of the variation in caffeine metabolism (>70%) appears to be down to genetics, with environmental and lifestyle factors accounting for the smaller remaining variation[23]. There is also evidence to suggest that variation in this gene can influence the ergogenic effect of caffeine use on performance[29].

Caffeine and sleep

Consuming caffeine before bed can delay *sleep onset* and impair *sleep quality*[37]. How late you can consume caffeine and how much you can consume *without* impacting on your sleep quality varies wildly between individuals. This is due to the high variability between people in the ability to break down and remove caffeine from the body[23,37]. Self-reported caffeine *"sensitive"* individuals display greater symptoms of poor sleep[37]. One person may be able to have several cups of coffee in the late afternoon and sleep well. Another person may only have one small coffee in the morning that keeps them awake at night. Your own sensitivity can be gauged by determining at what time of day you find that any caffeine consumption impairs your sleep.

Caffeine can improve focus, reduce perceptions of effort and improve performance across a range of anaerobic performance markers[29]. Such benefits may make resistance training sessions more productive, possibly facilitating greater adaptations[12]. However, *no* studies have formally assessed caffeine intake on muscle growth.

Whether you use caffeine prior to a workout is up to you. How much you consume and how late you can consume caffeine to benefit a workout later in the day, without any detrimental effect on your sleep is highly individual and requires personal experimentation.

Creatine monohydrate

Strong evidence shows creatine monohydrate can promote increased muscle mass.

Creatine monohydrate is the most researched nutritional supplement to date. It is completely safe with no side-effects, and with significant benefit to performance and body composition.

If you want a *magic pill* for muscle growth, creatine monohydrate is about as close as it gets. Few supplements have received as much attention as creatine monohydrate. A wide range of research bodies support the use of creatine monohydrate supplementation to increase muscle mass alongside progressive resistance training[2,38–40]. The International Society of Sports Nutrition (ISSN) have conducted a review on creatine monohydrate consumption and exercise[38].

Creatine is naturally found in meat and fish. It forms part of the energy pathway found in the cells of the body, including muscle cells. During intense physical activity, *adenosine triphosphate* (ATP) becomes depleted (see chapter 16 regarding energy pathways). If supplies are not quickly restored, fatigue sets in and there is a failure to continue the exercise and perform at maximum intensity. Creatine provides an emergency source of energy by donating the *phosphate* from *phosphocreatine* (PCr) to *adenosine diphosphate* (ADP) to regenerate adenosine triphosphate (ATP), which can be used to maintain high intensity anaerobic exercise for a fraction longer[38]. Creatine also has other important roles in the muscle cell relating to metabolism[38]. Normal creatine stores without supplementation are maintained through diet (red meat and fish are rich sources), which can provide half of the daily requirement for creatine. The other half is generated from the liver and kidneys[38]. Creatine monohydrate supplementation further increases intramuscular creatine stores by 20-40%[38,41]. Increasing the amount of phosphocreatine and creatine within the muscle increases the amount of ATP that can be resynthesized at a given instant. As such, creatine monohydrate supplementation increases the amount of available

ATP for the muscle to use, which benefits high intensity performance. This facilitates increased adaptions from training, such as muscle growth[38].

Current evidence shows that:

- A very large body of scientific evidence (>1000 studies) shows that creatine monohydrate supplementation is safe and has no short-term or long-term adverse effects in healthy individuals[42].
- Creatine monohydrate can improve physical performance by increasing high intensity exercise capacity[2].
- Creatine monohydrate can increase muscle size, strength and endurance alongside a resistance training programme[41,42].
- Creatine monohydrate may also help with recovery and reducing muscle damage from exercise[38].
- To increase muscle creatine stores rapidly to maximum levels, recommendations are to 'load' by consuming 5g, four times per day for 5-7 days, and then to consume 3-5g/day to maintain the elevated creatine stores. However, creatine 'loading' is not necessary. Consuming 3-5g/day will saturate creatine stores in around 4 weeks[41].
- Supplemented creatine stores can be maintained with 3-5g/day of creatine monohydrate[38].
- There may be a slight benefit to consuming creatine monohydrate after a workout, rather than before a workout[43]. However, pre-workout consumption is still effective[32].
- Of the different forms of creatine, creatine monohydrate is the most effective. Other forms of creatine are more expensive and/or less effective.
- Supplementation will be particularly beneficial to individuals who do not eat red meat or fish. Vegetarians and vegans have lower creatine levels than meat eaters[38].

Creatine monohydrate is the most studied supplement available and is the most effective form of creatine available. Other forms of creatine exist, such as creatine phosphate or creatine ethyl ester. These forms of creatine have been studied less extensively. It is inconclusive as to whether they are more or less effective than creatine monohydrate. However, there is no evidence that they may increase creatine retention in muscles compared to creatine monohydrate, which is a main feature used to market them[38].

Many of the anecdotally reported side effects of creatine monohydrate supplementation have also been refuted in controlled scientific studies:

- Weight gain during creatine monohydrate supplementation is not all from water retention.

- Creatine monohydrate supplementation does not lead to kidney problems in healthy individuals[38].
- Creatine monohydrate supplementation does not cause cramping, electrolyte imbalance, gastrointestinal distress nor dehydration[38].

In fact, due to the wide range of benefits from creatine monohydrate supplementation, its use can benefit a wide range of sports including football, tennis, basketball, rugby and tennis to name a few (essentially, any sport that involves high intensity intervals would benefit)[2]. Research is also underway assessing the potential benefit of creatine monohydrate in certain health conditions.

Creatine monohydrate has extensively been shown to be safe and effective across a wide range of sports and exercise disciplines, and effective across a wide range of ages. Creatine monohydrate is also a relatively cheap supplement. There are very few contraindications or reasons why it may not be worthwhile to supplement with creatine. Any minor benefit outweighs any theoretical detrimental effect, which studies have currently demonstrated to be non-existent.

Greg Nuckols has written a publicly available article about creatine, which covers the supplement in more depth[44].

Beta-hydroxy-beta-methylbutyrate (HMB)

Strong evidence shows HMB can promote increased muscle mass in untrained people.

The main benefit is in untrained beginners, in a caloric deficit or when there is greater muscle damage. There is limited benefit in trained individuals.

Beta-hydroxy-beta-methylbutyrate (HMB) is a product of leucine metabolism (leucine is one of the three branched-chain amino acids). It is naturally found in both humans and animals[45]. Typically, only 5% of consumed leucine is metabolised into HMB. Therefore, a very high amount of protein would need to be consumed to obtain enough leucine to produce the amounts of HMB shown to be beneficial in human studies. Therefore, supplementation with HMB is preferential. There are two forms of HMB, calcium-HMB and HMB-free acid. HMB-free acid has been studied most recently, with initial research focussing on calcium-HMB[2]. It is inconclusive as to whether one form is better than the other[46,47].

The International Society of Sports Nutrition (ISSN) conducted a review on HMB consumption and exercise in 2013[47].

Current evidence shows that:

- Long term consumption of HMB is safe in both young and old individuals[42,45–47].
- A systematic review from 2017 has shown that HMB supplementation may benefit muscle growth[46]. HMB supplementation is mainly beneficial to increase muscle mass in untrained individuals[2,48].
- HMB supplementation may be beneficial to increase muscle mass in trained individuals, but over a longer duration. This will be of greater benefit when training is high volume and induces greater muscle damage. This may be useful when implementing advanced training techniques (chapter 23) or high volume training phases (chapter 19), which can increase muscle damage[45].
- HMB can improve recovery by reducing exercise-induced muscle damage in mainly untrained, but also resistance trained individuals[46,49].
- It is beneficial to consume HMB near to the resistance training session, and to consume for a long duration (for at least 2 weeks).
- HMB alongside a structured progressive resistance training regime may aid lean mass retention during a calorie deficit.
- The recommended dose is 1-3g/day, or adjusted to 38mg per kg of body weight per day[45].
- It has been suggested that 1g consumed 3 times per day is beneficial to maximise retention and minimise the effects of muscle damage from training[2,45].
- The benefits of HMB may be achieved through optimum dietary protein intake alone (via leucine metabolism)[3].

There have been some highly contentious studies of HMB supplementation, with one lab reporting results as effective or better than steroid use for muscle growth in trained individuals[46,50]. As such, many researchers have called into question these findings, and suggested there may have been data manipulation[3,51]. Greg Nuckols recently wrote a publicly available article about the potentially flawed research in HMB[52]. This also reiterates the point that not all research can be held in the same regard.

HMB promotes a more positive net protein balance (the difference between muscle protein synthesis and muscle protein breakdown) by both stimulating protein synthesis and reducing protein breakdown[47]. It has a greater effect on preventing protein breakdown (a greater anti-catabolic effect). In untrained lifters, muscle protein synthesis is high after a novel workout as a result of high levels of muscle damage. Such that, acute post-workout elevations in muscle protein synthesis do not correlate with muscle growth[53]. As such, it would be expected that HMB might benefit individuals new to resistance training or where there is a large amount of muscle damage. In experienced lifters, muscle damage is lower and less influential on training performance. Day-to-day variations in muscle protein synthesis begin to correlate with muscle growth with training experience[53]. The benefit of HMB in trained individuals appears to only be when exercise is sufficiently intense and of high volume to induce large amounts of muscle damage.

HMB may therefore benefit beginners, but its utility in trained individuals still needs to be confirmed.

Beta-alanine

Strong evidence shows beta-alanine can enhance performance, but evidence for any benefit on muscle growth is lacking.

Beta-alanine supplementation raises muscle carnosine levels, which is a pH buffer. This may delay fatigue during short term, high intensity anaerobic exercise. It is safe to use in healthy people, but it can cause a tingling side-effect.

Beta-alanine is a non-essential amino acid. The theory behind beta-alanine supplementation is that it is involved in the metabolism of carnosine[3]. Carnosine is found in skeletal muscle. It has a role in buffering changes in pH (how acid or alkaline something is). Carnosine can buffer changes in acidity and alkalinity inside cells. Bicarbonate and phosphate are two other pH buffers found in the body (discussed next). Carnosine levels can be increased by consuming carnosine-rich foods including meat, chicken and fish[54]. During intense exercise, the pH of the working muscle can change, which can affect performance. Increased carnosine levels can in theory prevent changes in pH and maintain performance. Supplementing with beta-alanine can increase muscle carnosine levels above natural levels and aid intense exercise performance[3,41,54].

The International Society of Sports Nutrition (ISSN) conducted a review on beta-alanine consumption and exercise in 2013[54].

Current evidence shows that:

- Beta-alanine is safe in healthy people[2,54].
- A meta-analysis of 15 studies assessing beta-alanine supplementation has shown it can provide a small, but significant benefit to intense exercise performed to exhaustion. This is primarily in the range of 60 seconds to 4 minutes, but also over longer durations[54,55]. Earlier studies found beta-alanine did not benefit exercise shorter than 1 minute in

length. Increased acidity is unlikely to be the limiting factor for shorter duration muscular performance. However, since the publication of the meta-analysis, studies have found a benefit to beta-alanine supplementation with exercise under 60 seconds[56]. This involved several bouts of 30 second exercise. As the authors noted, the benefit was seen in the latter bouts, where fatigue and acid accumulation would be greater.

- Beta-alanine does not appear to benefit strength, despite its ability to increase training volume[54].
- Beta-alanine may promote increases in lean mass[42,57,58]. But, studies have also shown no increase in muscle mass[59].
- Beta-alanine appears to benefit performance by increasing muscle carnosine levels[54].
- Consuming 4-6g of beta-alanine daily for at least 4 weeks can elevate muscle carnosine levels by 40-60%, and result in performance improvements[3,54]. Consuming beta-alanine with a meal can also further increase muscle carnosine levels[32,54].
- Supplementation can result in short-term paraesthesia (skin tingling). This tingling presents no risk, but it can be discomforting. Usually the tingling lasts up to 60-90 minutes[3]. This can occur from consuming 4-6g in one dose. Splitting daily doses across the day appears to be more ergogenic and can limit the tingling effect.
- Vegetarians and vegans may have lower muscle carnosine levels and may benefit to a greater extent from supplementation[54].

However, further research is needed as a relationship between muscle carnosine levels and improvements in performance (a dose-response relationship) is yet to be shown[3]. The proposed benefit of beta-alanine supplementation is via increasing muscle carnosine levels; therefore, such a relationship would be expected[54].

Primarily consider using beta-alanine to improve high intensity performance if you have other training goals besides hypertrophy[32]. Whether such performance improvements lead to greater muscle growth is unclear[41]. The evidence for a benefit of beta-alanine on muscle growth requires further study. However, considering the only negative effects appear to be the harmless tingling sensation (which can be minimised by splitting the dosage across the day) and cost, it could be argued that for some individuals, it could be used to 'cover all bases'[12].

Sodium bicarbonate (baking soda)

Mixed evidence shows sodium bicarbonate can enhance performance. No evidence shows it can benefit muscle growth.

Bicarbonate is another pH buffer found in muscles and blood, like carnosine and phosphate. The benefit of sodium bicarbonate will be similar to the benefit of beta-alanine and phosphate. Sodium bicarbonate may benefit high intensity exercise, mainly between 60 to 180 seconds but also up to 10 minutes in length[2,3]. Current evidence is inconclusive as to whether sodium bicarbonate improves performance. Some authorities such as the International Olympic Committee (IOC) and the International Society of Sports Nutrition (ISSN) suggest it is beneficial, however some reviews have not found any benefit[3,60]. The benefit of sodium bicarbonate is unlikely to translate into improved muscle growth. There are *no* studies assessing sodium bicarbonate on muscle growth and very few on resistance training[60]. Studies on a single resistance training session are inconclusive as to whether sodium bicarbonate improves performance (the number of reps completed in a set to failure)[61-63]. Sodium bicarbonate is more likely to benefit short to middle distance events such as 400-800m runs, 200m swims and 3km cycling time trials, rather than resistance training[32,62,63]. Even so, some studies have shown a negative effect in some individuals[64]. It is unclear from current studies whether consuming sodium bicarbonate with beta-alanine has an additive benefit on performance[2].

Current evidence shows that:

- Sodium bicarbonate is safe.
- Sodium bicarbonate ingestion can cause gut distress[3].
- Consume 0.2-0.4g/kg of body weight, 1 to 2 ½ hours before exercise[2,3]. If consumption causes gut distress, split the dose over a 30 to 180 minute period before exercise, or consume sodium bicarbonate with a carbohydrate-rich meal[3,32].

Although inconclusive, sodium bicarbonate can improve performance, but it can also have negative effects on some people[64]. There is little evidence to support using sodium bicarbonate to increase muscle growth and therefore little reason to support its use for hypertrophy. Any benefit of sodium bicarbonate would primarily be in short-middle distance exercise, and more applicable for sports involving intermittent high intensity periods (such as football or rugby)[2].

Sodium phosphate

Strong evidence shows that sodium phosphate can enhance performance, but evidence for any benefit on muscle growth is lacking.

Phosphate is another pH buffer in the body, like carnosine and bicarbonate[54]. Phosphate may also have other ergogenic mechanisms, such as the role of phosphate in the ATP-phosphocreatine system[65]. The benefit of sodium phosphate will be similar to the benefit of beta-alanine and sodium bicarbonate. Sodium phosphate can benefit aerobic exercise and intermittent exercise performance[2,65-68]. However, not all studies show a benefit[2]. Any benefit of sodium phosphate is unlikely to translate into improved muscle growth. There are no studies assessing sodium phosphate on muscle growth.

Current evidence shows that:

- Sodium phosphate is safe with no side effects[65].
- Consume 1g of sodium phosphate, 4 times per day for 3-6 days[2,65].

Sodium phosphate can improve aerobic capacity and, in some studies, endurance performance[65]. There is currently no evidence to support using sodium phosphate to increase muscle growth and therefore little reason to support its use for hypertrophy.

Energy Drinks

The International Society of Sports Nutrition (ISSN) conducted a review on energy drink consumption and exercise in 2013[69]. In typical energy drinks, the main active ingredients are caffeine and carbohydrate (in the form of sugar)[69]. Caffeine has a proven ergogenic effect. The effects of caffeine have already been discussed on page 505. Whether the carbohydrate is of utility depends on the activity being performed and the carbohydrate content of the individual's diet. The long-term influence of frequent energy drink consumption can promote greater energy intake and therefore weight gain, and hence the associations between consumption of sugar-sweetened drinks and obesity. Less evidence has been conducted on the other ingredients (such as *taurine*, another amino acid) found in typical energy drinks on body composition and performance.

In *sugar-free* (*diet*) energy drinks, the main active ingredient is just caffeine (and possibly other vitamins and minerals) with water and non-sugar sweetener (see chapter 14 regarding artificial sweeteners). Meaning, diet energy drinks do not actually provide any energy at all. Sugar-free (diet) energy drinks therefore primarily just act as a source of caffeine supplementation and water, and provide very little else[3].

Arginine

Little to no evidence suggests arginine can promote muscle growth or enhance performance.

Arginine is an amino acid, and the pre-cursor to form *nitric oxide* (NO). Nitric oxide helps with dilating blood vessels and increasing blood flow. However, arginine supplementation has little effect on exercise performance[70]. Arginine appears to be useful in diseased states with impaired blood vessel function, but in normal individuals, it does not appear to provide any benefit[70]. The lack of supportive evidence means arginine is not recommended for use as a supplement[2,41].

"The available information does not support the use of l-arginine, either alone or in combination with caffeine, creatine, or both, to enhance athletic performance or improve recovery from exhaustion."
Brooks et al., 2016[71].

"As it stands, most of the published literature that has examined the ability of arginine to operate in an ergogenic fashion has failed to report positive outcomes. While more research is certainly indicated, consumers should exercise caution when using arginine to enhance exercise performance."
Kerksick et al., 2018[2].

Citrulline malate

Mixed evidence shows citrulline malate may enhance performance. The evidence for any benefit on muscle growth is lacking.

Citrulline forms part of the pathway to generate nitric oxide (via arginine), which is involved in blood vessel dilation and improved blood flow[2]. Citrulline and malate may also provide benefit through other mechanisms. Because of a lack of any evidence supporting a benefit of arginine supplementation, it is proposed that citrulline malate exerts its benefit through these other mechanisms, but this is still inconclusive[41,42]. The long-term safety of citrulline malate is yet to be confirmed, and studies are still fairly limited in humans[42].

A systematic review and meta-analysis of 12 studies shows that citrulline malate has a small, but significant effect on high intensity strength and power outcomes compared to a placebo, increasing the number of reps performed[41,72]. However, the analysis was not specific and only considered the effects on any form of high intensity exercise performance. The meta-analysis did not assess muscle growth. Studies of citrulline malate on body composition are limited.

As a beginner or intermediate trainer, the lack of evidence means it is probably unnecessary to supplement with citrulline malate. Citrulline malate supplementation to promote muscle growth cannot be recommended at this stage[41]. But, considering the equivocal or potentially beneficial findings on strength, advanced trainers might consider supplementing to 'cover all bases'[2].

Nitrate

Mixed evidence shows nitrates may enhance performance. There is no evidence to show that nitrates can increase muscle mass.

Nitrates have been suggested to improve performance by a range of mechanisms, such as blood flow (increasing levels of nitric oxide, promoting dilation of blood vessels), muscle contractility and cellular energy use. However, the mechanism by which nitrates exert their ergogenic effect is unclear, but different theories exist[73].

Current evidence shows that:

- Nitrates are safe for consumption and can be found in leafy greens and vegetables such as spinach, celery and beetroot[3].
- There are few side effects associated with nitrates.
- Most evidence has been demonstrated with endurance exercise[41].
- Nitrates are beneficial for a range of disciplines, from longer duration endurance exercise to shorter duration high intensity exercise performance, such as sprinting[3,32,73,74].
- These benefits appear to be greater in untrained compared to trained individuals[2,3,73].
- Nitrates are proposed to improve type II fibre function, which results in improvements in high intensity exercise performance[3].
- Consuming 3-5g, 2-3 hours before exercise can provide performance benefits[2,32]. Supplements include concentrated beetroot juice and nitrate salts. 200g of beetroot or spinach can achieve similar nitrate concentrations[73].
- A systematic review and meta-analysis of 29 randomised controlled trials assessing nitrates show that they result in an acute reduction in metabolic rate during moderate intensity exercise and increase the time to failure during high intensity exercise, but do not affect resting metabolic rate[75,76]. Nitrates result in a reduction in the oxygen cost of exercise by around 10-20% at a given intensity of effort (based on heart rate)[76,77]. The amount of fat and carbohydrate used during exercise are not altered. Nitrates appear to result in less energy being used to produce the same work output from exercise, potentially from improvements in the efficiency of muscle cells to use energy[2,76]. A reduction in the oxygen cost during exercise from nitrates has been shown to reduce the energy cost of performing exercise[76,77]. This may *reduce* the total number of calories burnt during exercise. If the aim is to expend additional calories through aerobic exercise, this improvement in muscle economy may not be beneficial[73].

One downside to nitrate supplementation (and many supplements for that fact) is that what is stated on the nutrition label is not necessarily is what is in the bottle. There is high variability in the nitrate content of nitrate supplements, despite what is claimed on the label[78]. Few products contain more than the minimal dose of nitrate for ergogenic benefit.

Nitrates can improve performance across a wide range of disciplines from muscular power and strength, to endurance[73]. There is evidence to suggest a mechanism by which nitric oxide may allow for muscle growth from lab studies in rodents[41]. But, whether nitrate supplements can specifically promote muscle growth has *not* been studied and is therefore inconclusive. Nitrate supplementation to promote muscle growth cannot be recommended at this stage[41].

Essential and branched-chain amino acids (EAAs and BCAAs)

Mixed evidence shows EAAs or BCAAs or may promote muscle growth and enhance performance. EAAs may have greater utility than BCAAs.

There are 20 amino acids. Of which 9 are essential amino acids (EAAs), including the 3 branched-chain amino acids (BCAAs): isoleucine, leucine and valine[79]. The theoretical rationale for EAAs and BCAAs for promoting muscle growth is that they are implicated in muscle protein synthesis and can prevent muscle breakdown. In particular, leucine (a BCAA) has been identified as being important (see chapter 9 regarding the leucine threshold)[2]. The theory is that consumption of these specific amino acids may help to minimise muscle breakdown and promote muscle retention or growth[2]. EAAs are found in incomplete and complete protein sources, with all 9 in sufficient proportions in complete sources. Evidence shows that protein sources that achieve the greatest elevations in muscle protein synthesis are those that are rich in EAAs, such as whey protein. As such, attention has turned to whether consuming isolated BCAAs or EAAs (as opposed to intact protein sources containing these amino acids) can benefit muscle growth.

There is limited evidence to suggest BCAA supplementation is beneficial for muscle growth[79]. Most evidence assesses differences in acute post-workout muscle protein synthesis. As discussed in chapter 9, acute changes in muscle protein synthesis do not appear to correlate with long-term muscle growth. There are actually very few long-term studies of BCAA supplementation in trained individuals. *No* studies have assessed whether supplementing with BCAAs between meals during a calorie deficit has a favourable effect on body composition, despite this being one of their most common uses. Most evidence currently originates from rats that have been given BCAAs. Human and rodent metabolisms can differ significantly, and rodent findings are not directly applicable to humans[42].

Most studies showing evidence of a benefit have been when EAAs or BCAAs are consumed after a fast, compared to a placebo control[2]. However, BCAA supplementation is inferior to a complete protein supplement (e.g. whey) for stimulating muscle protein synthesis[2,80,81]. BCAAs *can elevate* muscle protein synthesis, but *cannot maximise* muscle protein synthesis in the absence of other EAAs[79]. Leucine by itself does not increase muscle mass over a placebo with 8 weeks of resistance training[82]. Supplementing with 10g of leucine per day did not increase muscle mass over the course of a 12 week training programme in individuals who were consuming 1.8g/kg of body weight of protein per day[83]. Similarly, there is no evidence that BCAA supplementation in a calorie deficit is of greater benefit to preserve muscle than just consuming sufficient daily protein[84].

Emerging evidence suggests BCAAs may have a role in reducing muscle damage and soreness, and improving recovery, despite not improving performance[2,85,86]. This may have use when the primary goal is maximising training frequency and volume for sport, but not muscle growth. However, this benefit may actually just be due to the sub-optimal daily protein intakes of the participants in these studies[87].

A lack of EAAs can limit muscle protein synthesis. Because non-essential AAs can be made in the body, it has been suggested that EAA supplementation can therefore maximally stimulate muscle protein synthesis[2,79]. However again, the literature is inconclusive with few studies assessing EAAs.

If there is a benefit from consuming isolated BCAAs or EAAs, it has *yet* to be proven. BCAAs are less effective than complete protein (e.g. whey) for stimulating muscle protein synthesis. Based on the current evidence, EAA supplementation would be at best as effective, and at worst less effective than complete protein supplementation for muscle growth. Bearing in mind that a 20g dose of whey protein which is rich in EAAs can already maximise post-workout muscle protein synthesis, the benefit of consuming specific amino acids seems limited[88]. Current recommendations are to focus on consuming intact proteins (e.g. meat, dairy and plant-based sources) instead of isolated amino acid protein sources (e.g. BCAAs or EAAs)[2,12]. Daily protein intakes are calculated for whole protein sources, not for EAAs. It is not known whether EAA supplementation influences the recommended protein intake for muscle growth. Again, the primary focus should be on meeting total daily protein intake (1.6g/kg of body weight per day for muscle growth).

Glutamine

Little to no evidence shows glutamine enhances performance. The evidence for any benefit on muscle growth is lacking.

Glutamine is a non-essential amino acid with a wide range of uses in the body. It has been theorised to help promote muscle protein synthesis and help with recovery[2]. Limited evidence suggests there is *no* ergogenic benefit from its supplementation in healthy people[42,89]. A review shows that there is little evidence to suggest that glutamine can increase muscle mass, support the immune system or have anti-catabolic effects[89]. As such, glutamine is not recommended[42].

L-Carnitine

Little to no evidence shows l-carnitine enhances performance. The evidence for any benefit on muscle growth is lacking.

L-carnitine is produced by the liver and is involved in the metabolism of fat. As such, it has been suggested that increasing carnitine levels can increase fat loss[2]. However, most of the evidence shows no effect of carnitine supplementation on changes in fat metabolism, performance, or fat loss[2].

As such, there is little evidence to support using l-carnitine for any benefit on body composition.

Omega-3 fatty acids

Omega-3 fatty acids are a type of polyunsaturated fatty acid that are essential[90]. The omega-3 refers to the structure of the fatty acid (see chapter 6 regarding types of fat).

Omega-3s (in particular *eicosapentaenoic acid* (EPA) and *docosahexaenoic acid* (DHA)) can be obtained in the diet from oily fish. However, *Western* diets tend to be low in omega 3. As such, it has been suggested that using supplements (usually fish oils) can be of benefit to health, in particular in relation to cardiovascular disease[90].

Furthermore, it has been suggested that omega-3 supplements can have muscle building effects*. Some studies have been conducted on omega-3 and muscle growth, but most are inconclusive[12]. Current observational and experimental evidence does not show a benefit to their use for muscle growth[90]. There is also little evidence to suggest omega-3 supplementation can aid fat loss[3]. However, the evidence for muscle gain and fat loss is still limited and more studies are needed.

The current evidence on omega-3 supplementation and muscle growth is limited. The effect of omega-3 will probably depend on how much omega-3 people already consume, how well their diet and training are designed for muscle growth, and what research studies compare omega-3 supplementation to (e.g. comparing omega-3 to omega-6 fatty acids, saturated fat, another macronutrient or placebo).

However, the utility of omega-3 supplementation has been implicated for cardiovascular health. The health benefit of omega-3 supplementation from randomised controlled trials is not conclusive and may depend on habitual omega-3 intake[91]. As such, from a general health perspective, recommendations are to consume omega-3 rich oily fish twice per week, rather than to use an omega-3 supplement[3,4,12,90].

This is different to the saturated fat and polyunsaturated fat study discussed in chapter 8. In that study, people were in a calorie surplus and given either muffins with saturated fatty acids, or muffins with polyunsaturated fatty acids. Both groups gained the same amount of weight, but more weight was gained as muscle and less as fat in the polyunsaturated fat muffin group compared to the saturated fat group. In that study, different types of fatty acids were being compared in people eating more food than they need, without any resistance training for muscle growth. Also, a different type of polyunsaturated fat used in that study (omega-6, not omega-3), a subtle difference. Here, we are looking at whether consuming more omega-3 fatty acids can increase muscle growth regardless of the habitual diet.

Summary

Supplements at best have a minor role in benefitting body composition.

Many companies claim their supplements have beneficial effects, but any supporting evidence is mainly from lab studies or a theoretical consideration.

There is a lack of research directly assessing the effect of a given supplement on body composition outcomes. Most supplements have very little evidence to support their use.

References

1   Kårlund A, Gómez-Gallego C, Turpeinen AM, Palo-oja O-M, El-Nezami H, Kolehmainen M. Protein Supplements and Their Relation with Nutrition, Microbiota Composition and Health: Is More Protein Always Better for Sportspeople? *Nutrients* 2019; 11. Available from: doi:10.3390/nu11040829.

2   Kerksick CM, Wilborn CD, Roberts MD, Smith-Ryan A, Kleiner SM, Jäger R et al. ISSN exercise & sports nutrition review update: research & recommendations. *J Int Soc Sports Nutr* 2018; 15. Available from: doi:10.1186/s12970-018-0242-y.

3   Maughan RJ, Burke LM, Dvorak J, Larson-Meyer DE, Peeling P, Phillips SM et al. IOC consensus statement: dietary supplements and the high-performance athlete. *Br J Sports Med* 2018; 52: 439–455.

4   Valavanidis A. Dietary Supplements: Beneficial to Human Health or Just Peace of Mind? A Critical Review on the Issue of Benefit/Risk of Dietary Supplements. *Pharmakeftiki* 2016; 28: 60–83.

5   Centre for Evidence-Based Medicine. *Weight loss supplements.* 2014. Available from: https://www.cebm.net/2014/05/weight-loss-supplements-dont-work/ (accessed 13 Feb 2020).

6   Onakpoya IJ, Wider B, Pittler MH, Ernst E. Food Supplements for Body Weight Reduction: A Systematic Review of Systematic Reviews. *Obesity* 2011; 19: 239–244.

7   Pittler MH, Ernst E. Dietary supplements for body-weight reduction: a systematic review. *Am J Clin Nutr* 2004; 79: 529–536.

8   O'Bryan KR, Doering TM, Morton RW, Coffey VG, Phillips SM, Cox GR. Do multi-ingredient protein supplements augment resistance training-induced gains in skeletal muscle mass and strength? A systematic review and meta-analysis of 35 trials. *Br J Sports Med* 2019. Available from: doi:10.1136/bjsports-2018-099889.

9   Rodriguez NR, DiMarco NM, Langley S, American Dietetic Association, Dietitians of Canada, American College of Sports Medicine: Nutrition and Athletic Performance. Position of the American Dietetic Association, Dietitians of Canada, and the American College of Sports Medicine: Nutrition and athletic performance. *J Am Diet Assoc* 2009; 109: 509–527.

10   Morton R, Murphy K, McKellar S, Schoenfeld B, Henselmans M, Helms E et al. A systematic review, meta-analysis and meta-regression of the effect of protein supplementation on resistance training-induced gains in muscle mass and strength in healthy adults. *Br J Sports Med* 2018; 52(6):376-384.

11   Cermak NM, Res PT, de Groot LC, Saris WH, van Loon LJ. Protein supplementation augments the adaptive response of skeletal muscle to resistance-type exercise training: a meta-analysis. *Am J Clin Nutr* 2012; 96: 1454–1464.

12   Iraki J, Fitschen P, Espinar S, Helms E. Nutrition Recommendations for Bodybuilders in the Off-Season: A Narrative Review. *Sports* 2019; 7: 154.

13   Jakubowski JS, Wong EPT, Nunes EA, Noguchi KS, Vandeweerd JK, Murphy KT et al. Equivalent Hypertrophy and Strength Gains in β-Hydroxy-β-Methylbutyrate- or Leucine-supplemented Men. *Med Sci Sports Exerc* 2019; 51: 65–74.

14   Paulsen G, Hamarsland H, Cumming KT, Johansen RE, Hulmi JJ, Børsheim E et al. Vitamin C and E supplementation alters protein signalling after a strength training session, but not muscle growth during 10 weeks of training. *J Physiol* 2014; 592: 5391–5408.

15   Bryer SC, Goldfarb A. Effect of High Dose Vitamin C Supplementation on Muscle Soreness, Damage, Function, and Oxidative Stress to Eccentric Exercise. *Int J Sport Nutr Exerc Metab* 2006; 16: 270–80.

16   Avery NG, Kaiser JL, Sharman MJ, Scheett TP, Barnes DM, Gómez AL et al. Effects of vitamin E supplementation on recovery from repeated bouts of resistance exercise. *J Strength Cond Res* 2003; 17: 801–809.

17   Dutra MT, Alex S, Silva AF, Brown LE, Bottaro M. Antioxidant Supplementation Impairs Changes in Body Composition Induced by Strength Training in Young Women. *Int J Exerc Sci* 2019; 12: 287–296.

18   Dutra MT, Alex S, Mota MR, Sales NB, Brown LE, Bottaro M. Effect of strength training combined with antioxidant supplementation on muscular performance. *Appl Physiol Nutr Metab Physiol Appl Nutr Metab* 2018; 43: 775–781.

19   Green NR, Ferrando AA. Plasma boron and the effects of boron supplementation in males. *Environ Health Perspect* 1994; 102 Suppl 7: 73–77.

20   Ferrando AA, Green NR. The effect of boron supplementation on lean body mass, plasma testosterone levels, and strength in male bodybuilders. *Int J Sport Nutr* 1993; 3: 140–149.

21   Campbell WW, Joseph LJO, Anderson RA, Davey SL, Hinton J, Evans WJ. Effects of resistive training and chromium picolinate on body composition and skeletal muscle size in older women. *Int J Sport Nutr Exerc Metab* 2002; 12: 125–135.

22   Volpe SL, Huang HW, Larpadisorn K, Lesser II. Effect of chromium supplementation and exercise on body composition, resting metabolic rate and selected biochemical parameters in moderately obese women following an exercise program. *J Am Coll Nutr* 2001; 20: 293–306.

23   Magkos F, Kavouras SA. Caffeine Use in Sports, Pharmacokinetics in Man, and Cellular Mechanisms of Action. *Crit Rev Food Sci Nutr* 2005; 45: 535–562.

24   Goldstein ER, Ziegenfuss T, Kalman D, Kreider R, Campbell B, Wilborn C et al. International society of sports nutrition position stand: caffeine and performance. *J Int Soc Sports Nutr* 2010; 7: 5.

25   Fusar-Poli P, Radua J. Ten simple rules for conducting umbrella reviews. *Evid Based Ment Health* 2018; 21: 95–100.

26   Grgic J, Grgic I, Pickering C, Schoenfeld BJ, Bishop DJ, Pedisic Z. Wake up and smell the coffee: caffeine supplementation and exercise performance—an

umbrella review of 21 published meta-analyses. *Br J Sports Med* 2019. Available from: doi:10.1136/bjsports-2018-100278.

27   Grgic J, Trexler ET, Lazinica B, Pedisic Z. Effects of caffeine intake on muscle strength and power: a systematic review and meta-analysis. *J Int Soc Sports Nutr* 2018; 15: 11.

28   Grgic J, Pickering C. The effects of caffeine ingestion on isokinetic muscular strength: A meta-analysis. *J Sci Med Sport* 2019; 22: 353–360.

29   Grgic J, Mikulic P, Schoenfeld BJ, Bishop DJ, Pedisic Z. The Influence of Caffeine Supplementation on Resistance Exercise: A Review. *Sports Med Auckl NZ* 2019; 49: 17–30.

30   European Food Safety Authority. *Safety of caffeine.* 2015. Available from: https://www.efsa.europa.eu/en/efsajournal/pub/4102 (accessed 13 Feb 2020).

31   Robertson D, Frölich JC, Carr RK, Watson JT, Hollifield JW, Shand DG et al. Effects of caffeine on plasma renin activity, catecholamines and blood pressure. *N Engl J Med* 1978; 298: 181–186.

32   Stecker R, Harty P, Jagim A, Candow D, Kerksick C. Timing of ergogenic aids and micronutrients on muscle and exercise performance. *J Int Soc Sports Nutr* 2019; 16: 37.

33   Apostolidis A, Mougios V, Smilios I, Rodosthenous J, Hadjicharalambous M. Caffeine Supplementation: Ergogenic in Both High and Low Caffeine Responders. *Int J Sports Physiol Perform* 2019; 14: 650–657.

34   Blanchard J, Sawers SJ. The absolute bioavailability of caffeine in man. *Eur J Clin Pharmacol* 1983; 24: 93–98.

35   Teekachunhatean S, Tosri N, Rojanasthien N, Srichairatanakool S, Sangdee C. Pharmacokinetics of Caffeine following a Single Administration of Coffee Enema versus Oral Coffee Consumption in Healthy Male Subjects. *ISRN Pharmacol.* 2013. Available from: doi:https://doi.org/10.1155/2013/147238.

36   Roser M, Appel C, Ritchie H. *Human Height. Our World Data.* 2013. Available from: https://ourworldindata.org/human-height (accessed 13 Feb 2020).

37   Clark I, Landolt HP. Coffee, caffeine, and sleep: A systematic review of epidemiological studies and randomized controlled trials. *Sleep Med Rev* 2017; 31: 70–78.

38   Kreider R, Kalman D, Antonio J, Ziegenfuss T, Wildman R, Collins R et al. International Society of Sports Nutrition position stand: Safety and efficacy of creatine supplementation in exercise, sport, and medicine. *J Int Soc Sports Nutr* 2017; 14. Available from: doi:10.1186/s12970-017-0173-z.

39   Thomas DT, Erdman KA, Burke LM. Position of the Academy of Nutrition and Dietetics, Dietitians of Canada, and the American College of Sports Medicine: Nutrition and Athletic Performance. *J Acad Nutr Diet* 2016; 116: 501–528.

40   Rodriguez NR, DiMarco NM, Langley S, American Dietetic Association, Dietitians of Canada, American College of Sports Medicine: Nutrition and Athletic Performance. Position of the American Dietetic Association, Dietitians

of Canada, and the American College of Sports Medicine: Nutrition and athletic performance. *J Am Diet Assoc* 2009; 109: 509–527.

41   Roberts BM, Helms ER, Trexler ET, Fitschen PJ. Nutritional Recommendations for Physique Athletes. *J Hum Kinet* 2020. Available from: doi:http://dx.doi.org/10.2478/hukin-2019-0096.

42   Helms ER, Aragon AA, Fitschen PJ. Evidence-based recommendations for natural bodybuilding contest preparation: nutrition and supplementation. *J Int Soc Sports Nutr* 2014; 11: 20.

43   Antonio J, Ciccone V. The effects of pre versus post workout supplementation of creatine monohydrate on body composition and strength. *J Int Soc Sports Nutr* 2013; 10: 36.

44   Nuckols G. *Not Another Boring Creatine Guide: Answers to FAQs and Lesser-Known Benefits*. 2019. Available from: https://www.strongerbyscience.com/creatine/ (accessed 13 Feb 2020).

45   Kaczka P, Michalczyk MM, Jastrząb R, Gawelczyk M, Kubicka K. Mechanism of Action and the Effect of Beta-Hydroxy-Beta-Methylbutyrate (HMB) Supplementation on Different Types of Physical Performance - A Systematic Review. *J Hum Kinet* 2019; 68: 211–222.

46   Silva VR, Belozo FL, Micheletti TO, Conrado M, Stout JR, Pimentel GD et al. β-hydroxy-β-methylbutyrate free acid supplementation may improve recovery and muscle adaptations after resistance training: a systematic review. *Nutr Res* 2017; 45: 1–9.

47   Wilson J, Fitschen P, Campbell B, Wilson G, Zanchi N, Taylor L et al. International Society of Sports Nutrition Position Stand: Beta-hydroxy-beta-methylbutyrate (HMB). *J Int Soc Sports Nutr* 2013. Available from: doi:10.1186/1550-2783-10-6.

48   Gallagher PM, Carrithers JA, Godard MP, Schulze KE, Trappe SW. Beta-hydroxy-beta-methylbutyrate ingestion, Part I: effects on strength and fat free mass. *Med Sci Sports Exerc* 2000; 32: 2109–2115.

49   Albert F, Morente-Sánchez J, Ortega F, Castillo M, Gutiérrez A. Usefulness of β-hydroxy-β-methylbutyrate (HMB) supplementation in different sports: An update and practical Implications. *Nutr Hosp Organo Of Soc Espanola Nutr Parenter Enter* 2015; 32: 20–33.

50   Wilson JM, Lowery RP, Joy JM, Andersen JC, Wilson SMC, Stout JR et al. The effects of 12 weeks of beta-hydroxy-beta-methylbutyrate free acid supplementation on muscle mass, strength, and power in resistance-trained individuals: a randomized, double-blind, placebo-controlled study. *Eur J Appl Physiol* 2014; 114: 1217–1227.

51   Phillips SM, Aragon AA, Arciero PJ, Arent SM, Close GL, Hamilton DL et al. Changes in body composition and performance with supplemental HMB-FA+ATP. *J Strength Cond Res* 2017; 31: e71–e72.

52   Nuckols G. *The HMB Controversy: Better than Steroids?* 2016. Available from: https://www.strongerbyscience.com/hmb/ (accessed 13 Feb 2020).

53   Damas F, Phillips SM, Libardi CA, Vechin FC, Lixandrão ME, Jannig PR et al. Resistance training-induced changes in integrated myofibrillar protein synthesis are related to hypertrophy only after attenuation of muscle damage. *J Physiol* 2016; 594: 5209–5222.

54   Trexler ET, Smith-Ryan AE, Stout JR, Hoffman JR, Wilborn CD, Sale C et al. International society of sports nutrition position stand: Beta-Alanine. *J Int Soc Sports Nutr* 2015; 12. Available from: doi:10.1186/s12970-015-0090-y.

55   Hobson RM, Saunders B, Ball G, Harris RC, Sale C. Effects of β-alanine supplementation on exercise performance: a meta-analysis. *Amino Acids* 2012; 43: 25–37.

56   de Salles Painelli V, Saunders B, Sale C, Harris RC, Solis MY, Roschel H et al. Influence of training status on high-intensity intermittent performance in response to β-alanine supplementation. *Amino Acids* 2014; 46: 1207–1215.

57   Hoffman J, Ratamess N, Kang J, Mangine G, Faigenbaum A, Stout J. Effect of creatine and beta-alanine supplementation on performance and endocrine responses in strength/power athletes. *Int J Sport Nutr Exerc Metab* 2006; 16: 430–446.

58   Smith AE, Walter AA, Graef JL, Kendall KL, Moon JR, Lockwood CM et al. Effects of β-alanine supplementation and high-intensity interval training on endurance performance and body composition in men; a double-blind trial. *J Int Soc Sports Nutr* 2009; 6: 5.

59   Kendrick IP, Harris RC, Kim HJ, Kim CK, Dang VH, Lam TQ et al. The effects of 10 weeks of resistance training combined with beta-alanine supplementation on whole body strength, force production, muscular endurance and body composition. *Amino Acids* 2008; 34: 547–554.

60   Hadzic M, Eckstein ML, Schugardt M. The Impact of Sodium Bicarbonate on Performance in Response to Exercise Duration in Athletes: A Systematic Review. *J Sports Sci Med* 2019; 18: 271–281.

61   Duncan MJ, Weldon A, Price MJ. The Effect of Sodium Bicarbonate Ingestion on Back Squat and Bench Press Exercise to Failure. *J Strength Cond Res* 2014; 28: 1358–1366.

62   Carr B, Webster M, Boyd J, Hudson G, Scheett T. Sodium bicarbonate supplementation improves hypertrophy-type resistance exercise performance. *Eur J Appl Physiol* 2012; 113. Available from: doi:10.1007/s00421-012-2484-8.

63   Webster MJ, Webster MN, Crawford RE, Gladden LB. Effect of sodium bicarbonate ingestion on exhaustive resistance exercise performance. *Med Sci Sports Exerc* 1993; 25: 960–965.

64   Peart DJ, Siegler JC, Vince RV. Practical Recommendations for Coaches and Athletes: A Meta-Analysis of Sodium Bicarbonate Use for Athletic Performance. *J Strength Cond Res* 2012; 26: 1975–1983.

65   Buck CL, Wallman KE, Dawson B, Guelfi KJ. Sodium phosphate as an ergogenic aid. *Sports Med Auckl NZ* 2013; 43: 425–435.

66   Kreider RB, Miller GW, Williams MH, Somma CT, Nasser TA. Effects of phosphate loading on oxygen uptake, ventilatory anaerobic threshold, and run performance. *Med Sci Sports Exerc* 1990; 22: 250–256.

67   Kreider RB, Miller GW, Schenck D, Cortes CW, Miriel V, Somma CT et al. Effects of phosphate loading on metabolic and myocardial responses to maximal and endurance exercise. *Int J Sport Nutr* 1992; 2: 20–47.

68   Cade R, Conte M, Zauner C, Mars D, Peterson J, Lunne D et al. Effects of phosphate loading on 2,3-diphosphoglycerate and maximal oxygen uptake. *Med Sci Sports Exerc* 1984; 16: 263–268.

69   Campbell B, Wilborn C, La Bounty P, Taylor L, Nelson M, Greenwood M et al. International Society of Sports Nutrition position stand: Energy drinks. *J Int Soc Sports Nutr* 2013. Available from: doi:10.1186/1550-2783-10-1.

70   McConell GK. Effects of L-arginine supplementation on exercise metabolism. *Curr Opin Clin Nutr Metab Care* 2007; 10: 46–51.

71   Brooks JR, Oketch-Rabah H, Low Dog T, Gorecki DKJ, Barrett ML, Cantilena L et al. Safety and performance benefits of arginine supplements for military personnel: a systematic review. *Nutr Rev* 2016; 74: 708–721.

72   Trexler ET, Persky AM, Ryan ED, Schwartz TA, Stoner L, Smith-Ryan AE. Acute Effects of Citrulline Supplementation on High-Intensity Strength and Power Performance: A Systematic Review and Meta-Analysis. *Sports Med Auckl NZ* 2019; 49: 707–718.

73   Jones AM, Thompson C, Wylie LJ, Vanhatalo A. Dietary Nitrate and Physical Performance. *Annu Rev Nutr* 2018; 38: 303–328.

74   McMahon NF, Leveritt MD, Pavey TG. The Effect of Dietary Nitrate Supplementation on Endurance Exercise Performance in Healthy Adults: A Systematic Review and Meta-Analysis. *Sports Med Auckl NZ* 2017; 47: 735–756.

75   Pawlak-Chaouch M, Boissière J, Gamelin FX, Cuvelier G, Berthoin S, Aucouturier J. Effect of dietary nitrate supplementation on metabolic rate during rest and exercise in human: A systematic review and a meta-analysis. *Nitric Oxide* 2016; 53: 65–76.

76   Bailey SJ, Winyard P, Vanhatalo A, Blackwell JR, Dimenna FJ, Wilkerson DP et al. Dietary nitrate supplementation reduces the O2 cost of low-intensity exercise and enhances tolerance to high-intensity exercise in humans. *J Appl Physiol Bethesda* 2009; 107: 1144–1155.

77   Lansley KE, Winyard PG, Fulford J, Vanhatalo A, Bailey SJ, Blackwell JR et al. Dietary nitrate supplementation reduces the O2 cost of walking and running: a placebo-controlled study. *J Appl Physiol Bethesda* 2011; 110: 591–600.

78   Gallardo EJ, Coggan AR. What Is in Your Beet Juice? Nitrate and Nitrite Content of Beet Juice Products Marketed to Athletes. *Int J Sport Nutr Exerc Metab* 2019; 29: 345–349.

79   Santos C de S, Nascimento FEL. Isolated branched-chain amino acid intake and muscle protein synthesis in humans: a biochemical review. *Einstein* 2019; 17:3. Available from: doi:10.31744/einstein_journal/2019RB4898.

80   Churchward-Venne TA, Burd NA, Mitchell CJ, West DWD, Philp A, Marcotte GR et al. Supplementation of a suboptimal protein dose with leucine or essential amino acids: effects on myofibrillar protein synthesis at rest and following resistance exercise in men. *J Physiol* 2012; 590: 2751–2765.

81   Churchward-Venne TA, Breen L, Di Donato DM, Hector AJ, Mitchell CJ, Moore DR et al. Leucine supplementation of a low-protein mixed macronutrient beverage enhances myofibrillar protein synthesis in young men: a double-blind, randomized trial. *Am J Clin Nutr* 2014; 99: 276–286.

82   Aguiar AF, Grala AP, da Silva RA, Soares-Caldeira LF, Pacagnelli FL, Ribeiro AS et al. Free leucine supplementation during an 8-week resistance training program does not increase muscle mass and strength in untrained young adult subjects. *Amino Acids* 2017; 49: 1255–1262.

83   de Andrade IT, Gualano B, Hevia-Larraín V, Junior JN, Cajueiro M, Jardim F et al. Leucine Supplementation Has No Further Effect on Training-induced Muscle Adaptations. *Med Sci Sports Exerc* 2020. Available from: doi:10.1249/MSS.0000000000002307.

84   Dieter BP, Schoenfeld BJ, Aragon AA. The data do not seem to support a benefit to BCAA supplementation during periods of caloric restriction. *J Int Soc Sports Nutr* 2016; 13: 21.

85   Jackman SR, Witard OC, Jeukendrup AE, Tipton KD. Branched-chain amino acid ingestion can ameliorate soreness from eccentric exercise. *Med Sci Sports Exerc* 2010; 42: 962–970.

86   Howatson G, Hoad M, Goodall S, Tallent J, Bell PG, French DN. Exercise-induced muscle damage is reduced in resistance-trained males by branched chain amino acids: a randomized, double-blind, placebo controlled study. *J Int Soc Sports Nutr* 2012; 9: 20.

87   VanDusseldorp TA, Escobar KA, Johnson KE, Stratton MT, Moriarty T, Cole N et al. Effect of Branched-Chain Amino Acid Supplementation on Recovery Following Acute Eccentric Exercise. *Nutrients* 2018; 10. Available from: doi:10.3390/nu10101389.

88   Witard OC, Jackman SR, Breen L, Smith K, Selby A, Tipton KD. Myofibrillar muscle protein synthesis rates subsequent to a meal in response to increasing doses of whey protein at rest and after resistance exercise. *Am J Clin Nutr* 2014; 99: 86–95.

89   Gleeson M. Dosing and efficacy of glutamine supplementation in human exercise and sport training. *J Nutr* 2008; 138: 2045S-2049S.

90   Rossato LT, Schoenfeld BJ, de Oliveira EP. Is there sufficient evidence to supplement omega-3 fatty acids to increase muscle mass and strength in young and older adults? *Clin Nutr* 2020; 39: 23–32.

91   Wang DD, Hu FB. Dietary Fat and Risk of Cardiovascular Disease: Recent Controversies and Advances. *Annu Rev Nutr* 2017; 37: 423–446.

26. Conclusion

If there is one message to take from this whole book, it is that the number one priority for maintaining weight or changing weight is *consistency* and *adherence*. It isn't about what can be achieved in 2 weeks, or 4 weeks with extreme measures, but what can be achieved as a sustainable, long-term, lasting change over the course of a lifetime. Finding the elements of diet and exercise that *you* find most *enjoyable* and therefore most likely to *adhere* to should drive any decision making.

We have looked at why the current approaches to diet and training for building muscle and losing fat are outdated and lack evidential support. Not all research is equal, some studies can be more useful than others. There are many factors that influence our body weight and body composition, some of which are within our control, and some of which are not. We have seen how changing body weight has consequences in terms of our energy intake and energy expenditure; we cannot return to our original energy intake if any weight change is to be maintained. Many different diets can be incredibly successful, depending on how people like to live their lives.

Resistance exercise and aerobic exercise both have important and unique health benefits and should be incorporated into any lifestyle. Resistance exercise is important to build muscle. Most resistance training variables have very little influence on muscle growth. Aerobic exercise does not appear to interfere with how much muscle you can build. Aerobic exercise is not necessary to lose weight, but it can aid weight loss or weight maintenance. There is no superior form of aerobic or resistance exercise for weight loss or energy burning. Exercise choice should be dictated by which is the most enjoyable to perform.

Considering the diversity of individuals, one size does *not* fit all when it comes to diet and exercise to influence body composition. There are only a few *basic* principles to achieve changes in body composition. But, these basic principles are very important. As a base, get a good night of sleep (7-9 hours), consume a nutritionally complete diet with no deficiencies, and avoid excessive life stress. To lose weight, consume less energy than you expend. To gain weight, consume more energy than you expend. To lose weight mostly as fat and not as muscle, and to gain weight mostly as muscle and not as fat, consume only slightly less than you expend or slightly more than you expend. Also, partake in some form of resistance training and consume at least a certain amount of protein per day. With resistance training, performing at least a certain number of sets per week, but not too many sets per week is best to build or maintain muscle. Sets should be performed with a high enough effort, but not too much effort. Being consistent and adhering to these few principles will make up the vast *majority* of any successful weight change. Beyond this, any other factors are either down to *personal preference*, or are largely a *minor* consideration.

I hope you have found this book to be useful, whether that be in thinking about your own dietary pattern and training, having an insight into the world of research or aiding your understanding of the factors that can influence body weight and body composition.

Printed in Great Britain
by Amazon